Genitourinary Pathology

Cristina Magi-Galluzzi •
Christopher G. Przybycin
Editors

Genitourinary Pathology

Practical Advances

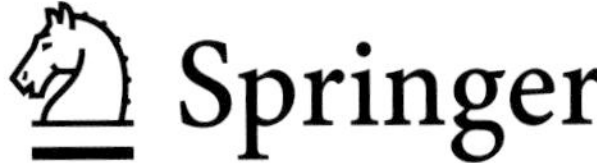

Springer

Editors
Cristina Magi-Galluzzi
Department of Pathology
Cleveland Clinic
Cleveland
Ohio
USA

Christopher G. Przybycin
Department of Pathology
Cleveland Clinic
Cleveland
Ohio
USA

ISBN 978-1-4939-2043-3 ISBN 978-1-4939-2044-0 (eBook)
DOI 10.1007/978-1-4939-2044-0

Library of Congress Control Number: 2015931952

Springer New York Heidelberg Dordrecht London

Printed on acid-free paper

Springer is part of Springer Science+Business Media (www.springer.com)

To my friend and charming husband Jean-Jacques Beaussart for his encouragement, forbearance, and love.

Cristina Magi-Galluzzi

To my wife Jennifer and my son Thomas, the two best things that ever happened to me.

Christopher G. Przybycin

Preface

Our understanding of urologic pathology has dramatically evolved over time. The field has undergone significant changes, particularly since the International Society of Urological Pathology (ISUP) has led numerous conferences to standardize specimen processing, reporting, and staging of urological malignancies and has recently published guidelines and recommendations regarding best practice approaches to the use of immunohistochemistry in differential diagnosis of tumors of the bladder, prostate, kidney, and testis.

Since the introduction of the Gleason grading system more than 40 years ago, many aspects of prostate cancer have changed, necessitating the modification of grading system to include new variants and subtypes of acinar adenocarcinoma of the prostate. Recently, researchers have gained new insights into the roles and function of the androgen receptors and the newly identified gene rearrangement involving the ETS family of transcription factors in prostate cancer and their clinical implications.

Histological grading of bladder cancer according to the modern principles of classification established in the World Health Organization (WHO) (2004)/ISUP system is crucial due to its prognostic significance, despite the limitations and opportunities for refinement inherent in all grading systems. Accurate tumor reporting and staging in transurethral resection and cystectomy specimens are critical to subsequent clinical management.

A new classification system, the ISUP/Vancouver classification of renal tumors, has been developed to include many recently described histological subtypes of adult renal epithelial neoplasms. A new nucleolar grading system for renal cell carcinoma has also been developed to better predict patients outcome. New advancements in genetics and molecular medicine have helped to better classify renal tumors into distinct clinicopathologic entities with different clinical outcomes and have improved our current understanding of familial syndromes of renal cell carcinoma.

Given the significant differences in treatment regimens and prognosis for the various testicular germ cell tumor types, particular emphasis has been placed on recently described patterns of overlapping morphology among germ cell tumors, on the important diagnostic pitfalls that could affect patient management, and on the utility of newly described immunomarkers in resolving challenging differential diagnosis.

This textbook of genitourinary pathology does not merely focus on diagnostic issues, important as they are, but also provides a single concise encapsulation of practical advances in the genitourinary tumor pathology field and the most contemporary thought regarding specimen processing, grading, staging, new insights on histologic morphology, prognostic and management implications of unusual morphologic entities, and molecular markers with diagnostic and/or prognostic values. This textbook will guide the reader through the intricacies of prostate, bladder, kidney, and testicular tumor pathology; diagnosis and reporting; associated familial and hereditary syndromes; and genetic and epigenetic alterations playing a key role in the understanding of tumor biology. A chapter underlining intraoperative consultation challenges and implications for treatment is included for each organ to emphasize the pathologist's role as a consultant during surgical procedures.

Although practicing anatomic pathologists represent the logical audience, this text includes facts useful to urologists, pathology residents, basic scientists, and translational researchers with an interest in genitourinary tumor pathology. This book assumes that the reader has a working knowledge of diagnostic genitourinary pathology.

The authors in this textbook have been carefully chosen as they represent the highest level of expertise in the field of uropathology. We are grateful to all contributors for believing in this project and for their effort to reach the final goal.

We hope that the readers of this volume will find this format friendly and helpful in the identification of practical advances in urological pathology.

Cristina Magi-Galluzzi, MD, PhD
Christopher G. Przybycin, MD

Contents

Part I Update on Prostate Tumor Pathology

1 Anatomy of the Prostate Revisited: Implications for Prostate Biopsy and Zonal Origins of Prostate Cancer 3
Samson W. Fine and Rohit Mehra

2 Contemporary Gleason Grading System 13
Kiril Trpkov

3 Contemporary Prostate Cancer Staging 33
Christopher G. Przybycin, Sara M. Falzarano and Cristina Magi-Galluzzi

4 Prostate Cancer Reporting on Biopsy and Radical Prostatectomy Specimens 45
Samson W. Fine

5 Unusual Epithelial and Nonepithelial Neoplasms of the Prostate 65
Adeboye O. Osunkoya and Cristina Magi-Galluzzi

6 Management Implications Associated with Unusual Morphologic Entities of the Prostate 79
Viraj A. Master, Jonathan Huang, Cristina Magi-Galluzzi and Adeboye O. Osunkoya

7 Nomograms for Prostate Cancer Decision Making 93
Cesar E. Ercole, Michael W. Kattan and Andrew J. Stephenson

8 Genetic Determinants of Familial and Hereditary Prostate Cancer 113
Jesse K. McKenney, Christopher G. Przybycin and Cristina Magi-Galluzzi

9 New Molecular Markers of Diagnosis and Prognosis in Prostate Cancer 123
Rajal B. Shah and Ritu Bhalla

10 **Intraoperative Consultation for Prostate Tumors: Challenges and Implications for Treatment** 145
Hiroshi Miyamoto and Steven S. Shen

11 **Genomics and Epigenomics of Prostate Cancer** 149
Juan Miguel Mosquera, Pei-Chun Lin and Mark A. Rubin

Part II Update on Bladder Tumor Pathology

12 **Anatomy of the Urinary Bladder Revisited: Implications for Diagnosis and Staging of Bladder Cancer** 173
Victor E. Reuter

13 **Classification and Histologic Grading of Urothelial Neoplasms by the WHO 2004 (ISUP 1998) Criteria** 189
Jesse K. McKenney

14 **Reporting of Bladder Cancer in Transurethral Resection of Bladder Tumor and Cystectomy Specimens** 201
Jesse K. McKenney

15 **Urothelial Carcinoma Variants: Morphology and Association with Outcomes** 205
Gladell P. Paner and Donna E. Hansel

16 **Independent Predictors of Clinical Outcomes and Prediction Models on Bladder and Upper Urinary Tract Cancer** 223
Maria Carmen Mir, Andrew J. Stephenson and Michael W. Kattan

17 **Familial Urothelial Carcinomas** 231
Christopher G. Przybycin and Jesse K. McKenney

18 **New Molecular Markers with Diagnostic and Prognostic Values in Bladder Cancer** 235
Hikmat A. Al-Ahmadie and Gopa Iyer

19 **Intraoperative Consultation for Bladder Tumors: Challenges and Implications for Treatment** 247
Hiroshi Miyamoto and Steven S. Shen

20 **Genetic and Epigenetic Alterations in Urothelial Carcinoma** 253
Hikmat A. Al-Ahmadie and Gopa Iyer

21 **Urine Cytology** 261
Jordan P. Reynolds

Part III Update on Renal Tumor Pathology

22 Anatomy of the Kidney Revisited: Implications for Diagnosis and Staging of Renal Cell Carcinoma 271
Stephen M. Bonsib

23 Classification of Adult Renal Tumors and Grading of Renal Cell Carcinoma 285
William R. Sukov and John C. Cheville

24 Tumor Staging for Renal Pathology 299
Stephen M. Bonsib

25 Surgical Pathology Reporting of Renal Cell Carcinomas 315
Christopher G. Przybycin, Angela Wu and Lakshmi P. Kunju

26 Newly Described Entities in Renal Tumor Pathology 321
Angela Wu, Christopher G. Przybycin and Lakshmi P. Kunju

27 Clinical and Management Implications Associated with Histologic Subtypes of Renal Cell Carcinomas 341
Maria Carmen Mir, Brian I. Rini and Steven C. Campbell

28 Independent Predictors of Clinical Outcomes and Prediction Models for Renal Tumor Pathology 355
Nils Kroeger, Daniel Y. C. Heng and Michael W. Kattan

29 Pathology of Inherited Forms of Renal Carcinoma 373
Maria J. Merino

30 The Utility of Immunohistochemistry in the Differential Diagnosis of Renal Cell Carcinomas 383
Ming Zhou and Fang-Ming Deng

31 Intraoperative Consultation for Renal Masses: Challenges and Implications for Treatment 401
Hiroshi Miyamoto and Steven S. Shen

32 Genetic and Epigenetic Alterations in Renal Cell Carcinoma 407
Fang-Ming Deng and Ming Zhou

33 Role of Needle Biopsy in Renal Masses: Past, Present, and Future 417
Ying-Bei Chen

Part IV Update on Testicular Tumor Pathology

34 **Anatomy of the Testis and Staging of its Cancers: Implications for Diagnosis** 433
Daniel M. Berney and Thomas M. Ulbright

35 **Classification of Testicular Tumors** 447
Cristina Magi-Galluzzi and Thomas M. Ulbright

36 **Testicular Cancer Reporting on Radical Orchiectomy and Retroperitoneal Lymph Node Dissection After Treatment** 463
Daniel M. Berney

37 **Difficult or Newly Described Morphologic Entities in Testicular Neoplasia** 471
Daniel M. Berney and Thomas M. Ulbright

38 **Clinical Implications of the Different Histologic Subtypes of Testicular Tumors** 483
Timothy Gilligan

39 **Familial Syndromes Associated with Testicular Tumors** 491
Jesse K. McKenney, Claudio Lizarralde and Cristina Magi-Galluzzi

40 **Molecular and Immunohistochemical Markers of Diagnostic and Prognostic Value in Testicular Tumors** 501
Victor E. Reuter

41 **Intraoperative Consultation for Testicular Tumors: Challenges and Implications for Treatment** 517
Hiroshi Miyamoto and Steven S. Shen

42 **Genetic and Epigenetic Alterations in Testicular Tumors** 521
Pallavi A. Patil and Cristina Magi-Galluzzi

Index 529

Contributors

Hikmat A. Al-Ahmadie Department of Pathology, Memorial Sloan Kettering Cancer Center, New York, NY, USA

Daniel M. Berney Dept of Molecular Oncology, Barts Cancer Inst., Bartshealth NHS Trust and Queen Mary University of London, London, Charterhouse Sq, UK

Department of Molecular Oncology, Barts Cancer Institute, Bartshealth NHS Trust and Queen Mary University of London, London, UK

Ritu Bhalla Department of Pathology, LSU Health Sciences Center, New Orleans, LA, USA

Stephen M. Bonsib Nephropath, Little Rock, 10810 Executive Center Drive, Suite 100AR, USA

Nephropath, Little Rock, AR, USA

Steven C. Campbell Department of Urology, Cleveland Clinic, Cleveland, OH, USA

Ying-Bei Chen Department of Pathology, Memorial Sloan Kettering Cancer Center, New York, NY, USA

John C. Cheville Department of Pathology, Mayo Clinic, Rochester, MN, USA

Fang-Ming Deng Department of Pathology, New York University Langone Medical Center, New York, NY, USA

Cesar E. Ercole Department of Urology, Cleveland Clinic, Cleveland, OH, USA

Sara M. Falzarano Department of Pathology, Cleveland Clinic, Robert J. Tomsich Pathology and Laboratory Medicine Institute, Cleveland, OH, USA

Samson W. Fine Department of Pathology, Memorial Sloan-Kettering Cancer Center, New York, NY, USA

Timothy Gilligan Cleveland Clinic, Cleveland, OH, USA

Donna E. Hansel Department of Pathology, University of California at San Diego, La Jolla, CA, USA

Daniel Y. C. Heng Department of Medical Oncology, Tom Baker Cancer Center, Calgary, AB, Canada

Jonathan Huang Department of Surgery, Emory University School of Medicine, Atlanta, GA, USA

Gopa Iyer Department of Medicine, Memorial Sloan Kettering Cancer Center, New York, NY, USA

Michael W. Kattan Department of Quantitative Health Sciences, Cleveland Clinic, Cleveland, OH, USA

Nils Kroeger Tom Baker Cancer Centre, Calgary, AB, Canada

University Medicine Greifswald, Greifswald, Germany

Lakshmi P. Kunju Department of Pathology, University of Michigan Medical Center, Ann Arbor, MI, USA

Department of Pathology, University of Michigan, Ann Arbor, MI, USA

Pei-Chun Lin Innovative Genomics Initiative, University of California, Berkeley, CA, USA

Claudio Lizarralde Department of Pathology, Cleveland Clinic, Robert J. Tomsich Pathology and Laboratory Medicine Institute, Cleveland, OH, USA

Cristina Magi-Galluzzi Department of Pathology, Cleveland Clinic, Robert J. Tomsich Pathology and Laboratory Medicine Institute, Cleveland, OH, USA

Viraj A. Master Department of Urology, Emory University School of Medicine, Atlanta, GA, USA

Jesse K. McKenney Department of Pathology, Cleveland Clinic, Robert J. Tomsich Pathology and Laboratory Medicine Institute, Cleveland, OH, USA

Rohit Mehra Department of Pathology, University of Michigan Hospital and Health Systems, Ann Arbor, MI, USA

Maria J. Merino Department of Pathology, National Cancer Institute, Bethesda, MD, USA

Maria Carmen Mir Cleveland Clinic, Glickman Urologic and Kidney Institute, Cleveland, OH, USA

Hiroshi Miyamoto Department of Pathology and Urology, The Johns Hopkins Medical Institutions, Baltimore, MD, USA

Juan Miguel Mosquera Department of Pathology and Laboratory Medicine, Institute for Precision Medicine, Weill Medical College of Cornell University, New York, NY, USA

Adeboye O. Osunkoya Department of Pathology, Emory University School of Medicine, Atlanta, GA, USA

Gladell P. Paner Department of Pathology, University of Chicago Medical Center, Chicago, IL, USA

Pallavi A. Patil Department of Pathology, Cleveland Clinic, RJ Tomsich Pathology and Laboratory Medicine Institute, Cleveland, OH, USA

Christopher G. Przybycin Department of Pathology, Cleveland Clinic, Robert J. Tomsich Pathology and Laboratory Medicine Institute, Cleveland, OH, USA

Victor E. Reuter Department of Pathology, Memorial Sloan Kettering Cancer Center, New York, NY, USA

Jordan P. Reynolds Department of Pathology, Cleveland Clinic, Robert J. Tomsich Pathology and Laboratory Medicine Institute, Cleveland, OH, USA

Brian I. Rini Department of Oncology, Cleveland Clinic, Cleveland, OH, USA

Mark A. Rubin Department of Pathology and Laboratory Medicine, Institute for Precision Medicine, Weill Medical College of Cornell University, New York, NY, USA

Rajal B. Shah Department of Pathology, Miraca Life Sciences, Irving, TX, USA

Steven S. Shen Department of Pathology and Genomic Medicine, Houston Methodist Hospital, Houston, TX, USA

Andrew J. Stephenson Center for Urologic Oncology, Cleveland Clinic, Glickman Urological and Kidney Institute, Cleveland, OH, USA

William R. Sukov Department of Pathology, Mayo Clinic, Rochester, MN, USA

Kiril Trpkov Department of Pathology and Laboratory Medicine, General Hospital, Calgary, AB, Canada

Thomas M. Ulbright Department of Pathology and Laboratory Medicine, Indiana University School of Medicine, Indianapolis, IN, USA

Angela Wu Department of Pathology, University of Michigan Medical Center, Ann Arbor, MI, USA

Ming Zhou Department of Pathology, New York University Langone Medical Center, New York, NY, USA

Part I

Update on Prostate Tumor Pathology

1 Anatomy of the Prostate Revisited: Implications for Prostate Biopsy and Zonal Origins of Prostate Cancer

Samson W. Fine and Rohit Mehra

Abbreviations

PZ	Peripheral zone
TZ	Transition zone
PSA	Prostate-specific antigen
PIN	Prostatic intraepithelial neoplasia

Topographic Relationships in McNeal's Zonal Anatomy

The body of knowledge regarding prostatic anatomy stems from McNeal's pioneering work, which demonstrated the human prostate to be a composite organ, composed of three glandular zones and a nonglandular zone, termed the anterior fibromuscular stroma [1, 2]. The in vivo three-dimensional spatial organization of these zones is best demonstrated by visualizing the prostate in the sagittal, coronal, and oblique coronal planes. These zones cannot be grossly dissected from one another, but rather are tightly fused within a common sheath of fibromuscular tissue known as the "prostatic capsule."

McNeal defined the relationship of these zones to the prostatic urethra and specified their location along the proximal/distal urethral axis. When visualized in the sagittal plane, the prostatic urethra is divided into proximal and distal segments by an anterior angulation at the midpoint between the prostate apex (distal) and bladder neck (proximal) [3]. The verumontanum protrudes from the posterior urethral wall at the point of angulation and is the point at which the ejaculatory ducts empty into the prostatic urethra. The ejaculatory ducts then extend toward the base (proximally), following a course that is nearly a direct extension of the long axis of the distal (apex to mid-gland) urethral segment (Fig. 1.1).

Coronal sections along the course of the ejaculatory ducts and distal (apex to mid-gland) urethral segment demonstrate the anatomic relationships between the two major glandular zones of the prostate, the peripheral and central zones [1]. The peripheral zone (PZ) comprises about 65 % of glandular prostatic mass and its ducts exit bilaterally from the posterior urethral wall at the verumontanum to the prostate apex with branches that curve anteriorly and posteriorly. The central zone (CZ) comprises about 30 % of the glandular prostate, with ducts branching from the verumontanum (mid-gland) and fanning out toward the base, in a flattened conical arrangement, to surround the ejaculatory duct orifices. Oblique coronal sections along the proximal (mid to base) prostatic urethra from verumontanum to bladder neck best define the transition zone (TZ), which normally encompasses about 5 % of the prostatic glandular tissue [2]. This zone is formed by two

S. W. Fine (✉)
Department of Pathology, Memorial Sloan-Kettering Cancer Center, New York, NY, USA
e-mail: fines@mskcc.org

R. Mehra
Department of Pathology, University of Michigan Hospital and Health Systems, Ann Arbor, MI, USA
e-mail: mrohit@med.umich.edu

C. Magi-Galluzzi, C. G. Przybycin (eds.), *Genitourinary Pathology*, DOI 10.1007/978-1-4939-2044-0_1,

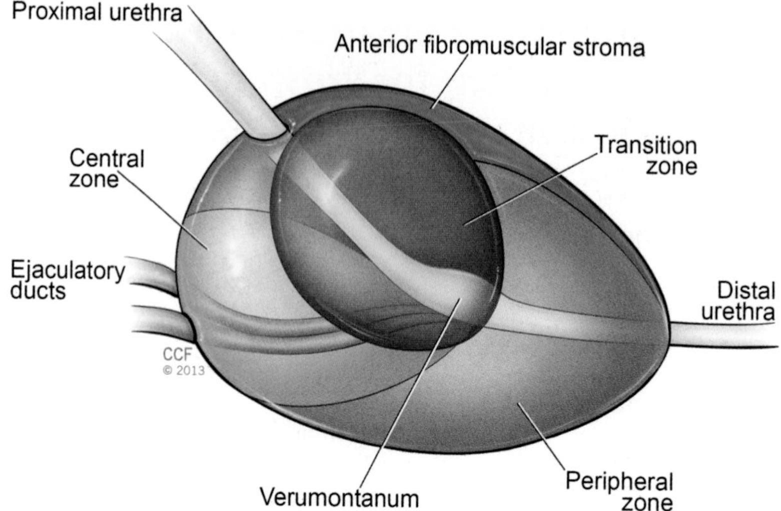

Fig. 1.1 Sagittal plane view of the prostate gland. (Reprinted with permission, Cleveland Clinic Center for Medical Art & Photography © 2014, all rights reserved)

small lobes whose ducts leave the posterolateral urethral wall and curve anteromedially. The main nonglandular tissue of the prostate is the anterior fibromuscular stroma, which overlies the urethra in the anteromedial prostate. Its bulk and consistency vary considerably from apex to base. McNeal considered this stroma as a wedge-shaped stromal barrier, shielding the prostatic urethra and glandular zones from overlying structures [4].

As McNeal's dissections in various planes were conducted in autopsy specimens, they likely reflect the cone-shaped organ seen in vivo. In contrast, radical prostatectomy specimens are typically spherical, owing to surgical manipulation, tissue contraction at removal and subsequent processing. Sectioning from apex to base in the anterior-posterior fashion common in surgical pathology practice yields topography that varies from McNeal's descriptions. Recent studies of whole mounted, serially sectioned and totally embedded radical prostatectomy specimens have highlighted underappreciated histopathologic features of glandular and stromal prostatic anatomy [5, 6].

Anatomy of the Prostate Gland in Surgical Pathology Specimens: Histologic Variation by Anatomic Region

Apical One Third of the Prostate (Apex)

In a surgical pathology specimen sectioned from anterior to posterior, the apical (distal) urethra is located near the center of the section (Fig. 1.2). Tissue shrinkage due to formalin fixation and processing artifactually shortens the distance from prostatic apex to verumontanum and everts the posterior peri-urethral tissue into the urethral space. These effects create an artificial "promontory" in the apical portions of the gland. The urethra is immediately surrounded by a thin stroma and variable number of peri-urethral glands, which intermingle anteriorly with a semicircular band ("sphincter") of compactly arranged and vertically oriented muscle fibers. This semicircular band is incomplete posterior to the urethra, appearing as a densely eosinophilic, aglandular, muscular column extending posteriorly from the urethra and serving as an important histopathologic landmark for apical prostatic tissue.

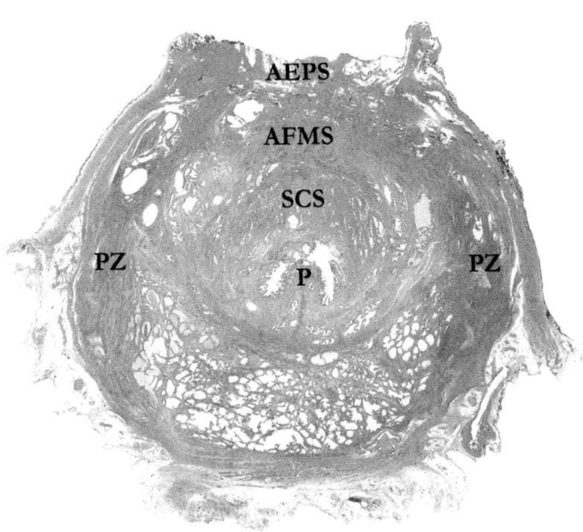

Fig. 1.2 Whole mount section from apex of prostate. The urethra and promontory (*P*) are central and proceeding anteriorly, the semicircular sphincter (*SCS*) and anterior fibromuscular stroma (*AFMS*) are visualized. The posterior, lateral, and anterolateral portions of the apex are composed of peripheral zone (*PZ*) tissue. Most anteriorly, the anterior extraprostatic space (*AEPS*) contains vascular and adipose remnants of the dorsal vascular complex

Further anterior to the semicircular muscle, the anterior fibromuscular stroma, intertwined at the apex with skeletal muscle fibers of the urogenital diaphragm, traverses horizontally and laterally and extends to the anterior- and apical-most aspects of the prostate. Unlike in the posterior and posterolateral prostate, the "prostatic capsule" is incomplete at the prostatic apex, anterior and anterolaterally, lacking a definitive border. Hence, the task of separating prostatic from extraprostatic tissue can be challenging in these regions of the gland. While heightened intraprostatic pressure may cause bulging of hypertrophic TZ acini, no normal TZ tissue is located in the prostatic apex. The bilateral PZ, which composes essentially all of the glandular tissue at the apex, occupies the posterior, lateral, and anterolateral prostate, abuts the anterior fibromuscular stroma medially and forms a nearly complete ring [5].

Middle One Third of the Prostate (Mid-Gland)

The key anatomic landmark in the mid-gland is the verumontanum, the exaggerated area of glandular-stromal tissue, located subjacent to the posterior urethral wall, into which the ejaculatory ducts insert and from which the glandular zones arise [4]. The verumontanum was identified by McNeal as the point of a 35° angulation, which divides the urethra into proximal (toward the base) and distal (toward the apex) segments. At mid-gland, the TZ emerges as bilateral lobes in the anteromedial region. In whole mount sections, the TZ ducts can be identified coursing anterolaterally from the posterior urethra to serve as a boundary between transition and PZs. In prostates without significant benign prostatic hypertrophy, the PZ still composes the posterior, lateral, and the majority of anterolateral tissue at the mid-gland (Fig. 1.3a). When benign processes including hypertrophy and adenosis prominently involve the TZ, the anterolateral "horns" of the PZ may be significantly compressed toward the lateral-most portions of the gland (Fig. 1.3b). In the mid-prostate, the anterior fibromuscular stroma may be fused with skeletal muscle fibers (of levator ani origin) as well, but may be less evident due to increased glandular density and the effects of organ contraction [5, 6].

Basal One Third of the Prostate (Base)

From mid-gland to base, the urethra is progressively invested by a thick layer of short smooth muscle fibers, constituting the "preprostatic sphincter," thought to function during ejaculation to prevent retrograde flow of seminal fluid and to maintain resting tone that ensures closure of the proximal urethral segment [2]. At the base, TZ glands gradually recede and few remaining PZ acini once again comprise the anterior glandular tissue. Unlike at the apex, PZ glands rarely extend anteromedially due to the vast stroma in this region. This stroma appears as an expansive swath of tissue comprised of both preprostatic sphincter and anterior fibromuscular stroma, with the latter often merging anteriorly with large smooth muscle bundles located in the anterior extraprostatic space (Fig. 1.4). With increasing angulation, the prostatic urethra is identified

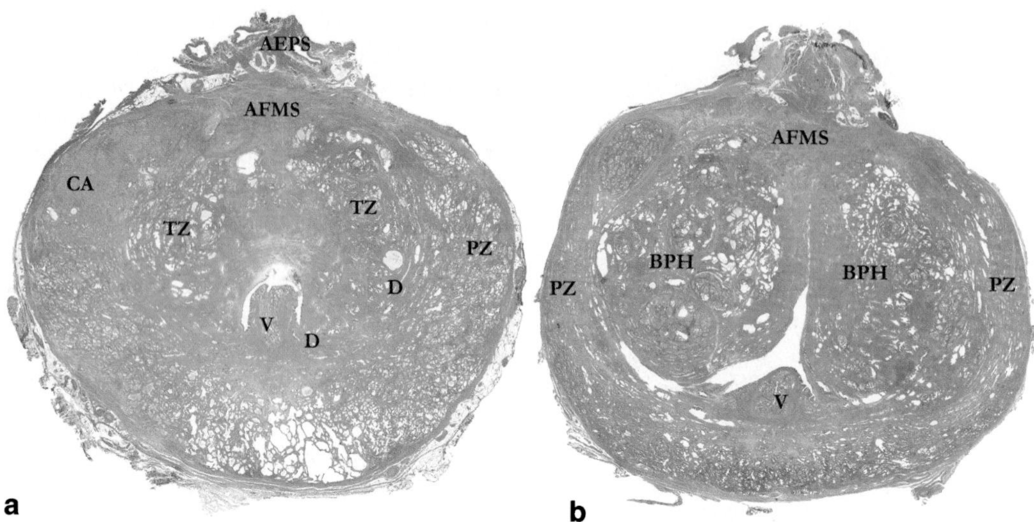

Fig. 1.3 **a** Whole mount section from mid-prostate at the level of the verumontanum (*V*). Note the bilobed transition zone (*TZ*) arising from elongated ducts (*D*), which course anteromedially. The peripheral zone (*PZ*) still occupies the posterior, lateral, and anterolateral portions of the gland, with a cancer nodule (*CA*) evident in the right anterior peripheral zone. In the mid-prostate, the anterior fibromuscular stroma (*AFMS*) is much condensed and the anterior extraprostatic space (*AEPS*) largely retains its apical content. **b** Whole mount section from mid-prostate at the level of the verumontanum (*V*) in a gland with extensive benign prostatic hypertrophy (*BPH*). Anterolateral "horns" of the peripheral zone (*PZ*) are compressed laterally by the expanded transition zone tissue and the anterior fibromuscular stroma (*AFMS*) is diminished in extent

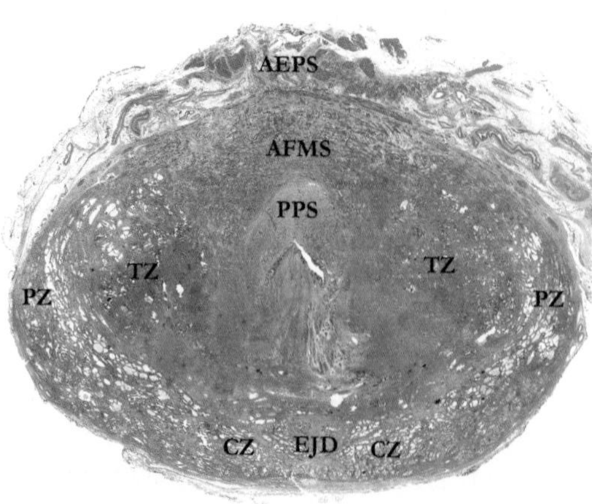

Fig. 1.4 Whole mount section from base of prostate. The preprostatic sphincter (*PPS*) is evident as a pale area surrounding the proximal urethra. The transition zone (*TZ*) shows abortive small acini and is covered anteriorly by a vast anterior fibromuscular stroma (*AFMS*), which merges with smooth muscle bundles in the anterior extraprostatic space (*AEPS*). Posteriorly, the expansive central zone (*CZ*) surrounds the ejaculatory duct complex (*EJD*), while some peripheral zone (*PZ*) is still apparent laterally

further anteriorly in histologic sections, eventually breaching the anterior-most border of tissue sections at the level of the bladder neck, a region which also contains no clear "capsule." Posterior to the urethra, the ejaculatory ducts emerge and are immediately encircled by a sheath of fibrous tissue with abundant lymphovascular spaces. Posterolaterally, central zone glands surround the ejaculatory duct sheath. In the most basal portions of the gland, the distinct muscular coat at the base of the seminal vesicles forms and separates from the bulk of the prostatic tissue creating a fibroadipose tissue septum. The last vestiges of the central zone are present at the most lateral aspects of the emerging seminal vesicles [5, 6].

Extraprostatic Tissue

In vivo, the tissue immediately anterior to the prostate is the dorsal venous or vascular complex, a series of veins and arteries set in fibroadipose tissue that runs over the anterior prostate and continues distally to supply/drain the penis. At radical prostatectomy, the complex is ligated and divided, with a portion of the blood vessels and fibroadipose tissue adhering to the prostate specimen. These are identified in the anterior extraprostatic tissue from apex through mid-gland (Fig. 1.3a, 1.3b), while the most proximal (basal) 2–3 sections reveal medium- to large-sized smooth muscles' bundles admixed with adipose tissue [5, 6]. These fibers are morphologically identical to those of the muscularis propria (detrusor muscle) of the bladder and probably represent a detrusor muscle extension over the prostatic base to mid-gland (Fig. 1.4).

Over the medial half of the posterior surface of the prostate, the "capsule" is thickened by its fusion to Denonvilliers' fascia, a thin collagenous membrane whose smooth posterior surface rests directly against the muscle of the rectal wall. The prostatic "capsule" is fused to the fascia with an interposed adipose layer containing a variable number of smooth muscle fibers. These smooth muscle fibers may cause confusion in determining the presence of extraprostatic extension as they complicate assessment of the outer border of the prostate [6].

Clinical and Diagnostic Significance of Prostatic Anatomy and Histomorphology

Clinicopathologic Features and Pathologic Outcomes of Anterior Prostate Cancers

Since the late 1980s, a number of authors have argued that TZ tumors could be identified using distinctive histomorphologic criteria [7]. McNeal and colleagues described "clear cell" histology [8] as discrete glands of variable size and contour, composed of tall cuboidal to columnar cells with clear-to-pale pink cytoplasm, basally oriented nuclei, and occasional eosinophilic luminal secretions (Fig. 1.5). In a small series, McNeal et al. demonstrated that this morphology predominated in up to two thirds of TZ-dominant cancers and nearly 75 % of incidental small TZ tumors diagnosed on transurethral resection specimens and was associated with a high percentage of Gleason pattern 1–2 cancer foci. It was concluded that this "clear cell" appearance was a marker of TZ tumors and more globally, of low-grade lesions [8].

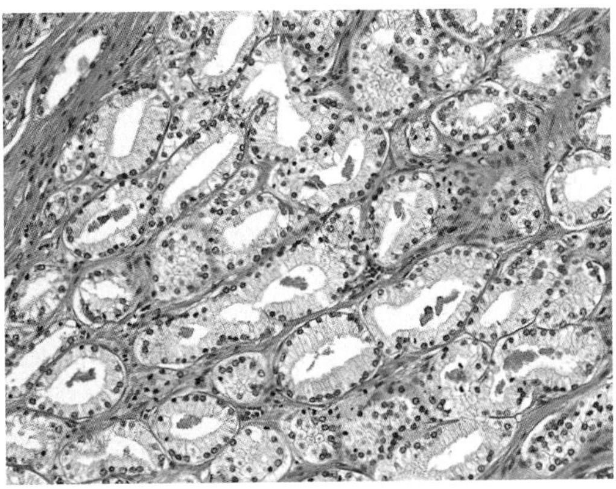

Fig. 1.5 Clear cell histology with variably shaped glands displaying pale cytoplasm and basally oriented nuclei

Nearly two decades later, Garcia et al. studied dominant prostatic lesions from both the peripheral and TZs and confirmed that this tumor appearance is present to some extent in the majority of TZ tumors and was more commonly the predominant morphology in TZ tumors than in PZ tumors (ratio >5:1). However, they also found that "clear cell" histology is the predominant morphology in only 50 % of TZ-dominant tumors [9]. A careful look at McNeal's original work reveals that 51 % of PZ-dominant tumors exhibited some "clear cell" histology, with 21 % of these showing ≥20 % [8]. Garcia et al. similarly found that 43 % of PZ-dominant tumors displayed some "clear cell" histology and that 35 % of these showed >25 % [9].

The finding of nonfocal "clear cell" morphology in peripheral-zone dominant prostate cancers is relevant to assignment of zonal origin for prostate cancer. The significant degree of variability in anterior prostatic anatomy described earlier—specifically, the proportions of PZ and TZ tissues in this region from apex to base—may engender difficulty in assessing zone of origin.

In such cases with anatomic complexity, finding 25–50% (nonfocal) "clear cell" histology in an anterior tumor will not help establishing its zonal origin. It has also been shown that the presence or absence of "clear cell" histology in needle biopsy specimens does not correlate with the presence of TZ tumor at radical prostatectomy [10].

Most studies that have compared tumors of TZ and PZ origin have ascribed a more indolent course, higher cure rate, and overall more favorable prognosis for TZ tumors when compared with PZ tumors [7, 11–13]. Although larger volumes and higher serum prostate-specific antigen (PSA) values have been described for TZ tumors, most reports have maintained that TZ tumors show significantly lower Gleason scores. However, classification of TZ cancers was often founded upon recognizing "clear cell" histology and these TZ tumors were compared with posterior PZ cancers. Until recently, few studies have compared TZ tumors with those arising in the anterior PZ, the predominant glandular tissue of the apical prostate.

In line with the contemporary anatomic analysis presented in this chapter, Al-Ahmadie et al. undertook a detailed analysis of 197 anterior-dominant tumors, emphasizing the variability of anterior prostatic anatomy from apex through base in determining zone of origin and pathological staging. They showed that the majority of anterior-dominant tumors are actually of anterior PZ origin (49 vs 36%; the remainder involved both zones equally). In comparing cases of anterior PZ origin and TZ origin, no significant differences in Gleason scores, incidence of extraprostatic extension or overall surgical margin positivity rate were observed [14]. This anatomy-sensitive approach (a) revealed the propensity of anterior PZ tumors to involve the apical one third of the prostate; (b) demonstrated that invasion of the anterior fibromuscular stroma may be seen in ~50% of anterior PZ tumors, reflecting the nearly complete ring that this tissue forms in the surgically resected prostate; and (c) allowed for an "apples to apples" comparison of exclusively anterior-dominant tumors which may show differences in pathologic stage compared with posterior tumors due to significant differences in nerve density [15] and difficulties in assessing extraprostatic extension in a region without a definitive "capsule." In the future, it is hoped that accurate histoanatomic classification of anterior prostatic tumors will enable more meaningful long-term clinical outcome and molecular analyses to assess differences in biology and behavior between tumors of differing zonal origin.

Biopsy Sampling Strategies for the Anterior Prostate

Among multiple changes to the diagnostic armamentarium for prostate cancer over the past two decades, systematic needle biopsies—now routinely 12-core—combined with aggressive PSA screening protocols have led to a profound clinical and pathologic stage migration toward nonpalpable tumors (cT1c), organ-confined disease (pT2), and improved clinical outcomes. Consequently, early detection of lower volume posterior tumors has increased, as these cancers are most readily biopsied with the standard transrectal approach. As a result, a trend toward dominant anterior prostatic tumors has been reported [14]. A significant percentage is located in the prostatic TZ and are typically more difficult to detect by digital rectal examination, poorly visualized on imaging and require more biopsy sessions to establish a diagnosis. Even when diagnosed, biopsies usually yield fewer involved cores and less total tumor length, complicating the assessment of cancer volume [16]. Therefore, the need for a needle biopsy technique that can adequately sample the anterior prostate is crucial [6].

The value of transrectal needle biopsies directed at the TZ in prostate cancer detection has been most extensively examined, with conflicting results. While some have shown utility for such biopsies in patients with previous negative biopsy sessions or "gray-zone" (4.0–9.9 ng/ml) PSA levels [17], most have argued against using TZ-directed biopsies in routine protocols, due to relatively low rates of cancer detection over traditional transrectal biopsy alone [18]. Few studies have correlated cancer seen in TZ-directed needle biopsies with that seen in prostatectomy specimens and/or the clinical relevance of these tumors. Haarer et al., working in an environment with routine sampling of TZ in needle biopsies, compared prostate cancers detected in TZ-directed needle biopsies with those seen in corresponding radical prostatectomy specimens. Among 61 patients in whom cancer was present on a TZ-directed needle biopsy, 80 % had either no tumor in the TZ or nondominant and clinically insignificant TZ cancer at radical prostatectomy. Similarly, nearly 50 % of cases with cancer in left or right TZ-directed needle biopsy, respectively, showed either no TZ tumor or tumor in the contralateral TZ only at radical prostatectomy. These collective findings suggest that TZ-directed needle biopsies do not adequately characterize TZ tumors and therefore care should be taken in their interpretation [10].

Beyond TZ-directed biopsies, a litany of biopsy strategies that may more accurately target the anterior prostate have been proposed, including anterior lateral horn biopsy, "extreme" anterior apical biopsy, transperineal biopsy with or without template mapping, and "saturation" biopsy. These techniques are worthy of consideration due to the increasing prevalence of anterior-dominant lesions.

Moussa et al. have shown that a scheme adding two extreme anterior apical biopsies to a standard 12-core biopsy achieves both the highest rates of both cancer detection when compared with ≤12-core schemes and the highest rate of unique cancer detection (i.e., in these cores only) when all regions were considered [19]. Among the largest studies of patients undergoing transperineal template mapping biopsy, Taira et al. studied 373 men (median: 57 cores), including 79 patients for whom this was the initial biopsy. They found a very high cancer detection rate of 76 % in the initial biopsy group, as well as a high rate of positive cancer cores in the anterior and apical regions both in this group and more prominently in patients with one or more previous negative biopsies [20]. Moreover, Patel et al., in a study of 539 patients using transperineal template mapping biopsy (median: 58 cores), determined that of 287 patients with cancer, 130 (45 %) had cancer in a transperineal TZ-directed biopsy. Of these, only 4 of 130 were clinically insignificant [21]. "Saturation" biopsy is a somewhat loosely applied term indicating biopsy schema with 20 or more transrectal cores taken in a systematic fashion. Although attempted by many, a systematic review has demonstrated that no significant cancer detection benefit accrues by taking greater than 12 cores [22]. Regarding anterior prostatic tumor detection, Falzarano and colleagues conducted a study which compared 72 patients with saturation biopsy (median: 21 cores) who underwent subsequent radical prostatectomy. Thirty-five of 39 patients with unilateral cancer on saturation biopsy showed bilateral cancers at prostatectomy. Eleven of these 35 had a clinically significant cancer in the lobe that was benign on saturation biopsy, with 10 of 11 located in the anterior-apical or TZ regions [23].

Taken together, these findings offer some hope that more precise detection of anteriorly localized prostatic tumors is possible. The majority of studies, however, have been performed in repeat biopsy or multiple negative prior biopsy settings with most arguing that such efforts do not improve cancer detection in the initial biopsy setting [6]. As in the case of TZ-directed needle biopsies, the true focus has been on cancer detection, rather than localization of tumor and therefore, relatively little correlative data with radical prostatectomy specimens exists. At this time, therefore, the ideal methodology for adequately sampling the anterior prostate awaits further study.

Prostatic Central Zone in Needle Biopsy Specimens

The prostatic central zone is a cone-like region running from the mid to the base of the prostate, where its glands surround the ejaculatory duct complex and lie adjacent to the seminal vesicles at the base in routine surgical pathology sections. Recent radiologic and pathologic studies have demonstrated that prostate cancers involving central zone are associated with more aggressive disease—higher PSA values, Gleason scores, and rates of extracapsular extension and seminal vesicle invasion—than those without central zone involvement [24]. While some have considered these tumors "central zone cancers," this phenomenon is probably better explained by large and high-grade PZ tumors near the base of the prostate invading adjacent local structures such as the seminal vesicles.

As opposed to the glandular component of the peripheral and TZs, central zone glands are thought to be of Wolffian origin, similar to the ejaculatory ducts/seminal vesicles. This is reflected in the morphologic appearance of central zone glands which are characterized by complex glands with papillary to cribriform architecture at low magnification and extensive epithelial bridging, often with classic "Roman arches." At higher power, these glands have pseudo-stratified columnar epithelium composed of cells with eosinophilic cytoplasm and an underlying prominent basal cell layer [25] (Fig. 1.6).

In needle biopsy specimens, central zone histology is one of the most common mimics of high-grade prostatic intraepithelial neoplasia (PIN) due to their ample low-power architectural overlap. As the dark cytoplasm of high-grade PIN may range from basophilic to eosinophilic depending on the histologic preparation, the eye is easily drawn to central zone glands at low magnification as foci suspicious for high-grade PIN. The lack of cytologic atypia and the prominent basal cell layer in central zone glands are two features aiding their distinction from PIN glands which exhibit at least some degree of macronucleoli and focal, patchy basal cells on H & E. Given the localization of the central zone, caution must be applied in diagnosing high-grade PIN in mid-base biopsies. In practice, an increased threshold for evaluation of nuclear and nucleolar atypia should be considered in this setting [6].

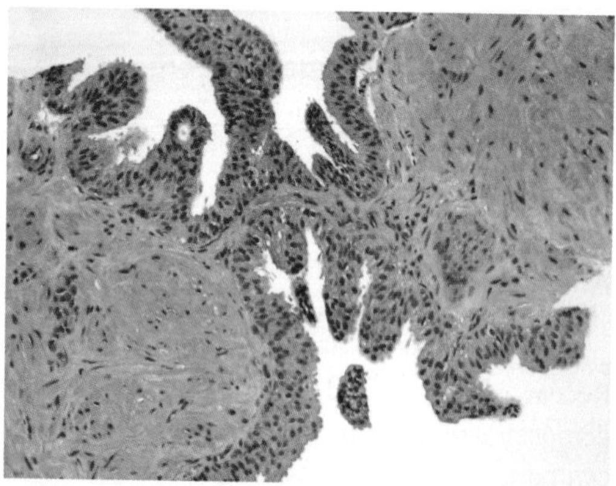

Fig. 1.6 Central zone epithelium in prostate needle biopsy displaying eosinophilic cytoplasm, prominent basal cell layer, and an intraepithelial bridge ("Roman arch")

Cancer Involving Skeletal Muscle on Needle Biopsy

The apical-anterior portions of the prostate contain smooth muscle which interdigitates with skeletal muscle fibers of the urogenital diaphragm in the context of the anterior fibromuscular stroma [5]. These regions may also contain benign and/or malignant glands and hence, it is important to recognize that finding glands within or adjacent to skeletal muscle is not diagnostic of carcinoma (for benign-appearing glands) or diagnostic of extraprostatic extension (for malignant-appearing glands). The one significant study comparing radical prostatectomy outcomes between biopsies with Gleason score 6 cancer involving one core with skeletal muscle involvement and similar cases without skeletal muscle involvement highlighted the lack of statistically significant differences in rates of Gleason score >6, extraprostatic extension or surgical margin positivity between the two groups at subsequent radical prostatectomy [26]. Hence, prostate cancers demonstrating skeletal muscle involvement on needle biopsy (Fig. 1.7) may not be more aggressive than other cases. Patients with skeletal muscle involvement on needle biopsy often showed positive surgical margins located at the apex and surgeons may choose to extend their apical dissection to avoid a positive margin.

Extraprostatic Extension on Needle Biopsy

Although peri-prostatic tissue, in the form of neural, lymphovascular, and adipose tissue, may be found in up to three-quarters of prostatic

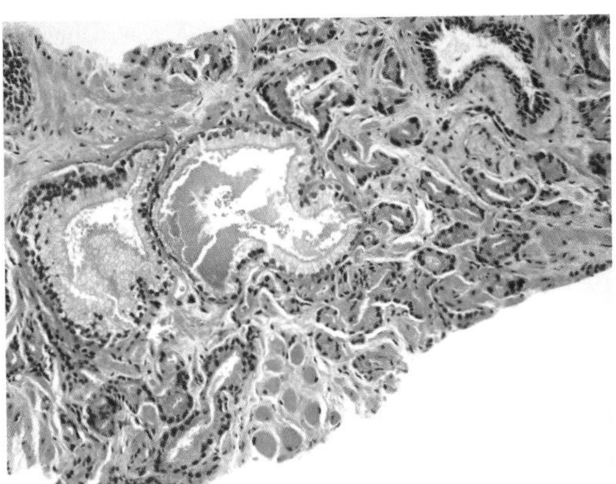

Fig. 1.7 Small acinar carcinoma involving skeletal muscle (lower portion of core) on needle biopsy

needle biopsies, the finding of carcinoma in peri-prostatic adipose tissue is exceedingly rare. Whether fat cells may be present within the prostatic parenchyma has been debated and is at most exceptionally rare. Hence, tumor infiltrating fat in a needle biopsy specimen should be diagnosed as extraprostatic extension. When present, this fat is typically found at the tips of needle cores. The single formal study of extraprostatic extension detected on biopsy found a strong association with extensive, high-grade carcinoma in the needle biopsy specimen and a high incidence of ≥pT3a disease in patients who underwent radical prostatectomy [27]. For biopsies with a low magnification appearance of abundant high-grade disease, it is a useful practice to survey any available adipose tissue to exclude the possibility of extraprostatic extension [6].

Seminal Vesicle/Ejaculatory Duct on Needle Biopsy

Seminal vesicle tissue or, more commonly, ejaculatory duct tissue may be seen in needle biopsies from the mid or base of the prostate, occasionally as a result of specific sampling. The seminal vesicle is characterized by a coat of smooth muscle encircling a central lumen with branching glands. Tangential sampling of these branching glands on needle biopsy may produce a small gland pattern architecturally reminiscent of acinar carcinoma. Enlarged, often bizarre hyperchromatic nuclei, small nuclear pseudoinclusions, and a variable amount of cytoplasmic golden-brown lipofuscin are helpful features to distinguish seminal vesicle-type epithelium. However, when the epithelial atypia and pigmentation are not prominent, a diagnostic challenge may result. In problematic cases, negative labeling for PSA and prostatic acid phosphatase, coupled with basal cell labeling with high molecular weight cytokeratin or p63 is helpful in distinguishing seminal vesicle glands from acinar carcinoma.

Ejaculatory duct epithelium is similar to that of the seminal vesicle. Ejaculatory ducts, however, are more typically surrounded by a band of loose fibrovascular connective tissue and lack the well-formed muscular coat of seminal vesicle. If detected, this distinction may be of clinical importance since the presence of carcinoma in ejaculatory duct tissue does not indicate extraprostatic disease whereas carcinomatous involvement of seminal vesicle proper indicates high-stage disease and an adverse prognosis [28].

Conclusion

In this chapter, we have provided a modern update of our understanding of prostatic anatomy and its clinical implications for identifying and classifying prostatic tumors. We have highlighted an anatomy-sensitive approach for assigning zonal origin, various biopsy strategies proposed for detecting anterior tumors, and instances in which recognition of normal anatomic variation may influence needle biopsy interpretation.

References

1. McNeal JE. Regional morphology and pathology of the prostate. Am J Clin Pathol. 1968;49:347–57.
2. McNeal JE. Origin and evolution of benign prostatic enlargement. Invest Urol. 1977;15:340–45.

3. McNeal JE, Stamey TA, Hodge KK. The prostate gland: morphology, pathology, ultrasound anatomy. Monogr Urol. 1988;9:36–54.
4. McNeal JE. The zonal anatomy of the prostate. Prostate. 1981;2:35–49.
5. Fine SW, Al-Ahmadie HA, Gopalan A, Tickoo SK, Scardino PT, Reuter VE. Anatomy of the anterior prostate and extraprostatic space: a contemporary surgical pathology analysis. Adv Anat Pathol. 2007;14:401–7.
6. Fine SW, Reuter VE. Anatomy of the prostate revisited: implications for prostate biopsy and zonal origins of prostate cancer. Histopathology. 2012;60:142–52.
7. Greene DR, Wheeler TM, Egawa S, Weaver RP, Scardino PT. Relationship between clinical stage and histological zone of origin in early prostate cancer: morphometric analysis. Br J Urol. 1991;68:499–509.
8. McNeal JE, Redwine EA, Freiha FS, Stamey TA. Zonal distribution of prostatic adenocarcinoma: correlation with histologic patterns and direction of spread. Am J Surg Pathol. 1988;12:897–906.
9. Garcia JJ, Al-Ahmadie HA, Gopalan A, et al. Do prostatic transition zone tumors have a distinct morphology? Am J Surg Pathol. 2008;32:1709–14.
10. Haarer CF, Gopalan A, Tickoo SK, et al. Prostatic transition zone directed needle biopsies uncommonly sample clinically relevant transition zone tumors. J Urol. 2009;182:1337–41.
11. Noguchi M, Stamey TA, McNeal JE, Yemoto C. An analysis of 148 consecutive transition zone cancers: clinical and histologic characteristics. J Urol. 2000;163:1751–5.
12. Shannon BA, McNeal JE, Cohen RJ. Transition zone carcinoma of the prostate gland: a common indolent tumour type that occasionally manifests aggressive behavior. Pathology. 2003;35:467–71.
13. Andreoiu M, Cheng L. Multifocal prostate cancer: biologic, prognostic and therapeutic implications. Hum Pathol. 2010;41:781–93.
14. Al-Ahmadie HA, Tickoo SK, Olgac S, et al. Anterior-predominant prostatic tumors: zone of origin and pathologic outcomes at radical prostatectomy. Am J Surg Pathol. 2008;32:229–35.
15. Powell MS, Li R, Dai H, Sayeeduddin M, Wheeler TM, Ayala GE. Neuroanatomy of the normal prostate. Prostate. 2005;65:52–7.
16. Bott SRJ, Young MPA, Kellett MJ, Parkinson MC. Anterior prostate cancer: is it more difficult to diagnose? BJU Int. 2002;89:886–9.
17. Ishizuka O, Mimura Y, Oguchi T, Kawakami M, Nishizawa O. Importance of transition zone biopsies in patients with gray-zone PSA levels undergoing the ultrasounded-guided systematic ten-biopsy regimen for the first time. Urol Int. 2005;74:23–6.
18. Liu IJ, Macy M, Lai YH, Terris MK. Critical evaluation of the current indications for transition zone biopsies. Urology. 2001;57:1117–20.
19. Moussa AS, Meshref A, Schoenfield L, et al. Importance of additional "extreme" anterior apical needle biopsies in the initial detection of prostate cancer. Urology. 2010;75:1034–9.
20. Taira AV, Merrick GS, Galbreath RW, et al. Performance of transperineal template-guided mapping biopsy in detecting prostate cancer in the initial and repeat biopsy setting. Prostate Cancer Prostatic Dis. 2010;13:71–7.
21. Patel V, Merrick GS, Allen ZA, et al. The incidence of transition zone prostate cancer diagnosed by transperineal template-guided mapping biopsy: implications for treatment planning. Urology. 2011;77:1148–1154.
22. Eichler K, Hempel S, Wilby J, Myers L, Bachmann LM, Kleijnen J. Diagnostic value of systematic biopsy methods in the investigation of prostate cancer: a systematic review. J Urol. 2006;175:1605–12.
23. Falzarano S, Zhou M, Hernandez AV, Moussa AS, Jones JS, Magi-Galluzzi C. Can saturation biopsy predict prostate cancer localization in radical prostatectomy specimens: a correlative study and implications for focal therapy. Urology. 2010;76:682–8.
24. Vargas HA, Akin O, Franiel T, Goldman DA, Udo K, Touijer KA, Reuter VE, Hricak H. Normal central zone of the prostate and central zone involvement by prostate cancer: clinical and MR imaging implications. Radiology. 2012;262(3):894–902.
25. Srodon M, Epstein JI. Central zone histology of the prostate: a mimicker of high-grade prostatic intraepithelial neoplasia. Hum Pathol. 2002;33:518–23.
26. Ye HH, Walsh PC, Epstein JI. Skeletal muscle involvement by limited Gleason score 6 adenocarcinoma of the prostate on needle biopsy is not associated with adverse findings at radical prostatectomy. J Urol. 2010;184:2308–12.
27. Miller JS, Chen YB, Ye H, Robinson BD, Brimo F, Epstein JI. Extraprostatic extension of prostatic adenocarcinoma on needle core biopsy: report of 72 cases with clinical follow-up. BJU Int. 2009;106:330–3.
28. Srigley JR. Benign mimickers of prostatic adenocarcinoma. Mod Pathol. 2004;17:328–48.

Contemporary Gleason Grading System

2

Kiril Trpkov

Historical Background and Context

Nearly half a century ago, in 1966, the pathologist Donald Gleason developed a grading system (Fig. 2.1a, b) for prostatic adenocarcinoma [1], which has been embraced almost universally as an essential component of prostate adenocarcinoma grading and reporting. Over time, the system has been modified by Gleason and his collaborators and by others [1–5]. Despite the modifications in the past four decades, the Gleason grading system has been validated as a fundamental prognostic factor for prostate cancer, both on biopsy and on radical prostatectomy (RP), of patient outcomes, including biochemical failure, local recurrence, and lymph node or distant metastasis. Gleason score (GS) has also been incorporated in clinical tools, such as Partin tables and Kattan nomograms, which are used to predict pathologic stage and outcome following RP or radiotherapy. GS on needle biopsy is also utilized to determine treatment selection, such as active surveillance, RP, brachytherapy, lymph node dissection, and the extent of neurovascular bundle resection.

The Gleason system is based on low-power microscopic assessment (×4 or ×10) of the cancer architecture. The key principle of the grading is based on the use of two most common cancer grades (out of possible 5), primary plus secondary grade, to produce a GS, which theoretically ranges from 2 to 10. When only a single grade is identified, it is doubled to yield a GS. The terms "pattern" and "grade" have also been retained. Typically, pattern is used to describe one or more of the morphologic variations, while grade is used in a more encompassing way, to include all pattern variations within a certain grade.

In clinical practice, the diagnosis of prostate cancer and its management have also evolved over the last few decades, first by introduction of prostate-specific antigen (PSA) testing in the late 1980s, and the extensive use of RP. Prostate cancer incidence has also changed since the introduction of PSA testing, first demonstrating an increase and then a drop; more recently, mortality, primarily in the Western countries, has also decreased [6]. Thus, in current practice, patients are diagnosed earlier, at a younger age, with smaller cancer volumes and lower stage disease [7]. During the last two decades, the practice of thin-needle prostate biopsies (16–18 gauge) has also taken place, first as sextant (six core) biopsies, and then as systematic and extended prostate biopsies, with at least ten tissue cores sampled from different prostate sites (apex, mid, base). The biopsies are also commonly submitted in a site-specific fashion. In contrast, Gleason developed his system on tissue samples from large-bore biopsies (14 gauge) without a site-specific submission, and on transurethral resection of prostate and prostatectomy specimens. In addition, immunohistochemistry was not available in the era when the system was developed, variants

K. Trpkov (✉)
Department of Pathology and Laboratory Medicine, General Hospital, 7007 14th Street, Calgary, AB T2V1P9, Canada
e-mail: kiril.trpkov@cls.ab.ca

C. Magi-Galluzzi, C. G. Przybycin (eds.), *Genitourinary Pathology*, DOI 10.1007/978-1-4939-2044-0_2,

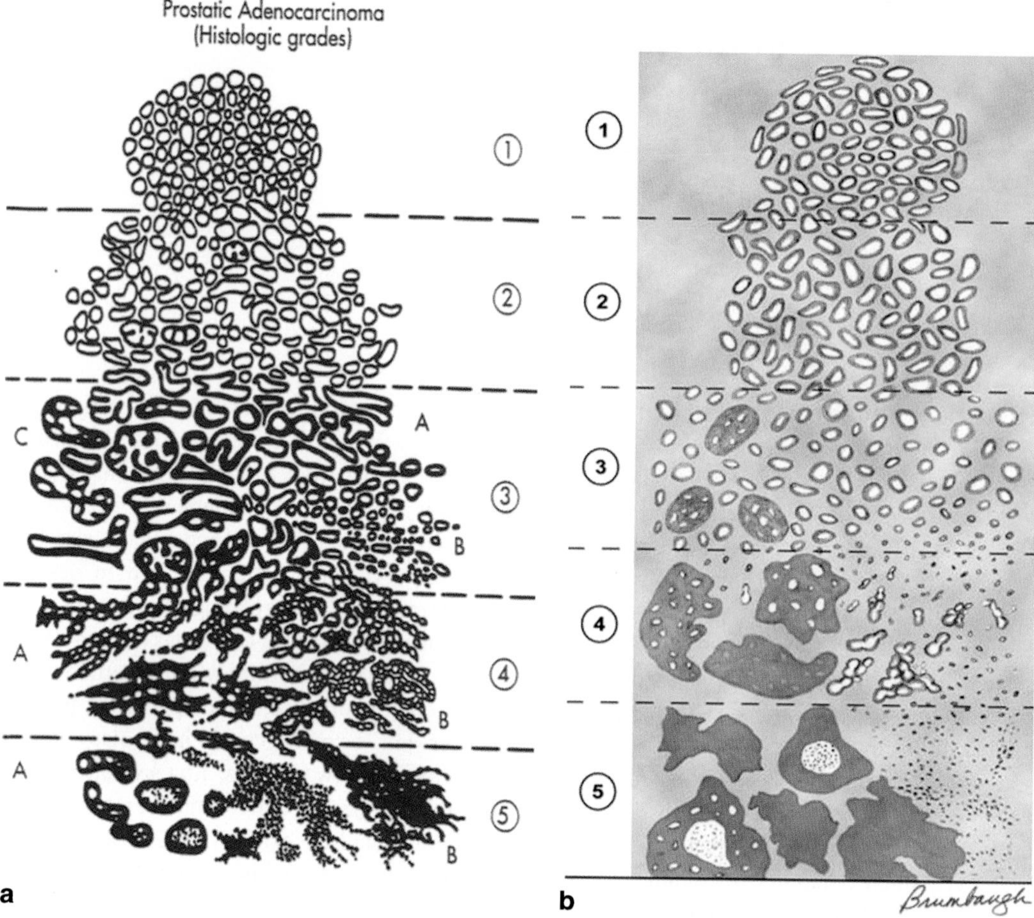

Fig. 2.1 Comparison of the diagrams of the original Gleason grading system (**a**) and the ISUP 2005 modified Gleason grading system (**b**). (**a** Used with permission from [5]. **b** Used with permission from [4])

of adenocarcinoma and certain morphologic patterns were not recognized, and the significance of the tertiary grade remained uncertain. Around the turn of the century, it also became evident that there are differences in the application of the Gleason system among pathologists (i.e., interobserver variability), particularly in the evolving needle biopsy practice. Pathologists used the Gleason system based on their own understanding, interpretation, or preference. Thus, it was necessary to establish a consensus and to codify the application of the Gleason system to correspond with the clinical practice in the twenty-first century.

International Society of Urologic Pathology 2005 Modification of the Gleason System

In March 2005, a consensus conference was convened by the International Society of Urologic Pathology (ISUP) in San Antonio, TX, USA, in an effort to standardize and unify the use of the Gleason grading system [4]. Specific areas of the original Gleason System reviewed at the 2005 ISUP conference are illustrated in Table 2.1. A "consensus" was defined when two third of the participants were in agreement on certain questions. This effort resulted in the 2005 ISUP modified Gleason system, which, similar to the original Gleason system, outlined the morphologic patterns 1–5

Table 2.1 Specific areas of the original Gleason grading system reviewed at the 2005 International Society of Urological Pathology (ISUP) conference

1	General applications of the Gleason grading system
2	Defining Gleason patterns 1–5
3	Grading variants and variations of acinar adenocarcinoma of the prostate
4	Reporting secondary patterns of lower grade when present to a limited extent
5	Reporting secondary patterns of higher grade when present to a limited extent
6	Tertiary Gleason patterns
7	Percentage of patterns 4–5
8	Radical prostatectomy specimens with separate tumor nodules
9	Needle biopsies with different cores showing different grades

Table 2.2 The architectural patterns 1–5 according to the 2005 International Society of Urologic Pathology modified Gleason system

Gleason Pattern	
1	Circumscribed nodule of closely packed, but separate, uniform, rounded to oval, medium-sized acini (larger glands than pattern 3)
2	Like pattern 1, fairly circumscribed, but at the edge of the tumor nodule, there may be minimal infiltration; glands are more loosely arranged and not quite as uniform as Gleason pattern 1
3	Discrete glandular units, typically smaller glands than seen in Gleason pattern 1 and 2; infiltrates in and amongst nonneoplastic prostate acini; marked variation in size and shape; smoothly circumscribed small cribriform nodules of tumor
4	Fused microacinar glands; ill-defined glands with poorly formed glandular lumina; large, cribriform glands; cribriform glands with an irregular border, hypernephromatoid
5	Essentially no glandular differentiation, composed of solid sheets, cords, or single cells; comedocarcinoma with central necrosis surrounded by papillary, cribriform, or solid masses

(shown in Table 2.2), which are accompanied by a diagram for the modified Gleason system (shown with the original Gleason system for comparison in Fig. 2.1a, b). The differences between the original Gleason system and the 2005 ISUP modified Gleason system are summarized in Table 2.3 [4, 8]. The 2005 ISUP modified Gleason system reiterated the following points (Table 2.4):

a. GS represents the sum of the primary (most predominant) Gleason grade and the secondary (second most predominant) Gleason grade. However, in needle biopsies, this principle was modified to include any component of higher grade than the second most predominant grade as the secondary grade. Thus, on needle biopsy the GS is derived based on the primary and the highest (worst) grade.
b. The reporting of the grade should be accompanied by using the words "pattern" or "grade," and it is therefore not acceptable to report only "Gleason 3" because it is unclear whether this represents grade (pattern) or score.
c. GS 1+1=2 on needle biopsy should rarely, if ever, be reported and should be carefully considered in practice, in any type of specimen. These cancers are extraordinarily rare in needle biopsies, although they can be infrequently seen in transurethral or RP specimens. There is a poor reproducibility even among experts in grading lower-grade tumors. Cancers that are assigned GS 2–4 on needle biopsy correlate poorly with RP GS and these "low" scores may misguide clinicians and misinform patients into considering these tumors as indolent.
d. Individual cells are not part of Gleason pattern 3.
e. Most cribriform glands are diagnosed as Gleason pattern 4. Only rare cribriform glands satisfy the stringent diagnostic criteria required for the diagnosis of cribriform pattern 3: rounded, well-circumscribed glands of the same size as the normal glands.

Table 2.3 Differences between the original Gleason system and the 2005 International Society of Urologic Pathology (ISUP) modified Gleason system

Original Gleason system	2005 ISUP modified Gleason system
Diagnosis of GS <4 can be made on NB	Diagnosis of GS <4 on NB specimens rarely, if ever, made
Cribriform glands with rounded and smooth contours as well as cribriform glands with an irregular outer border are diagnosed as Gleason pattern 3	Most cribriform glands would be diagnosed as Gleason pattern 4. Only rounded, well-circumscribed glands of the same size as normal ones, would be diagnosed as cribriform pattern
The same GS is used for NB and RP specimens	Different GS are used for NB and RP specimens
High-grade tumor of small quantity (<5 %) on NB should be excluded based on GS (5 % threshold rule)	High-grade tumor of any quantity on NB should be included within the GS
GS on NB based on the primary and the secondary patterns, with an exclusion of the tertiary one	If tertiary pattern is present on NB, GS is based on the primary pattern and the highest pattern
GS on RP specimens should be assigned based on the primary and secondary patterns (tertiary should not be included or mentioned)	GS on RP specimens is based on the primary and the secondary patterns; if tertiary, higher pattern is present, it is reported separately as a tertiary one
Separate or overall GS reported for all cores or tissue fragments on NB specimens	When NB specimens show different grades in separate cores, individual GS should be assigned to intact positive cores; overall GS is optional
The Gleason grade from the largest tumor nodule on RP should be assigned as GS, even if the second larger nodule is of higher grade	When RP specimens show different grades in separate tumor nodules, a separate GS should be assigned to each nodule, irrespective of the size

GS Gleason score, *NB* needle biopsy, *RP* radical prostatectomy

Table 2.4 Reporting recommendations for special Gleason grading scenarios

Scenario	Recommendation
Only one grade present (e.g., GG 3)	Double that grade (assign GS 3+3 = 6)
Abundant high-grade cancer (e.g., GG 4) with <5 % lower-grade cancer	Ignore the lower-grade cancer (assign GS 4+ 4 = 8)
Small focus with mostly GG 4 and few glands of GG 3	If GG 3 occupies >5 %, include lower-grade cancer (assign GS 4+3=7)
Abundant GG 3 with any extent of GG 4	Include the higher grade (assign GS 3 + 4 = 7)
Three grades (e.g., GG 3, 4, and 5) present	Classify as high grade (assign most common plus highest grade)
NB: multiple cores showing different grades—cores submitted separately and/or with designated location	Assign separate GS to each core
NB: multiple cores showing different grades—all cores were submitted in one container or cores are fragmented	Assign overall GS for the specimen

GG Gleason grade, *GS* Gleason score, *NB* needle biopsy

f. Morphologic variants of acinar adenocarcinoma, such as pseudohyperplastic and foamy adenocarcinoma, should be graded on the basis of the underlying architecture.
g. A secondary pattern of lower-grade cancer, when it occupies less than 5 % of tumor, should be ignored and not reported as part of the GS, both on needle biopsy and RP.
h. High-grade tumor of any quantity, even when occupying less than 5 % of the tumor, should always be included and reported within the GS on needle biopsy.
i. When a tertiary Gleason pattern is present, GS on biopsy should be derived by adding the primary and the highest (worst) pattern, whereas on RP, the tertiary pattern (the least common pattern), should be reported separately if it is of higher grade than the primary and the secondary patterns.

j. When separate tumor nodules with different Gleason patterns are encountered on RP, they should be scored and reported separately.
k. It remains optional to include the actual percentage of Gleason patterns 4 or 5 in a report.
l. For needle biopsies containing different cores with different cancer grades, separate GS should be assigned for individual positive cores, if they are submitted in separate containers or if the cores are in the same container, but have a designated location (for example, if marked by different ink color). An optional, overall GS can be provided at the end of the case for all positive biopsy cores. The overall (global) GS follows the general rule of primary (most predominant) Gleason grade and secondary (second most predominant) Gleason grade [9, 10]. When a container has multiple fragmented cores and it is unclear whether they represent intact cores or multiple cores, an overall score should be provided for all fragments in the container.

Changes and Trends in Practice in Interpreting Gleason Grades 1–5 After the 2005 ISUP Consensus Conference

The 2005 ISUP modified Gleason system was widely promoted and embraced in routine practice after the consensus conference and the subsequent publication, although certain issues remained unresolved. The main trends and changes in the use of individual grades in pathology practice after 2005 were as follows:

Gleason Grade 1

Since the 2005 ISUP consensus conference concluded that Gleason grade 1 tumors should be diagnosed "rarely, if ever," the use of pattern 1 after 2005 became vanishingly rare. Many uropathology experts maintain that pattern 1 in the original Gleason system likely represented adenosis (atypical adenomatous hyperplasia), a now well-recognized cancer mimicker. At that time, however, immunohistochemistry was not available and thus, adenosis may account for the great majority of cases considered traditionally as Gleason pattern 1. Many of the infrequently published images of Gleason pattern 1 can be critically questioned and accordingly it has been proposed that Gleason pattern 1 is completely abandoned in practice [11].

Gleason Grade 2

Similarly, the appropriateness of using pattern 2 in needle biopsies has also been questioned and pathologists have been advised not to use it in grading cancer on needle biopsies [12]. Cancers assigned GS 2–4 on needle biopsy correlate poorly with GS on RP, which almost always contain higher-grade cancer. Pattern 2 can be seen occasionally in transurethral resection and RP specimens, usually as part of multifocal cancer invariably showing a higher-grade component.

Gleason Grade 3

The general focus of the 2005 modifications pertained primarily to the most prevalent patterns 3 and 4. The 2005 ISUP modified Gleason system restricted the definitions of pattern 3 and broadened the spectrum of pattern 4 cancer [8, 13, 14]. As in the original Gleason system, pattern 3 in the 2005 ISUP modified Gleason system includes discrete well-formed individual glands, infiltrating in and among nonneoplastic prostate acini (Fig. 2.2a). Very small, well-formed glands are still considered Gleason pattern 3; however, in contrast to the original Gleason system, "individual cells" are not. The definition of grade 3, however, also stipulates "marked variation in glandular size and shape," which, unfortunately, was not well depicted in the 2005 diagram. It is still unclear, for example, which variations in glandular shape should be considered Gleason pattern 3 (Fig. 2.2b). Are individual glands showing branching and forming, for example, X, V, T, and Y glandular shapes (not illustrated in the 2005 diagram) still consistent with pattern

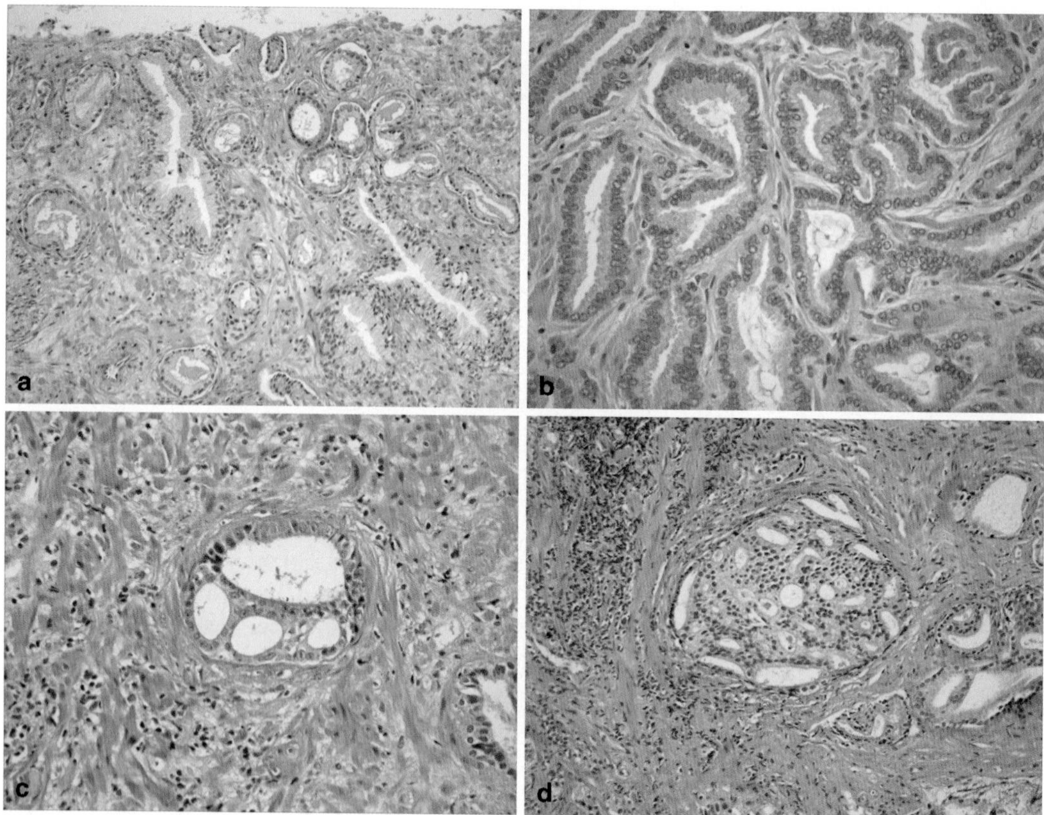

Fig. 2.2 Gleason grade 3 includes discrete infiltrative glands with well-formed lumina (a). Individual glands showing some modifications of size and shape such as branching (not illustrated in the 2005 diagram) are still interpreted as pattern 3, although some may interpret them as pattern 4 (b). Cribriform rounded, well-circumscribed glands of the same size as the normal glands are interpreted as pattern 3 (c). If they are with similar cribriform features but of larger size than a normal gland, they are currently interpreted as pattern 4. Using the original Gleason system, these would have been graded as pattern 3 (d)

3 or do they represent pattern 4? Indeed, many uropathologists would consider these common morphologies to represent pattern 3, but unfortunately this cannot be reconciled using the 2005 ISUP Gleason diagram.

More stringent criteria were established by the 2005 ISUP consensus conference concerning cribriform pattern 3 glands. Only rounded, well-circumscribed glands of the same size as the normal glands, with evenly spaced lumina and cellular bridges (Fig. 2.2c) are included as cribriform Gleason pattern 3. In essence, these types of cancers should morphologically resemble cribriform high-grade prostatic intraepithelial neoplasia (HGPIN), but lack basal cells. This definition was in contrast to the original Gleason illustrations of cribriform pattern 3, which included large, cribriform glands with rounded and smooth contours, exceeding the size of the normal glands (Fig. 2.2d). In the current practice, nearly all cribriform glands are being diagnosed as pattern 4 [13].

Gleason Grade 4

The scope of Gleason pattern 4 in the 2005 ISUP modified Gleason system was widened. A consensus was reached that ill-defined glands with poorly formed lumina, a pattern often seen in fused glandular structures, should also be included under Gleason pattern 4. This novel category was not described in the original Gleason system.

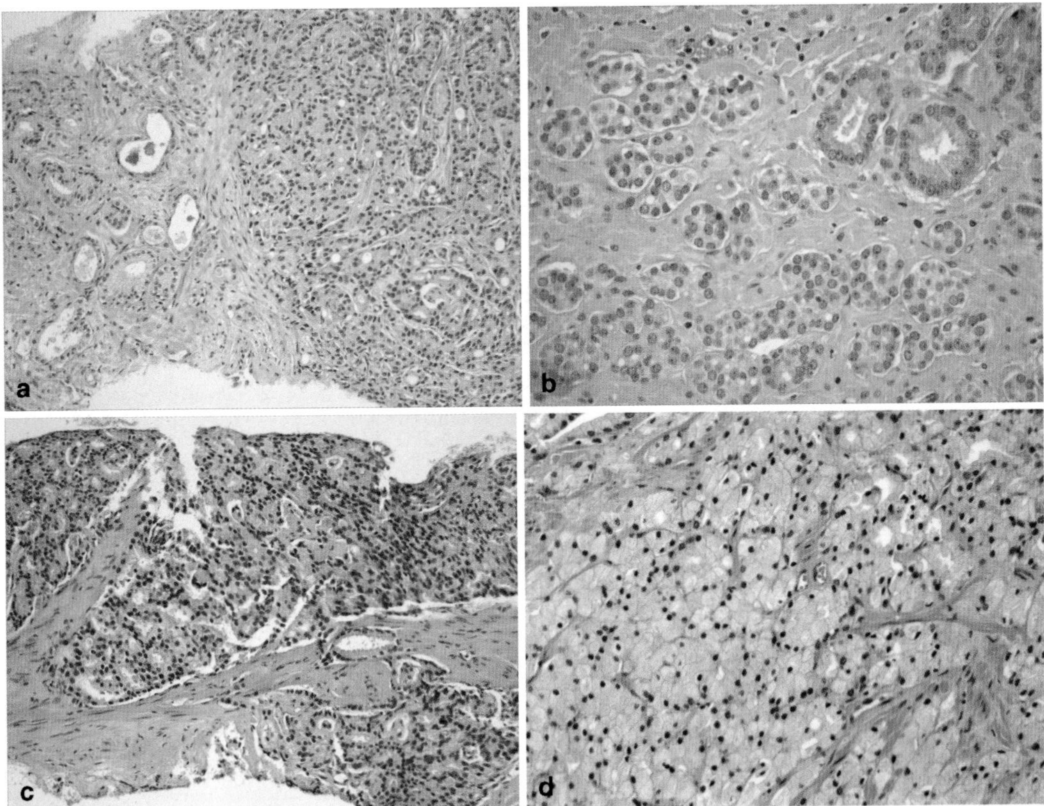

Fig. 2.3 Gleason grade 4 includes glands that are fused (represented on the *right*; contrast them with the individual glands on the *left*) (**a**), glands with ill-formed lumina (contrast them with a couple of individual glands with well-formed lumina in the *upper right*) (**b**), large cribriform glands (**c**), and hypernephromatoid glands (**d**)

Therefore, pattern 4 now includes: (a) fused microacinar glands; (b) ill-defined glands with poorly formed glandular lumina; (c) large, cribriform glands and cribriform glands with an irregular border, and (d) hypernephromatoid glands:

a. Fused glandular morphology implies that discrete glandular units are lost or are unrecognizable (unchanged from the original Gleason system) (Fig. 2.3a).
b. Ill-defined glands with poorly formed glandular lumina, a novel category, is now considered pattern 4 (Fig. 2.3b). The illustrations of this pattern remained sketchy and unclear in the literature, thus creating some confusion and leading to relatively open interpretation of this concept. Distinguishing, for example, between poorly formed glands (pattern 4) and tangentially sectioned glands (pattern 3) seems to be one of the most problematic issues of the current Gleason grading. This essentially requires two-dimensional interpretation of a three-dimensional complex glandular morphology, which can be subjective.
c. Cribriform glands, as previously outlined, are nearly uniformly diagnosed as Gleason pattern 4 in current practice, independently of the glandular contour (Fig. 2.3c). In a recent study, poor reproducibility was reported among urologic pathologists in defining Gleason pattern 3 cribriform glands; in addition, in 73 % of the cases there was a coexistent Gleason pattern 4 tumor [15]. Therefore, a proposal has been made by Epstein to alter the 2005 ISUP diagram and to delete the cribriform 3 morphology [13, 14].
d. Hypernephromatoid, an infrequent glandular morphology of fused glands with clear

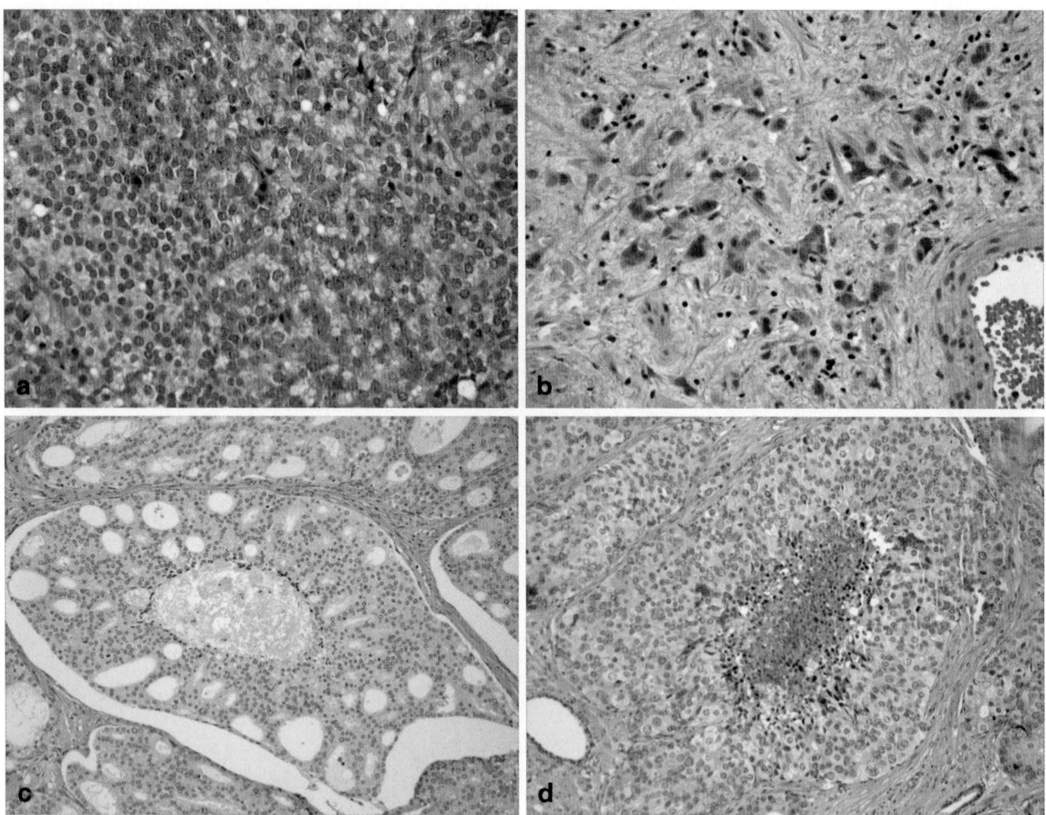

Fig. 2.4 Gleason grade 5 includes sheets of cells (**a**), single cells and single file cords (**b**), glands containing comedo-type necrosis surrounded by either cribriform (**c**), or solid masses (**d**)

or pale cytoplasm was retained as pattern 4 (Fig. 2.3d) (unchanged from the original Gleason system).

Gleason Grade 5

Pattern 5 remains almost unchanged from the original Gleason system and indicates absence of glandular differentiation, with neoplastic cells forming solid sheets, cords, or single cells (Fig. 2.4a, b). The presence of cords also includes single file cell formation. Solid nests, i.e., solid structures smaller than a "sheet" may potentially pose some problems, as smaller solid units may be interpreted as glands with ill-defined lumina (pattern 4). Comedocarcinoma with central necrosis surrounded by papillary, cribriform, or solid glands also represents pattern 5 (Fig. 2.4c, d).

Grading Variants of Prostate Adenocarcinoma in Contemporary Practice

Grading of different variants of prostatic adenocarcinoma is shown in Table 2.5 and illustrated in Fig. 2.5a–g):

Pseudohyperplastic Adenocarcinoma Cancers with pseudohyperplastic features (large

Table 2.5 Grading recommendations for prostate adenocarcinoma variants

Variant	Gleason grade
Pseudohyperplastic	3
Foamy	3 or 4 (depending on architecture)
Ductal	4 or 5 (if comedonecrosis present)
Mucinous (colloid)	3 or 4 (extract mucin/grade architecture)
Atrophic-cystic	3
PIN-like	3 (rarely 4)
Small cell (neuroendocrine)	Not graded
Squamous or adenosquamous	Not graded
Urothelial carcinomas	Not graded
Basaloid or adenoid-cystic	Not graded
Sarcomatoid	Not graded (same grade as 5, glandular component graded separately)

PIN prostatic intraepithelial neoplasia

individual glands resembling normal glands, but containing cytologically malignant nuclei), should be graded as Gleason grade 3, in large part based on the recognition that they are most often accompanied by more usual Gleason grade 3 adenocarcinoma (Fig. 2.5a).

Foamy Gland Carcinoma Although most cases of foamy (or xanthomatous) gland carcinoma would be graded as Gleason grade 3 (Fig. 2.5b), they can also show a higher-grade pattern and should be graded accordingly, usually as Gleason pattern 4.

Ductal Adenocarcinoma This is graded as Gleason pattern 4, but if comedonecrosis is present, it is graded as Gleason pattern 5 (Fig. 2.5c).

Colloid (mucinous) Carcinoma According to the 2005 ISUP consensus conference, mucin-containing adenocarcinoma can be graded as Gleason pattern 3, if individual round and discrete glands are floating within mucinous pools, or Gleason pattern 4, if irregular, cribriform or fused glands float within a mucinous background (Fig. 2.5d). In essence, the grade of the tumor should be based on the underlying architectural pattern, while the extracellular mucin should be ignored for grading purposes. Currently, however, there is no consensus on this issue. Both methods are acceptable until additional studies indicate which method is preferable.

Atrophic or Cystic/Microcystic Adenocarcinoma Both are graded as Gleason pattern 3 (Fig. 2.5e, f). They are often accompanied by usual acinar-type adenocarcinoma. Both atrophic and cystic/microcystic adenocarcinoma variants can be seen in association with PIN-like or pseudohyperplastic carcinoma, which usually represent pattern 3 [16].

PIN-like Adenocarcinoma This is graded as Gleason pattern 3 if discrete glandular units are present. It can be graded as Gleason pattern 4 if there is evidence of fusion (Fig. 2.5g).

The following types of prostatic carcinoma should not be graded:

Small cell (neuroendocrine) carcinoma
Squamous or adenosquamous carcinoma
Urothelial carcinoma of the prostate
Basaloid or adenoid cystic carcinoma
Sarcomatoid adenocarcinoma (some would grade as pattern 5)

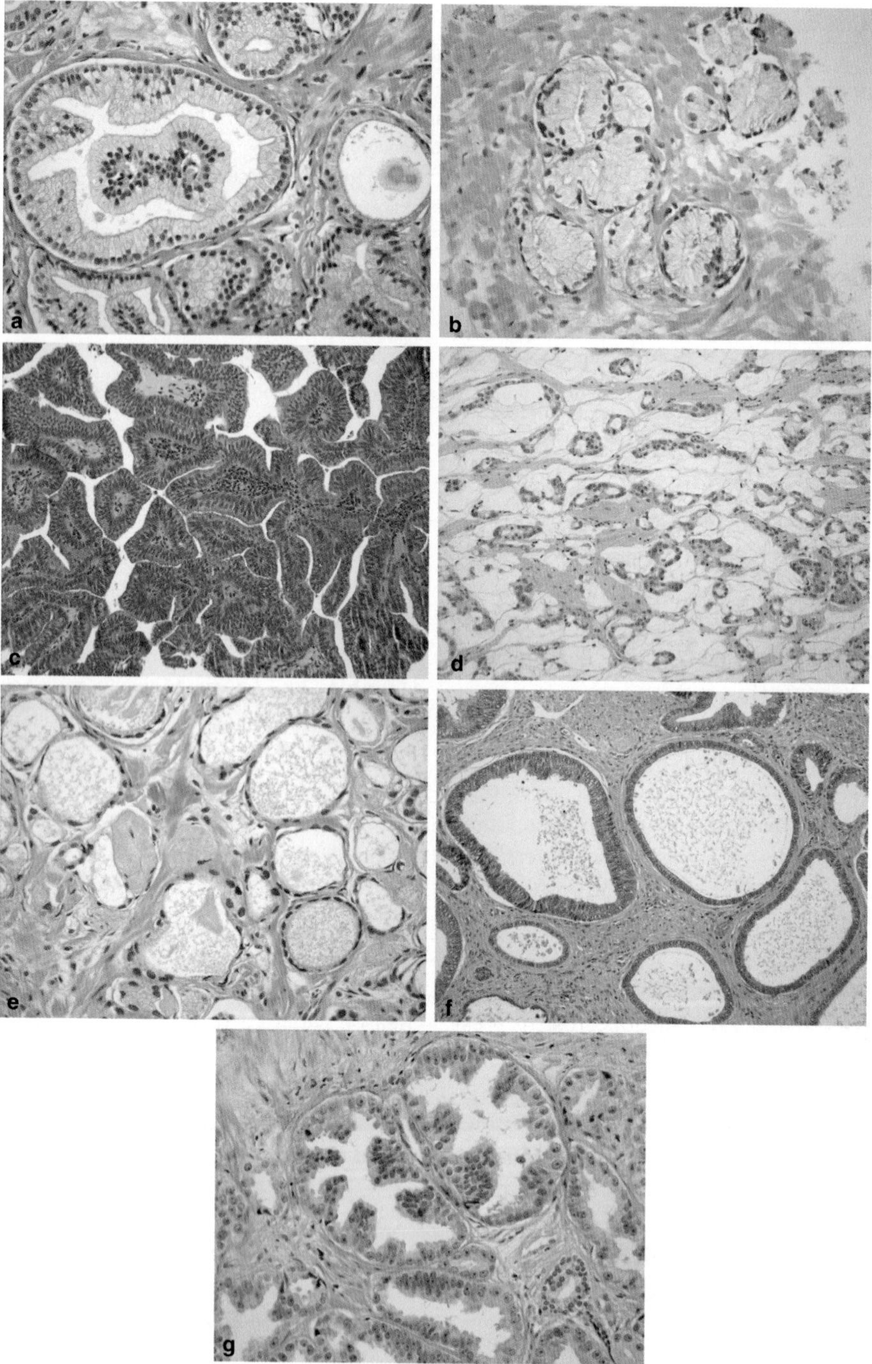

Fig. 2.5 Variants of prostatic carcinoma. Pseudohyperplastic carcinoma should be graded as pattern 3 (**a**). Foamy (or xanthomatous) carcinoma should be graded as pattern 4 if composed of individual glands (**b**) or pattern 4 if composed of fused or cribriform glands. Ductal adenocarcinoma is graded as pattern 4 (**c**); if comedonecrosis is present, it is graded as pattern 5. Colloid (mucinous) adenocarcinoma is graded as pattern 3 if individual discrete glands are floating within mucin (**d**) or pattern 4 if they appear irregular cribriform or fused (as rare glands on the image). Atrophic cancer is graded as pattern 3; note a collagenous micronodule slightly off to the *left of the center* (**e**); cystic and microcystic cancers are also graded as pattern 3 (**f**). PIN-like adenocarcinoma is graded as pattern 3 (**g**); if there is glandular fusion, it is graded as pattern 4

Grading-Specific Glandular Morphologies in Prostatic Adenocarcinoma

Glomerulations (Glomeruloid Structures)

Glomerulations are glands containing intraluminal, complex or cribriform structures, usually with a single point of attachment to the outer gland (Fig. 2.6a, b). Larger glomeruloid glands are almost uniformly accepted as Gleason pattern 4 by urologic pathologists. The opinions are divided whether all glomeruloid structures should be assigned Gleason pattern 4, or some smaller glomeruloid glands should be graded as Gleason pattern 3. Based on the ISUP consensus, either approach is currently acceptable until this issue is clarified.

Collagenous Micronodules (Mucinous Fibroplasia)

Glands containing collagenous micronodules (mucinous fibroplasia) present a grading challenge because glandular architecture is significantly altered. Collagenous micronodules are composed of collagen and scattered fibroblastic cells representing an organization of the intra- and extraluminal mucin associated with the neoplastic glands. Mucinous fibroplasia may also occur in fused or cribriform-appearing glands. In grading collagenous micronodules, it would be currently acceptable to grade the underlying glandular architecture and to subtract the mucinous fibroplasia, analogous to the scenario when grading neoplastic glands associated with mucinous adenocarcinoma (Fig. 2.6c, d).

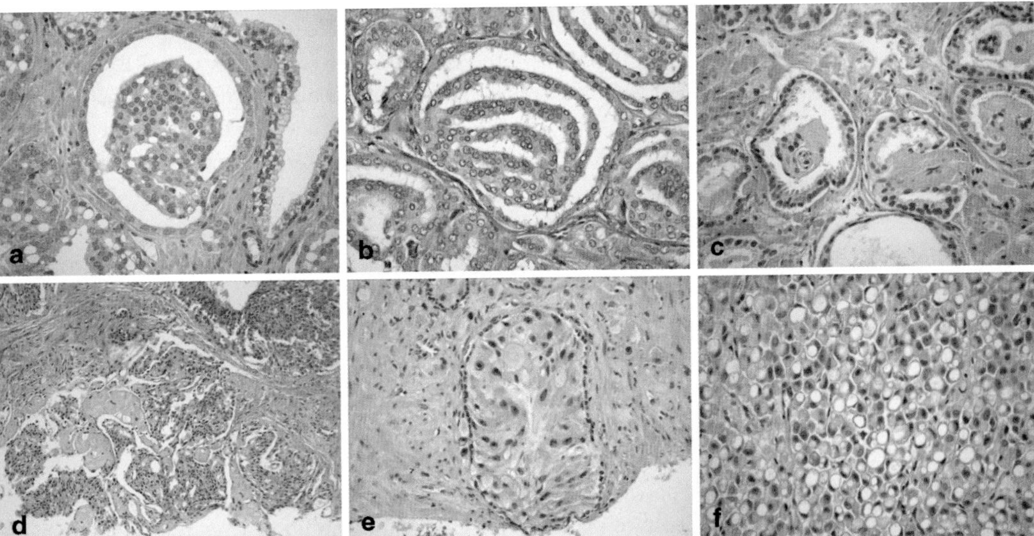

Fig. 2.6 Specific glandular morphologies are grades as follows: glomerulations which contain intraluminal cribriform (**a**) or complex structures (**b**) should be assigned pattern 4. Note the occasional vacuoles in (**a**); if vacuoles are present, the cancer should be graded based on the underlying morphology, by subtracting the vacuoles. In the case of collagenous micronodules (mucinous fibroplasia), the underlying glands are graded after subtracting the nodules; if the glands are individual, it is pattern 3 (**c**); if the background glands are fused, it is pattern 4 (**d**). Intraductal carcinoma is currently not graded, but a grade is assigned to the background invasive cancer; if single cells are present in the background (*top*), it is graded as pattern 5 (**e**). Signet ring-like as pattern is typically graded as pattern 5 (**f**)

Intraductal Carcinoma

Typically, intraductal carcinoma is not graded, but a grade is assigned to the background invasive cancer, which is present in the great majority of cases and is usually high grade (pattern 4 or 5) (Fig. 2.6e). Most experts currently do not assign a grade for intraductal carcinoma, but only include a note that intraductal carcinoma is present concomitantly with invasive carcinoma of a certain grade. Sometimes, however, no invasive carcinoma component is identified, particularly in limited needle biopsy specimens. Currently, there is no consensus how and if the isolated intraductal component should be graded. In these situations, it may be prudent to mention the frequent association with high-grade adenocarcinoma and suggest a repeat biopsy to clarify the diagnosis.

Vacuoles

Although vacuoles are usually seen in pattern 4, they may be seen in pattern 5 or even pattern 3 cancer. Cancer should be graded based on the underlying morphology, by subtracting the vacuoles (Fig. 2.6a).

Signet Ring-Like Pattern

Signet ring-like pattern is typically graded as Gleason pattern 5 (Fig. 2.6f). However, sometimes it is difficult to distinguish signet ring-like carcinoma from vacuoles, which can be seen in pattern 4 or even pattern 3. If only isolated or scattered vacuoles are present and there is absence of extensive signet ring formations, the vacuoles should not be graded as pattern 5, but rather the underlying cancer architecture should be evaluated.

Tertiary Gleason Pattern 5

Gleason reported in his original study that more than two tumor patterns occurred only rarely and noted that there were too few cases to permit meaningful analysis of the prognostic significance of a tertiary grade (3). More than two patterns are, however, often present in prostatectomy specimens, and also in needle biopsies. In RP specimens with three grades, it is currently recommended by the 2005 ISUP consensus that the tertiary pattern be reported separately when it is of higher grade than the primary and secondary grades. The incidence of a tertiary pattern varies greatly between series. Some studies consider tertiary pattern only if it is of higher grade than the primary and the secondary grades and if it represents <5 % of the whole tumor [17]. In other studies, if the tertiary component comprises >5 % of the tumor, this is considered to be a secondary pattern [18, 19]. One contemporary RP study, performed on a consecutive patient population from a single center, found a prevalence of tertiary Gleason pattern 5 of 22.5 % [20]. In this study, only the tertiary grade >5 % showed an independent and significant association with adverse pathology, but tertiary pattern ≤5 % did not demonstrate an association with adverse outcome [20]. Thus, there are variable approaches for considering the extent of tertiary pattern on RP, which potentially complicates comparisons of different study results. In several RP series, it has been clearly demonstrated that tertiary pattern 5 is a marker of more aggressive disease, which is associated more frequently with PSA recurrence, extraprostatic extension, surgical margin positivity, seminal vesicle infiltration, and lymph node metastasis [17, 19]. In practice, however, some pathologists report the GS, for example, GS 7 (either 3+4 or 4+3) with tertiary pattern 5, and specify the estimated percentages of primary, secondary, and tertiary grades, usually in a note. Other pathologists, however, maintain that tertiary grade should always represent <5 % of tumor, and if it exceeds 5 %, they automatically consider it to be a secondary pattern. Despite the recognition of these differences in practice, both approaches should be acceptable, provided it is clearly communicated in reports and in published studies which method was used in assigning the tertiary grade [18, 20, 21]. Currently, in RP reports, many pathologists include a note indicating the association of a tertiary grade 5 with adverse biologic behavior.

Some have recently proposed to account for the presence of tertiary grade 5 in RP specimens by reporting it as follows: GS 6 with tertiary 5 becomes GS 6.5; GS 3+4=7 with tertiary 5 becomes GS 7.25; Gleason 4+3=7 becomes GS 7.5; Gleason 4+3=7 with tertiary 5 becomes GS 8; and GS 8 with tertiary 5 becomes GS 8.5 [18]. While this proposal provides a rationale for stratification of cases which could potentially be used in prognostic nomograms, the practicality of its application remains questionable and awaits further confirmation [18].

Only a few studies have investigated the significance of tertiary Gleason grade on needle biopsy. For needle biopsies, the ISUP 2005 conference recommended that final GS should incorporate the highest (worst) pattern present, even if this was a tertiary one. Thus, GS on biopsy should be derived by adding primary and highest (worst) pattern. This question, however, required validation, with no good data available at the time of the consensus conference. Subsequently, it was demonstrated that in GS 7 cancers, those with tertiary pattern 5 on needle biopsy had a higher risk of PSA recurrence when compared to tumors without tertiary pattern 5 [22]. It has been also shown that tumors with GS 7 and tertiary pattern 5 had an intermediate time to PSA failure between GS 8 and GS 9/10 tumors [23]. In another study on biopsy, Gleason grade 5 was reported overall in 4.1% of all cancer-positive biopsies: 2.8% as primary or secondary pattern and 1.3% as tertiary pattern [24]. Trpkov et al. showed that tertiary pattern 5 on needle biopsy, particularly in nonsurgically treated patients, had a comparable all cause and cancer-specific mortality with secondary pattern 5, but much better outcome than patients with biopsy primary pattern 5 [24]. These findings supported the ISUP recommendation that tertiary pattern 5 found on biopsy is roughly equivalent to secondary pattern 5 and should be factored in the biopsy GS as such.

Grading Minute Foci of Prostate Cancer

Grading should be performed even on minute foci of prostatic carcinoma, which are often diagnostically challenging. Assignment of Gleason grade in this scenario can be problematic and often consists only of one Gleason pattern (Fig. 2.7a, b). If individual glands are present, it is recommended that even small foci of tumor be reported by doubling the pattern and reporting it as a primary and secondary (usually 3+3=6). The presence of small amounts of tumor in a biopsy does not

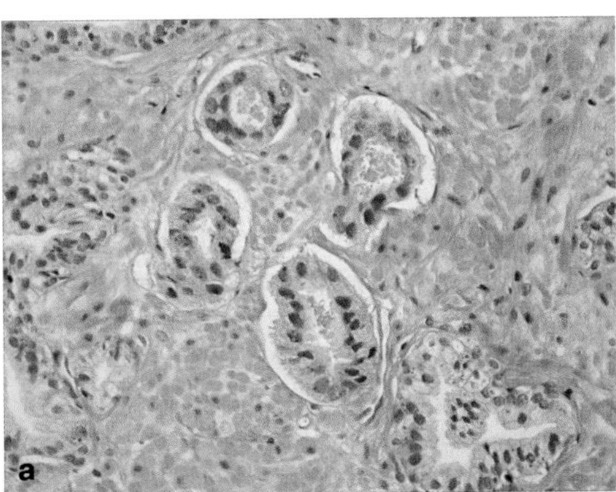

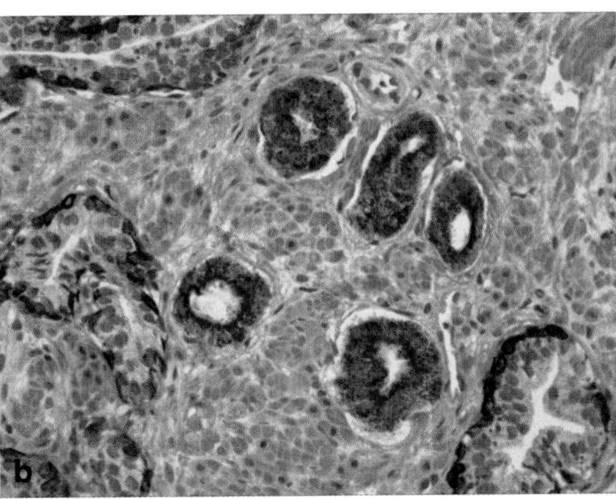

Fig. 2.7 Minute foci of prostate adenocarcinoma should be graded. A microfocus composed of 4–5 individual glands represents pattern 3 (**a**). Immunostains show complete absence of staining for high-molecular-weight keratin in the neoplastic glands, while the basal cells in the adjacent benign glands are positive. Neoplastic glands show diffuse cytoplasmic and luminal staining for racemase in contrast to the negative benign glands (**b**)

always correlate with small volume of tumor in the prostatectomy specimens, but this correlation has improved using extended prostate biopsies [12, 25].

Grading Prostate Cancer After Radiation and Other Treatments

Pathologists should also be familiar with the changes of normal and neoplastic prostate tissue occurring due to various treatments. If uncertain about the diagnosis or whether to grade or not, a pathologist should seek assistance from a uropathologist. Radiation therapy (external beam and brachytherapy, i.e., "seeds") is a widespread treatment for clinically localized or locally advanced prostate cancer. Cryotherapy ("freezing") of prostate has also been more widely used during the last decade [26]. A biopsy is typically performed when there is a rising PSA (usually no less than 12 months after radiation or cryotherapy) to distinguish local recurrence from metastatic disease and to determine whether additional treatment is needed. A history of radiation or other therapies is frequently not shared with the pathologist, and it may not be known even to the clinician, so it is essential to be familiar with the changes in benign and malignant glands that occur after various treatments.

Prostate cancers exhibiting marked radiation treatment changes typically display infiltrative, poorly formed glands or single cells with abundantly vacuolated and clear cytoplasm and small shrunken nuclei. Similar cancer morphology may also be seen after cryotherapy. When only cancer with radiation or cryotherapy treatment effect is seen in the specimen, the sign-out may include a statement such as "prostatic adenocarcinoma with extensive radiation/cryo treatment changes" and this cancer should not be Gleason graded. When prostatic adenocarcinoma does not demonstrate significant treatment changes and resembles the usual type adenocarcinoma, it should be graded. In these cases, GS can be assigned, with wording such as "prostatic adenocarcinoma, Gleason pattern 3+4=7, without significant radiation/cryo treatment changes." One may add an estimate of the proportion (or %) of the carcinoma exhibiting no treatment changes. Such a diagnosis is important for further clinical management, since patients with negative biopsies and patients whose cancers showed marked therapy changes on biopsy had similar 10-year PSA relapse-free survival outcomes (59%), and those outcomes were markedly different from patients with positive biopsies without treatment effect (3%) ($p < 0.001$). The 10-year Distant Metastasis-Free Survival rate in patients with negative/marked treatment effect biopsy outcomes was 90%, while corresponding outcome in patients with positive biopsies without treatment effect was 69% ($p = 0.0004$) [27].

Hormone-treated cancers exhibiting therapy effects also should not be graded because of the possibility of overgrading. One often encounters single and shrunken cells or lack of gland differentiation in this scenario. In summary, it is important to always report GS for cancers that do not exhibit appreciable treatment changes, because cancer in this setting most likely represents either de novo or recurrent disease (or possibly disease that has not been affected or has been missed by the treatment), which is usually associated with worse prognosis.

Concordance of Biopsy and Radical Prostatectomy Gleason Scores

One of the expected consequences of modifying the Gleason grading system has been an improvement in the agreement (concordance) between biopsy GS and RP GS. Before the 2005 Gleason modification, the agreement of the biopsy and RP GS ranged from approximately 30 to 70% in most studies. After 2005, some studies have indeed documented an improvement between needle biopsy and RP GS. One study showed that overall agreement between needle biopsy and RP specimens increased from 58 to 72% when the modified Gleason system was applied [28]. Other studies, however, failed to demonstrate significant improvement in the GS agreement between the biopsy and RP [29, 30]. In a study by Uemura et al., the biopsy-RP GS concordance using the original Gleason system and the ISUP modified system was 67 and 70 %, respectively [30]. Similarly, Zareba et al. showed that the biopsy-RP GS agreement did not improve significantly using the modified Gleason system (63.4 and 65.5 %, original vs modified Gleason, respectively). In current practice, RP GS upgrades are reported in 36 % (mean) cases (30 % in our practice) [29, 31]. The incidence of upgrading on biopsy is documented in current practice in fewer studies, and ranges between 5 and 15 % (5 % in our practice) [29].

There are several reasons for biopsy and RP GS discrepancies: sampling error, erroneous pattern interpretation, borderline grades, Gleason grade assignment on biopsy and clinician's interpretation of the biopsy GS. Extended biopsies (ten cores) are associated with less upgrading on RP than sextant biopsies. Prostate biopsy samples, however, represent only a fraction of a percentage of the whole gland (< 0.05 cc) and the chance to miss a limited higher-grade cancer on biopsy remains high. This typically occurs when a needle biopsy cancer is graded GS 3 + 3 = 6 and a limited pattern 4, which was not sampled in the biopsy becomes apparent in the RP specimen, resulting in RP upgrade of GS 3 + 4 = 7. Tumor multifocality may be another reason for possible discrepancies between biopsy and RP GS. With teaching and growing experience, pathologists also recognize the grading pitfalls and develop better accuracy and reproducibility in their grading. Common pathology errors in grading biopsy specimens include: (a) overcalling Gleason pattern 5 on tangentially sectioned small glands of pattern 3; (b) undercalling cribriform Gleason pattern 4 as pattern 3; and (c) undercalling small foci of Gleason pattern 5 (such as individual cells, cords, or solid nests). There are also common problems in assigning borderline grades between, for example, small glands of pattern 3 and poorly formed glands of pattern 4. Poorly formed glands (pattern 4) may also be interpreted as small foci of individual cells (pattern 5).

Undergrading on biopsy may also result from difficulty in recognizing small foci of glandular fusion. Another reason for apparent discrepancies between biopsy and RP GS is when the single highest (worst) GS in any positive core is considered to be the representative biopsy GS for the entire case. Using this approach in one study, a biopsy GS 8 could be reproduced as RP GS 8 in only 21.5 % cases and corresponded with RP GS < 8 in > 50 % of RP [31]. Similarly, the assignment of biopsy GS based on the primary and the highest (or the worst) grade may account for some discrepancies between the biopsy and RP GS. Although pathologists usually report Gleason grades of each site separately, clinicians often take the highest GS from any site when planning treatment, which may be a possible reason for biopsy-RP GS discrepancies [32].

Currently available prognostic tools, such as nomograms, have limited ability to predict clinically significant upgrading of biopsy GS and are not ready for clinical application. The predictive ability of various models to account for upgrades and downgrades between biopsy and RP GS has also been disappointing, which is also confounded by the differences in biopsy techniques, number of cores sampled, and indications for biopsy. Thus, GS upgrades and downgrades still remain an important issue in clinical practice after 2005.

Inter- and Intraobserver Reproducibility of the Modified Gleason System

The modified Gleason grading system has demonstrated good reproducibility along the entire spectrum of morphologic patterns. The improvement in reproducibility is likely due to the refined definitions of the individual grades and the decreased diagnosis of carcinomas with low GS (Gleason 2–5) on needle biopsy using the modified Gleason system. Exact intraobserver agreement on GS was reported in 43–78 % of cases, and agreement within ± 1 unit was reported in 72–87 % of cases [33, 34]. This is an improvement over Gleason's own performance, because he was able to exactly reproduce his previous scores approximately half of the times. Highly variable levels of interobserver agreement on GS have also been reported in another study (range of 36–81 % for exact agreement and 69–86 % within ± 1unit) [35].

Interobserver variability and reproducibility in applying the Gleason scoring system are due to various factors, including differences in training (various mentors, different institutions), familiarity with the system, varying personal experience, volume of practice, and inherent subjectivity, as in all grading systems. Problems still persist regarding the inter- and intraobserver variability and the threshold issues (particularly Gleason pattern 3 vs. Gleason pattern 4). These diagnostic variations could potentially have an effect on multi-institutional trials, for example, of active surveillance, because the population of patients at different centers may differ based on the thresholds of Gleason grading. A central, expert review may correct these problems, but even in this setting, the threshold issues may still persist. Providing a review by a specialized uropathologist in problematic cases, either in routine practice in each institution or through a single central review in a study setting may also mitigate the variations in reproducibility. Further improvements in the reproducibility of Gleason grading can be achieved by educational activities focusing on known problematic areas.

Clinical Impact of the ISUP Modified Gleason Grading System in Practice

The impact and consequences in clinical practice have been examined in several studies after the ISUP modified system was introduced in 2005 [14, 28–30, 36–39]. The summary result has been an upward migration of the GS. In clinical practice, Gleason pattern 3, which was previously the most common on biopsy, has become less common than pattern 4. Most of the studies, however, have been performed in retrospective fashion by reviewing previously scored cases [28, 39]. One retrospective study on matched biopsy and RP specimens documented a significant reduction of GS 6 from 48 to 22 % on biopsy and from 32 to only 6 % on RP [28]. This was accompanied by a significant increase in GS 7 from 25 to 68 % on biopsy and from 36 to 83 % on RP. In contrast, in routinely graded biopsy and RP cohorts before and after 2005, which included over 1300 cases, similar trends were observed both on biopsy and on RP [29]. There was a decline of GS 6 on biopsy from 68 to 55 % after 2005, which was reciprocated by an increase in GS 7 biopsies from 30 to 43 % after 2005. In the same fashion, there was a decline of RP GS 6 cancers from 47 to 32 % after 2005, accompanied by a corresponding increase of RP GS 7 cancers from 48 to 60 % after 2005. The most frequent change from biopsy to RP in patients after 2005 was an upgrade from biopsy GS 6 to RP GS 7 (3 + 4) (due to secondary pattern upgrades from pattern 3 to 4). This study also documented a trend towards better complete agreement for GS $\geq$ 7 [29).

Several changes in the ISUP 200 modified system may account for the upward migration in the Gleason grading. More strict definition of cribriform pattern reduced the morphologic spectrum of cribriform glands interpreted as Gleason pattern 3. Scoring of glands with poorly formed lumina has also been adopted in practice and uniformly interpreted as Gleason pattern 4. Although the morphologic spectrum of ill-defined glands (Gleason pattern 4) may include glands which can be interpreted either as Gleason pattern 3 or Gleason pattern 5, the creation of this category has allowed for routine and mainstream use of this morphologic pattern as Gleason pattern 4. Another reason for the Gleason upward migration after 2005 is the rule of excluding a lower Gleason pattern involving a minimal (< 5 %) proportion of cancer in a setting of extensive high-grade cancer. A sizable proportion of the upgrades on biopsy may be due to the rule to incorporate tertiary Gleason pattern (in practice, pattern 5) as a secondary pattern on biopsy specimens, when it is higher than the secondary pattern. Many pathologists also interpret glands with more or less complex branching (which was not explicitly discussed in the consensus paper) as part of "marked" variation in gland shape criteria, which was included in the text description of Gleason pattern 3. Some pathologists, however, tend to follow more closely the diagram and interpret the irregularities or gland branching as true gland fusion, and grade them as pattern 4, which may also account for some upgrades from pattern 3 to 4 after 2005. Some believe that Gleason pattern

5 is still underdiagnosed, particularly on needle biopsy, which may prompt some pathologists to call pattern 5 on biopsy more frequently [40]. In particular, the single cell pattern of Gleason grade 5, the most common biopsy pattern 5, may be potentially underdiagnosed and under-reported. Tangentially sectioned small-acinar pattern 3 glands may often exhibit a focal single cell pattern, or even glands with poorly formed lumina can sometimes appear as single cells. Thus, it is not unusual that diagnostic difficulties arise in interpreting single cell patterns. One approach in evaluating areas of possible pattern 5, particularly on biopsy, is to consider the background cancer morphology. If the background cancer demonstrates small-acinar pattern 3 or poorly formed glands, pattern 4, it would be prudent not to call these foci as pattern 5, but to interpret them as part of the background cancer morphology.

The significance of the upward shift of the Gleason grading in clinical practice and for patient management and prognosis is still uncertain. One possible consequence may be possible improvement in future patient outcomes for patients after 2005. This phenomenon of improved outcomes due to tumor grade (or stage) reclassification is well recognized and reflects a statistical artifact, known as the Will Rogers phenomenon [41]. This phenomenon occurs when changes are introduced in a classification system and an intermediate-risk group is moved from a low- to a higher-risk group, which improves the outcomes in both groups. Another possible consequence of the upward Gleason migration may be a change in treatment practices after 2005. Because GS is an important factor in treatment selection (i.e., active surveillance vs. RP), the proportion of patients reported as biopsy GS 6 may now be likely reduced, because their biopsy GS are more likely to be reported currently as GS≥7. This may result in exclusion of some patients from active surveillance. Similarly, in some institutions, only patients reported as GS≤6 on biopsy are considered for brachytherapy, and this patient population may now be also potentially reduced [29]. Pathology reviews of biopsies and RPs on specimens read before 2005 may result in GS regrading by using the modified Gleason, which clinicians and patients may not be aware of or familiar with, thus creating confusion. Thus, pathologists should clearly communicate these changes in review and consult reports and explain to clinicians and patients the reasons for GS upgrade.

Correlation of Gleason Score with Clinical Patient Outcomes

A true validation of the modified Gleason system will be demonstrating its correlation with the clinical outcomes. So far, only a few studies addressed clinical outcomes after 2005, mainly because the follow-up in these studies has been relatively short. Two relatively small studies demonstrated that the GS on needle biopsies using the modified system correlated better with progression after RP [30, 39]. Tsivian et al. found that modified GS, when analyzed in prognostic grade groups (<7 and >7), predicted biochemical recurrence after RP better than the original GS groups [42]. Berney et al. reported significant upgrading of biopsies, initially graded during 1990–1996 and subsequently regraded and published in 2007 [36]. Whereas the initial grades did not correlate with survival outcomes, the newly recorded grades, largely following the modified Gleason system, did. In the only study favoring the original over the modified Gleason system in predicting disease progression, Delahunt et al. reported that original Gleason system outperformed the modified system in predicting PSA nadir following external beam radiotherapy and hormone therapy [43]. Unfortunately, the use of PSA nadir, a suboptimal endpoint, limited the significance of the study results. Aiming to establish the risk of adverse outcome for patients with a GS 3+3=6, subsequently upgraded to GS 7 or 8 using the ISUP modified Gleason system, Dong et al. found that 34% of patients with classical GS 3+3=6 prostate cancer were upgraded to modified GS 7 or 8, using the ISUP criteria [37]. Compared to patients with modified GS 3+3=6 and patients with classical GS 3+4=7, the upgraded patients were at intermediate risk for biochemical progression and metastasis after RP

[37]. Another recent study has shown that presence of cribriform glands, now usually graded pattern 4, was more likely to be associated with biochemical failure [44].

After 2005, some studies also examined the clinical significance of specific prostate carcinoma variants and morphologies. While the early studies of mucinous carcinoma from the pre-PSA era showed adverse outcomes, more recent studies reported no deaths from disease and limited biochemical recurrence in patients with mucinous carcinoma treated by RP [45]. This supports the grading approach based on the architectural configuration, which needs confirmation in larger series. Another study examined glomeruloid features in needle biopsies to establish whether there is an association of this pattern with coexistent high-grade carcinoma [46]. In this study, glomerulations were associated with high-grade cancer on the same core, mostly Gleason pattern 4 (80 % of cases) and often appeared to represent a morphologic transition to larger cribriform glands. Only a minority of glomerulations were found to be associated with pattern 3 cancer (16 % of cases). Despite the limitations and the absence of clinical follow-up, this study supported the idea that glomerulations most likely represent an early stage of cribriform pattern 4 cancer and should be graded as such [46].

One of the most compelling testimonials, so far, of the prognostic ability of the ISUP modified grading system came from a large study from Johns Hopkins, which investigated pathologic and short-term outcomes after the Gleason system modifications in 2005 [38]. This study used multivariable models using preoperative and postoperative variables and demonstrated clearly separate prognostic groups based on GS both on biopsy and RP (≤6; 3+4; 4+3; 8; 9–10). These prognostic groups were among the strongest predictors of biochemical recurrence-free survival. Based on their results, they proposed adding a descriptive terminology, designated Prognostic Grade Groups (PGG) I–V: PGG I for GS≤6 (well-differentiated or low-grade), PGG II for GS 3+4 (moderately differentiated or intermediate low grade), PGG III for GS 4+3=7 (moderately–poorly differentiated or intermediate grade), PGG IV for GS 8 (poorly differentiated or high intermediate grade), and PGG V for GS 9–10 (undifferentiated or high grade) [38]. Interestingly, in contrast to previous studies, this study failed to show that adding the tertiary pattern enhanced the predictive value in multivariable analysis, which included a preoperative PSA, pathologic stage, margins, and Gleason grade on RP. Although it is currently recommended that tertiary patterns are noted in pathology reports for accurate grading, this study questioned whether the inclusion of tertiary patterns added significant prognostic information, in addition to the routinely reported parameters.

By adopting a system that starts with GS≤6 to represent a prognostic category 1 (PGG1), one would eliminate the current situation when Gleason grading essentially starts with GS 6. After 2005, GS≤6 category represents a more uniform and homogeneous category, reflecting a better patient prognosis. It has been demonstrated that virtually no pure GS 6 cancers are associated with progression after RP, using the ISUP modified Gleason system, whereas in the original Gleason system this occasionally occurred [47]. Of over 14,000 totally embedded RP from multiple institutions, there was not a single case of GS≤6 cancer with nodal metastasis [48]. Clearly defined prognostic groups would also obviate the need to potentially introduce decimal fractions to individual GS to better stratify patients [18, 49]. The proposals to consider these modifications arose from the fact that 2005 Gleason grading system introduced an upward migration, which required better prognostic separation in the current setting.

Future Perspectives

Although the 2005 ISUP modified grading system is still imperfect and somewhat subjective, there is no other marker or grading system that can be as quickly and reproducibly applied in practice, which underscores the pathologist's role in patient management. For a pathologist, the key issue remains to use consistent criteria for grading and to be attuned to the general and mainstream grading criteria. A consistent and reproducible grading approach will allow adaptation to future grading modifications. It is also desirable to establish a unified grading approach in a group practice with regular intradepartmental consultations or consultations with a uropathologist.

The 2005 ISUP modified Gleason grading has had an enormous impact on the evolving clinical practice of prostate cancer. It has achieved considerable acceptance and has been widely used. Certainly, further modifications and refinements of the criteria need to be carefully validated and confirmed in large or multi-institutional studies with well-defined outcomes, before additional changes are implemented. The ISUP modified Gleason system still remains one of the most powerful grading schemes in all of urologic oncology and a gold standard against which other prospective markers are and will be compared with and measured against in future studies. Although GS is a fundamental prognostic parameter for prostate cancer, additional biomarkers may either complement or replace GS in the future. Each biomarker aiming to replace Gleason, however, needs to be validated first head-to-head with Gleason in retrospective studies, with subsequent validation in independent and prospective data sets and cohorts.

References

1. Gleason DF. Classification of prostatic carcinomas. Cancer Chemother Rep. 1966;50(3):125–8.
2. Gleason DF, Mellinger GT. Prediction of prognosis for prostatic adenocarcinoma by combined histological grading and clinical staging. J Urol. 1974;111(1):58–64.
3. Gleason DF. Histologic grading and clinical staging of prostatic carcinoma. In: Teannenbaum M, editor. Urologic pathology: the prostate. the veterans administration cooperative urological research group. Philadelphia: Lea and Febiger; 1977. pp. 171–97.
4. Epstein JI, Allsbrook WC Jr., Amin MB, Egevad LL. The 2005 international society of urological pathology (ISUP) consensus conference on Gleason grading of prostatic carcinoma. Am J Surg Pathol. 2005;29(9):1228–42.
5. Gleason DF. Histologic grading of prostate cancer: a perspective. Hum Pathol. 1992;23(3):273–9.
6. Siegel R, Naishadham D, Jemal A. Cancer statistics. CA Cancer J Clin. 2012;62(1):10–29.
7. Stamey TA, Caldwell M, McNeal JE, Nolley R, Hemenez M, Downs J. The prostate specific antigen era in the United States is over for prostate cancer: what happened in the last 20 years?. J Urol. 2004;172(4 Pt 1):1297–301.
8. Egevad L, Mazzucchelli R, Montironi R. Implications of the international society of urological pathology modified Gleason grading system. Arch Pathol Lab Med. 2012;136(4):426–34.
9. Egevad L, Allsbrook WC, Jr., Epstein JI. Current practice of diagnosis and reporting of prostate cancer on needle biopsy among genitourinary pathologists. Hum Pathol. 2006;37(3):292–7.
10. Srigley JR, Amin MB, Epstein JI, Grignon DJ, Humphrey PA, Renshaw AA, et al. Updated protocol for the examination of specimens from patients with carcinomas of the prostate gland. Arch Pathol Lab Med. 2006;130(7):936–46.
11. Berney DM. The case for modifying the Gleason grading system. BJU Int. 2007;100(4):725–6.
12. Epstein JI. Gleason score 2–4 adenocarcinoma of the prostate on needle biopsy: a diagnosis that should not be made. Am J Surg Pathol. 2000;24(4):477–8.
13. Epstein JI. An update of the Gleason grading system. J Urol. 2010;183(2):433–40.
14. Lotan TL, Epstein JI. Clinical implications of changing definitions within the Gleason grading system. Nat Rev Urol. 2010;7(3):136–42.
15. Latour M, Amin MB, Billis A, Egevad L, Grignon DJ, Humphrey PA, et al. Grading of invasive cribriform carcinoma on prostate needle biopsy: an interobserver study among experts in genitourinary pathology. Am J Surg Pathol. 2008;32(10):1532–9.
16. Yaskiv O, Cao D, Humphrey PA. Microcystic adenocarcinoma of the prostate: a variant of pseudohyperplastic and atrophic patterns. Am J Surg Pathol. 2010;34(4):556–61.
17. Pan CC, Potter SR, Partin AW, Epstein JI. The prognostic significance of tertiary Gleason patterns of higher grade in radical prostatectomy specimens: a proposal to modify the Gleason grading system. Am J Surg Pathol. 2000;24(4):563–9.
18. Trock BJ, Guo CC, Gonzalgo ML, Magheli A, Loeb S, Epstein JI. Tertiary Gleason patterns and biochemical recurrence after prostatectomy: proposal for a modified Gleason scoring system. J Urol. 2009;182(4):1364–70.
19. Mosse CA, Magi-Galluzzi C, Tsuzuki T, Epstein JI. The prognostic significance of tertiary Gleason pattern 5 in radical prostatectomy specimens. Am J Surg Pathol. 2004;28(3):394–8.
20. Isbarn H, Ahyai SA, Chun FK, Budaus L, Schlomm T, Salomon G, et al. Prevalence of a tertiary Gleason grade and its impact on adverse histopathologic parameters in a contemporary radical prostatectomy series. Eur Urol. 2009;55(2):394–401.
21. Ikenberg K, Zimmermann AK, Kristiansen G. Re: tertiary Gleason patterns and biochemical recurrence after prostatectomy: proposal for a modified Gleason scoring system. Trock BJ, Guo CC, Gonzalgo ML, Magheli A, Loeb S, Epstein JI. J Urol 2009;182:1364–1370. J Urol. 2010;183(5):2100. Author reply-1.
22. Patel AA, Chen MH, Renshaw AA, D'Amico AV. PSA failure following definitive treatment of prostate

cancer having biopsy Gleason score 7 with tertiary grade 5. JAMA. 2007;298(13):1533–8.
23. Nanda A, Chen MH, Renshaw AA, D'Amico AV. Gleason Pattern 5 prostate cancer: further stratification of patients with high-risk disease and implications for future randomized trials. Int J Radiat Oncol Biol Phys. 2009;74(5):1419–23.
24. Trpkov K, Zhang J, Chan M, Eigl BJ, Yilmaz A. Prostate cancer with tertiary Gleason pattern 5 in prostate needle biopsy: clinicopathologic findings and disease progression. Am J Surg Pathol. 2009;33(2):233–40.
25. Rubin MA, Dunn R, Kambham N, Misick CP, O'Toole KM. Should a Gleason score be assigned to a minute focus of carcinoma on prostate biopsy? Am J Surg Pathol. 2000;24(12):1634–40.
26. Donnelly BJ, Saliken JC, Brasher PM, Ernst SD, Rewcastle JC, Lau H, et al. A randomized trial of external beam radiotherapy versus cryoablation in patients with localized prostate cancer. Cancer. 2010;116(2):323–30.
27. Zelefsky MJ, Reuter VE, Fuks Z, Scardino P, Shippy A. Influence of local tumor control on distant metastases and cancer related mortality after external beam radiotherapy for prostate cancer. J Urol. 2008;179(4):1368–73; discussion 73.
28. Helpap B, Egevad L. The significance of modified Gleason grading of prostatic carcinoma in biopsy and radical prostatectomy specimens. Virchows Arch. 2006;449(6):622–7.
29. Zareba P, Zhang J, Yilmaz A, Trpkov K. The impact of the 2005 international society of urological pathology (ISUP) consensus on Gleason grading in contemporary practice. Histopathology. 2009;55(4):384–91.
30. Uemura H, Hoshino K, Sasaki T, Miyoshi Y, Ishiguro H, Inayama Y, et al. Usefulness of the 2005 international society of urologic pathology Gleason grading system in prostate biopsy and radical prostatectomy specimens. BJU Int. 2009;103(9):1190–4.
31. Epstein JI, Feng Z, Trock BJ, Pierorazio PM. Upgrading and downgrading of prostate cancer from biopsy to radical prostatectomy: incidence and predictive factors using the modified Gleason grading system and factoring in tertiary grades. Eur Urol. 2012;61(5):1019–24.
32. Rubin MA, Bismar TA, Curtis S, Montie JE. Prostate needle biopsy reporting: how are the surgical members of the Ssociety of urologic oncology using pathology reports to guide treatment of prostate cancer patients? Am J Surg Pathol. 2004;28(7):946–52.
33. Griffiths DF, Melia J, McWilliam LJ, Ball RY, Grigor K, Harnden P, et al. A study of Gleason score interpretation in different groups of UK pathologists; techniques for improving reproducibility. Histopathology. 2006;48(6):655–62.
34. Melia J, Moseley R, Ball RY, Griffiths DF, Grigor K, Harnden P, et al. A UK-based investigation of inter-and intra-observer reproducibility of Gleason grading of prostatic biopsies. Histopathology. 2006;48(6):644–54.
35. Lopez-Beltran A, Mikuz G, Luque RJ, Mazzucchelli R, Montironi R. Current practice of Gleason grading of prostate carcinoma. Virchows Arch. 2006;448(2):111–8.
36. Berney DM, Fisher G, Kattan MW, Oliver RT, Moller H, Fearn P, et al. Major shifts in the treatment and prognosis of prostate cancer due to changes in pathological diagnosis and grading. BJU Int. 2007;100(6):1240–4.
37. Dong F, Wang C, Farris B, Wu S, Lee H, Olumi AF, et al. Impact on the clinical outcome of prostate cancer by the 2005 international society of urological pathology modified Gleason grading system. Am J Surg Pathol. 2012:36(6):838–43.
38. Pierorazio PM, Walsh P, Partin A, Epstein J. Prognostic Gleason grade grouping: data based on the modified Gleason scoring system. BJU Int. 2013;111(5):753–60.
39. Billis A, Guimaraes MS, Freitas LL, Meirelles L, Magna LA, Ferreira U. The impact of the 2005 international society of urological pathology consensus conference on standard Gleason grading of prostatic carcinoma in needle biopsies. J Urol. 2008;180(2):548–52; discussion 52–3.
40. Fajardo DA, Miyamoto H, Miller JS, Lee TK, Epstein JI. Identification of Gleason pattern 5 on prostatic needle core biopsy: frequency of underdiagnosis and relation to morphology. Am J Surg Pathol. 2011;35(11):1706–11.
41. Albertsen PC, Hanley JA, Barrows GH, Penson DF, Kowalczyk PD, Sanders MM, et al. Prostate cancer and the Will Rogers phenomenon. J Natl Cancer Inst. 2005;97(17):1248–53.
42. Tsivian M, Sun L, Mouraviev V, Madden JF, Mayes JM, Moul JW, et al. Changes in Gleason score grading and their effect in predicting outcome after radical prostatectomy. Urology. 2009;74(5):1090–3.
43. Delahunt B, Lamb DS, Srigley JR, Murray JD, Wilcox C, Samaratunga H, et al. Gleason scoring: a comparison of classical and modified (international society of urological pathology) criteria using nadir PSA as a clinical end point. Pathology. 2010;42(4):339–43.
44. Iczkowski KA, Torkko KC, Kotnis GR, Wilson RS, Huang W, Wheeler TM, et al. Digital quantification of five high-grade prostate cancer patterns, including the cribriform pattern, and their association with adverse outcome. Am J Clin Pathol. 2011;136(1):98–107.
45. Osunkoya AO, Nielsen ME, Epstein JI. Prognosis of mucinous adenocarcinoma of the prostate treated by radical prostatectomy: a study of 47 cases. Am J Surg Pathol. 2008;32(3):468–72.
46. Lotan TL, Epstein JI. Gleason grading of prostatic adenocarcinoma with glomeruloid features on needle biopsy. Hum Pathol. 2009;40(4):471–7.
47. Miyamoto H, Hernandez DJ, Epstein JI. A pathological reassessment of organ-confined, Gleason score 6 prostatic adenocarcinomas that progress after radical prostatectomy. Hum Pathol. 2009;40(12):1693–8.
48. Ross HM, Kryvenko ON, Cowan JE, Simko JP, Wheeler TM, Epstein JI. Do adenocarcinomas of the prostate with Gleason score (GS)</=6 have the potential to metastasize to lymph nodes? Am J Surg Pathol. 2012;36(9):1346–52.
49. Reese AC, Cowan JE, Brajtbord JS, Harris CR, Carroll PR, Cooperberg MR. The quantitative Gleason score improves prostate cancer risk assessment. Cancer. 2012;118(24):6046–54.

Contemporary Prostate Cancer Staging

3

Christopher G. Przybycin, Sara M. Falzarano and Cristina Magi-Galluzzi

Introduction

Stage remains the most important prognosticator of most cancers. Staging involves determination of the anatomic extent or spread of a disease at the time of diagnosis based on clinical and pathologic criteria. Cancer stage is based on the size and location of the primary tumor and whether the tumor has spread to other organs and/or areas of the body. According to the American Joint Committee on Cancer (AJCC) [1], these staging criteria are designed to serve several purposes: helping to predict patient's prognosis, assisting in planning of treatment strategies, providing a common language for practitioners to report extent of disease, and perform studies or clinical trials on homogeneous patient populations. The TNM staging is the most widely used system for prostate cancer (PCA) staging and assesses the extent of primary tumor (T stage), the absence or presence of regional lymph node involvement (N stage), and the absence or presence of distant metastases (M stage) (Table 3.1). Once the T, N, and M are determined, a stage of I, II, III, or IV is assigned, with stage I being early and stage IV being advanced disease (Table 3.2).

Several modifications have been made over time to the TNM staging system in an attempt to improve the uniformity of patient evaluation and to maintain a clinically relevant classification [2]. The ongoing critical evaluation of this staging system will indeed incorporate new evidence-based factors to secure future refinements to PCA staging. In the most recent AJCC text, Gleason score (GS) and prostate-specific antigen (PSA) have been incorporated in the anatomic stage/prognostic groups (Table 3.2) [1].

Clinical T Staging

Accurate clinical staging is crucial to provide adequate counseling for therapeutic treatment options, since risk stratification allows prediction of patient outcomes based on cancer characteristics. Clinical staging (cTNM) is performed by the urologist or referring physician during the initial evaluation of the patient, or when pathologic classification is not possible. All parameters available before the first definitive treatment may be used for clinical staging and remain unchanged even if pathologic findings differ. Primary tumor assessment includes digital rectal examination (DRE), transrectal ultrasound (TRUS), and histologic confirmation of PCA by prostate biopsy. DRE has been a cornerstone of staging; however, DRE is insufficient for determining accurate stage and extent of disease, since approximately half of tumors are understaged by DRE alone [3].

C. Magi-Galluzzi (✉) · C. G. Przybycin
Department of Pathology, Cleveland Clinic, Robert J. Tomsich Pathology and Laboratory Medicine Institute, Cleveland, OH, USA
e-mail: magic@ccf.org

C. G. Przybycin
e-mail: przybyc@ccf.org

S. M. Falzarano
Cleveland Clinic, Robert J. Tomsich Pathology and Laboratory Medicine Institute, Cleveland, OH, USA
e-mail: Falzars2@ccf.org

C. Magi-Galluzzi, C. G. Przybycin (eds.), *Genitourinary Pathology,* DOI 10.1007/978-1-4939-2044-0_3,

Table 3.1 Pathological staging. (Used with permission from [1])

Primary tumor (T)	
TX	Primary tumor cannot be assessed
T0	No evidence of primary tumor
a	
T2	Organ-confined disease
T2a	*Unilateral disease, one-half of one lobe or less*
T2b	*Unilateral disease, involving more than one-half of one lobe, but not both lobes*
T2c	*Bilateral disease*
T3	Extraprostatic extension
T3a	Extracapsular extension or microscopic bladder neck invasion
T3b	Seminal vesicle invasion
T4	Invasion of rectum levator muscles and/or pelvic wall
Regional lymph nodes (N)	
NX	Regional lymph nodes not sampled
N0	No positive regional lymph nodes
N1	Metastasis in regional lymph node(s)
Distant metastasis (M)	
MX	Distant metastasis status unknown
M0	No distant metastasis
M1	Distant metastasis
M1a	Nonregional lymph node(s)
M1b	Bone(s)
M1c	Other site(s) with or without bone disease

[a] There is no pathologic T1 classification

Table 3.2 Anatomic stage/prognostic groups. (Used with permission from [1])

Group	T	N	M	PSA	Gleason score (GS)
I	T1a–c	N0	M0	PSA<10	GS≤6
	T2a	N0	M0	PSA<10	GS≤6
	T1–2a	N0	M0	PSA x	GS x
IIA	T1a–c	N0	M0	PSA<20	GS 7
	T1a–c	N0	M0	PSA≥10<20	GS≤6
	T2a	N0	M0	PSA<20	GS≤7
	T2b	N0	M0	PSA<20	GS≤7
	T2b	N0	M0	PSA x	GS x
IIB	T2c	N0	M0	Any PSA	Any GS
	T1–2	N0	M0	PSA≥20	Any GS
	T1–2	N0	M0	Any PSA	GS≥8
III	T3a–b	N0	M0	Any PSA	Any GS
IV	T4	N0	M0	Any PSA	Any GS
	Any T	N1	M0	Any PSA	Any GS
	Any T	Any N	M1	Any PSA	Any GS

PSA prostate-specific antigen

Imaging modalities such as transrectal ultrasound (TRUS), CT, and MRI have also been utilized to improve staging accuracy. Transrectal ultrasonography of the prostate is the most commonly used imaging technique for staging as it is routinely used to direct initial prostate biopsies. Although the accuracy of TRUS for clinical staging has been questioned, in the current era of PSA screening with lower-risk tumors, TRUS may supplant DRE for the clinical staging of nonpalpable prostate cancer and add unique and important information when considering treatment options for men with early-stage prostate cancer [4].

The AJCC clinical staging stratifies patients according to the method of tumor detection, separating nonpalpable radiologically occult "incidental" prostate cancers detected during transurethral resection of the prostate for clinically benign prostatic hyperplasia (classified as stage cT1a or cT1b) from palpable cancers detected by DRE or imaging (classified as cT2a/cT2b for a unilateral palpable nodule and/or unilateral lesion on imaging). This staging system also recognizes nonpalpable cancer detected by an elevated serum PSA level or an abnormal TRUS image (stage T1c). It is generally accepted that biopsy results should not be incorporated into clinical stage assignment, otherwise, by definition no patient would be assigned to clinical T1c stage.

Substaging of clinical stage T2 prostate cancers is largely based on the extent of the abnormality palpated during a DRE or shown during TRUS in each half of the gland. Tumor extending beyond the boundary of the prostate gland is classified as stage T3; prostate cancer fixed or invading adjacent structures other than seminal vesicles, such as external sphincter, rectum, bladder, levator muscles, and/or pelvic wall is equivalent to clinical stage T4.

Clinical stage is included as a component of several frequently cited nomograms and prognostic tools [5]. However, in contemporary multivariable models incorporating powerful predictors such as PSA, GS, and percentage of positive biopsy cores, it appears that clinical staging criteria offer limited independent prognostic information in predicting recurrence of localized prostate cancer among radical prostatectomy patients [6–8].

Pathologic T Staging

Pathologic stage (pTNM) at radical prostatectomy remains one of the most important and accurate assignments, essential not only in determining the most appropriate choice of therapy of individual patients, but also in predicting the likelihood of local and distant disease recurrence. It is completely dependent on the pathologist's handling and reporting of the surgically resected specimen. Methods for the grossing and sampling of radical prostatectomy specimens have evolved over the years [9]. More recently the 2009 consensus conference sponsored by the International Society of Urological Pathology (ISUP) made recommendations regarding the standardization of pathology reporting of radical prostatectomy specimens and addressed controversies related to definitions of features such as extraprostatic extension (EPE), bladder neck involvement, and seminal vesicle invasion (SVI) [9–13].

Pathologic Stage T2

The TNM 2002 staging system subdivided pT2 disease into three categories as determined by involvement of less than one half of one side (pT2a), more than one half of one side (pT2b), and both sides of the prostate gland (pT2c), respectively, to mirror the clinical substaging and allow direct comparison of both. In contrast to clinical substaging of T2 cancers, pathological substaging does not convey prognostic information. Stage pT2 PCA seems to represent a homogeneous group with an overall excellent prognosis and a 5-year biochemical progression-free survival (BPFS) over 90%. Several recent studies, including very large cohorts of patients, have failed to demonstrate a significant prognostic difference for intermediate-term outcomes between pathological stage T2a versus T2b versus T2c disease [14, 15], suggesting that the pathological T2 substages may not confer any prognostic value for predicting biochemical recurrence after radical prostatectomy. The 2009 ISUP consensus conference recommendation was that reporting of pT2 substages should, at present, be optional [13].

Pathologic Stage T3

Stage T3 disease is subdivided into two categories, as determined by the presence of EPE in any location (pT3a) and presence of SVI with or without EPE (pT3b).

Extraprostatic Extension (pT3a)

EPE is the preferred terminology to indicate the extension of tumor beyond the confines of the prostate gland. However, the definition is complicated by the anatomy of the gland that in many areas does not possess a well-defined histologic capsule, particularly in the apical region and along the anterior and posterior surface. Tumor admixed with periprostatic fat is the most easily recognized manifestation of EPE (Fig. 3.1). Current definitions of EPE include "tumor abutting on or admixed with fat" and "tumor involving loose connective tissue or perineural spaces of

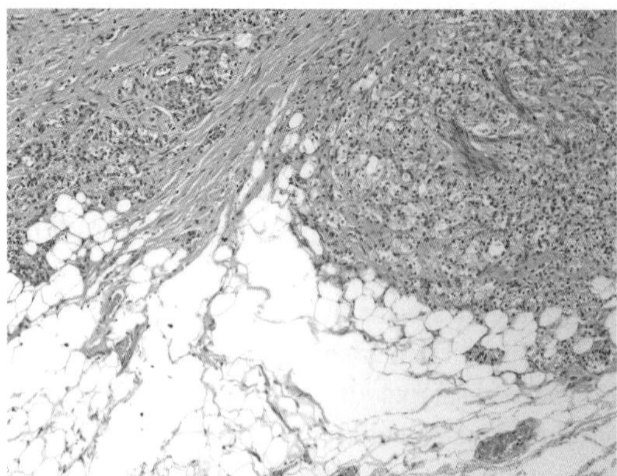

Fig. 3.1 Prostate cancer admixed with periprostatic fat is the most easily recognized manifestation of extraprostatic extension (×10)

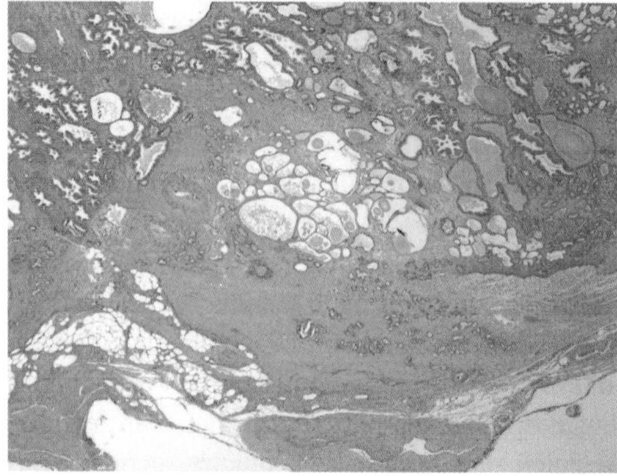

Fig. 3.3 A distinct tumor nodule within desmoplastic stroma bulging beyond the normal rounded contour of the gland represents another example of extraprostatic extension (×2)

the neurovascular bundles" even in the absence of direct contact between tumor cells and adipocytes (Fig. 3.2).

Posterolaterally, EPE may also be recognized as a distinct tumor nodule within desmoplastic stroma that bulges beyond the normal rounded contour of the gland (Fig. 3.3) or beyond the condensed smooth muscle of the prostate. Scanning magnification should be used to look for a protuberance of tumor from the normal smooth contour of the prostate, followed by higher magnification to confirm the absence of condensed smooth muscle in the desmoplastic stroma [11]. Although in the apex, anterior, and bladder neck regions, there is a paucity of fat and the histological boundary of the prostate is poorly defined, EPE may also be identified anteriorly when tumor touches an inked surgical margin, where benign glands have not been similarly cut across or when malignant glands extend beyond the contour of the normal glandular prostate (Fig. 3.4).

Finding malignant glands within striated muscle in the apex does not constitute EPE, since benign glands are frequently admixed with striated muscle in this location (Fig. 3.5).

However, it is important to keep in mind that variability among reviewers concerning the diagnosis of EPE has been reported in different

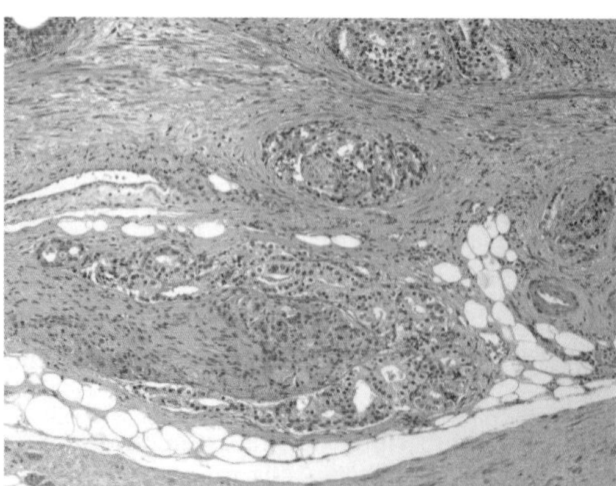

Fig. 3.2 Extraprostatic extension includes prostate cancer involving perineural spaces of the neurovascular bundle (×10)

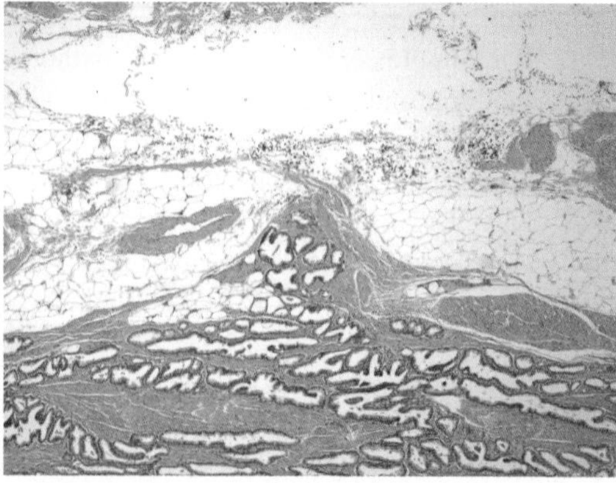

Fig. 3.4 Anterior extraprostatic extension with malignant glands extending beyond the normal contour of the prostate gland (×4)

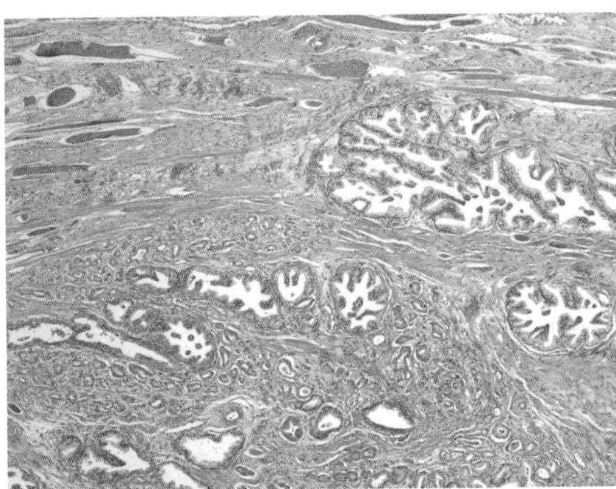

Fig. 3.5 The presence of prostate cancer glands within striated muscle in the apex does not constitute extraprostatic extension, since benign glands are frequently admixed with striated muscle in this location (×4)

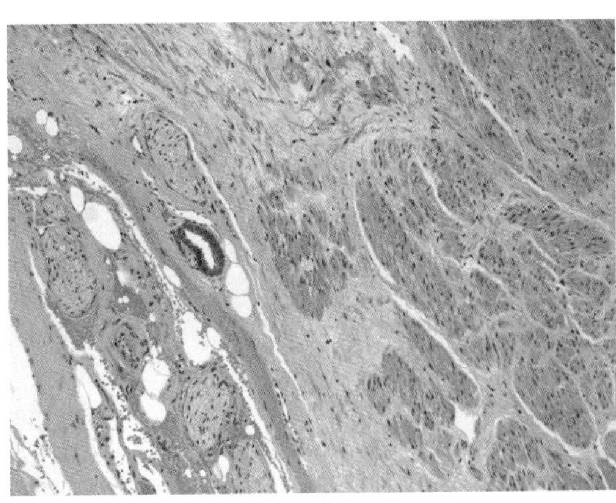

Fig. 3.7 Example of focal extraprostatic extension with a single prostate cancer gland within periprostatic fat. Notice the presence of perineural invasion (×10)

studies and robust interpretation of EPE is not always possible, due to the difficulty pathologists can encounter in identifying the boundary of the gland in some cases (Fig. 3.6).

Once EPE is diagnosed, there is good evidence that the amount of tumor beyond the prostate is prognostically significant. At the 2009 consensus conference, an overwhelming majority of the voting delegates supported the suggestion that EPE should be quantitated; however, no single method has emerged as objective, practical, and accurate in terms of its ability to predict cancer progression and biochemical failure. On the basis of the survey, pathologists appeared to prefer the subjective approach (focal, Fig. 3.7, vs. nonfocal, Fig. 3.8) suggested by either Epstein et al. (focal is defined as "only a few neoplastic glands") or Wheeler et al. (focal is defined as "tumor outside the prostate to a depth of <1 high power field in ≤ 2 separate sections") over quantitative methods (greatest linear dimension, radial dimension, volumetric measurements), and a slightly higher number of delegates seemed to prefer Epstein's method over Wheeler's one [11].

Reporting of the location of any EPE present is recommended, despite the lack of published evidence for its relevance on staging, prognosis, and treatment.

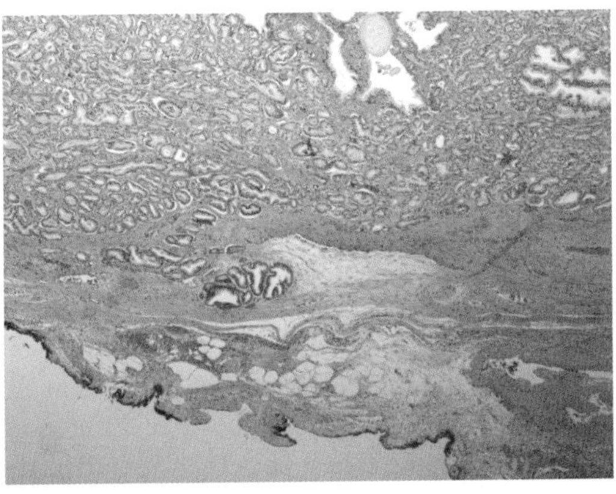

Fig. 3.6 Despite the fact that a group of malignant glands extends beyond the bulk of the tumor, it is difficult to identify the boundary of the prostate gland. No involvement of the periprostatic fat is identified (×4)

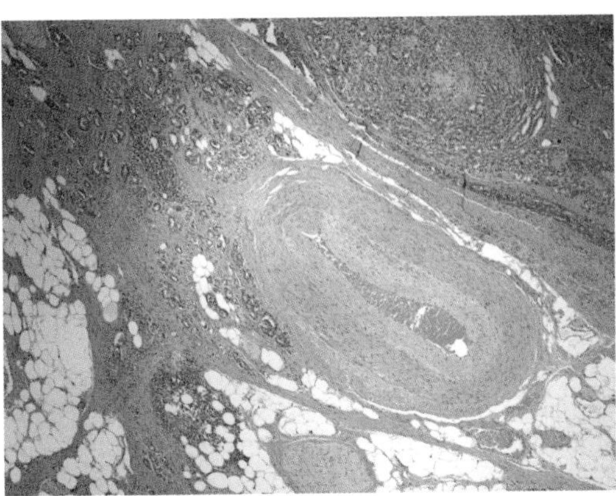

Fig. 3.8 Example of nonfocal extraprostatic extension with numerous clusters of prostate cancer glands within periprostatic fat (×4)

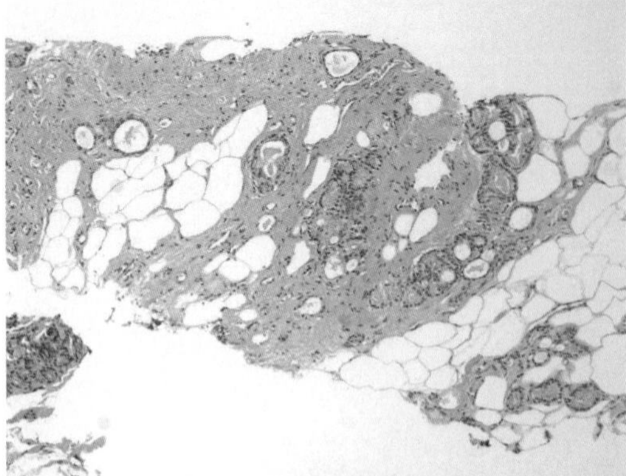

Fig. 3.9 Extraprostatic extension of prostatic adenocarcinoma on needle core biopsy (×10)

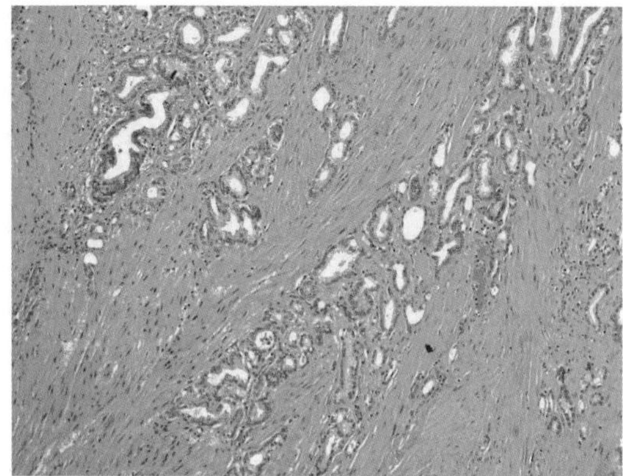

Fig. 3.10 Microscopic bladder neck involvement is defined as the presence of neoplastic cells within smooth muscle bundles of the bladder neck in the absence of benign prostatic glandular tissue on the corresponding slide (×10)

EPE of prostatic adenocarcinoma is exceedingly rare (<2 %) on needle core biopsy, but is frequently associated with extensive high-grade tumors with very poor prognosis [16]. In a recent study from our institution, EPE was detected in 95 of 4291 (2 %) patients who underwent prostate biopsy between 2004 and 2012 (Fig. 3.9). Most patients with EPE on needle biopsy were treated using a multimodality approach. Follow-up was available for 89 patients. Radiographic evidence of bone metastasis was present in 28/89 (31 %) men. Seven (8 %) patients died of disease [17].

Microscopic Bladder Neck Invasion (pT3a)

The stage classification of PCA invading bladder neck has been controversial for the last few years. In the 2002 AJCC TNM staging system, bladder neck invasion was designated as pT4 disease, whereas in the 2009 TNM scheme, microscopic bladder neck invasion was categorized as pT3a cancer. In the past, the diagnosis of prostate cancer with bladder neck invasion was based upon the urologist finding gross invasion of the bladder neck and considered as advanced disease, similar to external sphincter and/or rectal involvement [11].

Currently most PCA patients with bladder neck invasion are detected incidentally during microscopic evaluation of the radical prostatectomy specimen. Microscopic bladder neck involvement is defined as the presence of neoplastic cells within smooth muscle bundles of the coned bladder neck in absence of benign prostatic glandular tissue on the corresponding slide (Fig. 3.10) [11]. Microscopic involvement of bladder neck muscle fibers indicates pT3a disease, and gross involvement of the bladder neck is required for pT4 stage. Several recent studies have shown that bladder neck invasion carries a risk of progression similar to EPE and lower than that of SVI [18, 19], supporting the concept that bladder neck invasion should be considered as pT3a disease.

During the 2009 ISUP consensus meeting, there was consensus that the presence of prostate cancer glands intermixed with benign prostatic glands at the bladder neck should be considered equivalent to capsular incision. It was also recommended that if tumor is present at the inked resection margin at the bladder neck, this should be stated in the report [11].

Seminal Vesicle Invasion (pT3b)

SVI by PCA has generally been shown to be a poor prognostic factor after radical prostatectomy and is commonly associated with EPE. However, the considerable variation in the pathological handling and sampling of seminal vesicles in RP specimens is responsible for the large differences reported in major series, in both the percentages of cases with SVI (5–10 %) and in the 5-year BPFS (5–60 %). At the 2009 ISUP conference, there was a consensus that only muscular wall invasion of the extraprostatic portion of the

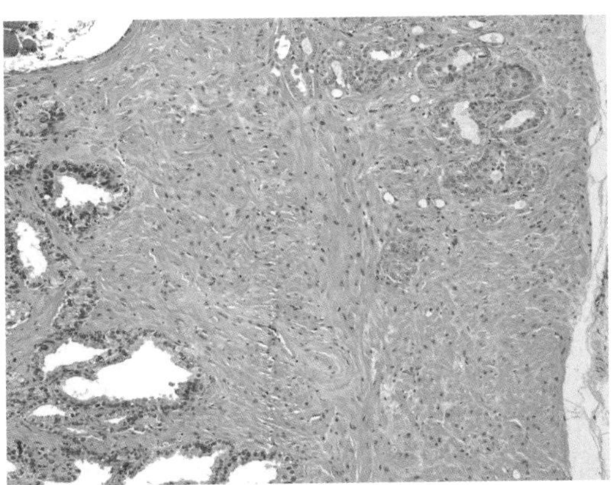

Fig. 3.11 Seminal vesicle invasion is defined as invasion of the muscular wall of the extraprostatic portion of the seminal vesicle (×10)

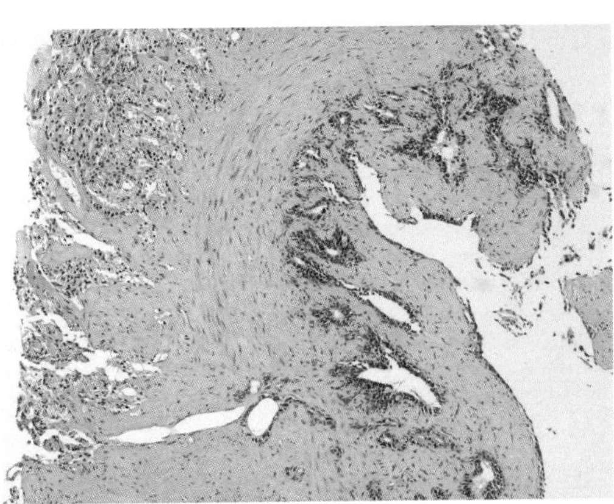

Fig. 3.12 Seminal vesicle invasion detected on needle biopsy (×10)

seminal vesicle should be regarded as SVI [10] (Fig. 3.11). It was recommended that the junction between seminal vesicle and prostate should always be assessed for contiguous spread. This should be considered the minimum necessary to adequately sample seminal vesicles.

Seminal vesicles are not routinely biopsied for evaluation of PCA; however, some clinicians choose to include seminal vesicles biopsies (SVB) along with prostate biopsies in certain clinical scenarios. In a recent study from our institution, of the 170 (0.8%) men with targeted SVB, 164 (96%) had SV tissue present in the biopsy specimen. Eighty-three (51%) men with SVB had been previously diagnosed with PCA and 77 (47%) had been formerly treated for PCA. In 16 (10%) cases only SV were sampled, of which 3 (19%) showed SVI (Fig. 3.12). Positive SVB results can aid in the selection of treatment options and in the prediction of outcome for individual patients by providing confirmation of locally advanced disease [20].

Pathologic Stage T4

Stage pT4 prostate cancer is defined by direct invasion of rectum or gross invasion of urinary bladder, external sphincter, levator muscles, and/or pelvic wall, with or without fixation [11]. Patients with large bulky masses involving the above-mentioned structures are not typically candidates for RP; however, it is reasonable to assign a pT4 stage to a RP specimen if an associated biopsy of rectum, urinary bladder (that is not microscopic invasion of bladder neck), or pelvic side wall is positive for PCA that is directly invading these structures, as assessed by clinical and/or radiological means.

Rectal involvement by prostate cancer (Fig. 3.13a, b) is now a clinically late event usually associated with wide EPE and frequent distant metastases, and carries a dismal prognosis despite multimodality treatment. The median survival is reported to be 15 months, with only few patients surviving more than 30 months [21].

Urinary bladder and rectum involvement by prostatic carcinoma can also occur via lymphovascular invasion (LVI), without contiguous spread; for these cases an M1 designation may be more appropriate than pT4.

Surgical Margin Status

Surgical margin status in RP specimens is a known prognostic parameter for postoperative biochemical recurrence and PCA disease progression.

Positive surgical margin on pathologic evaluation is defined as cancer cells touching the inked surgical margin of resection of the RP specimen (Fig. 3.14a, b). In recent studies, the positive surgical margin rate ranges from 13 to 26%.

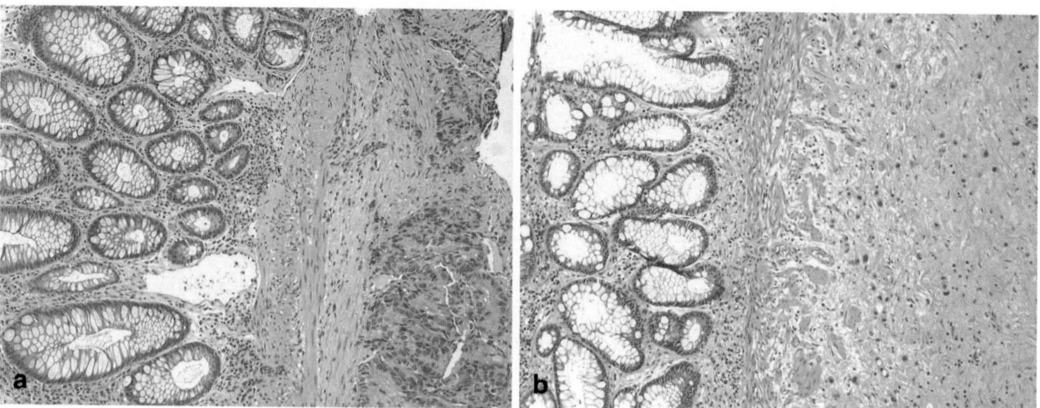

Fig. 3.13a and **b** Examples of rectal involvement by prostate cancer (×10). In **b,** the tumor shows marked treatment effect

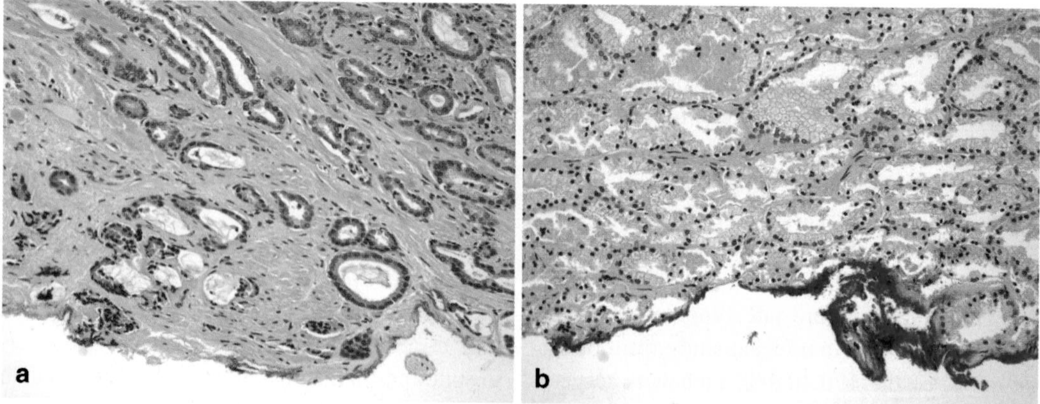

Fig. 3.14a and **b** Positive surgical margin on pathologic evaluation is defined as cancer cells touching the inked surgical margin of resection of the radical prostatectomy specimen (×20)

Progression free probability for men with positive surgical margins on RP ranges from 58 to 64% in contrast with 81–83% in patients with negative surgical margin.

Despite general consensus of the importance and clinical relevance of RP surgical margin status, marked variability still exists in the interpretation of surgical margins by pathologists practicing in different institutions.

The acceptance of considering a surgical margin as negative as long as cancer cells and/or glands do not reach the inked surface of the specimen, despite microscopically close distances (<0.1 mm) (Fig. 3.15a, b), is supported by absence of residual tumor and lack of postoperative disease progression in such patients [22, 23].

Several studies have shown that the extent of tumor at the surgical margin correlates with postoperative disease recurrence [22, 24].

Lymphovascular Invasion

LVI is a well-established prognostic factor in a number of human malignancies, and is among the histological variables that the Association of Directors of Anatomic and Surgical Pathology recommends to be reported in RP specimens [25].

LVI has been defined as the unequivocal presence of tumor cells within endothelial-lined spaces with no underlying muscular walls or as the

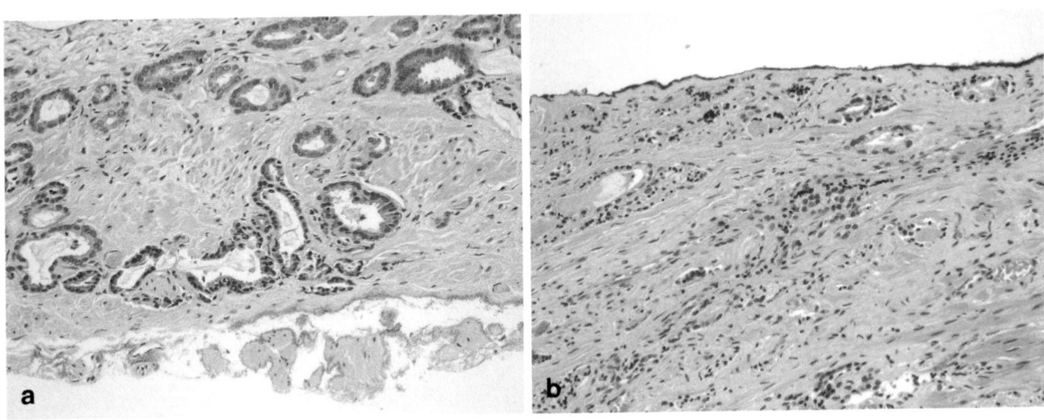

Fig. 3.15a and **b** Surgical margin is considered negative as long as cancer cells and/or glands do not reach the inked surface of the specimen, despite microscopically close distances (×20)

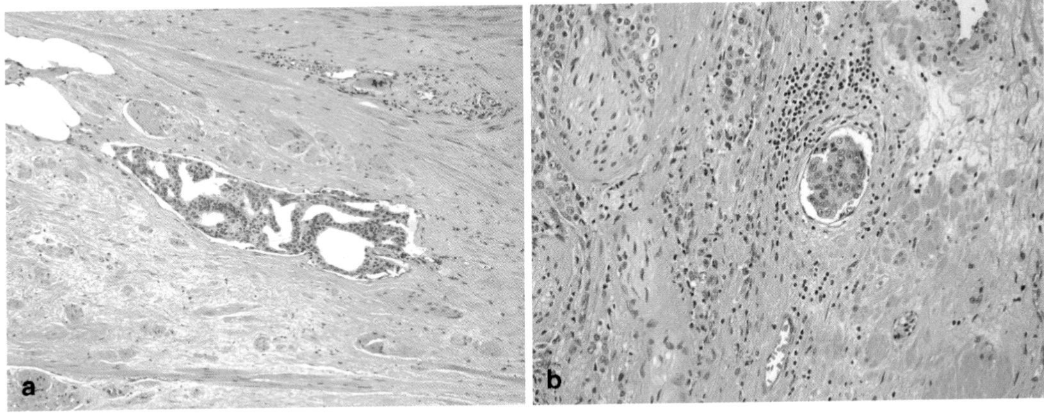

Fig. 3.16a and **b** Lymphovascular invasion is defined as the unequivocal presence of tumor cells within endothelial-lined spaces with no underlying muscular walls (×10, ×20)

presence of tumor emboli in small intraprostatic vessels [11] (Fig. 3.16a, b).

The prognostic significance of LVI in prostate cancer has been investigated by different groups with conflicting findings. LVI has been significantly associated with regional lymph node metastases and with adverse pathologic features in RP specimens, such as higher GS, positive surgical margins, EPE, and SVI. Multivariate analyses have confirmed that LVI is an independent predictor of disease recurrence when controlling for other pathologic variables known to influence clinical outcome [26, 27].

At the 2009 ISUP conference, there was consensus that LVI should be reported in the routine examination of radical prostatectomy specimens.

Regional Lymph Nodes

The spread of tumor to lymph nodes (Fig. 3.17) is a means of tumor dissemination with important impact on management and prognosis. For PCA, the regional lymph nodes are the nodes of the true pelvis, located below the bifurcation of the common iliac arteries.

As radical prostatectomy is generally reserved for men at low risk of metastatic disease, the rate of lymph node involvement is generally

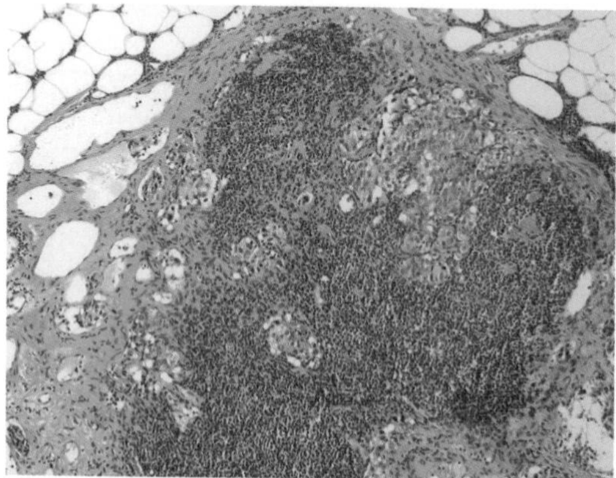

Fig. 3.17 Metastatic prostate cancer involving regional lymph nodes (×10)

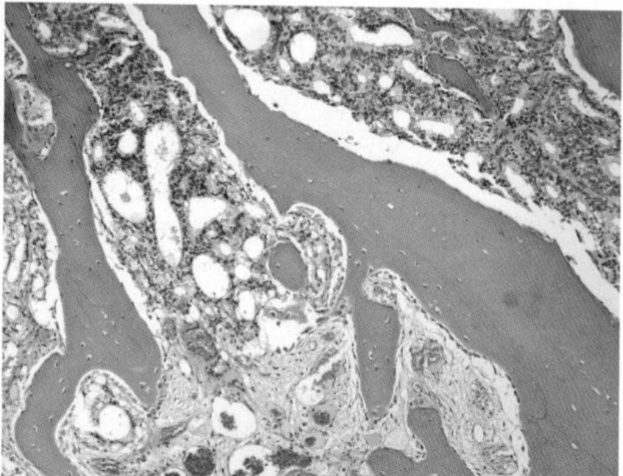

Fig. 3.18 Metastatic prostate cancer involving the head of femur (×10)

low. The number of lymph nodes obtained in a lymphadenectomy dissection varies widely among centers, which is a function of surgical technique as well as pathological practice. Quantitation of the number of lymph nodes seen on microscopy was considered necessary information for a pathology report by the 2009 consensus conference survey respondents [10]. The diameter of the largest metastasis appears to be more predictive of cancer-specific survival than the number of positive nodes alone, whereas the presence of extranodal extension has been shown not to be predictive on multivariate analysis. At the 2009 conference, there was consensus that the diameter of the largest lymph node metastasis should be included in the final pathology report [10].

Metastasis

Prostate cancer tends to spread to regional lymph nodes and bone (Fig. 3.18), and, to a lesser degree, to lung, liver, and brain. Metastases in other locations are exceptional. Involvement of lymph nodes lying outside the boundaries of the true pelvis is classified as M1a disease. Osteoblastic metastases are the most common nonnodal site of PCA metastasis with more than 50% of patients with advanced PCA having identifiable bone lesions (M1b) [28]. Lung and liver metastases are usually identified late in the course of the disease and classified as M1c category (Tables 3.1 and 3.2).

Imaging Techniques Used in Prostate Cancer Staging

Multiparametric magnetic resonance imaging (MP-MRI), which includes both high-resolution anatomic and functional pulse sequences and positron emission tomography–computed tomography (PET/CT) with targeted tracers, has begun to play a major role in the detection and staging of localized prostate cancer [29, 30]. T2-weighted MRI is the most commonly used component of MP-MRI of the prostate. It can be used to assess whether a prostate tumor is organ-confined or extending beyond the boundary of the gland [31], although the reported sensitivity and specificity for prostate cancer staging vary widely (14–100% and 67–100%, respectively) [32]. Diffusion-weighted MRI (DW-MRI), proton magnetic resonance spectroscopic imaging (MRSI), and dynamic contrast-enhanced MRI (DCE-MRI) have limited spatial resolution, which is critical for staging, and must be combined with T2-weighted MRI to improve local prostate cancer staging [32]. PET/CT has not yet made a clinical impact in localized prostate cancer.

References

1. Edge SBBD, Comptom CC, Fritz AG, Greene FL, Trotti A, editors. AJCC cancer staging. 7th ed. New York: Springer-Verlag; 2010. p. 525e38.
2. Falzarano SM, Magi-Galluzzi C. Staging prostate cancer and its relationship to prognosis. Diagn Histopathol. 2010;16:432–8.
3. Reese AC, Sadetsky N, Carroll PR, Cooperberg MR. Inaccuracies in assignment of clinical stage for localized prostate cancer. Cancer. 2011;117(2):283–9.
4. Eisenberg ML, Cowan JE, Davies BJ, Carroll PR, Shinohara K. The importance of tumor palpability and transrectal ultrasonographic appearance in the contemporary clinical staging of prostate cancer. Urol Oncol. 2011;29(2):171–6.
5. Shariat SF, Karakiewicz PI, Roehrborn CG, Kattan MW. An updated catalog of prostate cancer predictive tools. Cancer. 2008;113(11):3075–99.
6. Armatys SA, Koch MO, Bihrle R, Gardner TA, Cheng L. Is it necessary to separate clinical stage T1c from T2 prostate adenocarcinoma? BJU Int. 2005;96(6):777–80.
7. Billis A, Magna LA, Watanabe IC, Costa MV, Telles GH, Ferreira U. Are prostate carcinoma clinical stages T1c and T2 similar? Int Braz J Urol. 2006;32(2):165–71.
8. Reese AC, Cooperberg MR, Carroll PR. Minimal impact of clinical stage on prostate cancer prognosis among contemporary patients with clinically localized disease. J Urol. 2010;184(1):114–9.
9. Samaratunga H, Montironi R, True L, Epstein JI, Griffiths DF, Humphrey PA, et al. International Society of Urological Pathology (ISUP) consensus conference on handling and staging of radical prostatectomy specimens. Working group 1: specimen handling. Mod Pathol. 2011;24(1):6–15.
10. Berney DM, Wheeler TM, Grignon DJ, Epstein JI, Griffiths DF, Humphrey PA, et al. International Society of Urological Pathology (ISUP) consensus conference on handling and staging of radical prostatectomy specimens. Working group 4: seminal vesicles and lymph nodes. Mod Pathol. 2011;24(1):39–47.
11. Magi-Galluzzi C, Evans AJ, Delahunt B, Epstein JI, Griffiths DF, van der Kwast TH, et al. International Society of Urological Pathology (ISUP) consensus conference on handling and staging of radical prostatectomy specimens. Working group 3: extraprostatic extension, lymphovascular invasion and locally advanced disease. Mod Pathol. 2011;24(1):26–38.
12. Tan PH, Cheng L, Srigley JR, Griffiths D, Humphrey PA, van der Kwast TH, et al. International Society of Urological Pathology (ISUP) consensus conference on handling and staging of radical prostatectomy specimens. Working group 5: surgical margins. Mod Pathol. 2011;24(1):48–57.
13. van der Kwast TH, Amin MB, Billis A, Epstein JI, Griffiths D, Humphrey PA, et al. International Society of Urological Pathology (ISUP) consensus conference on handling and staging of radical prostatectomy specimens. Working group 2: T2 substaging and prostate cancer volume. Mod Pathol. 2011;24(1):16–25.
14. Kordan Y, Chang SS, Salem S, Cookson MS, Clark PE, Davis R, et al. Pathological stage T2 subgroups to predict biochemical recurrence after prostatectomy. J Urol. 2009;182(5):2291–5.
15. van Oort IM, Witjes JA, Kok DE, Kiemeney LA, Hulsbergen-Van De Kaa CA. The prognostic role of the pathological T2 subclassification for prostate cancer in the 2002 Tumour-Nodes-Metastasis staging system. BJU Int. 2008;102(4):438–41.
16. Miller JS, Chen Y, Ye H, Robinson BD, Brimo F, Epstein JI. Extraprostatic extension of prostatic adenocarcinoma on needle core biopsy: report of 72 cases with clinical follow-up. BJU Int. 2010;106(3):330–3.
17. Falzarano S, Streator Smith K, Magi-Galluzzi C. Extraprostatic extension on prostate needle biopsy: uncommon finding with important implications. United States and Canadian Academy of Pathology; Baltimore, MD: Mod Pathol; 2013:208A.
18. Rodriguez-Covarrubias F, Larre S, Dahan M, De La Taille A, Allory Y, Yiou R, et al. Invasion of bladder neck after radical prostatectomy: one definition for different outcomes. Prostate Cancer Prostatic Dis. 2008;11(3):294–7.
19. Zhou M, Reuther AM, Levin HS, Falzarano SM, Kodjoe E, Myles J, et al. Microscopic bladder neck involvement by prostate carcinoma in radical prostatectomy specimens is not a significant independent prognostic factor. Mod Pathol. 2009;22(3):385–92.
20. Watts KE, Magi-Galluzzi C. Targeted seminal vesicles biopsies: incidence and clinicopathological finding. United States and Canadian Academy of Pathology; Baltimore, MD: Mod Pathol; 2013:257A.
21. Bowrey DJ, Otter MI, Billings PJ. Rectal infiltration by prostatic adenocarcinoma: report on six patients and review of the literature. Ann R Coll Surg Engl. 2003;85(6):382–5.
22. Emerson RE, Koch MO, Daggy JK, Cheng L. Closest distance between tumor and resection margin in radical prostatectomy specimens: lack of prognostic significance. Am J Surg Pathol. 2005;29(2):225–9.
23. Epstein JI, Amin M, Boccon-Gibod L, Egevad L, Humphrey PA, Mikuz G, et al. Prognostic factors and reporting of prostate carcinoma in radical prostatectomy and pelvic lymphadenectomy specimens. Scand J Urol Nephrol Suppl. 2005(216):34–63.
24. Babaian RJ, Troncoso P, Bhadkamkar VA, Johnston DA. Analysis of clinicopathologic factors predicting outcome after radical prostatectomy. Cancer. 2001;91(8):1414–22.
25. Epstein JI, Srigley J, Grignon D, Humphrey P. Recommendations for the reporting of prostate carcinoma: association of directors of anatomic and surgical pathology. Am J Clin Pathol. 2008;129(1):24–30.
26. Ito K, Nakashima J, Mukai M, Asakura H, Ohigashi T, Saito S, et al. Prognostic implication of

microvascular invasion in biochemical failure in patients treated with radical prostatectomy. Urol Int. 2003;70(4):297–302.

27. May M, Kaufmann O, Hammermann F, Loy V, Siegsmund M. Prognostic impact of lymphovascular invasion in radical prostatectomy specimens. BJU Int. 2007;99(3):539–44.
28. Rove KO, Crawford ED. Metastatic cancer in solid tumors and clinical outcome: skeletal-related events. Oncology (Williston Park). 2009;23(14 Suppl 5): 21–7.
29. Bouchelouche K, Turkbey B, Choyke P, Capala J. Imaging prostate cancer: an update on positron emission tomography and magnetic resonance imaging. Curr Urol Rep. 2010;11(3):180–90.
30. Turkbey B, Bernardo M, Merino MJ, Wood BJ, Pinto PA, Choyke PL. MRI of localized prostate cancer: coming of age in the PSA era. Diagn Interv Radiol. 2012;18(1):34–45.
31. Bloch BN, Genega EM, Costa DN, Pedrosa I, Smith MP, Kressel HY, et al. Prediction of prostate cancer extracapsular extension with high spatial resolution dynamic contrast-enhanced 3-T MRI. Euro Radiol. 2012;22(10):2201–10.
32. Turkbey B, Mena E, Aras O, Garvey B, Grant K, Choyke PL. Functional and molecular imaging: applications for diagnosis and staging of localised prostate cancer. Clin Oncol. 2013;25(8):451–60.

Prostate Cancer Reporting on Biopsy and Radical Prostatectomy Specimens

4

Samson W. Fine

Abbreviations

PCa Prostate cancer
GS Gleason score
NB Needle biopsy
PIN Prostatic intraepithelial neoplasia
RP Radical prostatectomy
LN Lymph node

Introduction

Prostate cancer (PCa) remains the most commonly diagnosed cancer in men in developed countries, although death from PCa has steadily declined over the past 10–15 years [1]. Currently, most men in whom PCa is detected will die with, rather than of the disease. Characterization, clinical management, and follow-up of patients with PCa are highly dependent on a combination of laboratory (prostate-specific antigen (PSA) measurement), clinical (digital rectal examination, DRE), and pathologic factors [2–5]. Pathologists play a significant role in evaluation of pathologic features in both prostatic needle biopsy (NB) and radical prostatectomy specimens, allowing for risk stratification. As the patient population diagnosed with PCa and the diagnostic material/pathologic criteria for PCa have evolved over the past 30 years, the current chapter provides a review of contemporary handling and reporting of PCa-bearing specimens.

S. W. Fine (✉)
Department of Pathology, Memorial Sloan-Kettering Cancer Center, New York, NY, USA
e-mail: fines@mskcc.org

Pathology Reporting for Prostate Cancer: Biopsy Specimens

Essential reporting elements for cancer-bearing prostatic NB specimens are summarized in Table 4.1.

Specimen Submission, Gross Description, and Site Designation

Concurrent with the rise of PSA screening and increasingly sensitive imaging techniques, the average number of prostate NB cores has risen from 2 to 6 to 12 over the past 20 years [6]. As such, the primary purpose of NB has shifted from targeting specific areas of concern on DRE to the systematic mapping of the gland for cancer involvement and quantification [6]. In practice, this information is routinely used to determine (a) whether any form of therapy or follow-up is

Table 4.1 Essential reporting elements for cancer-bearing prostatic needle biopsy specimens

Gleason grades/score
Usual scenario: primary + secondary patterns
Special scenarios: see Tables 4.2 and 4.3
Number of positive cores
Tumor quantitation/extent (percent involvement and/or linear extent in mm)
Treatment-related changes

C. Magi-Galluzzi, C. G. Przybycin (eds.), *Genitourinary Pathology*, DOI 10.1007/978-1-4939-2044-0_4,

indicated, (b) the type of therapeutic options offered to the patient, including active surveillance, (c) the extent of resection (i.e., nerve-sparing or not) for surgical patients, and (d) the nature and dosing of radiation therapy.

The import of these results conveys clinical significance to the submission, handling, and description of NB cores. Whether needle cores are submitted in two containers (right and left sides) or in separate containers with specific site designations (i.e., right lateral apex, right lateral mid, right lateral base, etc.) is nonuniform among urologists/institutions. However, the importance of knowing the specific location of the biopsy, and therefore the location of detected cancer, is well recognized, as it allows for detailed correlation with clinical and imaging studies and effective treatment planning [6, 7]. On a practical level, processing and pathologic assessment of NB is greatly facilitated if biopsies are separated. Less material is lost when cutting single biopsies, reading biopsies one by one is easier and facilitates identification of minimal foci of cancer [8]. Therefore, when cores are submitted separately or assigned a clear site designation by container, the pathology report should reflect this labeling [9].

Gleason Grading: Background and Historical Context

The modern system for grading PCa emerged from work in the 1960s by Dr. Donald F. Gleason, based on a specimen cohort from the Veterans Administration Cooperative Research Group [10]. Nearly 50 years later, Gleason grading remains novel in that it is based only on the tumor's architectural pattern (Gleason patterns 1–5) with the sum of the two most common patterns—Gleason score (GS)—conveying the most clinical meaning (see Chap. 2). While additional morphologic descriptors were added to patterns 3, 4, and 5 in subsequent publications, these observations emanate from the era before PSA screening, when most patients presented with palpable and/or advanced disease and prostatic tissue was typically obtained from transurethral resection [9].

Introduction of PSA screening, coupled with the advent of thin NB techniques and expanded sampling has necessitated the diagnosis and grading of PCa on smaller and better characterized samples. Concurrently, a rising case volume and the importance assigned to Gleason grading in modern predictive models [2–4] have led to increased experience in the application of the Gleason system and a gradual evolution in practice.

In 2005, the International Society of Urologic Pathology (ISUP) convened a conference on Gleason grading to address emerging issues based on existing data as well as the personal/institutional experience of a large international group of urologic pathologists. The resulting manuscript serves as a provisional diagnostic guide to modern Gleason grading [11]. Importantly, the modifications to Gleason grading codified in the 2005 ISUP paper represent collective changes introduced over the course of the 1990s and early 2000s based on much-expanded experience with assessment of prostatic NB and modern radical prostatectomy specimens (see Chap. 2) [9].

Needle Biopsy Gleason Grading: Usual Scenarios

Nearly all prostatic carcinomas seen in NB specimens are of the usual (acinar, conventional) type, to which the Gleason system may be applied. Gleason patterns 1–2 (scores 2–4), which require nodular circumscription as a diagnostic criterion, are not easily evaluable in the limited tissue of NB. Due to poor correlation with prostatectomy grade and reproducibility among experts, GS 2–4 should not be diagnosed in these specimens [11]. Conversely, Gleason pattern 5, including single cells, sheet of cells, and comedocarcinoma, is essentially unchanged from its original descriptions [10]. The 2005 ISUP recommendations convey a significant contraction of Gleason pattern 3 and consequent expansion of Gleason pattern 4, with Gleason pattern 3 typically the lowest assigned grade. The most profound impact of these changes has been on grading of prostatic NB, with GS 7 now being the most commonly assigned score [12].

In modern terms, discrete and well-formed, infiltrative glands—even when small—have been retained within Gleason pattern 3. In contrast, practice patterns have evolved with regard to grading of cribriform glands as well as ill-defined glands with poorly formed lumina, originally considered within Gleason pattern 3 [11]. While a percentage of small- to medium-sized cribriform lesions label with basal cell markers and are better recognized today as cribriform high-grade prostatic intraepithelial neoplasia (HGPIN), the remainder of cribriform glands regardless of size, are nearly always diagnosed as pattern 4 [13]. A related feature is glomerulations or glomeruloid structures, characterized by dilated glands with an intraluminal cribriform proliferation attached to the periphery by a "stalk." This morphology was not accounted for in the original Gleason system and the 2005 ISUP recommendations did not reach consensus on this histology. Nonetheless, a recent report showed that in 45 biopsies with glomerulations, >80% showed an association with Gleason pattern 4 cancers in the same biopsy core [14]. The significant morphologic overlap with and occasionally observed transitions to cribriform Gleason pattern 4 carcinoma also favor classifying glomerulations as pattern 4 (Fig. 4.1).

The 2005 ISUP conference highlighted the controversy surrounding classification of "ill-defined glands with poorly formed glandular lumina" (Fig. 4.2). While there is some consensus that such foci should be graded as pattern 4, this morphology represents a significant challenge for the Gleason system, with few instructive images in the existing literature. The ISUP panel cautioned that a "cluster of ill-defined glands in which a tangential section of pattern 3 glands cannot account for the histology" would be diagnosable as Gleason pattern 4 [11], a determination that necessitates evaluation of multiple levels and sections of such glands.

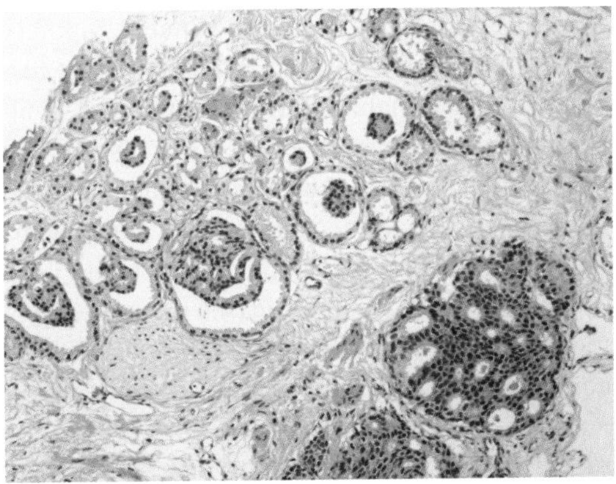

Fig. 4.1 Glomerulations demonstrating significant morphologic overlap with and transition to cribriform Gleason pattern 4 carcinoma

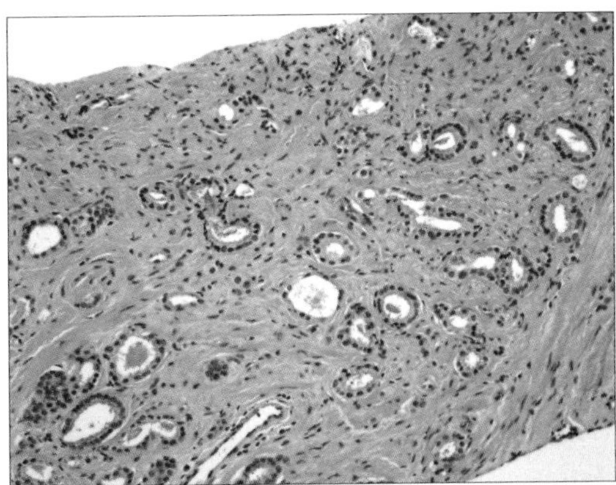

Fig. 4.2 Gleason score 3+4=7 carcinoma: note multiple poorly formed glands with ill-defined lumina and/or incomplete nuclear complement

Needle Biopsy Gleason Grading: Special Scenarios

Although Gleason grading is and always has been fundamentally based upon a sum of the first and second most common patterns, uropathologists have evolved reporting strategies for some specific scenarios in which (a) morphologic patterns are not well addressed within the original Gleason system, (b) the classic grading might not be clinically precise, and (c) the patient has received prior therapy. While some of these recommendations are consonant with the original Gleason system, the method of applying these rules has been clarified over time. Tables 4.2 and 4.3 summarize these recommendations.

Prostate Cancer Variants

The Gleason grading of a number of variants has been modified from the original system, as

Table 4.2 Reporting recommendations for prostate cancer variants

Variant	Gleason grade/pattern
Atrophic	3
Pseudohyperplastic	3
Foamy	3 or 4 (depending on architecture)
Vacuoles	3, 4 or 5 (extract vacuoles/ grade architecture)
Mucinous (colloid)	Either: 4 (based on extracellular mucin alone) or: 3 or 4 (extract mucin/grade architecture)
Ductal	4[a]
Sarcomatoid	5 (glandular component graded separately)
Signet ring cell	5
Small cell/ neuroendocrine	Not graded
Squamous	Not graded
Basaloid	Not graded

[a] Like a number of other variants, ductal carcinoma is typically associated with acinar (conventional) adenocarcinoma. Recently, ductal carcinomas with stratified or "high-grade prostatic intraepithelial neoplasia (PIN)-like" morphology have been described, typically associated with Gleason pattern 3. Finding ductal adenocarcinoma with comedonecrosis would warrant assigning Gleason pattern 5

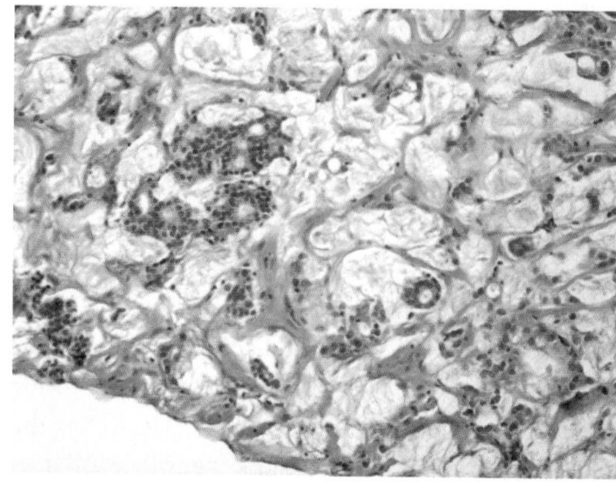

Fig. 4.3 Carcinoma with mucinous features: note that although some truly fused glands (pattern 4) are present, much of the cancer consists of discrete glands (pattern 3) with varying degrees of distortion by extravasated mucin

reflected in Table 4.2. While the unique clinical and histologic features of PCa variants are dealt with elsewhere in this text, a number of morphologies remain controversial with regard to Gleason grading [15]. Two examples are (a) the group of mucin-related tumors, including carcinomas associated with extravasated mucin (either focal or abundant) and/or mucinous fibroplasia and (b) prostatic ductal adenocarcinoma—especially those cases exhibiting "HGPIN-like" features.

In the NB context, it is difficult to evaluate true mucinous (colloid) carcinoma which requires the presence of >25 % mucin pools for its diagnosis. However, carcinomas with mucinous features may be diagnosed, typically comprised of irregular cribriform glands in a mucinous background. Such cases may also show individual glands in the same background or simulated "gland within gland" patterns representing single distorted acini and caused by encroachment of acellular mucin in and adjacent to neoplastic glands (Fig. 4.3). A similar finding is carcinoma with mucinous fibroplasia (collagenous micronodules), indicating the delicate ingrowth of fibrous tissue in and among glands, which may result in "fused-" or "cribriform-"appearing glands.

While mucinous (colloid) carcinoma with cribriform glands is routinely graded as GS 4+4=8 in radical prostatectomy specimens, there is no consensus regarding cases with discrete glands in a background of extravasated mucin or mucinous fibroplasia. At the 2005 ISUP conference, some suggested that the mucin or mucinous fibroplasia be extracted and the underlying architecture graded [11]. As such, a percentage of these cases would be assigned Gleason pattern 3. Such a designation may be supported by contemporary studies of mucinous carcinoma which have recognized the variability in the epithelial component and reported no death from disease and limited biochemical recurrence without clinical evidence of local or distant recurrence in patients who had mucinous carcinoma treated by RP [16].

The application of the Gleason grading system to prostatic ductal adenocarcinoma has also been controversial, with some initially advocating for not assigning a Gleason grade. The ISUP 2005 recommendations, recognizing that the majority of ductal adenocarcinoma displays complex papillary and/or cribriform morphology, advocated reporting such cases as Gleason pattern 4 with

Table 4.3 Reporting recommendations for special Gleason grading scenarios on needle biopsy specimens

Scenario	Recommendation
Only one grade present (e.g., GG 3)	Double that grade (assign GS 3+3=6)
Abundant high-grade cancer (e.g., GG 4) with <5% lower-grade cancer	Ignore the lower-grade cancer (assign GS 4+4=8)
Smaller focus with mostly GG 4 and few glands of GG 3	Since GG 3 occupies >5%, include lower-grade cancer (assign GS 4+3=7)
Abundant GG 3 with any extent of GG 4	Include the higher grade (assign GS 3+4=7)
Three grades (e.g., GG 3, 4 and 5) present	Classify as high grade (assign most common + highest grade)
NB: multiple cores showing different grades—cores submitted separately and/or with designated location	Assign separate GS to each core
NB: multiple cores showing different grades—all cores submitted in one container or cores are fragmented	Assign overall GS for the specimen

GG Gleason grade, *GS* Gleason score, *NB* needle biopsy

ductal features [11]. More recently, however, a significantly less frequent pattern of ductal adenocarcinoma, characterized by individual glands lined by tall pseudostratified columnar cells has been highlighted among a spectrum of PCa with nuclear stratification in single glands, so-called "prostatic intraepithelial neoplasia (PIN)-like" carcinoma [17]. As these cases may be more frequently associated with usual Gleason pattern 3 PCa and behave in a more indolent fashion than classic ductal adenocarcinoma, some have advocated assigning Gleason grade 3.

Increasing Clinical Precision with Gleason Grading on Needle Biopsy

There are circumstances in which reporting primary + secondary Gleason grade, may be inexact as traditional Gleason grading is unlikely to be representative of cancer in the gland (Table 4.3). In the context of abundant high-grade cancer, for example, lower-grade patterns should not be incorporated in the GS. Hence, a 15 mm core with 13 mm of cancer in which 0.5 mm displays Gleason pattern 3 and the remainder is Gleason pattern 4, should be diagnosed as GS 4+4=8 [16]. Conversely, any amount of high-grade tumor should be included, as it often reflects more significant high-grade tumor in the gland. As such, a 15 mm core with 13 mm of cancer in which 0.5 mm displays Gleason pattern 4 and the remainder is Gleason pattern 3, should be diagnosed as GS 3+4=7 [11]. Importantly, to apply the second rule correctly, the possibility of tangential sectioning of Gleason pattern 3 glands masquerading as fused or poorly formed glands must be excluded.

Although Gleason noted the presence of more than two patterns in ~50% of RP specimens, how to address tertiary Gleason patterns in the NB context is controversial, as incorporation of the third most common pattern is by definition contrary to Gleason's original approach [10]. Nonetheless, in 1.5–4% of cases, the pathologist encounters a core with three patterns of cancer, most typically, patterns 3, 4, and 5 (e.g., 3+4=7 or 4+3=7 with a minor component of 5) [9]. The 2005 ISUP group recommended that such cases be overall classified as high grade (primary grade + highest grade), due to the possibility that the highest grade is a more significant component in the gland and so that the highest grade would be utilized by clinicians when assessing risk using a variety of predictive models, which only allow for two grades. For example, a core with 10 mm of cancer comprised of 65% pattern 3, 25% pattern 4, and 10% pattern 5, would be diagnosed as GS 3+5=8 [11]. A subsequent NB study has supported this "first + worst" approach, finding earlier time to and percentage of patients with biochemical recurrence in patients with GS 7 with tertiary pattern 5 compared with GS 7 alone [18].

When NB cores are submitted in separate containers and/or have a clearly designated location, the pathologist should assign a separate GS to each sampled core, rather than an overall or averaged score for the entire biopsy session [11, 19]. Such practice avoids weakening the predictive power of the highest GS (e.g., one core showing 4+4=8 and multiple cores showing 3+3=6; overall GS would assign 3+4=7) and is buoyed by studies demonstrating that the highest GS in a specimen correlates with grade and stage at RP [20]. There is no uniform manner of grading cores of differing GS when multiple cores are submitted in one container without site designations. These settings are problematic as the relationship of each core/fragment to another is unclear and the potential for over-grading is increased. So as not to impose a seemingly precise assessment in an inherently imprecise scenario, logic dictates that the pathologist would assign an overall GS in these cases.

Grading Irradiated Cancer

Radiation therapy (external beam and/or brachytherapy ["seeds"]) is commonly used to treat clinically localized or locally advanced PCa . In the setting of a rising PSA postradiation therapy, a biopsy is performed to distinguish local recurrence from metastatic disease and for histological confirmation if salvage RP is to be attempted. Occasionally, the pathologist is not informed of a radiation therapy history and it is therefore essential to recognize the changes in benign and malignant glands that occur with this intervention, which have been well-described elsewhere [21].

While in the past, benign tissue with marked therapeutic effect may have been diagnosed as atypical, increased recognition that these changes are therapy-related has aided their correct identification. Cancerous foci exhibiting profound treatment effect secondary to radiation typically display infiltrative poorly formed glands or single cells with moderate-to-abundant vacuolated clear cytoplasm and prominent nucleoli [21] (Fig. 4.4). When only irradiated cancer is seen, the case may be signed out as "adenocarcinoma with profound treatment effect" and not graded. When usual-type PCa is solely present post-therapy, such that the observed cancer is indistinguishable from that of a patient who had not received radiation, the cancer is graded. In cases in which both gradable cancer and cancer with treatment effect are seen, a reasonable approach is to assign a GS and add a note stating that "the assigned Gleason score reflects the gradable portion of the carcinoma (%); the remaining cancer shows profound treatment effect" [9].

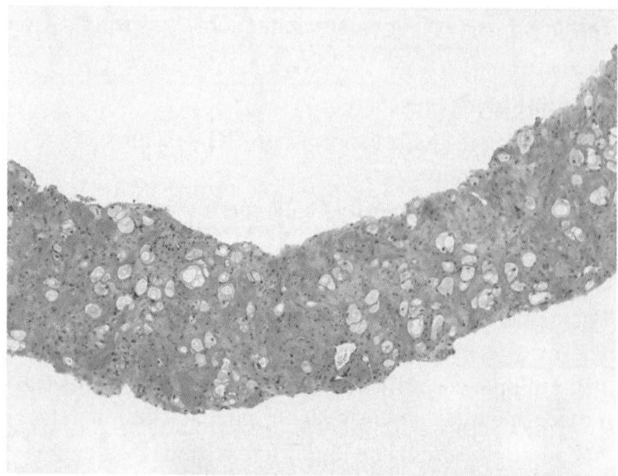

Fig. 4.4 Adenocarcinoma with profound radiation treatment effect: note poorly formed glands and single cells with vacuolated clear cytoplasm

Determining whether "gradable" cancer is present is crucial for clinical management as studies of postradiation NB with 10 years follow-up indicate that the biochemical recurrence-free and distant failure rates for patients having only cancer with profound treatment effect are similar to those with benign NB as opposed to patients with gradable cancer [22]. In other words, the presence or absence of gradable cancer in a postradiation therapy NB is a major indicator of clinical outcome.

Needle Biopsy Gleason Grade as a Measure of Risk

Accumulated evidence from over 40 years of application has shown the biopsy GS to be the most significant predictor of pathologic outcomes at RP, as well as one of the key predictors of clinical outcomes post-RP and radiation therapy [2–5, 23, 24]. GS on NB may also be used to determine therapeutic choices, the extent of neurovascular bundle resection or performance of a pelvic lymph node (LN) dissection. Consequent with the evolution described above, the value of grouping GS (i.e., GS≤6, 7, 8–10), such that each group behaved worse than the group below it, was recognized. Further substratification of GS 7 based on primary grade (i.e., GS 3+4=7 vs. 4+3=7) has also been shown to influence pathologic and clinical outcomes [25] and is routinely reported. More controversy exists as to whether GS 8–10 should be considered a homogenous group, as one study suggests that PCa with NB GS 9–10 are associated with a much worse prognosis than GS 8 [26]. Since GS is incorporated into every predictive tool [2–4] that has been designed for PCa, the accurate and reproducible application of this system has clinical meaning. Major educational efforts in the past two decades have resulted in significantly better correlation for GS on biopsy between community and academic pathologists [23].

Since the 2005 ISUP conference, few formal studies have evaluated its impact [12, 27] and these have been small cohorts with limited follow-up. As many of the "changes" represent modifications by groups of pathologists over time, such an exercise may not be fruitful, as using 2005 as a dividing line between an "old" and "new" system may be biased and inaccurate [9]. These studies have generally documented a higher percentage of NB specimens with GS≥7 in post-2005 cohorts, as well as somewhat improved biopsy–prostatectomy GS correlation and prediction of biochemical-free progression after RP.

Extent of Tumor Involvement

For core biopsy specimens, the absolute number of cores examined and involved is routinely reported. In cases with one core submitted per container, this assessment is simple. In the event of multiple cores per container, the degree to which tissue fragmentation has taken place will impact this determination.

Once a diagnosis of cancer has been rendered for a given NB core, there are multiple measures of tumor quantification which have been reported to correlate with pathologic grade and stage as well as to predict biochemical recurrence [28, 29]. However, many of these evaluations are tedious, not routinely used in contemporary practice and may add little to the predictive accuracy of more simple measurements. On the other hand, there is overwhelming consensus that in addition to the number of cores involved, some quantitation of tumor extent on a per core basis should occur, whether by visual estimation of linear extent in millimeters, percentage of core involvement, or both. When multiple cores are submitted in the same cassette, there is a higher likelihood of fragmentation [8] and it may be most prudent to report the percentage of the overall fragmented specimen involved by cancer in these cases.

Within a given NB core, foci of cancer may be present continuously or discontinuously along the length of the specimen. In the former case, length in millimeters and/or percentage of core involvement is readily assessed. When multiple foci of carcinoma are separated by intervening benign prostatic glands and stroma some pathologists will "collapse" the tumor by disregarding the intervening tissue [28] while others will measure the farthest distance between the outer-most foci and report the entire length or percentage as if it was one unbroken focus (e.g., three small foci of carcinoma discontinuously involving 80% of the core) [29]. This may result in vastly differing tumor quantitation, which may impact nomogram predictions or eligibility for active surveillance. Two contemporary studies of this specific issue convey different findings. The first study showed that in cores with discontinuous foci of cancer, stratifying the cancer lengths by various cutoffs of intervening stroma, below which discontinuous foci would be measured as one focus, yielded equal prognostic significance [28]. In contrast, another report has suggested that for cancer-bearing cores in which the NB GS is reflective of the entire tumor in the RP specimen, quantitating discontinuous foci as one unbroken focus correlates better with pathologic outcomes [29]. Given the limited evidence, it is not possible to draw a definitive conclusion at this time.

Perineural Invasion

Perineural invasion—defined as cancer tracking along or circumferentially around a nerve—is a relatively ubiquitous finding in RP specimens. In NB, an incidence between 11 and 38% has been reported [30]. There appears to be functional bidirectional communication between nerves and prostatic carcinoma cells accounting, at least in part, for perineural growth which is a major route of extraprostatic extension. Significant controversy exists as to whether this finding on NB predicts extraprostatic spread at RP and/or biochemical recurrence post-therapy (surgical or radiation). Reviews by Bismar et al. and Harnden et al. reveal that while most studies find perineural invasion to be predictive of extraprostatic extension in univariate analysis, its importance is not retained once PSA, clinical stage, and biopsy GS (common preoperative parameters) are considered in multivariate analysis [30, 31]. Similarly, there are conflicting data as to whether perineural invasion predicts for recurrence after surgery or radiation therapy. Importantly, studies which analyzed perineural invasion in specific patient groups stratified by PSA levels, clinical stage, GS, and/or NB tumor extent have found it to be an independent prognostic factor [30].

Urologic surgeons react in different ways to a report of perineural invasion on NB, with some considering this an indication to abandon nerve-sparing surgery. Recent data, however, suggest that bilateral nerve sparing may be performed without compromising oncologic efficacy in the majority of patients [32]. Taking into account the relative ease of identifying perineural invasion and its proposed significance in at least some patient groups, this finding is routinely reported.

High-Risk Lesions and Putative Precursors

Small Foci of Atypical Glands, Suspicious for Carcinoma

"Atypical small acinar proliferation" (ASAP) and "small focus of atypical glands suspicious for carcinoma (ATYP)" are terms that refer to a focus of acini that is suspicious for cancer but lacks sufficient architectural and/or cytological atypia for a definitive diagnosis. If used correctly, these terms reflect the pathologist's uncertainty as to whether a given glandular focus can be assigned a cancer diagnosis. It is therefore important that ASAP/ATYP not become a "wastebasket" diagnosis, subsuming a large spectrum of lesions. Rather, it should be a diagnosis of last resort, one in which the pathologist, after careful consideration using H&E criteria and ancillary immunohistochemical studies as appropriate, is unable to arrive at a definitive benign or cancer diagnosis [9].

There are many reasons for a finding of ASAP. Some of the more common struggles include: atypical glands that are few in number, foci with procedural-related crush or fragmentation artifact, crowded glands with minimal cytological atypia, glandular foci associated with significant inflammation, and small acinar foci in which outpouching/tangential sectioning of HGPIN cannot be distinguished from limited cancer adjacent to HGPIN [33].

It is important to recognize atypical foci suspicious for cancer in prostatic needle biopsies due to their association with cancer on repeat biopsies [34]. In this sense, ASAP may be seen as a risk factor for the subsequent finding of cancer, with the existing literature reporting an average 40 % risk of cancer following this diagnosis, a rate has been stable for nearly two decades [34]. In some cases, a focus of atypical glands is closely associated with a focus of high-grade PIN, a phenomenon which seems to carry a risk of cancer on repeat biopsy similar to ASAP. It is incumbent upon the pathologist to communicate to his/her colleagues the clinical import of these findings, so that appropriate follow-up, in the form of early repeat NB, may be performed [9].

High-Grade Prostatic Intraepithelial Neoplasia

Although PIN was first described in the 1960s by McNeal, formal characterization did not occur until the late 1980s when it was first termed "intraductal dysplasia" and quickly evolved to "PIN" [35]. Current evidence from a variety of sources has rendered high-grade PIN the only well-established precursor to prostatic adenocarcinoma [33, 34].

Morphologically, PIN describes architecturally benign prostatic glands lined by atypical cells. After initially being divided into three grades,

PIN was more concisely classified as either low grade (approximating grade 1) or high grade (approximating grades 2–3), with prominent nucleoli being the primary distinguishing factor [35]. In the past two decades, however, it has become evident that (a) there is low interobserver reproducibility for a diagnosis of low-grade PIN, with even urologic pathologists having difficulty separating this entity from slight variations of normal prostatic glandular architecture, and (b) low-grade PIN does not convey a significantly increased risk of cancer in follow-up biopsy when compared with an initial benign diagnosis [34]. As a result, the diagnosis of low-grade PIN has largely faded from the pathology-reporting spectrum, such that a diagnosis of PIN today refers to high-grade PIN.

Recent reviews reveal a large range of incidence, from 0 to 24.6% on initial NB, with no apparent relationship between PIN detection and number of cores sampled, year of sampling or academic versus community practice settings [33, 34]. This wide variation may be partially explained by the subjective nature of evaluating "cytologic atypia," specifically the presence of prominent nucleoli (how prominent? how many?), as well as multiple histological artifacts (thick sections; fixatives that enhance nucleolar detail). The difficulty in defining "atypia" is highlighted in the responses to a survey of urologic pathologists that inquired as to how prominent/how many nucleoli are required for a PIN diagnosis. "Any visible at ×40 magnification," "any visible at ×20 magnification," "any visible regardless of magnification," "in >10% of secretory cells at ×40 magnification," "in >10% of secretory cells at ×20 magnification," and "in >10% of secretory cells regardless of magnification" garnered 16, 17, 19, 11, 9, and 13% of replies, respectively, demonstrating great variability [36] and indicating the need for more specific diagnostic criteria to increase the reproducibility of a PIN diagnosis.

While the incidence of high-grade PIN does not appear to be dependent on the number of cores sampled, with studies in the 6-core and 12-core eras showing similar variability in PIN detection [34], a significantly decreased incidence of cancer detection following a high-grade PIN diagnosis has been observed [34, 37]. Although the literature reveals a large range of cancer incidence post-high-grade PIN diagnosis (from 2.3 to 100%), a more careful look reveals an incidence of ~50% in 1990s studies which has dropped to ~20% post-2000. This change approximates the shift toward more extended NB schema, which is now routine practice. Furthermore, recent studies which examine the risk of cancer on re-biopsy following a diagnosis of high-grade PIN compared with that following a benign diagnosis have shown no statistically significant differences [37]. This has led some to propose that early repeat NB is not required for men within 1 year of a PIN diagnosis, especially if there is only one core with high-grade PIN. When the initial biopsy has multifocal (>1 core with PIN), the risk of cancer on immediate repeat biopsy is about 40% and justifies repeat NB within the first year [38]. However, the long-term risk of cancer with unifocal HGPIN on initial biopsy remains unknown.

Intraductal Carcinoma

Intraductal carcinoma of the prostate is characterized by a malignant proliferation of epithelial cells conforming to the contours of often-expanded native ducts and/or acini displaying basal cells. Early descriptions from RP specimens drew attention to the fact that in contradistinction to high-grade PIN, intraductal carcinoma is rare in areas away from carcinoma [39]. This dichotomy is also reflected in needle biopsies, where it is rarely seen in the absence of invasive cancer. Further studies revealed associations with high GS and tumor volume, as well as increased rates of extraprostatic extension, seminal vesicle invasion, and recurrence after RP [40, 41]. Based on this evidence, most have argued that intraductal carcinoma is part of the evolution of PCa (a late event) or alternatively an aggressive precursor (which may or may not arise from PIN). Recent follow-up series of NB containing exclusively intraductal carcinoma have shown that the overwhelming number has invasive cancer with

GS≥7 and pT3 disease at subsequent RP [40]. These associations reveal the critical importance of separating high-grade PIN from intraductal carcinoma on NB.

Diagnosing intraductal carcinoma may be difficult, as its description may overlap with that of high-grade PIN in a given case. Additionally, it should be recognized that unlike ductal carcinoma, a morphologic phenotype/variant, intraductal carcinoma is a growth pattern of cancer, the morphology of which can be acinar or ductal. The most commonly agreed upon distinguishing criteria are those of intraductal foci with dense cribriform to solid masses with or without comedonecrosis. Though not always present, marked nuclear atypia, in the form of striking nucleomegaly, hyperchromasia, and/or overt pleomorphism, has been repeatedly associated with intraductal carcinoma (Fig. 4.5). In practice, identifying rounded or circumscribed masses of malignant cells with complex architecture and/or obvious nuclear atypia and a preserved basal cell layer should raise the diagnostic possibility of intraductal carcinoma [9]. Given the well-established correlation with high-grade, high-stage disease at RP, when detected, the presence of intraductal carcinoma should be noted in NB reports.

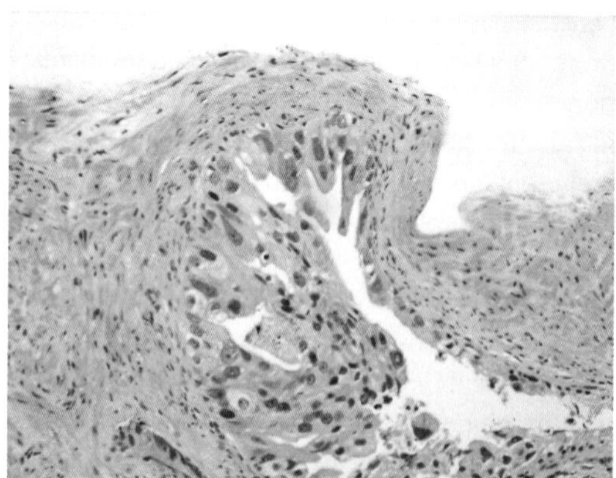

Fig. 4.5 Intraductal carcinoma: solid growth of malignant cells with marked nuclear atypia; note the evident basal cells at multiple points in the periphery of the duct

Table 4.4 Essential reporting elements for cancer-bearing radical prostatectomy specimens

Gleason grades/score
Primary + secondary patterns
Tertiary pattern
Location of tumor/dominant tumor mass
Extraprostatic extension
Present/absent
Extent (focal vs. established)
Location
Seminal vesicle invasion
Present/absent
Margin positivity
Present/absent
Location
Treatment-related changes
Lymphovascular invasion
pT stage
Lymph node metastasis

Pathology Reporting for Prostate Cancer: Radical Prostatectomy Specimens

Essential reporting elements for cancer-bearing radical prostatectomy specimens are summarized in Table 4.4.

Assessment of pathologic parameters, including GS, presence of extraprostatic extension, seminal vesicle invasion, LN metastasis, and surgical margin status, among others, are crucial in determining the prognosis following RP as precise characterization of these factors is the cornerstone of modern predictive models for biochemical recurrence and survival [2–5]. While a number of groups have published detailed recommendations regarding the handling, grading, and staging of RP specimens [42–48], in this segment the rationale and key considerations for the major reporting elements in this specimen type are highlighted.

Specimen Handling and Sectioning

Most pathology laboratories receive RP specimens in formalin. However, with expanded emphasis on tissue procurement and snap-freezing of fresh tissues for molecular and genomic studies, pathologists increasingly receive prostatectomies without fixative [44]. This condition raises the possibility of altered protein, DNA, RNA, or gene expression depending on the length of ischemia [9].

Once received, RP specimens are measured in vertical (apex to base), transverse (right to left), and sagittal (anterior to posterior) dimensions. A specimen weight is also determined which most commonly conveys the weight of the prostate with attached seminal vesicles, although at the recent ISUP conference on handling and staging of radical prostatectomy specimens there was consensus that the prostate weight should be recorded without the seminal vesicles [44]. Specimens are routinely inked to enable (a) accurate assessment of surgical margins and (b) accurate identification of laterality—when more than one color ink is used.

While prostates from which fresh tissue will be harvested may be sectioned in the fresh state, sectioning is clearly facilitated when the gland is fixed, allowing for more uniform slicing. At the prostatic apex, evaluation of prognostically significant features, including the presence of tumor at the margin, necessitates evaluation of the entire convexity of the apical surface. The most effective method to accomplish this is by taking an approximately 3 mm section of the most apical portion of the gland and then "coning" the resultant disk to submit the entire apex. At the ISUP conference, it was found that most urologic pathologists preferred sagittal coning (to ensure blocks of uniform thickness) as opposed to the radial cone method employed in the cervix [44]. In this way, each coned fragment has one inked surface that reflects the true apical margin.

Assessment of the bladder neck margin has clinical import, yet the optimal method for evaluation is much less clear. In order to report tumor in "bladder neck" tissue at RP, one must see cancer glands in thick muscle bundles (detrusor muscle- or muscularis propria-like) outside the prostate (see Chap. 3). However, the degree of bladder neck tissue resected with the specimen by the urologic surgeon may vary and is not easily visualized due to tissue contraction upon removal from the patient. Moreover, it had been demonstrated that detrusor-like muscle bundles continue over the anterior and lateral aspects of the prostate from base to mid-gland [49]. Hence, while most laboratories employ a similar sectioning and coning method as in the apex [44], this protocol may not truly reflect the bladder neck margin.

Sampling of the seminal vesicles is likewise vital to PCa staging. While there is general agreement that sections should be taken at the junction of the prostate and seminal vesicles bilaterally [47] to exclude the possibility of tumor invasion by direct extension, there is wide variability in how much of the remainder should be sampled. As other routes of tumor spread to seminal vesicles by lymphovascular invasion or in conjunction with extraprostatic extension have been reported [50], it may be reasonable to consider some degree of enhanced sampling, e.g., one additional section from the mid-seminal vesicle, in addition to the junctional section.

Whether one partially or totally embeds the prostate is largely dependent on the nature of the institution and its investment in research, tissue harvesting, and/or correlation with imaging studies. Regardless of the approach, the most diagnostically and clinically useful method is one that provides maximal information on grade, stage, and margin status. While there are many approaches for subtotal sampling, Sehdev et al. compared ten sampling techniques in patients with cT1c tumors with one or more adverse pathologic findings (e.g., GS$\geq$7, extraprostatic extension, margin positivity) and described a method with comparable results to whole gland submission. This entailed embedding every posterior section and one mid-anterior section from both right and left. If either anterior section had potentially dominant (by size) tumor, all anterior sections were submitted. This method detected >95% of adverse features [51] and represents a practical alternative for institutions not wishing to submit the entire gland. Centers opting for subtotal submission of the gland should balance its benefits against the additional effort expended in keeping track of remaining tissue, subsequent embedding of additional blocks, dictating amended reports, and/or a delayed final diagnosis [44].

Multifocality, Zonal Origin, and Defining the Index (Dominant) Tumor

Multifocality

The tendency of PCa to develop in a multifocal fashion is well established, with reported rates between 60 and 90% in surgically removed glands [52]. Although the biological basis for multifocality still requires clarification, this aspect of PCa has significant impact on RP reporting, especially in assigning zonal origin, identifying the index or dominant tumor nodule, as well as in grading and staging.

Zonal Origin

Numerous studies have claimed that transition zone tumors should be considered and reported separately from peripheral zone tumors. In part, these observations were based on a series of studies from the late 1980s and early 1990s in which investigators identified transition zone tumors by distinctive histology, including well-differentiated glands of variable size and contour, composed of tall cuboidal to columnar cells with clear-to-pale pink cytoplasm, basally oriented nuclei, and occasional eosinophilic luminal secretions [53]. These studies concluded that this "clear cell" appearance was a marker of transition zone tumors, which were associated with a more indolent course, higher cure rate, and overall more favorable prognosis. Few studies, however, compared tumors arising in the transition zone with those arising in the anterior peripheral zone, the predominant glandular tissue of the apical prostate.

A recent large-scale analysis of anterior dominant tumors, in which zone of origin was determined using an anatomy-sensitive approach emphasizing the variability in anterior prostatic anatomy from apex through base, showed that the majority of dominant anterior tumors in the prostate are actually of anterior peripheral zone origin. No significant differences in GS, incidence of extraprostatic extension, or overall surgical margin positivity rate were observed between anterior peripheral zone and transition zone tumors [53]. Therefore, while it is important to recognize the increasing percentage of anterior dominant prostatic tumors, there is less definitive evidence at this time to specify zone of origin in the pathology report [9].

Index or Dominant Tumor

The notion of an index or dominant tumor was originally proposed by McNeal and Stamey at Stanford, who measured the volume of the largest tumor nodule and correlated this with outcome [54]. While empiric experience and logic dictate that the dominant nodule by size will be associated with the highest GS and will be the stage-determining lesion, up to one third of cases may not conform to this rule [52]. While it is relatively easy to report a dominant nodule location in the former case, there is no consensus as to how the index lesion should be designated in those cases for which size, grade, and stage do not converge in a single tumor nodule [45]. This leads to diagnostic challenges in GS assignment and staging. Although there was no consensus at the 2009 ISUP conference as to the defining features of the dominant/index tumor in a radical prostatectomy specimen, there was great support for the concept that tumor size and Gleason grade are the two most important parameters to be considered. Slightly less support was obtained for the suggestion that the dominant/index tumor should be defined on the basis of pathologic stage. It was suggested that the tumor with the highest grade and/or stage might also be more appropriately considered to be the dominant/index tumor for the purpose of correlating imaging studies with subsequent prostatectomy findings.

Radical Prostatectomy Gleason Grading

Grading of Specimens with Separate Tumor Nodules

While the general principles, historical background, and recent modifications in morphology to Gleason grading are equally applicable to NB and RP specimens, there are a number of GS reporting elements specific to RP. The first is the grading of cases with separate tumor nodules, best illustrated using two examples: (1) a gland with multiple tumor nodules in which the largest nodule has GS 4+4=8, while multifocal smaller nodules with GS 3+3=6 are also present. Assigning an overall GS in such a case may result in a diagnosis of 4+3=7 or even 3+4=7 depending on the extent of the multifocal disease. In light of limited data, the 2005 and 2009 ISUP conferences [11, 45] recommended assigning a separate GS to each dominant tumor nodule. In this case, the reported GS would only reflect the dominant nodule by size, i.e., GS 4+4=8, without the need to record smaller foci of lower-grade tumor; (2) a gland with multiple nodules, in which the largest nodule has GS 3+3=6 while a smaller nodule shows GS 3+4=7. Here grading on the basis of the dominant nodule by size alone may underestimate the biologic potential of the tumor. Hence, the 2005 ISUP group recommended reporting two GSs, one for the largest nodule (i.e., GS 3+3=6) and one for the nodule with highest grade (i.e., GS 3+4=7). This approach would lead to separate GS for at most two nodules in the overwhelming majority of cases [11]. However, given the lack of evidence in the literature, it is also reasonable to assign one GS of 3+4=7 as this may be utilized in a more straightforward fashion by clinicians in prognostic nomograms. A similar strategy may be used when no dominant nodule is present and scattered small foci of GS 3+3=6 and 3+4=7 comprise the tumor [9].

Tertiary Gleason Grades

The definition of tertiary Gleason grade in RP specimens is not analogous to that of NB because (a) the entire tumor is available for examination and (b) the multifocal nature of PCa impacts its assessment [11]. Technically, the extent of a tertiary or "third most common" grade can vary from <1 to ~30%. While there is no consensus definition, a number of authors have used <5% higher-grade tumor (usually pattern 5) as a cut off, choosing to regard the highest pattern as the secondary pattern if more abundant than 5% [55]. A significant difficulty is imposed by the routine omission of tertiary grades in clinical management due to the presence of only two grades in existing nomograms. Nonetheless, recognition and assignment of tertiary grades in RP specimens is widely practiced, with data suggesting that GS 3+4=7 tumors with a minor component of pattern 5 have similar stage and risk of biochemical progression to GS 8 tumors. Interestingly, while RP with GS 4+3=7 and a minor component of pattern 5 fare worse than GS 4+3=7 tumors, they are not akin to GS 4+5=9 tumors [55], underscoring the impropriety of adopting a "first + worst" approach as in NB specimens. Whether it is appropriate to assign tertiary patterns in cases with, for example, overwhelming Gleason pattern 3 and <5% pattern 4 is more controversial.

Grading After Androgen Ablation (Hormonal) Therapy

Since the prostate is an androgen-responsive organ and the androgen pathway plays a key role in development of function of the gland, androgen-related molecules/enzymes are molecular targets for hormonal ablation therapy, especially in patients with advanced disease. Limited hormonal therapy may also be administered prior to radical prostatectomy to reduce gland size. Therefore, similar to biopsies' postradiation therapy, it is important to recognize changes in benign and malignant glands introduced by hormonal ablation.

While benign tissue may exhibit glandular atrophy in the form of cytoplasmic diminution resulting in glandular lining cells that appear cuboidal and flat, relative basal cell prominence and occasionally squamous metaplasia, stromal edema, and/or fibrosis [56], the profound treatment effect on cancer glands is more pronounced. Glands may have little cytoplasm and hyperchromatic, yet pyknotic nuclei in which only their infiltrative growth is indicative of cancer. Aggregates of cells with pyknotic nuclei and abundant xanthomatous cytoplasm, resembling histiocytes as well as largely acellular mucin pools with rare floating single cells may also be seen, such that positive immunohistochemical labeling for pancytokeratin and PSA as well as negative basal cell markers/positive racemase may be required to establish the diagnosis. Limited cancer with treatment effect may be a cause of understaging in such patients and careful evaluation of the margins and extraprostatic tissue should be undertaken [56]. Reporting recommendations for grading are similar to those for radiation therapy, though whether a tumor shows profound treatment effect or not is of less clinical consequence, as hormonal therapy does not negate adverse outcomes in the long term.

Organ-Confined Disease: pT2 Substaging

A controversial area of RP reporting, still in evolution, is substratification of organ-confined disease [45]. With the advent of the tumor-nodes-metastasis (TNM) staging in 1992, pathologic stage T2 PCas were assigned to one of three categories: (a) pT2a—tumors occupying less than one half of one lobe, (b) pT2b—tumors occupying greater than one half of one lobe, or (c) pT2c—tumors involving both lobes, to parallel the clinical staging system. However, differences between the staging systems (DRE vs. pathologic evaluation of RP specimens) were evident and using this substaging, few pT2b tumors were identified [9]. The pT system was simplified in 1997 to include pT2a: tumors confined to one lobe and pT2b: bilateral disease. This modification created the illogical circumstance in which bilateral small foci of disease could receive a higher stage than a unilateral large lesion [45]. Limited clinical utility and correlation with clinical staging led to reversal of the 1997 TNM in its 2002 and 2010 iterations, such that three subcategories are now listed. However, a number of studies in the past decade demonstrate that pathologic substaging of organ-confined disease by any of the above systems lacks prognostic import [9, 45]. While many still report pT2 substages at this time, a recent ISUP recommendation was that this practice was optional and should be modified in the future [45].

Extraprostatic Extension

In pathologic terms, extraprostatic extension refers to the presence of tumor beyond the borders of the gland. While this terminology may convey ease in application, the reality of determining extraprostatic extension in practice is highly dependent on anatomic location and the presence of desmoplastic reaction to tumor and/or biopsy-related changes. The basic boundary of the prostate is a condensed fibromuscular layer of prostatic stroma, rather than a true, epithelial-lined capsule. Early observations showed that although the boundary was usually intact in the posterior and posterolateral aspects of the gland, this was not the case in the apex, anterior, or bladder neck regions [57]. Not surprisingly, interobserver variability studies among pathologists targeting extraprostatic extension report the most variation in areas and cases without clear anatomic landmarks.

The most easily recognizable sign of extraprostatic extension is tumor admixed with periprostatic fat. In the posterolateral prostate, a pT3a stage may also be assigned to tumor identified within loose connective tissue and/or perineural spaces of the neurovascular bundles and, when present, to distinct tumor nodules within desmoplastic stroma that bulges beyond the prostatic contour [46]. There is debate as to whether extraprostatic extension can be diagnosed at the apex and how to separate this finding from apical margin positivity [57]. The current convention is to call tumor organ-confined at the apex as long as tumor is not at the inked margin. The presence of skeletal muscle (apex) and blood vessels (apex through base) both in the anterior prostatic stroma and in the anterior extraprostatic space, coupled with blending of the prostatic stroma with extraprostatic smooth muscle bundles (mid to base), leave invasion into or at the level of adipose tissue as the most reasonable diagnostic feature of extraprostatic extension in the anterior prostate [58].

Once the presence or absence of extraprostatic extension has been established, some method of quantitation is routine [46]. The two most common approaches are those of Epstein [59] and Wheeler [60], which both distinguish "focal" from "established" extraprostatic extension (see Chap. 3). Using these subjective, yet readily applicable criteria, clinically meaningful separation of pT3a patients can be achieved. Extraprostatic extension is a significant parameter in nearly all postoperative predictive tools in use today [2, 4]. Although pathologists typically report the

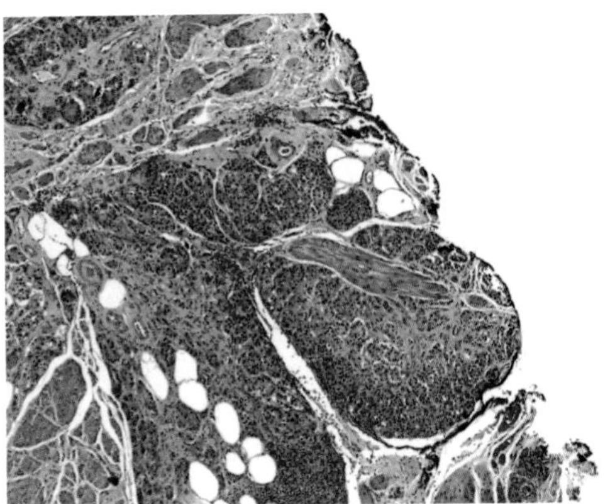

Fig. 4.6 Positive surgical margin in an area of extraprostatic extension

location(s) of extraprostatic extension, this parameter has no known prognostic significance in the absence of a positive margin at the site (Fig. 4.6).

Bladder Neck Invasion

In a significant change from prior versions, the 2010 TNM classification categorizes microscopic bladder neck invasion as pT3a, rather than together with gross invasion (pT4) (see Chap. 3). This change represents the culmination of a decade of work in which the clinical significance of microscopic bladder neck invasion was challenged [46]. The overwhelming number of studies found that usual grading and staging parameters, but not microscopic bladder neck invasion alone, were independent predictors of progression or that patients with this finding have a greater likelihood of 3- and 5-year progression-free survival than those with seminal vesicle invasion [61].

While this is now the consensus in the urologic pathologic community, there exists some variability in defining microscopic bladder neck invasion based on the specimen handling considerations highlighted above. All prior studies have called microscopic bladder neck invasion when malignant cells or glands invade thick smooth muscle bundles in the bladder neck section [46]. However, equating this with bladder neck margin positivity will depend on whether specimens are coned (not equated) or shaved (equated). Importantly, microscopic bladder neck invasion should be distinguished from tumor intermixed with benign prostatic glands in the bladder neck section; this may represent either a false positive margin due to the pathologist obtaining too thick a shave margin or a true positive margin in an area of intraprostatic incision by the surgeon [9].

Seminal Vesicle Invasion

Tumor infiltration of the muscular wall of the seminal vesicle is a well-established adverse prognostic feature in PCa [47, 50]. Two decades ago, Ohori et al. studied a cohort of patients with seminal vesicle invasion and described three routes of spread from the prostate: (a) direct spread along the ejaculatory ducts at the base, (b) extraprostatic extension into peri-seminal vesicle soft tissue with ensuing seminal vesicle invasion, and (c) discontinuous spread (in cases where no prostatic base tumor was identified) [50]. While it is possible that the latter may reflect lymphovascular invasion, the distinction of seminal vesicle invasion types is not routine reporting practice [47].

There are three significant caveats regarding assessment of seminal vesicle invasion. The first is in assessment and staging of tumor invading peri-seminal vesicle soft tissue. While early studies designated these tumors within the rubric of "seminal vesicle invasion," this finding is currently staged as pT3a (extraprostatic extension). Secondly, in the unusual case in which tumor is present in endothelial-lined lymphovascular spaces within the seminal vesicle wall alone, without overt muscular wall invasion, there is no consensus as to whether pT3a (tumor beyond the prostate) or pT3b (seminal vesicle invasion akin to muscular wall invasion) should be assigned. Similarly, whether to diagnose pT3b disease when tumor is seen at the ejaculatory duct-seminal vesicle junction in prostatic sections is controversial. Two approaches are (1) only diagnose pT3b when tumor is seen in the extraprostatic seminal vesicle or (2) allow for the diagnosis of tumor invading the "base of the seminal vesicle," but require that it has a well-formed muscular coat and be topographically separate from prostatic glandular tissue [47].

Lymph Node Metastasis

Pelvic LN dissection is the standard means for detecting LN metastasis in PCa [62] and LN metastasis is overwhelmingly associated with high-grade, high-stage, and large-volume disease [63]. Over the past three decades, the manner in which urologists and oncologists view the finding of LN positivity in relation to patient management has evolved. While finding LN metastasis on frozen section analysis was once an absolute contraindication to RP more recent studies have suggested the curative potential of LN dissection. Coinciding with the advent of risk stratification tools, which aid in selecting/avoiding intervention, and the increasing popularity of minimally invasive surgery, evidence from groups such as CaPSURE suggests a steady decline in the performance of LN dissection, especially for patients in low- and intermediate-risk groups [62]. However, great debate still exists in determining which risk categories warrant lymph node dissection and the extent of LN sampling that should be routinely performed. Two recent studies in large cohorts of LN-positive patients have shown that the typical limited sampling (external iliac LN only) detects only one third of positive LN and that 30–40% of LN metastases may occur contralateral to the dominant tumor in the prostate [63], suggesting that current trends in LN sampling may need reassessment.

As a result, some urologic surgeons still send frozen section LN samples, though studies have revealed a relatively high false-negative and pathologists may be asked to evaluate either no LN, a limited sampling (usually bilateral external iliac nodes) submitted as "right and left pelvic lymph nodes" or occasionally, more extensive sampling by LN packet (external iliac, obturator, and hypogastric) [63]. This leads to extreme variability in the average number of LNs identified [47]. While pathologists routinely report the number of LN and the number involved by tumor, there is significantly more variation in reporting diameter of largest LN, diameter of largest metastatic focus, and the presence of extranodal extension [47], the independent prognostic value of which is not well defined.

Surgical Margins

Surgical margin status is a known prognosticator for PSA recurrence and disease progression in PCa [48]. A positive surgical margin is defined as tumor cells at the inked margin of the prostatectomy specimen, with an incidence of 11–38% in large series. This finding may occur in a region of extraprostatic extension (pT3 R1 in 2010 TNM classification) or by intraprostatic incision into an otherwise organ-confined tumor (pT2 R1 in 2010 TNM classification or pT2+ in many institutions). While most have shown that it is predominantly positive surgical margins in pT3 disease (Fig. 4.6) that are relevant in terms of recurrence risk, the value of surgical margin positivity in otherwise organ-confined disease (pT2+) has also more recently been elucidated. Studies by Chuang et al. and Stephenson et al. have found worse progression-free probability for pT2+ patients than those with organ-confined/margin-negative disease [64, 65]. Hence, reporting of overall margin status as positive or negative should be uniform in pathology practice.

In many institutions, report of a positive margin is cause for initiating radiation therapy, as there is evidence to suggest that this reduces the rate of rising PSA after prostatectomy [66]. However, recognizing that a significant percentage of patients with positive margins never experience PSA recurrence, other clinicians apply for a more selective application of this adjuvant therapy, choosing instead to follow patients closely and treat only if biochemical recurrence occurs or there is clinical/radiological evidence of progression. A wealth of conflicting evidence attempting to substratify positive surgical margins by number, site, extent (including linear length in millimeters), or GS at a positive margin [67] has been reported in an attempt to find associations with biochemical recurrence. More recent analyses demonstrate that while many parameters are independently prognostic, no single parameter, including linear length and/or GS at the margin, improved the predictive accuracy of a standard nomogram in which surgical margin status was modeled as positive versus negative [65, 67]. Further evaluation of the range of features may be necessary to determine which, if any, is the most robust predictor of outcome, warrants routine reporting and helps select patients most likely to benefit from adjuvant radiation therapy [9].

Tumor Quantitation

It has been long known that PCa tumor volume correlates well with common adverse features such as high GS, extraprostatic extension, seminal vesicle invasion, and clinical outcomes. Although many have studied the independent prognostic value of tumor volume, wide differences exist within cohorts such that half of large series find association with biochemical recurrence and half find no association [45, 68]. These results can be explained by differences in quantification method, composition of the cohort and failure to demonstrate significance when added to commonly reported PSA and pathologic findings. Hence, whether overall tumor volume was calculated by estimation of tumor percentage, number of blocks with tumors, ratio of involved to uninvolved blocks, greatest length × greatest thickness or by one of these measures for the dominant nodule alone [68], significantly impacts the ability to compare one study with another. The intimate correlation with other prognostic factors leaves the independent value of tumor volume uncertain at this time. Though in practice many pathologists report some measure of tumor volume/size and this is widely advocated by a variety of professional groups, including a recent ISUP conference [45], given the lack of uniformity and definitive evidence, there is no one recommended method for doing so.

Lymphovascular Invasion

Identifying lymphovascular invasion requires the presence of tumor cells within endothelial-lined spaces conforming to the contour of the space and, when possible, attachment to the endothelium (Fig. 4.7) [46]. Care must be taken to exclude common artifacts including retraction around cancer glands or mechanical displacement of tumor cells [69]. The reported incidence of lymphovascular invasion ranges from 5 to 53 %, with most studies finding strong associations with high GS, positive surgical margins, extraprostatic extension, LN metastasis, and in univariate analysis, biochemical progression. Akin to the situation with tumor volume, the independent prognostic value of this marker is debatable due to differences between studies in specimen handling, definition of lymphovascular invasion, marked variation in number and follow-up between cohorts, inclusion of patients with LN involvement and whether specimens were rereviewed or garnered from the report [69]. While few investigators have stratified patients by stage and other features, Herman et al. and Yamamoto et al. have studied pT3aN0 patients, finding lymphovascular invasion in 35 and 28 % of cases and independent predictive value for PSA failure and clinical progression in multivariable analysis [70]. While further studies with standardized definitions and pathologic examination are needed, the relative ease of identification and reporting warrants the inclusion of lymphovascular invasion in routine pathology reports.

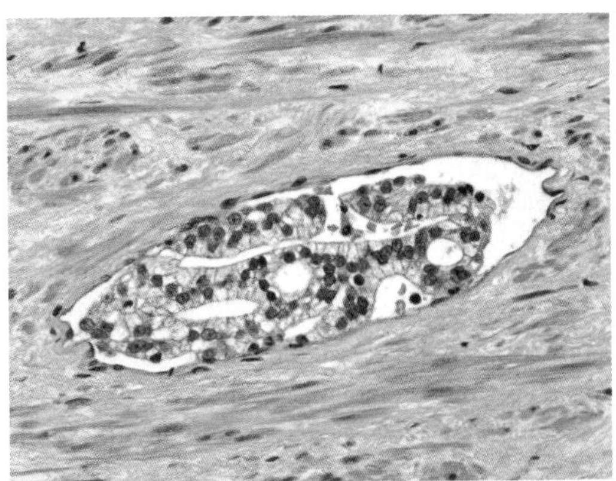

Fig. 4.7 Lymphovascular invasion by prostate cancer

References

1. Jemal A, Bray F, Center MM, Ferlay J, Ward E, Forman D. Global cancer statistics. CA Cancer J Clin. 2011;61:69–90.
2. Makarov DV, Trock BJ, Humphreys EB, et al. Updated nomogram to predict pathologic stage of prostate cancer given prostate-specific antigen level, clinical stage, and biopsy Gleason score (Partin tables) based on cases from 2000 to 2005. Urology. 2007;69:1095–101.
3. Stephenson AJ, Scardino PT, Eastham JA, et al. Preoperative nomogram predicting the 10-year probability of prostate cancer recurrence after radical prostatectomy. J Natl Cancer Inst. 2006;98:715–7.
4. Stephenson AJ, Scardino PT, Eastham JA, et al. Post-operative nomogram predicting the 10-year probability of prostate cancer recurrence after radical prostatectomy. J Clin Oncol. 2005;23:7005–12.
5. Eggener SE, Scardino PT, Walsh PC, et al. Predicting 15-year prostate cancer specific mortality after radical prostatectomy. J Urol. 2011;185:869–75.
6. Amin M, Boccon-Gibod L, Egevad L, et al. Prognostic and predictive factors and reporting of prostate carcinoma in prostate needle biopsy specimens. Scand J Urol Nephrol Suppl. 2005;216:20–33.
7. Touma NJ, Chin JL, Bella T, Sener A, Izawa JI. Location of a positive biopsy as a predictor of surgical margin status and extraprostatic disease in radical prostatectomy. BJU Int. 2006;97:259–62.
8. Fajardo DA, Epstein JI. Fragmentation of prostatic needle biopsy cores containing adenocarcinoma: the role of specimen submission. BJU Int. 2010;105:172–5.
9. Fine SW, Amin MB, Berney DM, et al. A contemporary update on pathology reporting for prostate cancer: biopsy and radical prostatectomy specimens. Eur Urol. 2012;62:20–39.
10. Mellinger GT, Gleason DF, Bailar JC 3rd. The histology and prognosis of prostate cancer. J Urol. 1967;97:331–7.
11. Epstein JI, Allsbrook WC Jr., Amin MB, Egevad LL. The 2005 International Society of Urological Pathology (ISUP) consensus conference on Gleason grading of prostatic carcinoma. Am J Surg Pathol. 2005;29:1228–42.
12. Zareba P, Zhang J, Yilmaz A, Trpkov K. The impact of the 2005 International Society of Urological Pathology (ISUP) consensus on Gleason grading in contemporary practice. Histopathology. 2009;55:384–91.
13. Latour M, Amin MB, Billis A, et al. Grading of invasive cribriform carcinoma on prostate needle biopsy: an interobserver study among experts in genitourinary pathology. Am J Surg Pathol. 2008;32:1532–9.
14. Lotan TL, Epstein JI. Gleason grading of prostatic adenocarcinoma with glomeruloid features on needle biopsy. Hum Pathol. 2009;40:471–7.
15. Fine SW. Variants and unusual patterns of prostate cancer: clinicopathologic and differential diagnostic considerations. Adv Anat Pathol. 2012;19:204–16.
16. Osunkoya AO, Nielsen ME, Epstein JI. Prognosis of mucinous adenocarcinoma of the prostate treated by radical prostatectomy: a study of 47 cases. Am J Surg Pathol. 2008;32:468–72.
17. Tavora F, Epstein JI. High-grade prostatic intraepithelial neoplasia-like ductal adenocarcinoma of the prostate: a clinicopathologic study of 28 cases. Am J Surg Pathol. 2008;32:1060–7.
18. Patel AA, Chen MH, Renshaw AA, D'Amico AV. PSA failure following definitive treatment of prostate cancer having biopsy Gleason score 7 with tertiary grade 5. JAMA. 2007;298:1533–8.
19. Kunju LP, Daignault S, Wei JT, Shah RB. Multiple prostate cancer cores with different Gleason grades submitted in the same specimen container without specific site designation: should each core be assigned an individual Gleason score? Hum Pathol. 2009;40:558–64.
20. Poulos CK, Daggy JK, Cheng L. Preoperative prediction of Gleason grade in radical prostatectomy specimens: the influence of different Gleason grades from multiple positive biopsy sites. Mod Pathol. 2005;18:228–34.
21. Gaudin PB, Zelefsky MB, Leibel SA. Histopathologic effects of three-dimensional conformal external beam radiation therapy on benign and malignant prostate tissues. Am J Surg Pathol. 1999;23:1021–31.
22. Zelefsky MJ, Reuter VE, Fuks Z, Scardino P, Shippy A. Influence of local tumor control on distant metastases and cancer related mortality after external beam radiotherapy for prostate cancer. J Urol. 2008;179:1368–73.
23. Fine SW, Epstein JI. A contemporary study correlating prostate needle biopsy and radical prostatectomy Gleason score. J Urol. 2008;179:1335–8.
24. Helpap B, Egevad L. Correlation of modified Gleason grading with pT stage of prostatic carcinoma after radical prostatectomy. Anal Quant Cytol Histol. 2008;30:1–7.
25. Stark JR, Perner S, Stampfer MJ, et al. Gleason score and lethal prostate cancer: does 3+4=4+3? J Clin Oncol. 2009;27:3459–64.
26. Pierorazio PM, Guzzo TJ, Han M, et al. Long-term survival after radical prostatectomy for men with high Gleason sum in pathologic specimen. Urology. 2010;76:715–21.
27. Uemura H, Hoshino K, Sasaki T, et al. Usefulness of the 2005 International Society of Urologic Pathology Gleason grading system in prostate biopsy and radical prostatectomy specimens. BJU Int. 2009;103:1190–4.
28. Brimo F, Vollmer RT, Corcos J, et al. Prognostic value of various morphometric measurements of tumour extent in prostate needle core tissue. Histopathology. 2008;53:177–83.
29. Karram S, Trock BJ, Netto GJ, Epstein JI. Should intervening benign tissue be included in the

measurement of discontinuous foci of cancer on prostate needle biopsy? Correlation with radical prostatectomy findings. Am J Surg Pathol. 2011;35:1351–5.
30. Harnden P, Shelley MD, Clements H, et al. The prognostic significance of perineural invasion in prostatic cancer biopsies: a systematic review. Cancer. 2007;109:13–24.
31. Bismar TA, Lewis JS Jr., Vollmer RT, Humphrey PA. Multiple measures of carcinoma extent versus perineural invasion in prostate needle biopsy tissue in prediction of pathologic stage in a screening population. Am J Surg Pathol. 2003;27:432–40.
32. Loeb S, Epstein JI, Humphreys EB, Walsh PC. Does perineural invasion on prostate biopsy predict adverse prostatectomy outcomes? BJU Int. 2010;105:1510–3.
33. Schlesinger C, Bostwick DG, Iczkowski KA. High-grade prostatic intraepithelial neoplasia and atypical small acinar proliferation: predictive value for cancer in current practice. Am J Surg Pathol. 2005;29:1201–7.
34. Epstein JI, Herawi M. Prostate needle biopsies containing prostatic intraepithelial neoplasia or atypical foci suspicious for carcinoma: implications for patient care. J Urol. 2006;175:820–34.
35. Bostwick DG, Qian J. High-grade prostatic intraepithelial neoplasia. Mod Pathol. 2004;17:360–79.
36. Egevad L, Allsbrook WC, Epstein JI. Current practice of diagnosis and reporting of prostatic intraepithelial neoplasia and glandular atypia among genitourinary pathologists. Mod Pathol. 2006;19:180–5.
37. Herawi M, Kahane H, Cavallo C, Epstein JI. Risk of prostate cancer on first re-biopsy within 1 year following a diagnosis of high grade prostatic intraepithelial neoplasia is related to the number of cores sampled. J Urol. 2006;175:121–4.
38. Merrimen JL, Jones G, Walker D, Leung CS, Kapusta LR, Srigley JR. Multifocal high grade prostatic intraepithelial neoplasia is a significant risk factor for prostatic adenocarcinoma. J Urol. 2009;182:485–90.
39. McNeal JE, Yemoto CE. Spread of adenocarcinoma within prostatic ducts and acini: morphologic and clinical correlations. Am J Surg Pathol. 1996;20:802–14.
40. Robinson BD, Epstein JI. Intraductal carcinoma of the prostate without invasive carcinoma on needle biopsy: emphasis on radical prostatectomy findings. J Urol. 2010;184:1328–33.
41. Epstein JI. Precursor lesions to prostatic adenocarcinoma. Virchows Arch. 2009;454:1–16.
42. Egevad L, Algaba F, Berney DM, et al. Handling and reporting of radical prostatectomy specimens in Europe: a web-based survey by the European Network of Uropathology (ENUP). Histopathology. 2008;53:333–9.
43. Kench J, Clouston D, Delahunt B, et al. Royal College of Pathologists of Australasia prostate cancer (radical prostatectomy) structured reporting protocol. 2010, p. 54.
44. Samaratunga H, Montironi R, True L, et al. International Society of Urological Pathology (ISUP) consensus conference on handling and staging of radical prostatectomy specimens. Working group 1: specimen handling. Mod Pathol. 2011;24:6–15.
45. van der Kwast TH, Amin MB, Billis A, et al. International Society of Urological Pathology (ISUP) consensus conference on handling and staging of radical prostatectomy specimens. Working group 2: T2 substaging and prostate cancer volume. Mod Pathol. 2011;24:16–25.
46. Magi-Galluzzi C, Evans AJ, Delahunt B, et al. International Society of Urological Pathology (ISUP) consensus conference on handling and staging of radical prostatectomy specimens. Working group 3: extraprostatic extension, lymphovascular invasion and locally advanced disease. Mod Pathol. 2011;24:26–38.
47. Berney DM, Wheeler TM, Grignon DJ, et al. International Society of Urological Pathology (ISUP) consensus conference on handling and staging of radical prostatectomy specimens. Working group 4: seminal vesicles and lymph nodes. Mod Pathol. 2011;24:39–47.
48. Tan PH, Cheng L, Srigley JR, et al. International Society of Urological Pathology (ISUP) consensus conference on handling and staging of radical prostatectomy specimens. Working group 5: surgical margins. Mod Pathol. 2011;24:48–57.
49. Fine SW, Al-Ahmadie HA, Gopalan A, Tickoo SK, Reuter VE. Defining the anterior extraprostatic space: anatomical considerations and clinical implications. Mod Pathol. 2008;21:156A.
50. Ohori M, Scardino PT, Lapin SL, Seale-Hawkins C, Link J, Wheeler TM. The mechanisms and prognostic significance of seminal vesicle involvement by prostate cancer. Am J Surg Pathol. 1993;17:1252–61.
51. Sehdev AE, Pan CC, Epstein JI. Comparative analysis of sampling methods for grossing radical prostatectomy specimens performed for nonpalpable (stage T1c) prostatic adenocarcinoma. Hum Pathol. 2001;32:494–9.
52. Andreoiu M, Cheng L. Multifocal prostate cancer: biologic, prognostic and therapeutic implications. Hum Pathol. 2010;41:781–93.
53. Al-Ahmadie HA, Tickoo SK, Olgac S, Gopalan A, Scardino PT, Reuter VE, Fine SW. Anterior-predominant prostatic tumors: zone of origin and pathologic outcomes at radical prostatectomy. Am J Surg Pathol. 2008;32:229–35.
54. McNeal JE, Price HM, Redwine EA, Freiha FS, Stamey TA. Stage A versus stage B adenocarcinoma of the prostate: morphological comparison and biological significance. J Urol. 1988;139:61–5.
55. Pan CC, Potter SR, Partin AW, Epstein JI. The prognostic significance of tertiary Gleason patterns of higher grade in radical prostatectomy specimens: a proposal to modify the Gleason grading system. Am J Surg Pathol. 2000;24:563–9.
56. Reuter VE. Pathological changes in benign and malignant tissue following androgen deprivation

therapy. Urology. 1997;49:16–22.
57. Ayala AG, Ro JY, Babaian R, Troncoso P, Grignon DJ. The prostatic capsule: does it exist? Its importance in the staging and treatment of prostatic carcinoma. Am J Surg Pathol. 1989;13:21–7.
58. Fine SW, Al-Ahmadie HA, Gopalan A, Tickoo SK, Scardino PT, Reuter VE. Anatomy of the anterior prostate and extraprostatic space: a contemporary surgical pathology analysis. Adv Anat Pathol. 2007;14:401–7.
59. Epstein JI, Carmichael MJ, Pizov G, Walsh PC. Influence of capsular penetration on progression following radical prostatectomy: a study of 196 cases with long-term followup. J Urol. 1993;150:135–41.
60. Wheeler TM, Dillioglugil O, Kattan MW, et al. Clinical and pathological significance of the level and extent of capsular invasion in clinical stage T1–2 prostate cancer. Hum Pathol. 1998;29:856–62.
61. Zhou M, Reuther AM, Levin HS, et al. Microscopic bladder neck involvement by prostate carcinoma in radical prostatectomy specimens is not a significant independent prognostic factor. Mod Pathol. 2009;22:385–92.
62. Kawakami J, Meng MV, Sadetsky N, et al. Changing patterns of pelvic lymphadenectomy for prostate cancer: results from CaPSURE. J Urol. 2006;176:1382–6.
63. Tokuda Y, Carlino LJ, Gopalan A, et al. Prostate cancer topography and patterns of lymph node metastasis. Am J Surg Pathol. 2010;34:1862–7.
64. Chuang AY, Nielsen ME, Hernandez DJ, Walsh PC, Epstein JI. The significance of positive surgical margin in areas of capsular incision in otherwise organ confined disease at radical prostatectomy. J Urol. 2007;178:1306–10.
65. Stephenson AJ, Wood DP, Kattan MW, et al. Location, extent and number of positive surgical margins do not improve accuracy of predicting prostate cancer recurrence after radical prostatectomy. J Urol. 2009;182:1357–63.
66. Thompson IM, Tangen CM, Paradelo J, et al. Adjuvant radiotherapy for pathological T3N0M0 prostate cancer significantly reduces risk of metastases and improves survival: long-term followup of a randomized clinical trial. J Urol. 2009;181:956–62.
67. Udo K, Cronin AM, Carlino LJ, et al. Prognostic impact of subclassification of radical prostatectomy positive margins by linear extent and Gleason grade. J Urol. 2013;189:1302–7.
68. Epstein JI. Prognostic significance of tumor volume in radical prostatectomy and needle biopsy specimens. J Urol. 2011;186:790–7.
69. Fine SW, Reuter VE. What is the prognostic significance of lymphovascular invasion in radical prostatectomy specimens? Nat Clin Pract Urol. 2007;4:128–9.
70. Yamamoto S, Kawakami S, Yonese J, et al. Lymphovascular invasion is an independent predictor of prostate-specific antigen failure after radical prostatectomy in patients with pT3aN0 prostate cancer. Int J Urol. 2008;15:895–9.

Unusual Epithelial and Nonepithelial Neoplasms of the Prostate

5

Adeboye O. Osunkoya and Cristina Magi-Galluzzi

Introduction

The vast majority of prostatic neoplasms are epithelial, and the most common is conventional acinar prostatic adenocarcinoma. This chapter will focus exclusively on unusual epithelial and non-epithelial neoplasms that may involve the prostate.

Unusual Epithelial Neoplasms of the Prostate

Although the vast majority of prostate cancers are conventional acinar prostatic adenocarcinoma, about 5–10 % of cases are considered to be unusual neoplasms or so-called variants [1, 2].

Mucinous Adenocarcinoma of the Prostate

Mucinous adenocarcinoma of the prostate (also referred to as colloid carcinoma), is a rare morphologic variant of prostate cancer. The incidence of mucinous adenocarcinoma of the prostate, defined by the presence of more than 25 % of the tumor composed of glands with extraluminal mucin (Fig. 5.1), is approximately 0.2 % [3–6]. Based on the strict definition, the diagnosis of this entity can only be made on radical prostatectomy specimens. Prostate cancer with extraluminal mucin in needle core biopsies or transurethral resection of prostate specimens should be diagnosed as "prostatic adenocarcinoma with mucinous features." The presence of intraluminal mucin, seen in up to one third of prostatic adenocarcinomas, should not be referred to as mucinous adenocarcinoma of the prostate. In the past, there was debate about whether to assign a Gleason score to these tumors. Recent data support grading mucinous prostate carcinomas on the basis of the underlying architectural pattern (well-formed glands, poorly formed glands, cribriform glands, etc.) rather than assuming that all of these tumors are aggressive [6]. Recent studies have also shown that mucinous adenocarcinoma of the prostate has a similar, and probably even better prognosis than conventional acinar prostatic adenocarcinoma [7].

Prostatic Ductal Adenocarcinoma

Prostatic ductal adenocarcinoma is a rare variant of prostate cancer that was previously referred to as endometrioid carcinoma, endometrial carcinoma, or papillary ductal carcinoma [8–11]. The incidence of the pure form of this variant is approximately 0.5–1.0 %; however, the incidence

A. O. Osunkoya (✉)
Department of Pathology, Emory University School of Medicine, Atlanta, GA, USA
e-mail: Adeboye.osunkoya@emory.edu

C. Magi-Galluzzi
Department of Pathology, Cleveland Clinic, Robert J. Tomsich Pathology and Laboratory Medicine Institute, Cleveland, OH, USA
e-mail: magic@ccf.org

C. Magi-Galluzzi, C. G. Przybycin (eds.), *Genitourinary Pathology,* DOI 10.1007/978-1-4939-2044-0_5,

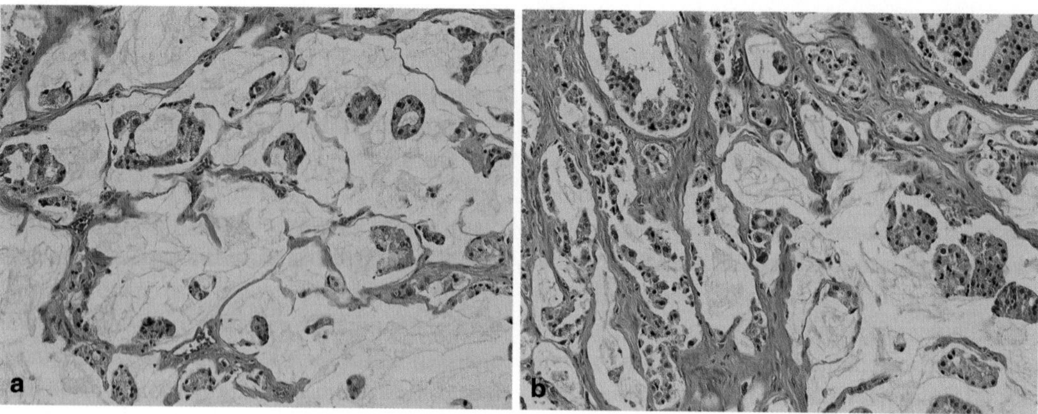

Fig. 5.1 **a** Radical prostatectomy, mucinous adenocarcinoma (low magnification). **b** Radical prostatectomy, mucinous adenocarcinoma (high magnification)

of the more common mixed prostatic ductal adenocarcinoma and conventional acinar adenocarcinoma is approximately 5% [1, 2, 12]. These tumors are composed of papillary fronds lined by pseudostratified columnar epithelial cells with amphophilic cytoplasm (Fig. 5.2). Basal cells are typically absent, but may be present focally as demonstrated by basal cell markers in a patchy distribution. Prostatic ductal adenocarcinoma typically arises from the periurethral region but can extend to the peripheral zone and extraprostatic tissue including the bladder, confirming the aggressive nature of the majority of these tumors. A Gleason score of 4+4=8 is assigned to tumors composed entirely of classic prostatic ductal adenocarcinoma. If comedonecrosis is present, then the Gleason score has to be increased accordingly. It should also be noted that a Gleason score of 3+3=6 should be assigned to tumors composed entirely of the recently described "High-grade prostatic intraepithelial neoplasia-like ductal adenocarcinoma of the prostate" [13, 14]. Although immunohistochemical stains are typically positive for prostate-specific antigen (PSA) and prostatic acid phosphatase (PSAP), serum PSA level may occasionally be normal.

Intraductal Carcinoma of the Prostate

Although there are some similarities between prostatic ductal adenocarcinoma and intraductal

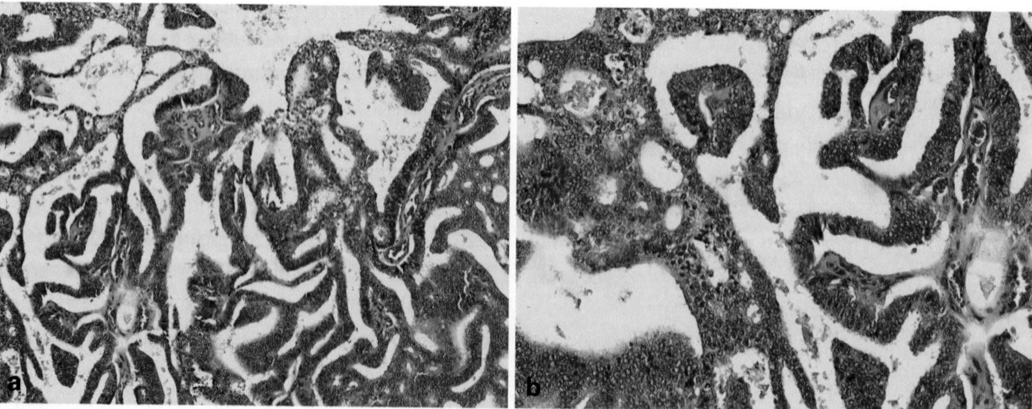

Fig. 5.2 **a** Transurethral resection of the prostate (TURP), prostatic ductal adenocarcinoma (low magnification). **b** TURP, prostatic ductal adenocarcinoma (high magnification)

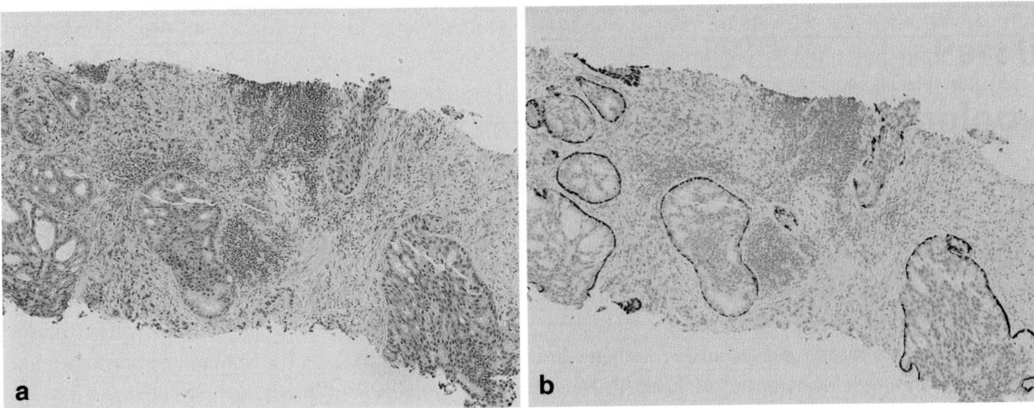

Fig. 5.3 a Needle core biopsy, intraductal carcinoma of the prostate (H & E). b Needle core biopsy, intraductal carcinoma of the prostate (p63/high-molecular-weight cytokeratin (HMWCK))

carcinoma of the prostate (including bad prognosis), they are somewhat distinct entities. Intraductal carcinoma of the prostate is composed of an expansile proliferation of malignant prostatic epithelial cells that spans the entire lumen of prostatic ducts or acini, while the normal architecture of ducts or acini are still maintained [15–19]. In contrast to prostatic ductal adenocarcinoma, in intraductal carcinoma of the prostate, basal cells are always present (Fig. 5.3) and distinguish this entity from conventional cribriform Gleason pattern/grade 4 cancer. Tumor cells are typically cuboidal, and may form cribriform structures with small rounded lumens and/or micropapillary tufts lacking fibrovascular cores. More importantly, intraductal carcinoma of the prostate should be distinguished from high-grade prostatic intraepithelial neoplasia and urothelial carcinoma. Most cases of intraductal carcinoma of the prostate have a Gleason score of 4+4=8 or higher.

Squamous Cell Carcinoma

Squamous cell carcinoma of the prostate may occur in a pure form, or may be intimately admixed with prostatic adenocarcinoma (Fig. 5.4). The tumors may arise from the prostatic ducts and acini, but it is important to also realize that these tumors may also arise from the prostatic urethra. It is well established that most cases of squamous

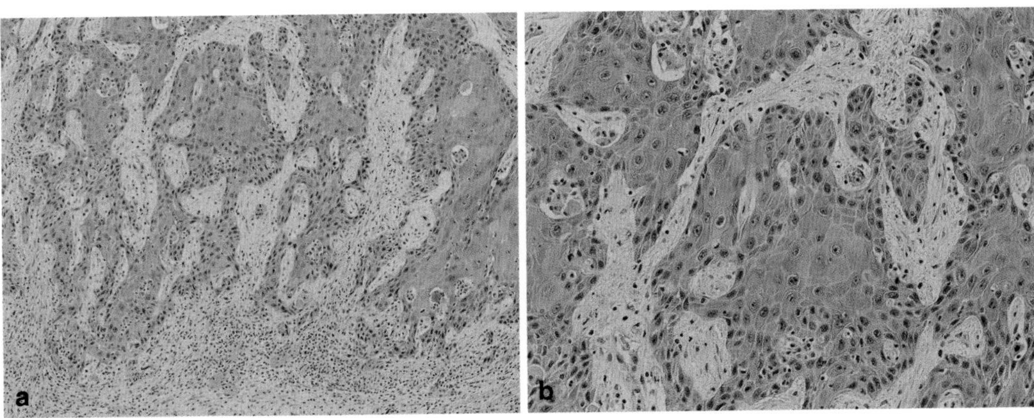

Fig. 5.4 a Transurethral resection of the prostate (TURP), squamous cell carcinoma (low magnification). b TURP, squamous cell carcinoma (high magnification)

cell carcinoma of the prostate occur in the setting of prior radiation therapy and/or androgen deprivation therapy [20–24]. Similar to other variants, squamous cell carcinoma of the prostate is more aggressive than conventional low-grade acinar prostatic adenocarcinoma. Florid squamous metaplasia secondary to prostatic infarcts, inflammation, prior radiation therapy, and/or androgen deprivation therapy, may be a potential mimicker of squamous cell carcinoma of the prostate. The absence of frank malignant features in squamous metaplasia, should exclude the possibility of squamous cell carcinoma of the prostate. Secondary involvement of the prostate by squamous cell carcinoma or urothelial carcinoma with extensive squamous differentiation of bladder origin should also be excluded. This is especially important in needle core biopsies in which the true site of origin of the tumor may not be appreciated.

Sarcomatoid Carcinoma

Sarcomatoid carcinoma (carcinosarcoma) is composed of both malignant epithelial (typically adenocarcinoma) and mesenchymal (typically sarcoma) elements (Fig. 5.5) [24–26]. Although there has been some debate regarding the origin of these tumors, both the epithelial and mesenchymal components are thought by most experts to be derived from a single cell of origin [27]. This variant of prostate cancer typically occurs in elderly patients, and may present with an expansile mass that may extend to the transition zone, subsequently resulting in obstructive symptomatology [26]. The sarcomatoid component may demonstrate a spectrum of histologic patterns, ranging from haphazardly arranged spindle cells with or without intimately admixed pleomorphic giant cells and numerous mitotic figures, to more distinct sarcomatous proliferations with heterologous elements, including osteosarcoma, chondrosarcoma, rhabdomyosarcoma, and angiosarcoma [24]. In the largest study to date, the vast majority of men had a prior history of prostatic adenocarcinoma and had been treated with either radiation or hormonal therapy [28]. The authors, however, found no correlation between either the prior grade of conventional prostatic adenocarcinoma, or the time to progression to sarcomatoid carcinoma and patient survival [28]. The current consensus is that the sarcomatoid component of these tumors should be designated as Gleason pattern 5. Primary high-grade prostatic stromal sarcoma (which typically does not have a malignant epithelial component) should be excluded. The prognosis of sarcomatoid carcinoma of the prostate is poor.

Prostatic Carcinoid Tumor and Prostatic Adenocarcinoma with Paneth Cell-Like Neuroendocrine Differentiation

True primary carcinoid tumors of the prostate are rare [29–32]. By definition, these tumors should be negative for PSA and PSAP, and must

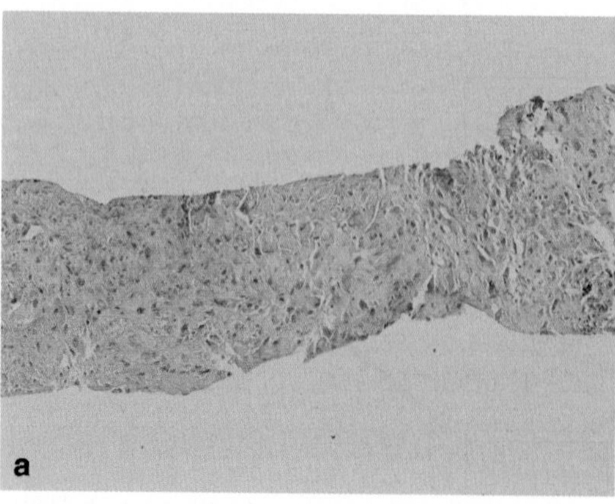

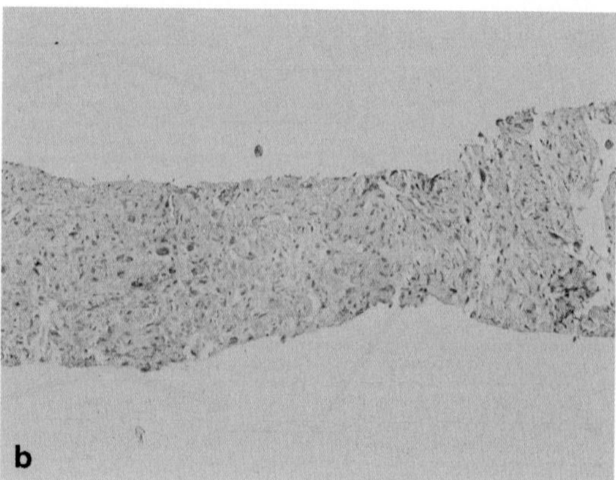

Fig. 5.5 **a** Needle core biopsy, sarcomatoid carcinoma of the prostate (H & E). **b** Needle core biopsy, intraductal carcinoma of the prostate (p63/high-molecular-weight cytokeratin (HMWCK)/P504S)

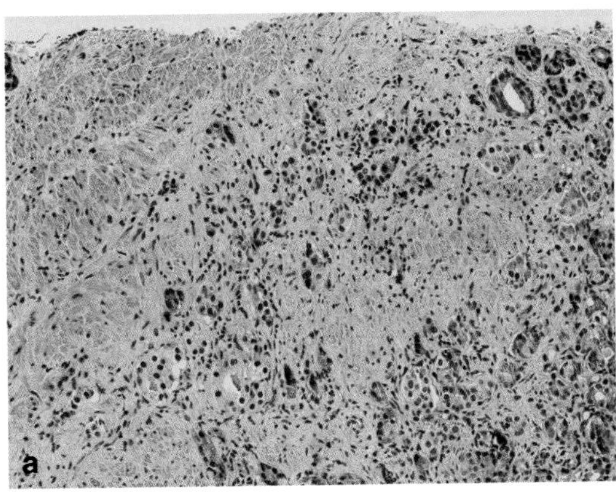

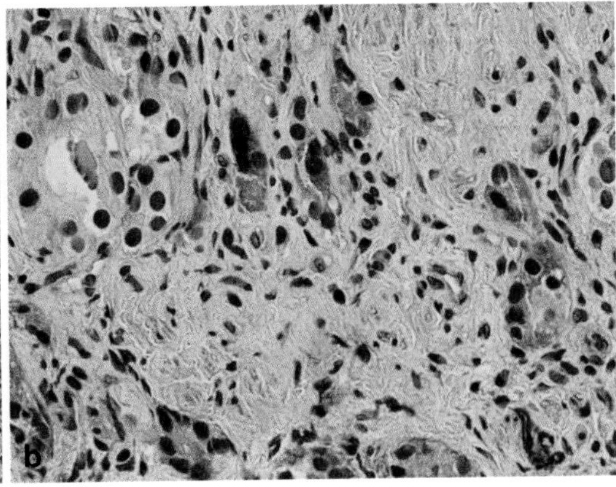

Fig. 5.6 **a** Needle core biopsy, prostatic adenocarcinoma with Paneth cell-like neuroendocrine differentiation (low magnification). **b** Needle core biopsy, prostatic adenocarcinoma with Paneth cell-like neuroendocrine differentiation (high magnification)

be characterized by typical morphologic and immunohistochemical profile of carcinoid tumor of any other site. What is more prevalent is the so-called prostatic adenocarcinoma with Paneth cell-like neuroendocrine differentiation (Fig. 5.6) [33]. Studies have shown that these tumors have a relatively good prognosis despite the fact that they may be composed predominantly of poorly formed glands or single cells [33]. It is therefore recommended that a Gleason score should not be assigned to these tumors. It is also important to note that high-grade prostatic intraepithelial neoplasia may also rarely have Paneth cell-like neuroendocrine differentiation.

Small Cell Carcinoma

Primary small cell carcinoma of the prostate is a rare and aggressive neoplasm with distinctive clinicopathologic characteristics, including disseminated metastasis [34–40]. Small cell carcinoma of the prostate was first described over three decades ago, and our understanding of the pathobiology of this aggressive tumor has improved over the years [41]. Small cell carcinomas irrespective of the site of origin have very similar morphologic features (Fig. 5.7). The determination of primary origin thus occasional poses a challenge in some cases, especially since

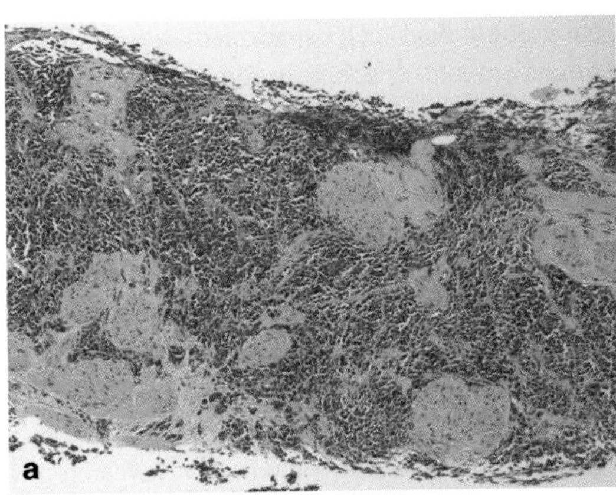

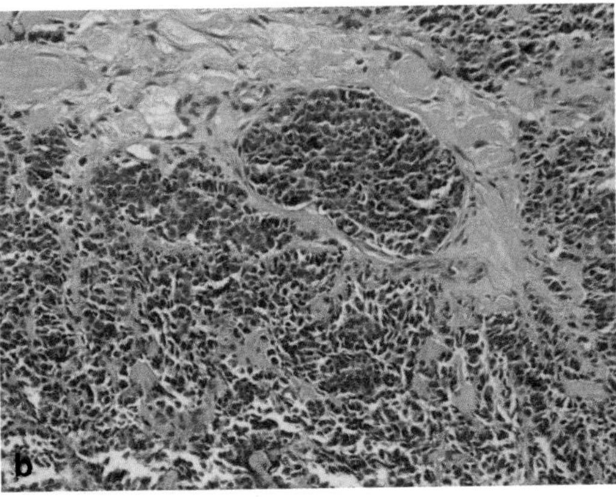

Fig. 5.7 **a** Needle core biopsy, small cell carcinoma (low magnification). **b** Radical prostatectomy, small cell carcinoma (high magnification)

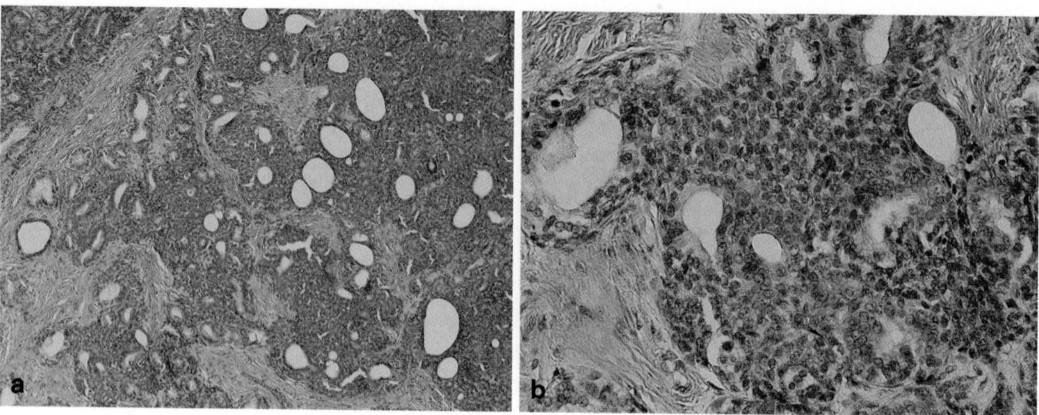

Fig. 5.8 **a** Transurethral resection of the prostate (TURP), basal cell carcinoma with (low magnification). **b** TURP, basal cell carcinoma with (high magnification)

immunohistochemical stains such as TTF-1, synaptophysin, chromogranin, and CD56 are positive in most small cell carcinomas irrespective of site of origin. A characteristic feature of pure primary small cell carcinoma of the prostate is the fact that patients typically have low serum PSA levels and a poor response to androgen deprivation therapy. Interestingly, a number of patients have developed small cell carcinoma of the prostate following androgen deprivation therapy for conventional prostatic adenocarcinoma [42–44]. One of the recent advances in our understanding of primary small cell carcinoma of the prostate, is the fact that gene fusions between members of the erythroblast transformation-specific (ETS)-related gene (*ERG*) and transmembrane protease, serine 2 (TMPRSS2), have been identified in a significant number of these tumors, compared to small cell carcinoma from other sites [45–49]. This finding confirms the fact that primary small cell carcinoma of the prostate likely represents de-differentiation of conventional prostatic adenocarcinoma. There is also agreement amongst experts that a Gleason score should not be assigned to pure small cell carcinoma of the prostate.

Basal Cell Carcinoma

Prostatic adenocarcinoma arises from the secretory cells of the prostatic glands and acini. In contrast, basaloid proliferations of the prostate including basal cell hyperplasia and basal cell carcinoma arise from basal cells of glands typically located in the transition zone, though in some cases peripheral zone involvement may be seen. The distinction between these two entities may occasionally be challenging [50–54]. Basal cell carcinoma is characterized by variably sized basaloid nests with anastomosing areas, eosinophilic luminal lining, and foci of necrosis. The nests typically have an infiltrative growth pattern, and may elicit a desmoplastic stromal response (Fig. 5.8). Cribriforming of the glands with adenoid cystic-like areas may also be seen. Immunohistochemical stains are positive for p63, high–molecular-weight cytokeratin (HMWCK), B-cell lymphoma 2 (Bcl2), CD10, Ki-67 (increased expression), and negative for PSA and PSAP [54, 55]. A Gleason score should not be assigned to basal cell carcinoma.

Urothelial Carcinoma

Primary urothelial carcinoma of the prostate is rare and typically arises from the prostatic urethra or prostatic ducts and acini (Fig. 5.9) [56–58]. Although a number of cases are composed of urothelial carcinoma in situ of the prostatic urethra or colonization of prostatic ducts and acini, a diligent search for possible foci of invasion into the periurethral soft tissue and prostatic stroma should be made. It is also important to note that prostatic stromal invasion due to primary

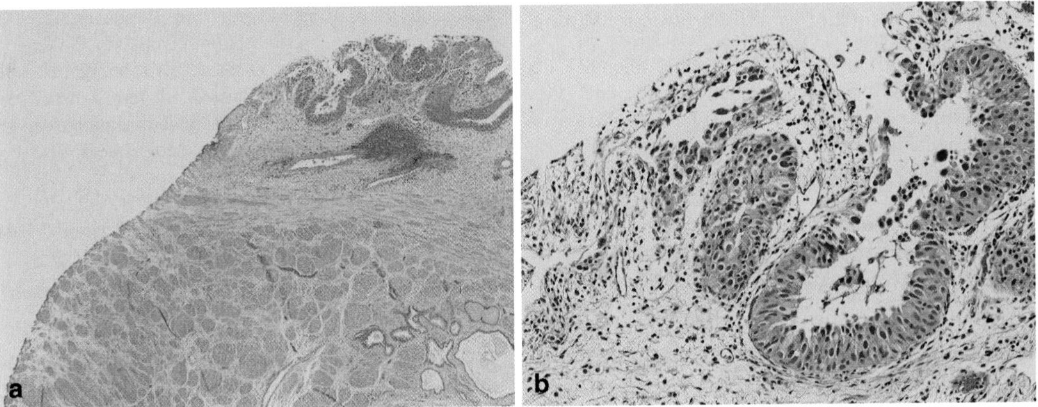

Fig. 5.9 **a** Radical prostatectomy, urothelial carcinoma of the prostatic urethra (low magnification). **b** Radical prostatectomy, urothelial carcinoma of the prostatic urethra (high magnification)

urothelial carcinoma of the prostate and prostatic stromal invasion due to transmural invasion of a bladder primary are staged as pT2 and pT4a, respectively [59].

Mucin-Producing Urothelial-Type Adenocarcinoma (Prostatic Urethral Adenocarcinoma)

Rarely, in situ and invasive tumors analogous to mucinous adenocarcinoma of the urinary bladder may arise from the prostatic urethra. These tumors are referred to as mucin-producing urothelial-type adenocarcinoma or prostatic urethral adenocarcinoma (Fig. 5.10) [5, 60–62]. Mean patient age at diagnosis of this aggressive tumor is 72 years (range 58–93 years). In view of the fact that urothelial-type adenocarcinoma of the prostate is identical in its morphology and histogenesis to mucinous adenocarcinoma of the bladder, the latter must be excluded before this diagnosis is rendered. Other tumors that should be considered in the differential diagnosis and excluded include mucinous prostatic adenocarcinoma and mucinous colorectal adenocarcinoma involving the prostate [5, 6, 63]. Immunohistochemical stains are typically positive in the tumor cells for CK7 and negative for PSA, PSAP, b-catenin, and CDX2.

Other primary epithelial and epithelial-like tumors involving the prostate include but are

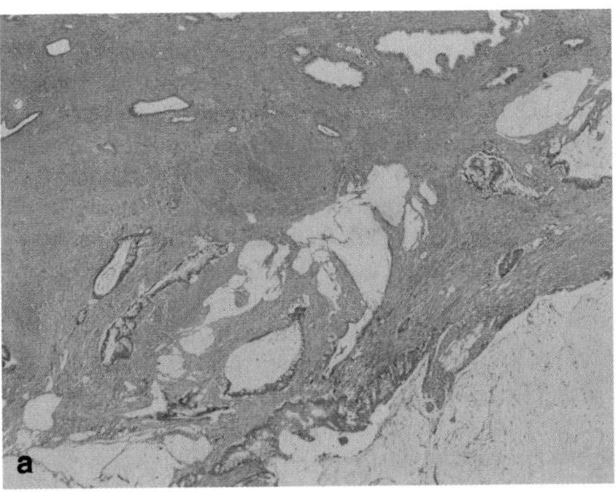

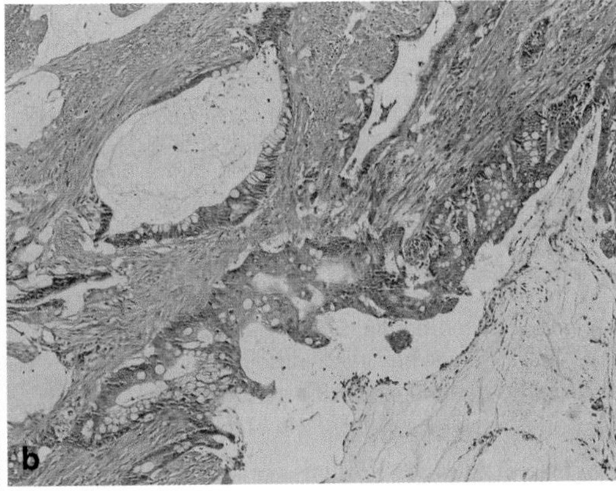

Fig. 5.10 **a** Radical prostatectomy, mucin-producing urothelial-type adenocarcinoma/prostatic urethral adenocarcinoma (low magnification). **b** Radical prostatectomy, mucin-producing urothelial-type adenocarcinoma/prostatic urethral adenocarcinoma (high magnification)

not limited to squamous cell carcinoma, Wilms' tumor, clear cell adenocarcinoma, neuroblastoma, and melanoma.

Secondary Epithelial Tumors

Secondary tumors involving the prostate excluding those from direct extension are rare. Metastasis from other sites to the prostate typically arise from the lung, gastrointestinal tract, skin (melanoma), kidney, testicle, and endocrine organs, with an incidence ranging from 0.1 to 6% depending on the series [64–66]. In view of the proximity to the prostate, the most common secondary tumor involving the prostate through direct extension is from the urinary bladder. Colorectal tumors including colorectal adenocarcinoma may also occasionally involve the prostate.

Urothelial Carcinoma

The incidence of prostatic involvement by urothelial carcinoma of the bladder in radical cystoprostatectomy specimens ranges from 12 to 48% [67, 68]. Prostatic stromal invasion in this setting typically occurs by direct transmural extension of urothelial carcinoma from the bladder primary, and is designated as stage pT4a (Fig. 5.11) [59, 69]. The challenge occurs if the tumor is detected first on needle core biopsy or transurethral resection of the prostate (TURP), in the absence of a known history of urothelial carcinoma. Making the distinction between urothelial carcinoma and prostatic adenocarcinoma is critical in view of the different therapeutic options and approaches for these tumors. In cases that are challenging on H & E, readily available immunohistochemical stains (PSA, PSAP, p63, HMWCK, uroplakin and thrombomodulin, GATA3) can aid in the distinction between these two entities in most cases. In the few cases in which the distinction can still not be made with the previous markers, additional immunohistochemical stains (P501S, PSMA, NKX3.1, and pPSA), which are typically positive even in advanced prostatic adenocarcinoma and negative in urothelial carcinoma, are useful [70].

Colorectal Adenocarcinoma

Despite the proximity of the colorectum to the prostate, involvement of the prostate from this site in clinical specimens is rare with only very few case reports and series in the literature (Fig. 5.12) [63]. Although most patients present with classic symptoms of colonic cancer, patients may present with obstructive uropathy due to involvement of the prostatic urethra, and may therefore be diagnosed for the first time following TURP [63]. Histologically, the two most common entities that are in the differential diagnosis of colorectal adenocarcinoma invading the prostate are prostatic ductal adenocarcinoma and adenocarcinoma of the bladder. In addition, the various patterns of infiltrating colorectal adenocarcinoma, including mucinous, enteric, and signet-ring cell type, may also be seen in prostatic adenocarcinoma. Most

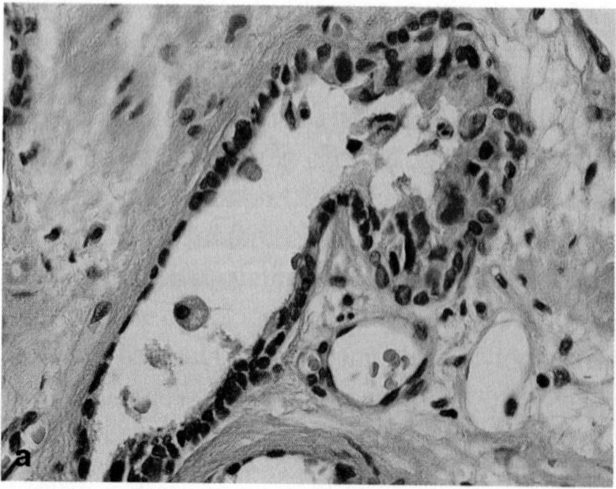

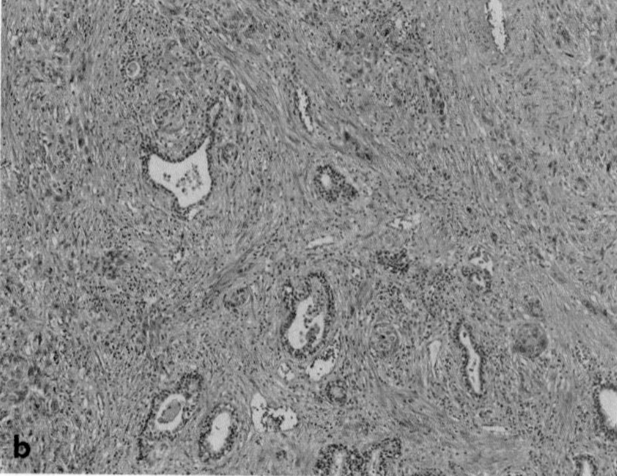

Fig. 5.11 **a** Radical cystoprostatectomy, urothelial carcinoma with colonization of prostatic ducts. **b** Radical cystoprostatectomy, urothelial carcinoma with prostatic stromal invasion

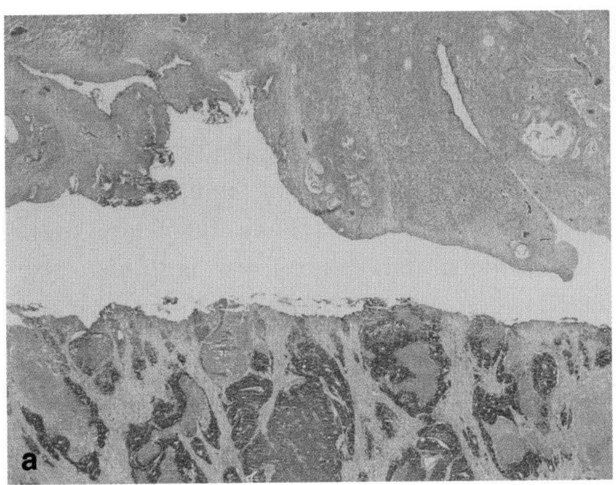

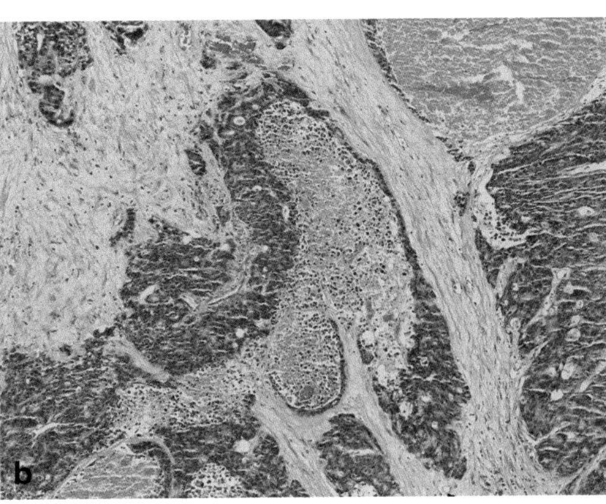

Fig. 5.12 **a** Transurethral resection of the prostate (TURP), colorectal adenocarcinoma with necrosis involving the prostate (low magnification). **b** TURP, colorectal adenocarcinoma with necrosis involving the prostate (high magnification)

colonic adenocarcinomas are positive for CDX2, villin, β-catenin, mucins (MUC1 and MUC3), CEA, and B72.3; and all are negative for prostate-specific markers.

Primary Mesenchymal Tumors of the Prostate

Benign or malignant mesenchymal neoplasms of the prostate are rare. Apart from smooth muscle tumors involving the prostate, another group of tumors which arise from the specialized prostatic stroma are also recognized as distinct entities. These tumors have been classified into prostatic stromal tumors of uncertain malignant potential (STUMP) and prostatic stromal sarcoma [71–73].

Stromal Tumors of Uncertain Malignant Potential (STUMP)

These tumors arise from the specialized hormonally responsive stroma of the prostate. There are at least four main histologic patterns of STUMP; hypercellular stroma with scattered atypical/degenerative cells, hypercellular stroma with bland stromal cells, myxoid pattern and "phyllodes"-like pattern, with the first two being the most common (Fig. 5.13). The various histologic patterns of

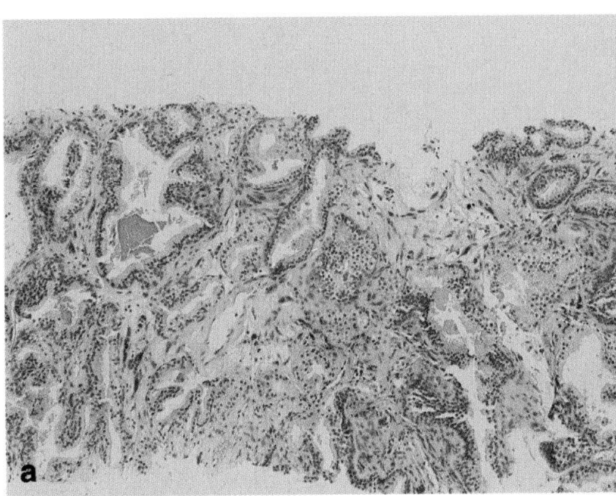

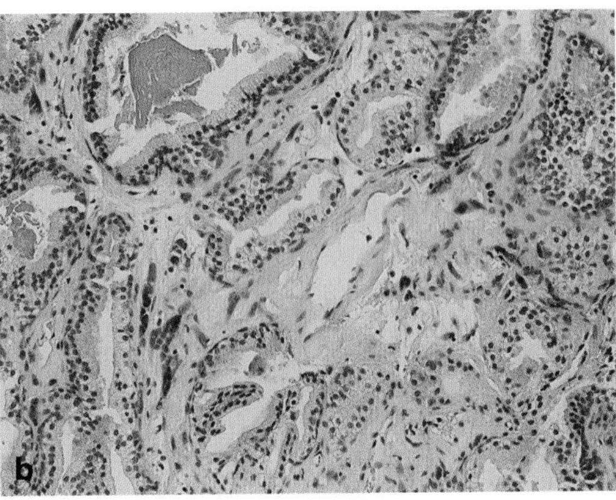

Fig. 5.13 **a** Needle core biopsy, stromal tumor of unknown malignant potential, with adjacent benign prostatic glands (low magnification). **b** Needle core biopsy, stromal tumor of unknown malignant potential, with adjacent benign prostatic glands (high magnification)

STUMP may be confused with benign prostatic hyperplasia (BPH). However, it should be noted that some cases of STUMP may have the potential to undergo malignant transformation, or may be intimately associated with stromal sarcoma, and thus should be recognized as a distinct entity from BPH. STUMP may be associated with various epithelial proliferations, and it is therefore thought that this may represent epithelial-mesenchymal crosstalk [74]. Prostatic adenocarcinoma may also occasionally be identified in cases of STUMP.

Stromal Sarcoma

These aggressive tumors also arise from the specialized hormonally responsive stroma of the prostate. However, unlike STUMP these tumors are characterized by increased mitotic activity, nondegenerate nuclear pleomorphism and necrosis (Fig. 5.14). Stromal sarcoma may also extend beyond the prostate and metastasize.

Other primary mesenchymal tumors of the prostate include but are not limited to inflammatory myofibroblastic tumor (IMT), solitary fibrous tumor (SFT), leiomyoma, leiomyosarcoma, and rhabdomyosarcoma.

Secondary Mesenchymal Tumors

Secondary mesenchymal tumors involving the prostate are rare, and are almost always from direct extension. In view of the proximity to the prostate, the most common secondary tumor mesenchymal tumors are from the urinary bladder and colorectal including gastrointestinal stromal tumor (GIST).

GIST

A challenging and well-described scenario is one in which a patient has a positive digital rectal examination (DRE) and on imaging appears to have a mass involving the prostate or extending in between the prostate and the colorectum. One of the entities to consider in this setting is GIST. Most cases of "prostatic" GIST are sampled on needle core biopsy, and one of the clues to the diagnosis is the absence of prostatic glands and stroma in the cores that are involved. This is due to the fact that the vast majority of these tumors arise from the colorectal wall and are not true GIST of prostatic origin. Unfortunately, if GIST is misdiagnosed as a sarcoma, patients may undergo unnecessary pelvic exenteration or chemoradiation therapy [75]. GISTs in this location are similar to those at other sites (Fig. 5.15), thus the tumors are typically positive for CD117, CD34, and DOG1.

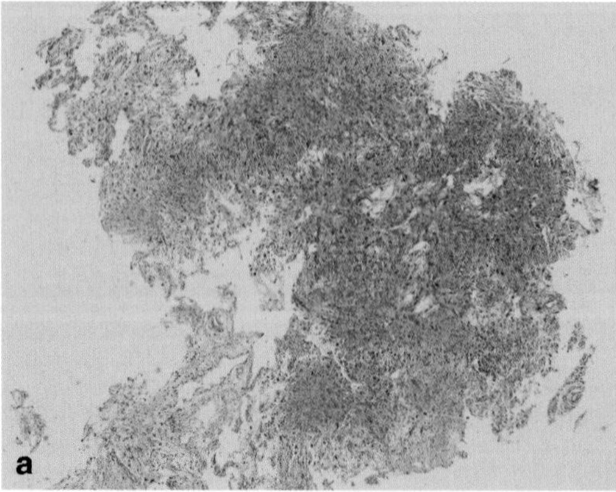

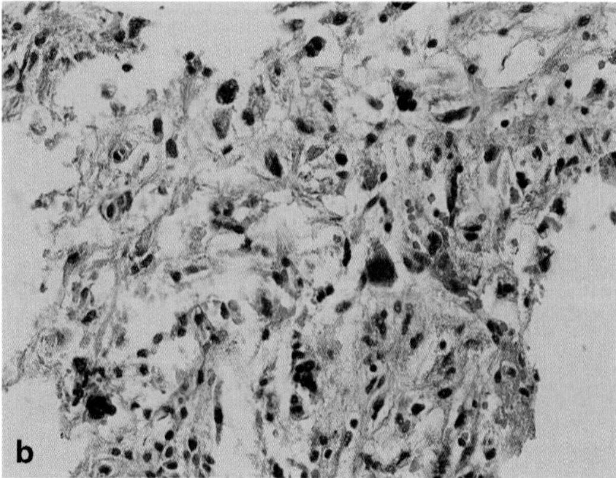

Fig. 5.14 **a** Transurethral resection of the prostate (TURP), high-grade prostatic stromal sarcoma (low magnification). **b** TURP, high-grade prostatic stromal sarcoma, note prominent mitotic figure (high magnification)

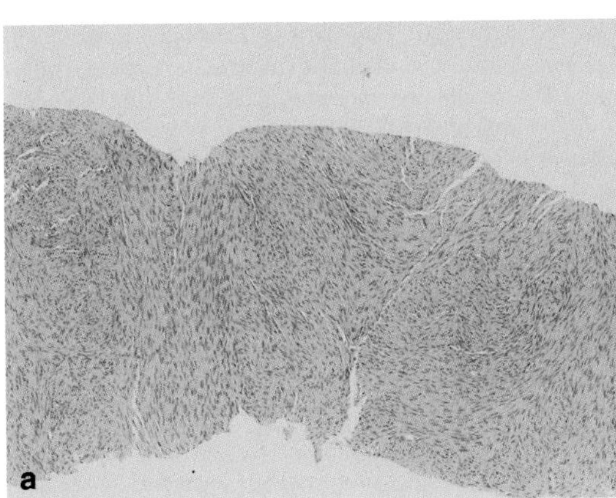
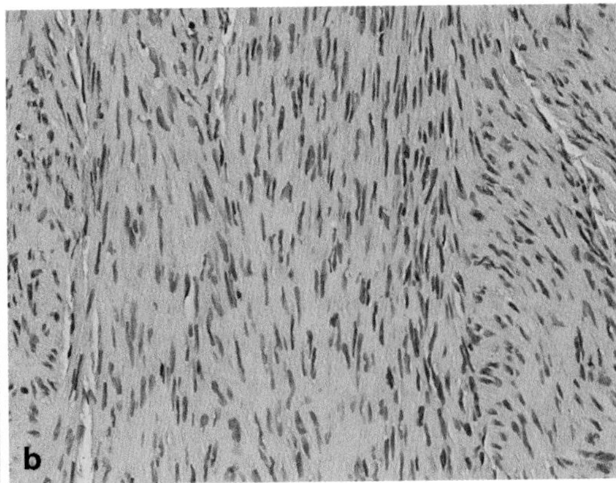

Fig. 5.15 **a** Needle core biopsy, gastrointestinal stromal tumor (low magnification). **b** Needle core biopsy, gastrointestinal stromal tumor (high magnification)

References

1. Grignon DJ. Unusual subtypes of prostate cancer. Mod Pathol. 2004;17(3):316–27.
2. Mazzucchelli R, Lopez-Beltran A, Cheng L, et al. Rare and unusual histological variants of prostatic carcinoma: clinical significance. BJU Int. 2008;102(10):1369–74.
3. Epstein JI, Lieberman PH. Mucinous adenocarcinoma of the prostate gland. Am J Surg Pathol. 1985;9:299–308.
4. Ro JY, Grignon DJ, Ayala AG, et al. Mucinous adenocarcinoma of the prostate: histochemical and immunohistochemical studies. Hum Pathol. 1990;21:593–600.
5. Osunkoya AO, Epstein JI. Primary mucin-producing urothelial-type adenocarcinoma of prostate: report of 15 cases. Am J Surg Pathol. 2007;31:1323–9.
6. Osunkoya AO, Nielsen ME, Epstein JI. Prognosis of mucinous adenocarcinoma of the prostate treated by radical prostatectomy: a study of 47 cases. Am J Surg Pathol. 2008;32(3):468–72.
7. Lane BR, Magi-Galluzzi C, Reuther AM, et al. Mucinous adenocarcinoma of the prostate does not confer poor prognosis. Urology. 2006;68(4):825–30.
8. Melicow MM, Pachter MR. Endometrial carcinoma of prostatic utricle (uterus masculinus). Cancer. 1967;20:1715–22.
9. Bostwick DG, Kindrachuk RW, Rouse RV. Prostatic adenocarcinoma with endometrioid features. Clinical, pathologic, and ultrastructural findings. Am J Surg Pathol. 1985;9(8):595–609.
10. Epstein JI, Woodruff JM. Adenocarcinoma of the prostate with endometrioid features. A light microscopic and immunohistochemical study of ten cases. Cancer. 1986;57:111–9.
11. Ro JY, Ayala AG, Wishnow KI, Ordonez NG. Prostatic duct adenocarcinoma with endometrioid features: immunohistochemical and electron microscopic study. Semin Diagn Pathol. 1988;5:301–11.
12. Amin A, Epstein JI. Pathologic stage of prostatic ductal adenocarcinoma at radical prostatectomy: effect of percentage of the ductal component and associated grade of acinar adenocarcinoma. Am J Surg Pathol. 2011;35(4):615–9.
13. Tavora F, Epstein JI. High-grade prostatic intraepithelial neoplasia like ductal adenocarcinoma of the prostate: a clinicopathologic study of 28 cases. Am J Surg Pathol. 2008;32(7):1060–7.
14. Lee TK, Miller JS, Epstein JI. Rare histological patterns of prostatic ductal adenocarcinoma. Pathology. 2010;42(4):319–24.
15. Kovi J, Jackson MA, Heshmat MY. Ductal spread in prostatic carcinoma. Cancer. 1985;56(7):1566–73.
16. McNeal JE, Yemoto CE. Spread of adenocarcinoma within prostatic ducts and acini. Morphologic and clinical correlations. Am J Surg Pathol. 1996;20(7):802–14.
17. Guo CC, Epstein JI. Intraductal carcinoma of the prostate on needle biopsy: histologic features and clinical significance. Mod Pathol. 2006;19(12):1528–35.
18. Cohen RJ, Wheeler TM, Bonkhoff H, Rubin MA. A proposal on the identification, histologic reporting, and implications of intraductal prostatic carcinoma. Arch Pathol Lab Med. 2007;131(7):1103–9.
19. Henry PC, Evans AJ. Intraductal carcinoma of the prostate: a distinct histopathological entity with important prognostic implications. J Clin Pathol. 2009;62(7):579–83.
20. Braslis KG, Davi RC, Nelson E, et al. Squamous cell carcinoma of the prostate: a transformation from adenocarcinoma after the use of a luteinizing hormone-releasing hormone agonist and flutamide. Urology. 1995;45:329–31.
21. Miller VA, Reuter V, Scher HI. Primary squamous cell carcinoma of the prostate after radiation

seed implantation for adenocarcinoma. Urology. 1995;46:111–3.

22. Nabi G, Ansari MS, Singh I, et al. Primary squamous cell carcinoma of the prostate: a rare clinicopathological entity—report of 2 cases and review of literature. Urol Int. 2001;66:216–9.
23. Parwani AV, Kronz JD, Genega EM, et al. Prostate carcinoma with squamous differentiation: an analysis of 33 cases. Am J Surg Pathol. 2004;28:651–7.
24. Fine SW. Variants and unusual patterns of prostate cancer: clinicopathologic and differential diagnostic considerations. Adv Anat Pathol. 2012;19(4): 204–16.
25. Ordonez NG, Ayala AG, von Eschenbach AC, et al. Immunoperoxidase localization of prostatic acid phosphatase in prostatic carcinoma with sarcomatoid changes. Urology. 1982;19:210–4.
26. Wick MR, Young RH, Malvesta R, et al. Prostatic carcinosarcomas: clinical, histologic, and immunohistochemical data on two cases with a review of the literature. Am J Clin Pathol. 1989;92:131–9.
27. Delahunt B, Eble JN, Nacey JN, et al. Sarcomatoid carcinoma of the prostate: progression from adenocarcinoma is associated with p53 over-expression. Anticancer Res. 1999;19:4279–83.
28. Hansel DE, Epstein JI. Sarcomatoid carcinoma of the prostate: a study of 42 cases. Am J Surg Pathol. 2006;30:1316–21.
29. Azumi N, Shibuya H, Ishikura M. Primary prostatic carcinoid tumor with intracytoplasmic prostatic acid phosphatase and prostate specific antigen. Am J Surg Pathol. 1984;8:545–50.
30. Almagro UA. Argyrophilic prostatic carcinoma: case report with literature review on prostatic carcinoid and "carcinoidlike" prostatic carcinoma. Cancer. 1985;55:608–14.
31. Ghannoum JE, DeLellis RA, Shin SJ. Primary carcinoid tumor of the prostate with concurrent adenocarcinoma: a case report. Int J Surg Pathol. 2004;12:167–70.
32. Zarkovic A, Masters J, Carpenter L. Primary carcinoid tumour of the prostate. Pathology. 2005;37(2):184–6.
33. Tamas EF, Epstein JI. Prognostic significance of paneth cell-like neuroendocrine differentiation in adenocarcinoma of the prostate. Am J Surg Pathol. 2006;30(8):980–5.
34. Grignon DJ. Unusual subtypes of prostate cancer. Mod Pathol. 2004;17:316–27.
35. Mazzucchelli R, Lopez-Beltran A, Cheng L, et al. Rare and unusual histological variants of prostatic carcinoma: clinical significance. BJU Int. 2008;102:1369–74.
36. Tetu B, Ro JY, Ayala AB, et al. Small cell carcinoma of the prostate. Part 1. A clinicopathologic study of 20 cases. Cancer. 1987;59:1803–9.
37. Christopher ME, Seftel AD, Sorenson K, Resnick MI. Small cell carcinoma of the genitourinary tract: an immunohistochemical, electron microscopic and clinicopathological study. J Urol. 1991;146:382–8.
38. Oesterling JE, Hauzeur CG, Farrow GM. Small cell anaplastic carcinoma of the prostate: clinical, pathological and immunohistological study of 27 patients. J Urol. 1992;147:804–7.
39. Nadig SN, Deibler AR, El Salamony TM, et al. Small cell carcinoma of the prostate: an underrecognized entity. Can J Urol. 2001;8:1207–10.
40. Wang W, Epstein JI. Small cell carcinoma of the prostate. A morphologic and immunohistochemical study of 95 cases. Am J Surg Pathol. 2008;32(1):65–71.
41. Wenk RE, Bhagavan BS, Levy R, et al. Ectopic ACTH, prostatic oat cell carcinoma, and marked hypernatremia. Cancer. 1977;40:773–8.
42. Valle J, von Boguslawsky K, Stenborg M, Andersson LC. Progression from adenocarcinoma to small cell carcinoma of the prostate with normalization of prostate-specific antigen (PSA) levels. Scand J Urol Nephrol. 1996;30(6):509–12.
43. Miyoshi Y, Uemura H, Kitami K, et al. Neuroendocrine differentiated small cell carcinoma presenting as recurrent prostate cancer after androgen deprivation therapy. BJU Int. 2001;88(9):982–3.
44. Nemoto K, Tomita Y. Neuroendocrine differentiation of localized prostate cancer during endocrine therapy. Scand J Urol Nephrol. 2007;41(6):558–60.
45. Han B, Mehra R, Suleman K, et al. Characterization of ETS gene aberrations in select histologic variants of prostate carcinoma. Mod Pathol. 2009;22(9):1176–85.
46. Scheble VJ, Braun M, Wilbertz T, et al. ERG rearrangement in small cell prostatic and lung cancer. Histopathology. 2010;56(7):937–43.
47. Guo CC, Dancer JY, Wang Y, et al. TMPRSS2-ERG gene fusion in small cell carcinoma of the prostate. Hum Pathol. 2011;42(1):11–7.
48. Lotan TL, Gupta NS, Wang W, et al. ERG gene rearrangements are common in prostatic small cell carcinomas. Mod Pathol. 2011;24(6):820–8.
49. Williamson SR, Zhang S, Yao JL, et al. ERG-TMPRSS2 rearrangement is shared by concurrent prostatic adenocarcinoma and prostatic small cell carcinoma and absent in small cell carcinoma of the urinary bladder: evidence supporting monoclonal origin. Mod Pathol. 2011;24(8):1120–7.
50. Grignon DJ, Ro JY, Ordonez NG, et al. Basal cell hyperplasia, adenoid basal cell tumor, and adenoid cystic carcinoma of the prostate gland: an immunohistochemical study. Hum Pathol. 1988;19:1425–33.
51. Iczkowski KA, Ferguson KL, Grier DD, et al. Adenoid cystic/basal cell carcinoma of the prostate: clinicopathologic findings in 19 cases. Am J Surg Pathol. 2003;27:1523–9.
52. McKenney JK, Amin MB, Srigley JR, et al. Basal cell proliferations of the prostate other than usual basal cell hyperplasia: a clinicopathologic study of 23 cases, including four carcinomas, with a proposed classification. Am J Surg Pathol. 2004;28:1289–98.
53. Hosler GA, Epstein JI. Basal cell hyperplasia: an unusual diagnostic dilemma on prostate needle biopsies. Hum Pathol. 2005;36:480–5.

54. Ali TZ, Epstein JI. Basal cell carcinoma of the prostate: a clinicopathologic study of 29 cases. Am J Surg Pathol. 2007;31(5):697–705.
55. Yang XJ, McEntee M, Epstein JI. Distinction of basaloid carcinoma of the prostate from benign basal cell lesions by using immunohistochemistry for bcl-2 and Ki-67. Hum Pathol. 1998;29:1447–50.
56. Greene LF, O'Dea MJ, Dockerty MB. Primary transitional cell carcinoma of the prostate. J Urol. 1976;116(6):761–3.
57. Algaba F, Santanlaria JM, Lamas M, Ayala G. Transitional cell carcinoma of the prostate. Eur Urol. 1985;11:87–90.
58. Cheville JC, Dundore PA, Bostwick DG, et al. Transitional cell carcinoma of the prostate: clinicopathologic study of 50 cases. Cancer. 1998;82(4):703–7.
59. Edge SB, Byrd DR, Carducci M, et al., editors. AJCC cancer staging manual. 7th ed. New York: Springer; 2010.
60. Tran KP, Epstein JI. Mucinous adenocarcinoma of urinary bladder type arising from the prostatic urethra. Distinction from mucinous adenocarcinoma of the prostate. Am J Surg Pathol. 1996;20(11): 1346–50.
61. Ortiz-Rey JA, Dos Santos JE, Rodríguez-Castilla M, Alvarez C, Fariña L. Mucinous urothelial-type adenocarcinoma of the prostate. Scand J Urol Nephrol. 2004;38(3):256–7.
62. Curtis MW, Evans AJ, Srigley JR. Mucin-producing urothelial-type adenocarcinoma of prostate: report of two cases of a rare and diagnostically challenging entity. Mod Pathol. 2005;18(4):585–90.
63. Osunkoya AO, Netto GJ, Epstein JI. Colorectal adenocarcinoma involving the prostate: report of 9 cases. Hum Pathol. 2007;38(12):1836–41.
64. Johnson DE, Chalbaud R, Ayala AG. Secondary tumors of the prostate. J Urol. 1974;112(4):507–8.
65. Zein TA, Huben R, Lane W, Pontes JE, Englander LS. Secondary tumors of the prostate. J Urol. 1985;133(4):615–6.
66. Bates AW, Baithun SI. Secondary solid neoplasms of the prostate: a clinico-pathological series of 51 cases. Virchows Arch. 2002;440(4):392–6.
67. Schellhammer PF, Bean MA, Whitmore WF Jr. Prostatic involvement by transitional cell carcinoma: pathogenesis, patterns and prognosis. J Urol. 1977;118:399–403.
68. Revelo MP, Cookson MS, Chang SS, et al. Incidence and location of prostate and urothelial carcinoma in prostates from cystoprostatectomies: implications for possible apical sparing surgery. J Urol. 2004;171:646–51.
69. Oliva IV, Smith SL, Chen Z, Osunkoya AO. Urothelial carcinoma of the bladder with transmural and direct prostatic stromal invasion: does extent of stromal invasion significantly impact patient outcome? Hum Pathol. 2011;42(1):51–6.
70. Chuang AY, DeMarzo AM, Veltri RW, et al. Immunohistochemical differentiation of high-grade prostate carcinoma from urothelial carcinoma. Am J Surg Pathol. 2007;31(8):1246–55.
71. Eble JN, Sauter G, Epstein JI, et al., editors. The world health organization classification of tumors of the urinary system and male genital organs. Lyon: IARC Press; 2004.
72. Herawi M, Epstein JI. Specialized stromal tumors of the prostate: a clinicopathologic study of 50 cases. Am J Surg Pathol. 2006;30(6):694–704.
73. Hansel DE, Herawi M, Montgomery E, Epstein JI. Spindle cell lesions of the adult prostate. Mod Pathol. 2007;20(1):148–58.
74. Nagar M, Epstein JI. Epithelial proliferations in prostatic stromal tumors of uncertain malignant potential (STUMP). Am J Surg Pathol. 2011;35(6):898–903.
75. Madden JF, Burchette JL, Raj GV, et al. Anterior rectal wall gastrointestinal stromal tumor presenting clinically as prostatic mass. Urol Oncol. 2005;23:268–72.

Management Implications Associated with Unusual Morphologic Entities of the Prostate

6

Viraj A. Master, Jonathan Huang, Cristina Magi-Galluzzi and Adeboye O. Osunkoya

Introduction

Although the vast majority of malignant neoplasms of the prostate clinicians manage are conventional acinar prostatic adenocarcinomas, this chapter focusses exclusively on the management implications associated with unusual morphologic entities involving the prostate gland.

Primary Urothelial Carcinoma of the Prostate

Primary urothelial carcinoma (UC) of the prostate is a relatively uncommon tumor. Historically, any UC involving the prostate was stage 4 disease, but, over the past two decades, further understanding has allowed for disease sub-stratification with important management differences.

A. O. Osunkoya (✉) · V. A. Master
Department of Urology, Emory University School of Medicine, Atlanta, GA, USA
e-mail: Adeboye.osunkoya@emory.edu

V. A. Master
e-mail: vmaster@emory.edu

J. Huang
Department of Surgery, Emory University School of Medicine, Atlanta, GA, USA
e-mail: Jonathan.hwaien.huang@emory.edu

C. Magi-Galluzzi
Department of Pathology, Cleveland Clinic, Robert J. Tomsich Pathology and Laboratory Medicine Institute, Cleveland, OH, USA
e-mail: magic@ccf.org

In 2012, the Second International Consultation on Bladder Cancer, sponsored by the World Health Organization, under the auspices of the European Association of Urology, had an expert consensus panel review the management of this disease process. Updated recommendations were assigned based on a systematic review of the literature [1]. The predominant guiding management principle is correct staging to detect prostatic stromal invasion, although current tools for detection are imperfect. A high degree of suspicion must also be entertained for those patients who have a diagnosis of high grade, or multicentric, or recurrent bladder cancer, as the rate of prostatic urethral involvement may be as high as 40 % [2].

Papillary noninvasive UC of the prostate, is uncommon, with an incidence of approximately 1–4 %, and is managed with local resection via a transurethral endoscopic approach. As discussed previously, this lesion may be present in the lumen of the prostatic urethra or in the prostatic ducts. Presentation is insidious and is usually silent. It is important to ensure that the bladder is completely surveyed, including biopsies of any suspicious lesions. The metastatic evaluation is initiated only if the lesion is a high-grade lesion, or if the lesion is invasive. In such circumstance, a cross-sectional imaging study [computed tomography (CT) or magnetic resonance imaging (MRI)] of the chest, abdomen, and pelvis is recommended. Importantly, imaging should contain delayed images as well, so that the urinary tract is well opacified by contrast, thus allowing for the

C. Magi-Galluzzi, C. G. Przybycin (eds.), *Genitourinary Pathology,* DOI 10.1007/978-1-4939-2044-0_6,

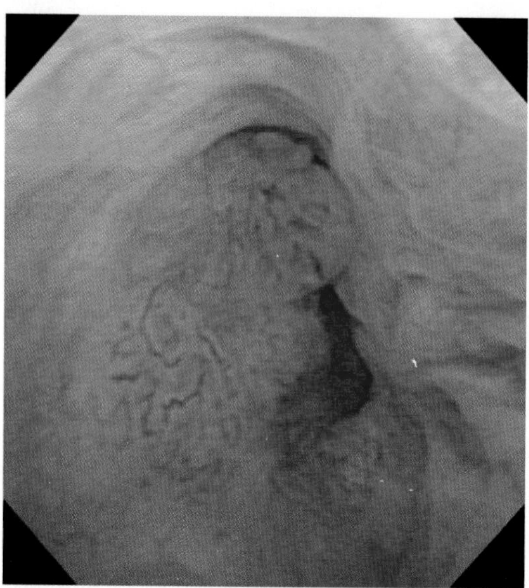

Fig. 6.1 Urethroscopic/cystoscopic appearance of primary papillary urothelial carcinoma of the prostatic urethra. Note the visual similarity to Fig. 6.2 depicting a prostatic ductal adenocarcinoma

radiographic detection of small urothelial lesions of the upper tract. Radiography is not currently sufficient to evaluate the lower urinary tract and thus endoscopy, namely cystourethroscopy, is mandatory (Fig. 6.1).

Carcinoma-in-situ (CIS) of the prostatic urethra is almost always associated with a bladder tumor. In a large study of over 1500 patients with primary bladder tumors, 2.5% had CIS in the prostatic urethra [3]. CIS of the prostatic urethra may evolve to stromal disease, which has a virulent course. CIS of the bladder is best managed with local resection and a full transurethral resection of the prostate (TURP). The TURP should certainly include the bladder neck as well. This procedure will allow for detection of stromal disease, and will also permit intravesical chemo/immunotherapy to come in contact with the prostatic epithelium [4]. The first line therapy is likely to be Bacillus Calmette-Guérin (BCG). If patients do get BCG to the prostate, transient elevations in prostate-specific antigen (PSA) will be noted, generally resolving in 3 months. The response rate to BCG is very good, with complete response noted in 70–100% of patients with prostate-only CIS [5]. It is vital to note that such patients will need to be followed closely, not only with cystourethroscopy, but also cytology, as lesions may not be visible. If a positive cytology is detected, but no obvious lesions are seen, random biopsies should be considered. If these biopsies are negative, attention should be given to upper tract evaluation. It is important to stress that the endoscopic evaluation of the bladder should be thorough, especially in the region of the trigone, as bladder trigone involvement is often predictive of prostate stromal involvement. A high proportion of patients, approximately one in three, will experience relapse and progression, requiring radical cystoprostatectomy [6].

Prostatic stromal invasion is a good surrogate marker of tumor virulence, and will help in the disease management to counsel patients that a very high degree of metastases would be found. Prostate stromal involvement mandates a radical operation to remove bladder and prostate, and management principles do not include transurethral operations. Shen et al. found that 3/4 patients with stromal involvement had malignant adenopathy, with a low 5-year survival rate of 32% [7]. Although there is little consensus in the literature, neoadjuvant chemotherapy and an extended lymph node dissection may be of benefit.

Mucin-Producing Urothelial-Type Adenocarcinoma of the Prostate

Mucin-producing urothelial-type adenocarcinoma of the prostate is a rare tumor that arises from the prostatic urethra, with the largest series consisting of 15 patients [8]. Patients often present with obstructive urinary symptoms. Some may have mucusuria, which is reported to be a specific finding, but is a sign also found in mucinous prostatic adenocarcinoma [8]. The histologic appearance, from TURP and prostate biopsy specimens, and clinical presentation can be similar to other diseases. As such, additional tests should be completed to ensure a definitive diagnosis. Cystoscopic evaluation may help to rule out a metastatic nonurachal adenocarcinoma of the bladder [8]. A colonoscopy, with immunohistochemical

(IHC) staining of tissue biopsies, can rule out metastatic colonic adenocarcinoma [9]. With regards to serological markers, PSA is usually within normal limits, as the cancer does not develop from prostatic acini [8, 9]. There may also be a potential benefit in looking for precursor lesions. In one study, only one third of specimens did not have precursor lesions, such cystitis glandularis and villous adenoma, and their absence was attributed to sampling issues and destruction of the surface components by the infiltrating tumor [8].

With such a small number of cases describing mucin-producing urothelial-type adenocarcinoma of the prostate, treatment has not been standardized. However, these tumors are reported to be refractory to hormonal therapy [8]. Most case reports present patients treated with surgery, with varying degrees of success. In one report, consisting of two patients, one patient had no signs of recurrence 1 year after radical prostatectomy, while the other patient had local recurrence 4 years after simple prostatectomy [10]. In a series of 15 patients, all eight patients treated with radical prostatectomy had extraprostatic extension of their disease. Furthermore, eight patients out of the cohort died at an average of 49.2 months from presentation [8]. Although information about this disease is limited, an accurate diagnosis is essential to distinguish it from conventional or mucinous prostatic adenocarcinomas which respond to androgen deprivation therapy.

Mucinous Adenocarcinoma of the Prostate

Mucinous adenocarcinoma (MC) of the prostate is a rare form of prostate cancer, with many large series reporting less than 0.5 % incidence among prostate specimens [11–14]. It can only be diagnosed with certainty on radical prostatectomy. However, it is important to realize that mucin staining on histology is a nonspecific finding, although many clinicians are not aware of this distinction. Conditions like benign prostatic hyperplasia, prostatic intraepithelial neoplasia (PIN), and signet ring cell prostatic adenocarcinoma often have positive mucin staining [15, 16]. It should be noted that careful examination of the specimen is necessary, as signet ring cell adenocarcinoma portends a worse prognosis than MC and may be less responsive to hormone therapy [17]. In the clinical evaluation of this form of prostate cancer, PSA values have been shown to be elevated in MC, with one series showing PSA elevations in 77.8 % of the patients [18]. One group hypothesized that MRI and MR spectroscopy could be useful in detecting mucin lakes and diagnosing MC. However, their results showed that these modalities could not distinguish mucin lakes, even when they comprised the majority of the tumor volume, and thus, currently, radiographic imaging is not used to make this diagnosis [19].

In a study published in 1999, most cases of MC were either stage C or D on the Whitmore–Jewett staging system [18]. Patients may often present with osteoblastic metastases. The clinical behavior of MC is still unclear. MC was once thought to be an aggressive disease, with one series reporting 8/12 patients presenting with at least stage C disease and all 12 patients developing metastases [13]. However, a recent study reports that MC has a similar, if not better, prognosis than conventional prostatic acinar adenocarcinoma, when treated with radical prostatectomy. The researchers reported a 5-year actuarial PSA progression-free risk of progression for mucinous and non-MC of the prostate of 97.2 and 85.4 %, respectively [20]. With the majority of MC presenting at an advanced stage, surgical therapy may not always be a feasible form of treatment. One case report detailed a patient with MC's response to hormonal therapy. The patient's elevated PSA, prostatic-specific acid phosphatase (PSAP), and gamma-seminoprotein returned to normal 2 months after therapy [21]. Furthermore, another study reported a 77.8 % (22/27) response rate for MC treated with endocrine therapy [18]. This study found the 3- and 5-year survival rate to be 50 and 25 %, respectively, in patient with MC. Most studies do not mention the use of chemotherapy in the treatment of MC. However, one study reports the use of chemotherapy, in addition to other modalities, in the treatment of five patients with Gleason score 6 and above MC.

Each one of these patients was reported to have expired. Multiple case reports have detailed long-term survival with both radical prostatectomy and hormonal therapy, but further investigation, with larger cohorts, will be necessary to determine which modality provides a better prognosis.

Prostatic Ductal Adenocarcinoma

Prostatic ductal adenocarcinoma comprises up to 6.3% of prostatic adenocarcinomas [22]. Patients often present complaining of obstructive symptoms. On urethroscopy/cystoscopy, this tumor may mimic papillary UC because of the presence of papillary fronds (Fig. 6.2). Transrectal ultrasound may also be helpful (Fig. 6.3) in the differential diagnosis. In a series of 55 patients, 7/8 patients with primary duct adenocarcinoma of the prostate and 44/47 patients with secondary duct adenocarcinoma reported obstructive urinary symptoms [22]. Since this tumor typically arises from the periurethral or occasionally the peripheral zone of the prostate, diagnosis of prostatic ductal adenocarcinoma is ascertained through examination of tissue specimens from TURP or prostatic needle biopsy [23]. This tumor is frequently mixed with prostatic acinar adenocarcinoma. Other entities can also resemble this disease, including prostatic urethral polyps, hyperplastic benign prostate glands, high-grade PIN, colorectal adenocarcinoma, and papillary UC [24]. As such, IHC staining can be utilized to provide a more accurate diagnosis. Serum PSA levels are often elevated in prostatic ductal adenocarcinoma, with a mean PSA of 12.5 in one series of 23 patients [25]. However, the increase in PSA may not adequately reflect the extent of this disease.

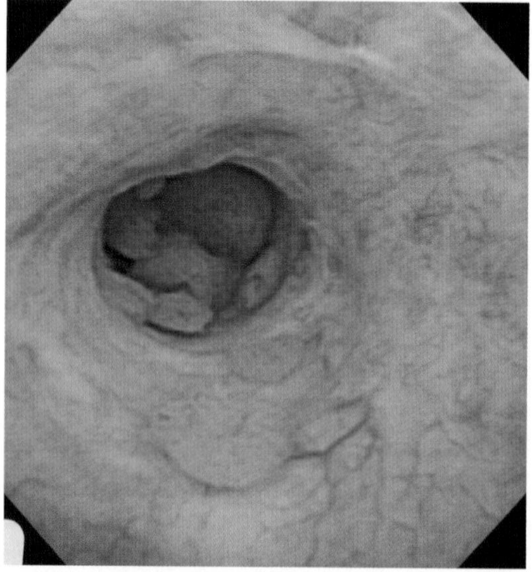

Fig. 6.2 Urethroscopic/cystoscopic appearance of prostatic ductal adenocarcinoma involving the prostatic urethra. Patient presented with hematuria and urinary obstruction, and the lesion was initially thought to be papillary urothelial carcinoma

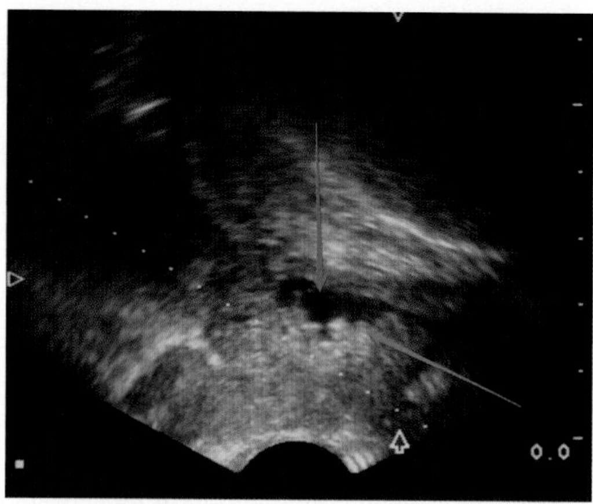

Fig. 6.3 Transrectal ultrasound. The patient has a hyperechoic posterior lesion (*red arrow*) creating an irregular border in the urethra (*blue arrow*)

Prostatic ductal adenocarcinoma has been reported to be an aggressive disease. In a series of 15 patients, who appeared to have a resectable tumor, treated with radical prostatectomy, 97% of the specimens showed extraprostatic extension [26]. Prognosis is dependent on multiple factors, including whether prostatic acinar adenocarcinoma is present and the depth of invasion [22, 27]. The presence of prostatic acinar adenocarcinoma in the specimen, when compared to pure prostatic ductal adenocarcinoma, decreases the median survival from 13.8 to 8.9 years [27]. The 5-year survival rate decreases from 42 to 22% when the secondary periurethral ducts, in addition to the primary periurethral ducts, are involved [22]. Early disease, if localized to the primary periurethral ducts, may be eradicated through TURP, although standard of care is radical prostatectomy [25]. However, a needle biopsy is recommended to determine if there are foci of disease in the peripheral zones of the prostate, warranting a radical prostatectomy or additional treatments. While radiotherapy has not been employed extensively in the treatment of prostatic ductal adenocarcinoma, one series showed that 4/6 patients were alive at 3.2 years after radiotherapy [28]. One case report documented a patient with metastatic prostatic ductal adenocarcinoma. The patient showed a partial biochemical response during nine cycles of palliative docetaxel, but expired soon after completion of chemotherapy [29]. Additional work may determine other effective treatments for this disease. Patients who have this disease warrant a complete evaluation for metastatic disease, including chest imaging. Of note, penile urethral recurrence may occur.

Intraductal Carcinoma of Prostate

Intraductal carcinoma of the prostate (IDC-P) is an aggressive form of prostate cancer, associated with high-grade disease and a poor prognosis. This form of prostate cancer is often associated with invasive cancer [30, 31]. When isolated IDC-P is diagnosed on prostate biopsies, a repeat biopsy is warranted to confirm the concomitance of invasive cancer. Other pathology, such as high-grade PIN, can resemble IDC-P [32]. It is important to note that IDC-P may or may not be associated with a high tumor volume or elevated PSA values. Instead, IDC-P has been associated with low serum PSA values [33]. Once IDC-P is confirmed, definitive therapy is warranted.

One group suggested that radical prostatectomy with extended lymph node dissection may be a feasible approach for treatment [34]. Furthermore, for patients with IDC-P on prostate biopsies, obturator node sampling, seminal vesicle biopsy, and a bone scan prior to prostatectomy may help determine the extent of the disease [35]. The reasoning is that patients with IDC-P on prostate biopsies and transurethral resections have been shown to have early biochemical relapse and metastatic failure when treated with radiotherapy [36]. Similarly, all 11 patients, in a series of 59 patients, with IDC-P on prostate biopsies had clinical relapse after prostatectomy [35]. Androgen ablation therapy, neoadjuvant chemotherapy, and radiation therapy are associated with poor results in the treatment of IDC-P. Another study analyzed a series of 115 patients who had androgen ablation, with or without chemotherapy, prior to radical prostatectomy. Of the 42 patients who had biochemical failure, 38 patients had either cribriform pattern or IDC-P [37]. In the EORTC 22863 phase 3 randomized clinical trial, one arm of the study assessed the response of external-beam radiation on patients with prostate cancer. The patients with IDC-P had a median time of 19.9 months to clinical progression, compared to 61.2 months in patients without IDC-P.

Currently, from a clinician standpoint, there has been effort to urge pathologist to report the presence of IDC-P, even when IDC-P comprises a fraction of the specimen. Doing so may help determine a patient's prognosis and treatment. The inclusion of IDC-P as a preoperative variable was shown to improve the predictive accuracy of post-prostatectomy nomograms in predicting biochemical recurrence [38].

Squamous Cell Carcinoma of the Prostate

Primary squamous cell carcinoma (SQCC) of the prostate accounts for less than 1 % of prostatic tumors [39]. This may even be an overestimate, as other pathology, including benign squamous metaplasia, UC with squamous differentiation of the bladder, and the prostatic urethra, may appear histologically similar on the specimens obtained by TURP and prostate biopsy [40]. Conventional prostate cancer can also have a malignant squamous component. A careful review of a patient's history, including cystoscopy, may provide details suggesting the presence of squamous metaplasia. This entity may arise secondary to prostatic infarct, prior radiation or androgen deprivation therapy, reactive changes after TURP, and granulomatous prostatitis due to BCG therapy [40, 41]. UC with squamous differentiation of the bladder and prostatic urethra must also be ruled out. Cystoscopy and imaging may help determine the presence of these diseases [42]. Symptoms of urinary obstruction and bone involvement, secondary to metastatic disease, are often the first clinical clues to this disease [40]. Serum levels of PSA and PSAP are usually normal, as SQCC does not typically develop from prostatic acini [40, 43]. The tumor often appears as a hypoechoic hypervascular lesion on transrectal ultrasonography (TRUS) and MRI often depicts low lesion signal intensities in the prostate on T2-weighted images [44].

With the low number of cases, treatment of SQCC of the prostate has not been standardized. Furthermore, the efficacy of treatments is currently based on anecdotal evidence. One study presents two patients, including one with positive periaortic and pelvic lymph nodes, who had a radical cystoprostatectomy, pelvic lymphadenectomy, and a urinary diversion. These patients had a survival rate between 25 and 40 months [40]. Another study presented a patient with metastatic osteolytic bone lesion who was treated with cobalt irradiation. This patient survived 8 months after presentation [45]. Hormonal therapy has been reported to be ineffective in the treatment of SQCC of the prostate [46]. From case reports, multimodal therapy appears to have the most benefits. A patient with pelvic relapse treated with cisplatin, 5-fluorouracil, and radiotherapy had a length of survival of 60 months [47]. Surgical treatment with negative margins is thought to be an effective form of treatment. However, the aggressive nature of SQCC of the prostate and metastatic osteolytic lesions at presentation often precludes this form of treatment. Thus, continued research is necessary to determine an effective therapeutic regimen for this form of prostate cancer.

Sarcomatoid Carcinoma of the Prostate

Sarcomatoid carcinoma of the prostate is a rare disease, described mostly in case reports and small series of patients. This disease is thought to arise secondary to radiation therapy or androgen deprivation, as many patients have had prostatic adenocarcinoma treated with these modalities [48, 49]. Diagnosis is made through evaluation of prostatic tissue specimens. A differential diagnosis of phyllodes tumor must be kept in mind. IHC staining can also help distinguish adenocarcinoma from sarcomatoid carcinoma. With the limited tissue specimen a prostate biopsy provides, both epithelial and mesenchymal components may not always be present. To ensure a correct diagnosis of sarcomatoid carcinoma, diseases such as a true prostatic sarcoma, leiomyosarcoma, and inflammatory myofibroblastic tumor need to be ruled out by characteristic microscopic features and IHC staining [49].

Treatment for sarcomatoid carcinoma of the prostate has not been standardized. TURP is often utilized to manage obstructive symptoms. At presentation, this aggressive disease may involve the urinary bladder or penis. Additionally, metastases to the bone, liver, and lungs are also present [49]. In one study, patients were treated with various forms of therapy, including surgery, radiation therapy, androgen deprivation therapy, and various adjuvant chemotherapy regimens, with no significant difference in length of survival. The 5- and 7-year survival rates were 41 and 14 %, respectively, and the median length of survival was 9.5 months. The patient with no evidence of disease at 85 months was treated with a pelvic exenteration and resection of the lung metastases [48]. In another study, nine patients with metastases or bulky local disease were treated with chemotherapy. Three of these patients died within a year and five patients had no response to the chemotherapy [49]. While many cases report the use of chemotherapy in treating patients with sarcomatoid carcinoma of the prostate, a regimen has not been standardized. The use of adriamycin, carboplatinum, cisplatinum, estramustine, etoposide, ifosfamide, taxotere, in various combinations, have been utilized [48–50]. Further work will be necessary to determine an effective form of treatment.

Prostatic Carcinoid

Primary carcinoid tumor, or low-grade neuroendocrine tumor, of the prostate is a rare disease, mostly documented in case reports. The diagnosis of this disease is based on microscopic examination of tissue specimens, acquired by TURP and prostate biopsies, and IHC staining [51, 52]. Prostatic acinar adenocarcinoma with carcinoid features can resemble a carcinoid tumor. An accurate diagnosis is important because prostatic adenocarcinoma is thought to be more aggressive than carcinoid tumor of the prostate [53]. An octreotide scan and 18F-fluorodeoxyglucose positron emission tomography can be utilized to determine whether the carcinoid tumor has metastasized [52]. One study reported that the tumor appeared as a hypoechoic irregularly shaped mass with increased irregularity on TRUS and a low attenuating mass with peripheral enhancement on CT [44].

Treatment for primary carcinoid tumor of the prostate has not been standardized. With surgical management being the only independent prognostic factor in prostatic small cell carcinoma, a high-grade neuroendocrine tumor, patients with prostatic carcinoid tumor may have the best outcome with surgery [54]. In two case reports, the patients were surgically treated with cystoprostatectomy [51, 52]. However, their outcomes were not reported. Another study reported two patients with metastatic disease to the bone marrow and bone. These patients were both managed by surgical castration. Both died within 10 months of initial diagnosis [55]. Reports about the prognosis of this disease are varied. Some reports have hypothesized that prostatic carcinoid tumor is an indolent disease and that aggressive forms of the disease are in actuality prostatic carcinoma with carcinoid features [51].

Small Cell Carcinoma of the Prostate

Small cell carcinoma of the prostate, a high-grade neuroendocrine tumor, is a rare disease, diagnosed by histologic examination and IHC staining. The most common clinical feature is urinary obstruction. However, symptoms due to metastatic disease and paraneoplastic syndromes may also be present [56]. Serum PSA levels are not usually elevated in pure small cell carcinoma of the prostate. At presentation, CT often reveals bone metastases and abdominal and pelvic lymphadenopathy [44].

This is an aggressive disease that is unresponsive to hormonal therapy. Surgical treatment is not often employed because of the metastatic nature of small cell carcinoma. In one study, 75 % of patient had metastases at presentation [56]. Chemotherapy has been shown to be an effective form of treatment, with 62–72 % of patients having some form of response [56, 57]. However, the chemotherapy regimen has not been standardized. Radiation therapy has also been employed for local control and palliation [58]. The median survival in patients with small cell carcinoma of the prostate is 9–10 months [56, 57]. Elevated serum lactate dehydrogenase (LDH) levels and low serum albumin were reported to be predictive of inferior disease-specific survival [59].

Basal Cell Carcinoma of the Prostate

Basal cell carcinoma of the prostate is a rare tumor that comprises less than 0.01 % of malignant tumors of the prostate. A TURP is often completed for obstructive urinary symptoms and examination of the tissue fragments leads to a diagnosis of basal cell carcinoma. While there have been cases of elevated serum PSA in pure basal cell carcinoma of the prostate, serum PSA and PSAP are not usually elevated, unless a component of prostate adenocarcinoma is present [60]. No imaging modality has been effective in diagnosing this disease [61].

Older studies have reported basal cell carcinoma of the prostate to maintain an indolent course [62, 63]. Recent studies indicate that basal cell carcinoma, notably of the adenoid cystic carcinoma histologic variant, may actually be more aggressive, recurring locally after surgery and metastasizing [60, 64]. Treatment for this disease usually involves surgery, including TURP, radical prostatectomy, and pelvic exenteration [60, 61, 64]. In one study, 6/7 patients treated with radical prostatectomy had no evidence of disease at

1 year follow-up [64]. However, the small number of cases does not provide enough evidence to standardize treatment. The type of surgery is usually determined based on the initial extent of the disease. Basal cell carcinoma is reported to be unresponsive to androgen deprivation therapy [65]. Lifelong follow-up is recommended, as this disease may recur locally or metastasize.

Urothelial Carcinoma with Secondary Prostate Involvement

In the USA, the standard of care of the management of muscle invasive UC of the bladder (muscle-invasive bladder cancer, MIBC) is radical cystoprostatectomy as an en bloc procedure, along with an extensive pelvic lymph node dissection. In other countries, definitive combination chemotherapy and radiation therapy are utilized, with the caveat that the failure rate requiring salvage radical cystoprostatectomy is approximately 30 % [66, 67]. There have been attempts at prostate-sparing radical cystectomy, with a view to ameliorating urinary continence, and erectile dysfunction postoperatively, but these should be considered treatments to be undertaken only in the context of a clinical trial [68, 69]. Thus, if a patient has invasive bladder cancer, neoadjuvant chemotherapy followed by radical cystoprostatectomy is performed.

Recent data have helped to clarify the issue that prostatic stromal invasion from bladder cancer is significantly more common than appreciated in previous series. This mode of invasion may be contiguous or noncontiguous, and happens in approximately equal proportions [70]. Several cystoprostatectomy series using whole-mount methods have shown that stromal invasion is present in approximately half of patients. Richards et al. studied a large series of 121 consecutive whole-mount specimens, and found that 48 % had prostate involvement [71]. Other groups detected stromal invasion in 37–64 % of men undergoing cystoprostatectomy for MIBC [70, 72]. However, stromal invasion is not only restricted to patients with MIBC. Herr and Donat, looking at a large series of 186 patients from Memorial Sloan Kettering with Ta/T1 bladder disease, found that 14 % of patients relapsed with prostatic stromal involvement. In patients with presumed bladder-only refractory CIS and those with multicentric UC, approximately 30 % had prostatic urethral involvement.

With the above data in mind, it is a prudent management principle to diligently inspect the prostatic urethra for lesions if the patient has any degree of bladder cancer, even noninvasive lesions. Biopsies should be taken of lesions, and if possible, underlying prostatic stroma should be evaluated as well with a cold loop resection that includes both the mucosal and the deeper layers. TRUS-guided biopsy is not accurate, and should not be performed to assess for prostate stromal invasion. In the latest edition of the AJCC staging manual (7 ed., 2010), prostate stromal invasion directly from bladder cancer represents a T4a lesion, but interestingly, this T-stage is still classified as Stage III, and the patient may have a 30 % 5-year survival. Subepithelial invasion of prostatic urethra will not constitute T4 staging status.

Colorectal Adenocarcinoma Involving the Prostate

Colorectal adenocarcinoma secondarily involving the prostate is a rare occurrence. Clinicians treating patients who have had colorectal adenocarcinoma or treatment for this disease, and presenting with obstructive urinary symptoms, should acknowledge that there may be direct extension to the prostate from the primary colonic tumor. Diagnosis of this disease is made through evaluation of prostatic tissue specimens, from TURP or prostate biopsies. Bladder and prostatic adenocarcinomas share other similar histologic characteristics with colorectal adenocarcinoma, which may necessitate the use of tests, such as IHC staining, to differentiate these diseases [73]. Serum PSA may also be elevated, even in the absence of prostatic adenocarcinoma, if the prostatic ducts are disrupted [73]. Radiographic evidence of tumor extension and patient presentation can also help in distinguishing these various diseases [73]. However, direct extension may not always be visualized on CT.

There has been a case of hematogenous metastasis to the prostate [74]. Distinguishing colorectal adenocarcinoma from other diseases will help determine the proper form of treatment.

Treatment of secondary colorectal adenocarcinoma involvement of the prostate has not been standardized. Hormonal therapy is known not to be effective in treating colorectal adenocarcinoma [73]. One patient was treated with cystoprostatectomy, partial urethrectomy, and ileal conduit urinary diversion. No metastases were noted during abdominal exploration. At 14 months postoperatively, the patient has been asymptomatic, with an elevated, but stable, CEA level [75]. Another study reported nine cases of colorectal adenocarcinoma involving the prostate, with treatment modalities including surgery, chemotherapy, and radiation therapy. Despite treatment, six of these patients died within 34 months [73]. Further work, including evaluating the role of antibody-based therapy, still needs to be accomplished in order to determine an optimal form of treatment [73].

Prostatic Stromal Tumor of Uncertain Malignant Potential

Prostatic stromal tumor of uncertain malignant potential (STUMP) is a rare disease that usually presents with urinary obstruction [76]. Diagnosis is made through analysis of tissue specimens, obtained from TURP or prostate biopsies. However, other diseases may have a similar appearance. Histologically, prostatic STUMP has been reported to appear similar to both prostatic stromal sarcomas (PSS) and benign prostatic hyperplasia (BPH), diseases that have disparate prognoses [76]. On TRUS, prostatic STUMP has a multicystic appearance, with thin septations [76]. The use of MRI has the potential to distinguish STUMP from prostatic adenocarcinoma and prostatic sarcoma. Prostatic adenocarcinoma has low signal intensity on T2-weighted images. PSS is often a solid lesion that has heterogeneous signal intensity on T2-weighted images. In contrast, one study reported that STUMP has diffuse heterogeneous signal intensity on T2-weighted images, due to cystic areas in the lesion [76]. Both STUMP and prostatic sarcoma may extend into or near adjacent organs. The cystic component may make distinguishing STUMP from cystoadenoma of the prostate difficult. Even though a diagnosis may be difficult to ascertain, proper diagnosis will help determine the appropriate treatment and prognosis for a patient.

Treatment for STUMP has not been standardized. The aggressiveness of these tumors have been shown to vary, some with only obstructive symptoms and others with frequent local recurrence and metastasis [76, 77]. Oftentimes, patients have multiple TURP or transurethral resection of bladder tumor to manage recurrent urinary obstruction [78, 79]. Despite management with these procedures or radical cystoprostatectomy, 46 % of patients will have recurrence of the tumor [78]. Furthermore, 5 % of patients have progression from STUMP to PSS [79, 80]. In deciding whether invasive surgery should be pursued, the patient's age, treatment choices, whether the lesion is palpable on digital rectal examination, extension of the lesion on the tissue specimen, and extension of the lesion on imaging should be considered [81]. More aggressive surgery has been suggested for younger patients and those with more extensive tumors on imaging [76].

Prostatic Stromal Sarcoma

PSS is a rare disease, documented mostly in case reports. Physical examination often reveals an enlarged prostate [82–84]. Diagnosis is made by microscopic examination and IHC staining of tissue specimens. Serum PSA in PSS is often normal [85]. There has been one report of increased serum PSA of 7.25 ng/mL in a patient diagnosed with PSS that contained hyperplastic glands [83]. One case report described images of PSS with CT as a solid lesion with a cystic wall and well-defined margins [84]. Another report described PSS on CT as lobulated, homogeneous without contrast, and heterogeneous with contrast [82]. In addition to an abdominal CT, a bone scan can be utilized to look for bony metastases. MRI is reported to show a multinodular mass, often in the central zone of the prostate, with heterogeneous high signal intensity and a low signal intensity pseudocapsule on T2-weighted imaging, and weak enhancement on dynamic contrast-enhanced MRI [86]. While these features on MRI may separate PSS from prostatic adenocarcinoma, many of these features are found in more common prostatic sarcomas, such as leiomyosarcoma and rhabdomyosarcoma.

Treatment for PSS has not been standardized. Patients often present with urinary retention. Further management, with modalities such as a TURP and imaging, may lead to a diagnosis of PSS [87]. Surgical treatment, with negative margins, is the suggested form of therapy, as prostatic sarcomas are aggressive diseases and prone to develop early metastases [85, 87]. Procedures such as radical prostatectomy, radical cystoprostatectomy, and enucleation have been employed [84]. One patient underwent a radical prostatectomy, with negative margins and no evidence of metastasis, and has had no recurrence after 8 years [85]. However, most cases present patients that have no evidence of disease at their limited follow-up of 1 year [80, 84]. The value of adjuvant radiation and chemotherapy are currently unknown. Investigation into the responsiveness of PSS to hormones may lead to further insight and therapies for this disease [85].

Gastrointestinal Stromal Tumor of the Prostate

The prostate is an uncommon location for gastrointestinal stromal tumors (GIST). In the literature, there have only been 20 cases of GIST involving the prostate [88]. As GIST usually arises from the gastrointestinal tract, patients may present with an array of gastrointestinal and genitourinary symptoms. Diagnosis of this disease is based on analysis of tissue specimens and IHC staining. Currently, there are only two cases of GIST thought to occur primarily in the prostate [89, 90]. Most other cases have originated from the rectum, which lies in close proximity to the prostate [88, 91]. CT and MRI can be of utility in distinguishing primary from secondary prostate GIST, as well as the location of secondary extension and the presence of metastases.

The importance in correctly diagnosing GIST cannot be overemphasized. Doing so will help guide treatment and may limit the extent of surgical intervention. Local recurrence is common after surgical resection of GIST, even in the presence of negative margins [92]. Recurrent and metastatic GIST is documented to be responsive to imatinib mesylate, a tyrosine kinase inhibitor [91, 93]. The use of imatinib mesylate can reduce the size of GIST lesions and maintain these lesions at the decreased size without surgery [90, 92]. Furthermore, analysis of an excisional prostate specimen that contained GIST, after treatment with imatinib mesylate, demonstrated no residual disease [94]. Patients treated with imatinib mesylate are documented to be stable 2 years after treatment [90]. Chemotherapy and radiation have minimal efficacy in treating GIST [95].

References

1. Palou J, Wood D, Bochner BH, van der Poel H, Al-Ahmadie HA, Yossepowitch O, et al. ICUD-EAU international consultation on bladder cancer 2012: urothelial carcinoma of the prostate. Eur Urol. 2013;63:81–7.
2. Herr HW, Donat SM. Prostatic tumor relapse in patients with superficial bladder tumors: 15-year outcome. J Urol. 1999;161:1854–7.
3. Millan-Rodriguez F, Chechile-Toniolo G, Salvador-Bayarri J, Palou J, Vicente-Rodriguez J. Multivariate analysis of the prognostic factors of primary superficial bladder cancer. J Urol. 2000;163:73–8.
4. Chibber PJ, McIntyre MA, Hindmarsh JR, Hargreave TB, Newsam JE, Chisholm GD. Transitional cell carcinoma involving the prostate. Br J Urol. 1981;53:605–9.
5. Taylor JH, Davis J, Schellhammer P. Long-term follow-up of intravesical bacillus Calmette-Guerin treatment for superficial transitional-cell carcinoma of the bladder involving the prostatic urethra. Clin Genitourin Cancer. 2007;5:386–9.
6. Arce J, Gaya JM, Huguet J, Rodriguez O, Palou J, Villavicencio H. Can we identify those patients who will benefit from prostate-sparing surgery? Predictive factors for invasive prostatic involvement by transitional cell carcinoma. Can J Urol. 2011;18:5529–36.
7. Revelo MP, Cookson MS, Chang SS, Shook MF, Smith JA Jr., Shappell SB. Incidence and location of

prostate and urothelial carcinoma in prostates from cystoprostatectomies: implications for possible apical sparing surgery. J Urol. 2004;171:646–51.
8. Osunkoya AO, Epstein JI. Primary mucin-producing urothelial-type adenocarcinoma of prostate: report of 15 cases. Am J Surg Pathol. 2007;31:1323–9.
9. Curtis MW, Evans AJ, Srigley JR. Mucin-producing urothelial-type adenocarcinoma of prostate: report of two cases of a rare and diagnostically challenging entity. Mod Pathol. 2005;18:585–90.
10. Tran KP, Epstein JI. Mucinous adenocarcinoma of urinary bladder type arising from the prostatic urethra. Distinction from mucinous adenocarcinoma of the prostate. Am J Surg Pathol. 1996;20:1346–50.
11. Lane BR, Magi-Galluzzi C, Reuther AM, Levin HS, Zhou M, Klein EA. Mucinous adenocarcinoma of the prostate does not confer poor prognosis. Urology. 2006;68:825–30.
12. Xie LP, Qin J, Zheng XY, Shen HF, Chen ZD, Cai SL, et al. Age and pathological features of 481 prostate cancer patients. Zhonghua Nan Ke Xue. 2005;11:428–30.
13. Ro JY, Grignon DJ, Ayala AG, Fernandez PL, Ordonez NG, Wishnow KI. Mucinous adenocarcinoma of the prostate: histochemical and immunohistochemical studies. Hum Pathol. 1990;21:593–600.
14. Epstein JI, Lieberman PH. Mucinous adenocarcinoma of the prostate gland. Am J Surg Pathol. 1985;9:299–308.
15. Pinder SE, McMahon RF. Mucins in prostatic carcinoma. Histopathology. 1990;16:43–6.
16. Remmele W, Weber A, Harding P. Primary signet-ring cell carcinoma of the prostate. Hum Pathol. 1988;19:478–80.
17. Gumus E, Yilmaz B, Miroglu C. Prostate mucinous adenocarcinoma with signet ring cell. Int J Urol. 2003;10:239–41.
18. Saito S, Iwaki H. Mucin-producing carcinoma of the prostate: review of 88 cases. Urology. 1999;54:141–4.
19. Westphalen AC, Coakley FV, Kurhanewicz J, Reed G, Wang ZJ, Simko JP. Mucinous adenocarcinoma of the prostate: MRI and MR spectroscopy features. AJR Am J Roentgenol. 2009;193:W238–43.
20. Osunkoya AO, Nielsen ME, Epstein JI. Prognosis of mucinous adenocarcinoma of the prostate treated by radical prostatectomy: a study of 47 cases. Am J Surg Pathol. 2008;32:468–72.
21. Ishizu K, Yoshihiro S, Joko K, Takihara H, Sakatoku J, Tanaka K. Mucinous adenocarcinoma of the prostate with good response to hormonal therapy: a case report. Hinyokika Kiyo. 1991;37:1057–60.
22. Dube VE, Farrow GM, Greene LF. Prostatic adenocarcinoma of ductal origin. Cancer. 1973;32:402–9.
23. Hertel JD, Humphrey PA. Ductal adenocarcinoma of the prostate. J Urol. 2011;186:277–8.
24. Epstein JI. Prostatic ductal adenocarcinoma: a mini review. Med Princ Pract. 2010;19:82–5.
25. Aydin H, Zhang J, Samaratunga H, Tan N, Magi-Galluzzi C, Klein E, et al. Ductal adenocarcinoma of the prostate diagnosed on transurethral biopsy or resection is not always indicative of aggressive disease: implications for clinical management. BJU Int. 2010;105:476–80.
26. Christensen WN, Steinberg G, Walsh PC, Epstein JI. Prostatic duct adenocarcinoma. Findings at radical prostatectomy. Cancer. 1991;67:2118–24.
27. Tu SM, Lopez A, Leibovici D, Bilen MA, Evliyaoglu F, Aparicio A, et al. Ductal adenocarcinoma of the prostate: clinical features and implications after local therapy. Cancer. 2009;115:2872–80.
28. Eade TN, Al-Saleem T, Horwitz EM, Buyyounouski MK, Chen DY, Pollack A. Role of radiotherapy in ductal (endometrioid) carcinoma of the prostate. Cancer. 2007;109:2011–15.
29. Paterson C, Correa PD, Russell JM. Ductal variant of adenocarcinoma prostate responding to docetaxel—a case report. Clin Oncol (R Coll Radiol). 2010;22:617.
30. Guo CC, Epstein JI. Intraductal carcinoma of the prostate on needle biopsy: histologic features and clinical significance. Mod Pathol. 2006;19:1528–35.
31. McNeal JE, Yemoto CE. Spread of adenocarcinoma within prostatic ducts and acini. Morphologic and clinical correlations. Am J Surg Pathol. 1996;20:802–14.
32. Robinson B, Magi-Galluzzi C, Zhou M. Intraductal carcinoma of the prostate. Arch Pathol Lab Med. 2012;136:418–25.
33. Cohen RJ, Haffejee Z, Steele GS, Nayler SJ. Advanced prostate cancer with normal serum prostate-specific antigen values. Arch Pathol Lab Med. 1994;118:1123–6.
34. Bonkhoff H, Wheeler TM, van der Kwast TH, Magi-Galluzzi C, Montironi R, Cohen RJ. Intraductal carcinoma of the prostate: precursor or aggressive phenotype of prostate cancer? Prostate. 2013;73:442–8.
35. Cohen RJ, Chan WC, Edgar SG, Robinson E, Dodd N, Hoscek S, et al. Prediction of pathological stage and clinical outcome in prostate cancer: an improved preoperative model incorporating biopsy-determined intraductal carcinoma. Br J Urol. 1998;81:413–8.
36. Van der Kwast T, Al Daoud N, Collette L, Sykes J, Thoms J, Milosevic M, et al. Biopsy diagnosis of intraductal carcinoma is prognostic in intermediate and high risk prostate cancer patients treated by radiotherapy. Eur J Cancer. 2012;48:1318–25.
37. Efstathiou E, Abrahams NA, Tibbs RF, Wang X, Pettaway CA, Pisters LL, et al. Morphologic characterization of preoperatively treated prostate cancer: toward a post-therapy histologic classification. Eur Urol. 2010;57:1030–8.
38. O'Brien BA, Cohen RJ, Wheeler TM, Moorin RE. A post-radical-prostatectomy nomogram incorporating new pathological variables and interaction terms for improved prognosis. BJU Int. 2011;107:389–95.
39. Wernert N, Goebbels R, Bonkhoff H, Dhom G. Squamous cell carcinoma of the prostate. Histopathology. 1990;17:339–44.
40. Little NA, Wiener JS, Walther PJ, Paulson DF, Anderson EE. Squamous cell carcinoma of the pros-

tate: 2 cases of a rare malignancy and review of the literature. J Urol. 1993;149:137–9.
41. Malik RD, Dakwar G, Hardee ME, Sanfilippo NJ, Rosenkrantz AB, Taneja SS. Squamous cell carcinoma of the prostate. Rev Urol. 2011;13:56–60.
42. John TT, Bashir J, Burrow CT, Machin DG. Squamous cell carcinoma of the prostate—a case report. Int Urol Nephrol. 2005;37:311–3.
43. Sarma DP, Weilbaecher TG, Moon TD. Squamous cell carcinoma of prostate. Urology. 1991;37:260–2.
44. Chang JM, Lee HJ, Lee SE, Byun SS, Choe GY, Kim SH, et al. Pictorial review: unusual tumours involving the prostate: radiological-pathological findings. Br J Radiol. 2008;81:907–15.
45. Mott LJ. Squamous cell carcinoma of the prostate: report of 2 cases and review of the literature. J Urol. 1979;121:833–5.
46. Nabi G, Ansari MS, Singh I, Sharma MC, Dogra PN. Primary squamous cell carcinoma of the prostate: a rare clinicopathological entity. Report of 2 cases and review of literature. Urol Int. 2001;66:216–9.
47. Munoz F, Franco P, Ciammella P, Clerico M, Giudici M, Filippi AR, et al. Squamous cell carcinoma of the prostate: long-term survival after combined chemoradiation. Radiat Oncol. 2007;2:15.
48. Dundore PA, Cheville JC, Nascimento AG, Farrow GM, Bostwick DG. Carcinosarcoma of the prostate. Report of 21 cases. Cancer. 1995;76:1035–42.
49. Hansel DE, Epstein JI. Sarcomatoid carcinoma of the prostate: a study of 42 cases. Am J Surg Pathol. 2006;30:1316–21.
50. Goto T, Maeshima A, Oyamada Y, Kato R. Solitary pulmonary metastasis from prostate sarcomatoid cancer. World J Surg Oncol. 2010;8:101.
51. Reyes A, Moran CA. Low-grade neuroendocrine carcinoma (carcinoid tumor) of the prostate. Arch Pathol Lab Med. 2004;128:e166–8.
52. Giordano S, Tolonen T, Tolonen T, Hirsimaki S, Kataja V. A pure primary low-grade neuroendocrine carcinoma (carcinoid tumor) of the prostate. Int Urol Nephrol. 2010;42:683–7.
53. Turbat-Herrera EA, Herrera GA, Gore I, Lott RL, Grizzle WE, Bonnin JM. Neuroendocrine differentiation in prostatic carcinomas. A retrospective autopsy study. Arch Pathol Lab Med. 1988;112:1100–5.
54. Freschi M, Colombo R, Naspro R, Rigatti P. Primary and pure neuroendocrine tumor of the prostate. Eur Urol. 2004;45:166–9; discussion 169–170.
55. Ketata S, Ketata H, Fakhfakh H, Sahnoun A, Bahloul A, Boudawara T, et al. Pure primary neuroendocrine tumor of the prostate: a rare entity. Clin Genitourin Cancer. 2006;5:82–4.
56. Abbas F, Civantos F, Benedetto P, Soloway MS. Small cell carcinoma of the bladder and prostate. Urology. 1995;46:617–30.
57. Stein ME, Bernstein Z, Abacioglu U, Sengoz M, Miller RC, Meirovitz A, et al. Small cell (neuroendocrine) carcinoma of the prostate: etiology, diagnosis, prognosis, and therapeutic implications—a retrospective study of 30 patients from the rare cancer network. Am J Med Sci. 2008;336:478–88.
58. Palmgren JS, Karavadia SS, Wakefield MR. Unusual and underappreciated: small cell carcinoma of the prostate. Semin Oncol. 2007;34:22–9.
59. Spiess PE, Pettaway CA, Vakar-Lopez F, Kassouf W, Wang X, Busby JE, et al. Treatment outcomes of small cell carcinoma of the prostate: a single-center study. Cancer. 2007;110:1729–37.
60. Iczkowski KA, Ferguson KL, Grier DD, Hossain D, Banerjee SS, McNeal JE, et al. Adenoid cystic/basal cell carcinoma of the prostate: clinicopathologic findings in 19 cases. Am J Surg Pathol. 2003;27:1523–9.
61. Ayyathurai R, Civantos F, Soloway MS, Manoharan M. Basal cell carcinoma of the prostate: current concepts. BJU Int. 2007;99:1345–9.
62. Frankel K, Craig JR. Adenoid cystic carcinoma of the prostate. Report of a case. Am J Clin Pathol. 1974;62:639–45.
63. Gilmour AM, Bell TJ. Adenoid cystic carcinoma of the prostate. Br J Urol. 1986;58:105–6.
64. Ali TZ, Epstein JI. Basal cell carcinoma of the prostate: a clinicopathologic study of 29 cases. Am J Surg Pathol. 2007;31:697–705.
65. Manrique JJ, Albores-Saavedra J, Orantes A, Brandt H. Malignant mixed tumor of the salivary-gland type, primary in the prostate. Am J Clin Pathol. 1978;70:932–7.
66. Eswara JR, Efstathiou JA, Heney NM, Paly J, Kaufman DS, McDougal WS, et al. Complications and long-term results of salvage cystectomy after failed bladder sparing therapy for muscle invasive bladder cancer. J Urol. 2012;187:463–8.
67. James ND, Hussain SA, Hall E, Jenkins P, Tremlett J, Rawlings C, et al. Radiotherapy with or without chemotherapy in muscle-invasive bladder cancer. N Engl J Med. 2012;366:1477–88.
68. Rozet F, Lesur G, Cathelineau X, Barret E, Smyth G, Soon S, et al. Oncological evaluation of prostate sparing cystectomy: the Montsouris long-term results. J Urol. 2008;179:2170–4; discussion 2174–2175.
69. Klotz L, Pinthus J. The case for prostate capsule-sparing radical cystectomy in selected patients. Can Urol Assoc J. 2009;3:S215–9.
70. Ayyathurai R, Gomez P, Luongo T, Soloway MS, Manoharan M. Prostatic involvement by urothelial carcinoma of the bladder: clinicopathological features and outcome after radical cystectomy. BJU Int. 2007;100:1021–5.
71. Richards KA, Parks GE, Badlani GH, Kader AK, Hemal AK, Pettus JA. Developing selection criteria for prostate-sparing cystectomy: a review of cystoprostatectomy specimens. Urology. 2010;75:1116–20.
72. Mazzucchelli R, Barbisan F, Santinelli A, Scarpelli M, Galosi AB, Lopez-Beltran A, et al. Prediction of prostatic involvement by urothelial carcinoma in radical cystoprostatectomy for bladder cancer. Urology. 2009;74:385–90.
73. Osunkoya AO, Netto GJ, Epstein JI. Colorectal adenocarcinoma involving the prostate: report of 9

cases. Hum Pathol. 2007;38:1836–41.
74. Schips L, Zigeuner RE, Langner C, Mayer R, Pummer K, Hubmer G. Metastasis of an ascending colon carcinoma in the prostate 10 years after hemicolectomy. J Urol. 2002;168:641–2.
75. Berman JR, Nunnemann RG, Broshears JR, Berman IR. Sigmoid colon carcinoma metastatic to prostate. Urology. 1993;41:150–2.
76. Muglia VF, Saber G, Maggioni G Jr., Monteiro AJ. MRI findings of prostate stromal tumour of uncertain malignant potential: a case report. Br J Radiol. 2011;84:e194–6.
77. Herawi M, Epstein JI. Specialized stromal tumors of the prostate: a clinicopathologic study of 50 cases. Am J Surg Pathol. 2006;30:694–704.
78. Klausner AP, Unger P, Fine EM. Recurrent prostatic stromal proliferation of uncertain malignant potential: a therapeutic challenge. J Urol. 2002;168:1493–4.
79. Wee HM, Ho SH, Tan PH. Recurrent prostatic stromal tumour of uncertain malignant potential (STUMP) presenting with urinary retention 6 Years after transurethral resection of prostate (TURP). Ann Acad Med Singapore. 2005;34:441–2.
80. Gaudin PB, Rosai J, Epstein JI. Sarcomas and related proliferative lesions of specialized prostatic stroma: a clinicopathologic study of 22 cases. Am J Surg Pathol. 1998;22:148–62.
81. Akin O, Sala E, Moskowitz CS, Kuroiwa K, Ishill NM, Pucar D, et al. Transition zone prostate cancers: features, detection, localization, and staging at endorectal MR imaging. Radiology. 2006;239:784–92.
82. Chang YS, Chuang CK, Ng KF, Liao SK. Prostatic stromal sarcoma in a young adult: a case report. Arch Androl. 2005;51:419–24.
83. Morikawa T, Goto A, Tomita K, Tsurumaki Y, Ota S, Kitamura T, et al. Recurrent prostatic stromal sarcoma with massive high-grade prostatic intraepithelial neoplasia. J Clin Pathol. 2007;60:330–2.
84. Probert JL, O'Rourke JS, Farrow R, Cox P. Stromal sarcoma of the prostate. Eur J Surg Oncol. 2000;26:100–1.
85. Osaki M, Osaki M, Takahashi C, Miyagawa T, Adachi H, Ito H. Prostatic stromal sarcoma: case report and review of the literature. Pathol Int. 2003;53:407–11.
86. Tamada T, Sone T, Miyaji Y, Kozuka Y, Ito K. MRI appearance of prostatic stromal sarcoma in a young adult. Korean J Radiol. 2011;12:519–23.
87. Huang YC, Wang JY, Lin PY, Chin CC, Chen CS. Synchronous prostate stromal sarcoma and gastrointestinal stromal tumor of rectum: case report and review of the literature. Urology. 2006;68:672 e611–73.
88. Anagnostou E, Miliaras D, Panagiotakopoulos V. Diagnosis of gastrointestinal stromal tumor (GIST) on transurethral resection of the prostate: a case report and review of the literature. Int J Surg Pathol. 2011;19:632–6.
89. Lee CH, Lin YH, Lin HY, Lee CM, Chu JS. Gastrointestinal stromal tumor of the prostate: a case report and literature review. Hum Pathol. 2006;37:1361–5.
90. Van der Aa F, Sciot R, Blyweert W, Ost D, Van Poppel H, Van Oosterom A, et al. Gastrointestinal stromal tumor of the prostate. Urology. 2005;65:388.
91. Madden JF, Burchette JL, Raj GV, Daly JT, Tannenbaum M. Anterior rectal wall gastrointestinal stromal tumor presenting clinically as prostatic mass. Urol Oncol. 2005;23:268–72.
92. Voelzke BB, Sakamoto K, Hantel A, Paner GP, Kash J, Waters WB, et al. Gastrointestinal stromal tumor: involvement in urologic patients and recent therapeutic advances. Urology. 2002;60:218–22.
93. Demetri GD, von Mehren M, Blanke CD, Van den Abbeele AD, Eisenberg B, Roberts PJ, et al. Efficacy and safety of imatinib mesylate in advanced gastrointestinal stromal tumors. N Engl J Med. 2002;347:472–80.
94. Herawi M, Montgomery EA, Epstein JI. Gastrointestinal stromal tumors (GISTs) on prostate needle biopsy: a clinicopathologic study of 8 cases. Am J Surg Pathol. 2006;30:1389–95.
95. Din OS, Woll PJ. Treatment of gastrointestinal stromal tumor: focus on imatinib mesylate. Ther Clin Risk Manag. 2008;4:149–62.

7 Nomograms for Prostate Cancer Decision Making

Cesar E. Ercole, Michael W. Kattan and Andrew J. Stephenson

Introduction

Patients should have a frank discussion with their physician to determine if screening for prostate cancer is a path they desire to embark upon. Those who opt for cancer screening will start by getting a blood test to measure their prostate-specific antigen (PSA) levels and a digital rectal examination (DRE). An elevated PSA (or a rising trend) and/or an abnormal prostate exam may lead to a transrectal ultrasound-guided prostate needle biopsy for a pathologic diagnosis. Should cancer be detected, it is in the hope to identify early organ-confined prostate adenocarcinoma. Having a diagnosis is only part of the subsequent decision-making process, as men with clinically localized prostate cancer are candidates for definitive therapy, which may be in the form of radical therapy or active surveillance for a cancer that may pose an uncertain threat to the patient's longevity [1]. Healthy men with long life expectancy may seek an aggressive treatment modality such as radical prostatectomy, external-beam radiation therapy, and brachytherapy. These are considered standard treatment alternatives (with the exception of brachytherapy as monotherapy for high-risk disease) and none has been definitively proven to be superior in terms of cancer control.

A major factor for the patient in deciding amongst these options is their impact on quality of life. From an oncological perspective long-term cancer control is the main goal, yet this may not prove to be the optimal therapy for that individual patient based on the therapy's potential to affect on his quality of life. He may be unwilling to accept the treatment option with the highest likelihood of cure if it is also associated with unacceptable morbidity. All treatments may negatively impact urinary, sexual, and bowel function to varying degrees which the patient must take into consideration. For example, radical prostatectomy is associated with a higher incidence of urinary incontinence, while external-beam radiotherapy and brachytherapy are associated with higher rates of bowel dysfunction and irritative bladder symptoms. Each of these therapies also affects sexual function to varying degrees. When balancing this information, the patient must also consider his values and priorities.

The final decision for the treatment choice is personal and individualized. The patient needs to consider the consequences of choosing one treatment over another, generally selecting the one that will have the least impact on his quality of life yet optimizing his chances for cure. He is the only one that can decide how much he

A. J. Stephenson (✉) · C. E. Ercole
Center for Urologic Oncology, Cleveland Clinic, Glickman Urological and Kidney Institute, Cleveland, OH, USA
e-mail: Stephea2@ccf.org

C. E. Ercole
e-mail: ercolec@ccf.org

M. W. Kattan
Department of Quantitative Health Sciences, Cleveland Clinic, Cleveland, OH, USA
e-mail: kattanm@ccf.edu

C. Magi-Galluzzi, C. G. Przybycin (eds.), *Genitourinary Pathology,* DOI 10.1007/978-1-4939-2044-0_7,

is willing to compromise long-term cancer control over treatment-related morbidity on quality of life. This is where the physician serves more as an advisor and guides the patient to make a decision that most suits his principles and lifestyle. Knowing how the patient feels about each treatment will make this easier, especially if the patient feels strongly one way or another in favor of a particular treatment modality. Some patients may opt for observation, whereas others may not be able to rest until the prostate is surgically removed. Ultimately, the decision needs to be made by the patient. In return this will limit any regret on his part, especially if he is to experience a bad outcome from the treatment.

Paramount to the patient's decision making are accurate probabilities of the potential outcomes of each treatment modality in terms of its success, complications, and long-term morbidity. This will promote a more positive environment allowing the patient to be more satisfied after treatment. A risk that leads to patient regret is failing to fully consider all the treatment options that are available to him. Equipped with accurate probabilities of the outcomes of each therapy, the physician can avoid being overly optimistic (which may lead to regret and disappoint on the part of the patient if he experiences a bad outcome) and pessimistic (which may have influenced a patient to forgo a treatment that he would otherwise have benefitted from). To have a well-informed patient and to make quality treatment decisions, the physician should endeavor to provide accurate probabilities of outcomes that could occur as a consequence of the decision to undergo (or forgo) a specific treatment. Subsequently, when a recommendation is made for or against a particular treatment modality, it is evidence based.

Historically, physicians used clinical judgment to assign risks when counseling patients about treatment. Unfortunately, it is human nature to incorporate bias into each stage of decision making. Personal experience clouds how events get transcribed and affects memory leading to inconsistency, allowing the physician to rely on heuristics when the decision process becomes difficult. This leads to bias for the preferred outcome rather than the outcome with the highest probability. Prognostic variables for prostate cancer progression have been defined to include PSA, clinical stage, biopsy Gleason score, and individual surgeon technique. The challenge for the physician is to figure out the relative importance of each of these factors and how they affect outcomes.

To assist the physician, researchers have developed prediction tools. By design, prediction models incorporate different variables and generally perform as well or better than clinical judgment to predict outcome probabilities [2]. Therefore, outcome prediction tools help personalize patient care by allowing the patient to see his likelihood of short- and long-term oncological and functional outcomes associated with each treatment modality when deciding upon his treatment for his cancer diagnosis.

Developing Prediction Models

One method to developing a prediction model is to assess patients and group them based on similarities, then make predictions for each group. One such method was used by D'Amico et al. to develop a model to predict cancer control for patients treated with radical prostatectomy, external-beam radiotherapy, or brachytherapy [3]. The model places patients into mutually exclusive risk groups based on pretreatment PSA level, biopsy Gleason score, and clinical stage. Grouping patients makes sense, yet it is limiting by not allowing to maximize the predictive accuracy of a prognostic model based on the available data. One needs to be careful with the evaluation of a subset of patients, as this ignores the relative importance of prognostic variables in another patient group. To accurately represent each risk factor and variable, one must not assign equal weight to each variable, as each does not exert an equal prognostic weight on the outcome. An additional limit in risk grouping is converting continuous variables into categorical variables, thus removing information about the actual value.

Another approach is the prognostic index, which is often based on a Cox or logistic regression model. A numerical score is assigned to an individual parameter in the model based on its parameter estimate or hazard ratio. The sum of each parameter's score gives a total score. One such index is the Cancer of the Prostate Risk Assessment (CAPRA) score [4]. When using this index, the patient is assigned a CAPRA score between 0 and 10 based on the points assigned for PSA (0–4), biopsy Gleason score (0–3), clinical stage (0–1), percentage of positive biopsy cores (0–1), and age (0–1). The patient's estimated 5-year recurrence-free probability after a radical prostatectomy is based on each point of the CAPRA score.

The nomogram serves an alternative to risk group or prognostic index prediction tool, as it is used to develop continuous multivariable models and predict a particular endpoint. It is a graphic representation of a mathematical formula or algorithm that incorporates several predictors modeled as continuous variables to predict the endpoint. A nomogram consists of sets of axes; each variable is represented by a scale, with each value of that variable corresponding to a specific number of points according to its prognostic significance. By using scales, nomograms calculate the *continuous* probability of a particular outcome. This is shown by the nomogram in Fig. 7.1, where each PSA level is assigned a unique point

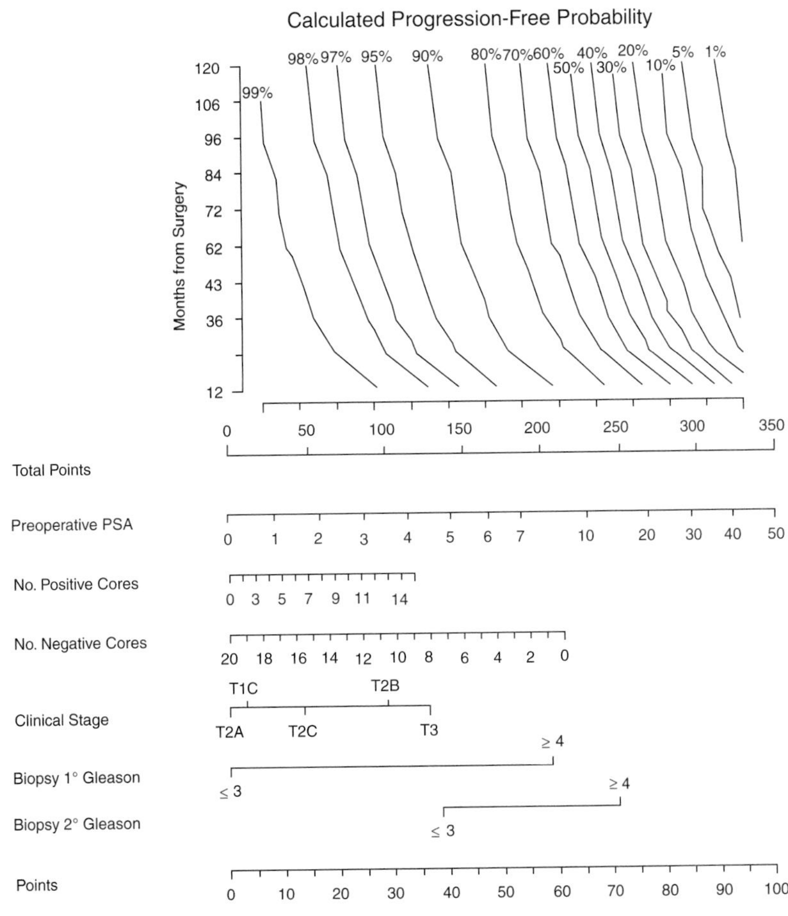

Fig. 7.1 Preoperative nomogram based on 1978 patients treated by two high-volume surgeons between 1987 and 2003 for predicting the 10-year probability of freedom from prostate-specific antigen (*PSA*) recurrence after radical prostatectomy using preoperative *PSA* level, number of positive and negative biopsy cores, clinical stage, and primary and secondary biopsy Gleason grade. The predictions of the model are adjusted for the year of surgery and the model assumes patients are treated in 2003 (the most recent year of treatment of patients included in this model). (Used with permission from [15])

value that represents its prognostic significance. The final pair of axes is used to obtain a total point value from all the variables and converted into the probability of reaching the endpoint.

The advantage of nomograms is that they incorporate all relevant continuous predictive factors for individual patients, thus providing a more accurate prediction than models based on risk grouping. They usually also surpass clinical experts at outcome's prediction by calculating probabilities in a uniform fashion. The superior performance has been shown by several studies comparing nomograms to risk-grouping schemata, in part, due to substantial heterogeneity within risk group categories. A good example of the heterogeneity inherent in risk groups is shown in Fig. 7.2 where the 5-year progression-free probability (PFP) after radical prostatectomy was calculated for patients classified as low-, medium-, and high-risk using the criteria by D'Amico et al. [5]. The graph shows a substantial distribution of intermediate- and high-risk patients across the spectra of nomogram probabilities; clearly, it would be incorrect to call a patient "high-risk" if their likelihood of being free of cancer progression at 5 years exceeded 90%. This highlights the substantial heterogeneity within risk group's categories and as such, is useful for gauging the prognosis for that specific group of patients, not necessarily the individual patient. A nomogram should be able to be tailored to an individual patient, as this is what is most important to the patient, that is his individual prognosis not that of a group.

A nomogram can be used to personalize the prediction of outcomes for an individual based on his unique characteristics. The complexity of nomograms over risk groups enhances the predictive

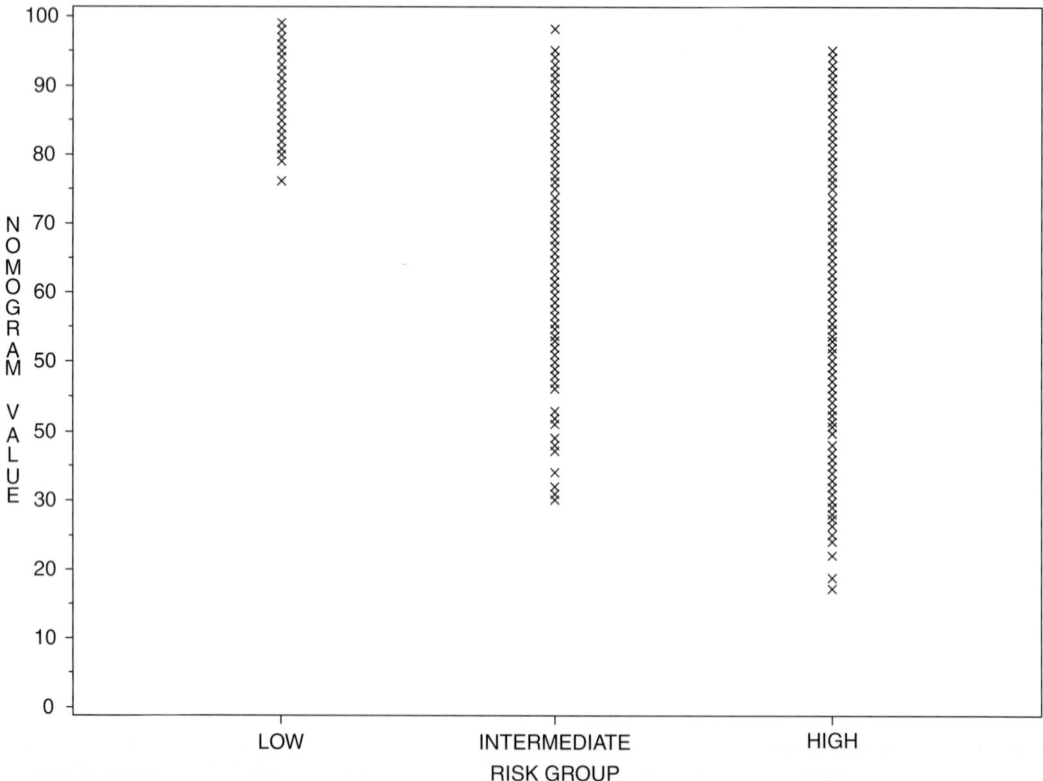

Fig. 7.2 Five-year progression-free probability after radical prostatectomy calculated by preoperative nomogram for patients classified as low-, intermediate-, and high-risk by D'Amico et al. based on an analysis of patients from the CaPSURE database. (Used with permission from [5])

accuracy for both the patient and the physician. While cumbersome to use in paper form (and nearly impossible to calculate in one's head!), the availability of the nomograms in on-line web format in the public domain facilitates their use in the setting of a busy clinic (http://www.nomograms.org or htttp://www.clinicriskcalculators.org).

One way to illustrate the superior predictive performance of nomograms relative to risk groups is to compare several staging nomograms to the "Partin Tables." The Partin tables take into account serum PSA (four categories), clinical stage (seven categories), and biopsy Gleason sum (five categories) to predict pathological stage of prostate cancer. Then the patient is assigned to one of the four mutually exclusive groups (organ confined, established extraprostatic extension (EPE), seminal vesicle invasion (SVI), or lymph node involvement (LNI)). In a review of our institution's prostate cancer database, the predictive accuracy of the "Partin Tables" for predicting organ-confined disease, SVI, and LNI was 0.71, 0.72, and 0.74, respectively [6]. These tables underestimate the probability of EPE, since a substantial proportion of patients with lymph node metastases and SVI will also have EPE. A more accurate predictive model is done with having each variable as a continuous variable. Thus, PSA, clinical stage, and Gleason sum when modeled as a continuous variable had a concordance index for predicting organ-confined disease, SVI, and LNI of 0.74, 0.84, and 0.76, respectively (Bianco FJ Jr et al., unpublished data).

Some general principles need to be taken into consideration with designing a predictive model. First is *discrimination*, the model should accurately predict which patients will and will not reach the endpoint. Next *calibration*, the model should be able to make predictions that reflect actual outcomes. And finally, *validation*, the model should perform consistently when applied to different data sets. Careful consideration should be taken when determining the patient population that the model will be based on. The model should have an index patient that is representative of the general population to whom the model will be applied. The treatments being received by the cohort population should mirror those of the general population. There should be a built-in broad applicability to the model. Trying to define a very specific population or to model after a population with uncommon treatment modalities will limit the model's application to future patients. A good predictive model should not only be based on enough cases to be able to reach specific endpoints, but also have an appropriate number of variables. The model should include variables that are statistically significant and those that are not statistically significant (if there is a strong clinical rationale for including them). Including only significant variables will result in falsely narrowed confidence intervals (CI) that make the model appear more accurate than it is, secondary to the inappropriately large influence exerted by these variables. A well-constructed model will repeatedly perform with similar accuracy when applied to *heterogeneous* novel populations, hence exemplify *generalizability*. Factors that diminish this concept are when a prognostic model's data set is too small, not all the variables are recorded correctly or large portions missing, or too many variables are used. In the clinical setting, the value of a nomogram is when it is easy to use and it uses parameters that are routinely employed and reliable. The ease of use is important, because even though a model may be very accurate, if it proves cumbersome to use, then it loses its practicality in the clinical setting.

Kattan and colleagues developed nomograms based on Cox proportional hazards or logistic regression analysis modified by restricted cubic splines. The use of cubic splines has the benefit of being able to use continuous variable while maintaining a nonlinear relationship. When using unmodified regression models, they require variables to assume linear relationships, which is not ideal because it assumes that the weight assigned to incremental changes is the same across the spectrum. For example, a rise in PSA from 3 to 6 ng/mL would have the same impact as a rise from 303 to 306 ng/mL. In theory, machine learning modeling methods (e.g., artificial neural networks) may lead to enhanced predictive accuracy as they offer greater flexibility than traditional statistical methods. This is especially true if data sets contain highly predictive nonlinear or interactive effects. In spite of this, traditional statistical methods seem to perform as well as machine learning methods and provide the added advantage of reproducibility and interpretability through the generation of hazard ratios and tests of significance for the predictors.

A benefit of nomograms is that they maximize the available information in a data set, in return obtaining the most value out of each variable. An example is when looking at a Gleason score, as it may be further defined by the primary and secondary Gleason grades and then each may be used as independent variables, rather than using the Gleason score alone, especially since various combinations of primary/secondary Gleason grades can result in the same Gleason score (e.g., 3+4=7 and 4+3=7) yet reflect quite different disease states with different prognoses [7].

Many nomograms that predict cancer recurrence incorporate an important concept of how patients who receive secondary treatment before demonstrating disease progression are classified as treatment failures. As the secondary treatment was most likely triggered by an adverse feature associated with a high risk of recurrence or some evidence of recurrence, therefore it is presumed that the treatment is given shortly before the recurrence would have declared itself [8]. One could exclude these patients from the nomogram, but censoring (or excluding) them would bias the nomogram towards improved outcomes. Including these patients but assigning treatment failure at the time of adjuvant therapy may lead to overly pessimistic predictions. A different and favored approach is to view the use of secondary therapy as a time-dependent covariate instead of as a fixed parameter like pathological stage.

Rather than the area under the receiver operator characteristic curve (AUC), the discrimination of these nomograms is measured using the concordance index (or *c*-index). The *c*-index functions in the presence of case censoring and is more appropriate for analyzing survival or time-to-event data, while the AUC requires binary outcomes (e.g., yes/no).

Nomograms are calibrated and then validated to determine accuracy. If an external validation (i.e., the gold standard) is not possible for evaluating accuracy and reproducibility, then internal validation methods may be used, such as jackknife, leave-one-out cross-validation, and bootstrapping. These are considered legitimate alternatives that can be used alone or together with external validation to assess the nomograms accuracy.

Clinical States of Prostate

A patient-centric as opposed to treatment-centric way of thinking about prostate cancer is achieved by using a multistate model as proposed by Scher and Heller [9]. In the clinical states' model, prostate cancer is assessed by a series of clinical states with the spectrum ranging from diagnosis to death from prostate cancer (or death from competing causes) which reflects its treated natural history (Fig. 7.3) [9]. At each state, the patient is faced with different prognoses in terms of the risk of progressing from one clinical state to the next (and ultimately dying from his disease) versus dying from competing causes. Different treatment decisions about the need of further therapy and the nature, risks, and benefits of those treatment alternatives need to be addressed. As previously discussed, accurate estimates of treatment success and side effects (and informed decision making) will determine what an appropriate treatment is for the patient at each clinical state. To our benefit, there are published validated nomograms for some of the endpoints of interest at each clinical state to help guide the clinical decision-making process in the clinical states' model. At this time, there are well over 100 published prediction tools of various accuracy that have been developed for use in risk estimation for all clinical states of prostate cancer. We sought to review some of the prediction models in the literature for each of these clinical states with an emphasis on those focused on localized prostate cancer.

Clinically Localized Disease

The first patient we will evaluate is a man with localized prostate cancer, who is interested in

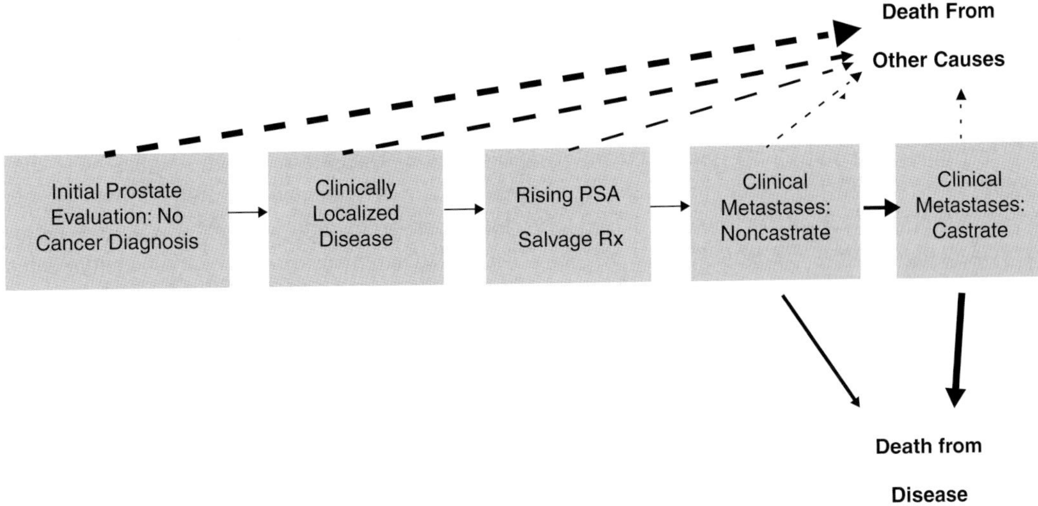

Fig. 7.3 Clinical states' model of prostate cancer progression. *Dashed line arrows* indicate pathways from a clinical state to a nonprostate cancer-related mortality; *solid line arrows* indicate pathways from a clinical state to a prostate cancer-related mortality. *PSA* prostate-specific antigen. (Used with permission from [9])

knowing the risk of developing symptoms and/or dying from his disease, with or without definitive local therapy. He would also determine the likelihood of treatment success with radical therapy and the short- and long-term complications of therapy. Several nomograms have been developed for prostate cancer recurrence after definitive local therapy [10]. The management of prostate cancer carries with it treatment-related morbidity. There is a need for nomograms that estimate the likelihood of treatment-related morbidity (e.g., urinary incontinence, sexual dysfunction, bowel dysfunction). The scope of this discussion will be limited to contemporary models that predict the continuous risk of disease progression, developing distant metastasis, and/or prostate cancer-specific mortality (PCSM) after definitive therapy with radical prostatectomy, external-beam radiotherapy, transperineal brachytherapy, and with expectant management. Models that evaluate PFP are mostly based on biochemical recurrence (rising PSA) posttreatment. Considering that at 15 years the risk of death from prostate cancer for men with biochemical recurrence is 33 %, just about equal to risk of death from competing causes, it is imprecise to use it as a substitute for distant metastasis and PCSM [11]. The physician can use both pretreatment and posttreatment nomograms to help decide between the various treatment alternatives for clinically localized prostate cancer and/or the need for multimodal therapy. They can also be used to determine the need for adjuvant therapy and/or the appropriate level of monitoring for posttreatment surveillance testing or imaging.

Radical Prostatectomy

Nomograms for pretreatment and posttreatment have been developed to predict the continuous probability of disease progression and PCSM after radical prostatectomy.

Pretreatment

Risk stratification based on clinical stage, biopsy Gleason score, and pretreatment serum PSA level, are known pretreatment variables associated with disease progression after radical prostatectomy. Along with the Partin et al. tables, these factors may be combined to predict the pathological stage of the prostatectomy specimen. The limit of this process is that the model is useful for surgical planning, but it often does not correlate with the risk of disease progression. It has been noted that 50 % of patients with nonorgan-confined disease were free from disease recurrence at 15 years after radical prostatectomy, confirming that the presence of extraprostatic disease does not imply definite disease progression.

The radical prostatectomy pretreatment nomogram developed by Kattan and colleagues predicts the 5-year PFP for patients based on clinical stage, biopsy Gleason score, and pretreatment PSA level. This model was designed on data from 983 patients with clinically localized prostate cancer treated by a single surgeon. The definition of disease progression was (1) an initial PSA rise to ≥0.4 ng/mL followed by any further rise above this level, (2) evidence of clinical recurrence (local, regional, or distant), (3) administration of adjuvant therapy, or (4) death from prostate cancer. Patients who had positive lymph nodes at the start of the prostatectomy resulting in an aborted procedure were classified as treatment failures at the time of surgery. For this cohort the overall 5-year PFP was 73 %. This model is accurate and discriminating with a concordance index (*c*-index) of 0.75 when applied to an international external validation cohort [12]. It also showed good validation when taking into consideration ethnicity with a *c*-index of 0.74 observed with the African-American population [13].

A substantial number of patients are at risk for disease progression after 5 years; therefore, a 5-year endpoint is insufficient to predict the likelihood of cure after radical prostatectomy. However, when evaluating patients after 10 years, recurrence is rare. For patients in our series treated with radical prostatectomy, disease progression was noted in 1 % of patients who had an undetectable PSA at 10 years or later after RP [14]. Therefore, a more appropriate endpoint to estimate cure from a radical prostatectomy alone, would be the 10-year PFP.

The original model designed by Kattan et al. was updated by extending the predictions to 10 years. The model was also adjusted for the stage migration of prostate cancer which occurred since the introduction of mass PSA screening (by including year of treatment as a predictor), and including information from a systematic prostate biopsy in terms of the number of positive and negative cores (Fig. 7.1) [15]. The nomogram is based on 1978 patients treated by two high-volume surgeons and externally validated with a cohort of 1545 patients treated at a separate institution. Data from several studies state that the results of systematic prostate biopsy provide important prognostic information, yet the inclusion of the number of positive and negative cores resulted in only a mild improvement in predictive accuracy over stage, grade, and PSA in independent validation (*c*-index 0.79 vs. 0.78). The model also has the ability to predict the probability of disease progression at any time point after radical prostatectomy between years 1 and 10.

Recently, we developed a pretreatment nomogram that predicts the 15-year PCSM after radical prostatectomy based on PSA, clinical stage, biopsy Gleason score, and the year of treatment (Fig. 7.4) [16]. The nomogram is based on a cohort consisting of 6398 patients treated between 1987 and 2005 by surgeons at Memorial Sloan-Kettering Cancer Center (MSKCC) and then the model was externally validated on 6279 patients treated at Cleveland Clinic and University of Michigan during the same period. The statistically significant predictors in the nomogram were the primary and secondary Gleason grade of the biopsy, PSA, and year of treatment, with the *c*-index of the model being 0.84. For those patients with a risk of biochemical recurrence greater than 50 % the PCSM was predicted to be less than 20 %, and overall it was noted to be 12 %. This means that the prognosis for patients with clinically localized prostate cancer is very favorable in terms of PCSM at 15 years, with only 1980 (17 %) patients having a predicted 15-year PCSM greater than 5 %, and 467(4 %) having a probability greater than 30 %. Another variable that has been evaluated as a predictor of PCSM is pretreatment PSA velocity, yet the predictive accuracy of the nomogram was not improved when including this variable.

Posttreatment

For posttreatment, we elaborated a nomogram to determine patients at high risk for developing disease progression after radical prostatectomy. This model uses the pretreatment PSA level, and

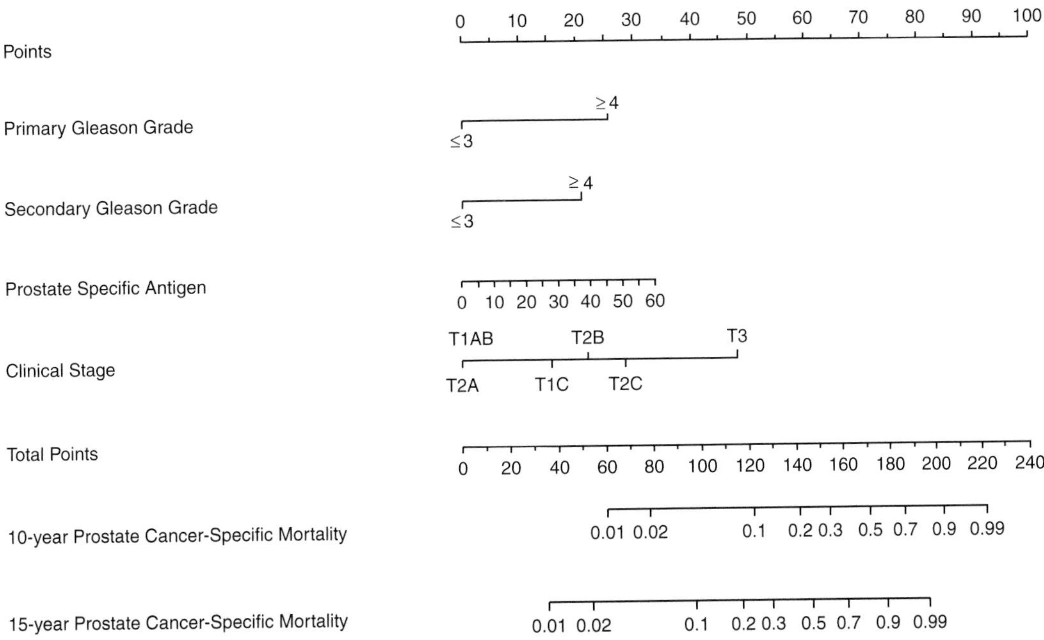

Fig. 7.4 Preoperative nomogram predicting 10- and 15-year prostate cancer-specific mortality after radical prostatectomy based on primary and secondary biopsy Gleason grade, preoperative PSA level, and clinical stage. The predictions of the model are adjusted for the year of surgery and the model assumes the patient is treated in 2005 (the most recent treatment year of patients included in the model). (Used with permission from [16])

then information from the pathology report, including: Gleason score, extraprostatic extension, margin status, SVI, and lymph node status to predict the 7-year probability of disease progression. The cohort used included 996 men with clinically localized prostate cancer treated by a single surgeon. Failure after treatment was defined as an initial PSA rise to ≥0.4 ng/mL followed by any further rise above this level, clinical evidence of disease progression (local or distant), initiation of adjuvant therapy, or death from prostate cancer. The 7-year PFP for this population was 73 %. The *c*-index for the nomogram was 0.80 when validated with an international cohort and 0.83 when validated with an African-American cohort [13].

This nomogram was also updated and improved to calculate the 10-year probability of prostate cancer recurrence after radical prostatectomy (Fig. 7.5) [17]. Just as for the pretreatment nomogram, treatment year was also included to adjust for the stage migration caused by widespread PSA screening. Special consideration was given to adjuvant radiotherapy, where in previous models it was considered treatment failure, in this model it was used as a time-dependent parameter. Taking into account that a patient's prognosis improves over time, the longer he stays disease-free, the nomogram was adjusted to reflect this in the 10-year PFP. The cohort for this nomogram consisted of 1881 patients treated by two high-volume surgeons between 1987 and 2003. The model was demonstrated to be accurate and discriminating (*c*-index 0.81 and 0.79) when used in two independent validation cohorts of 1782 and 1357 patients.

Similar to the preoperative nomogram, we developed a postoperative nomogram that predicts the 15-year PCSM after radical prostatectomy based on PSA, year of treatment, and the pathological features of prostate cancer in terms of grade, stage, and surgical margin status [16]. The model was developed with the clinical information of 11,521 patients treated by radical prostatectomy at four US academic centers from 1987 to 2005 and externally validated on 12,389 patients treated at a separate institution during

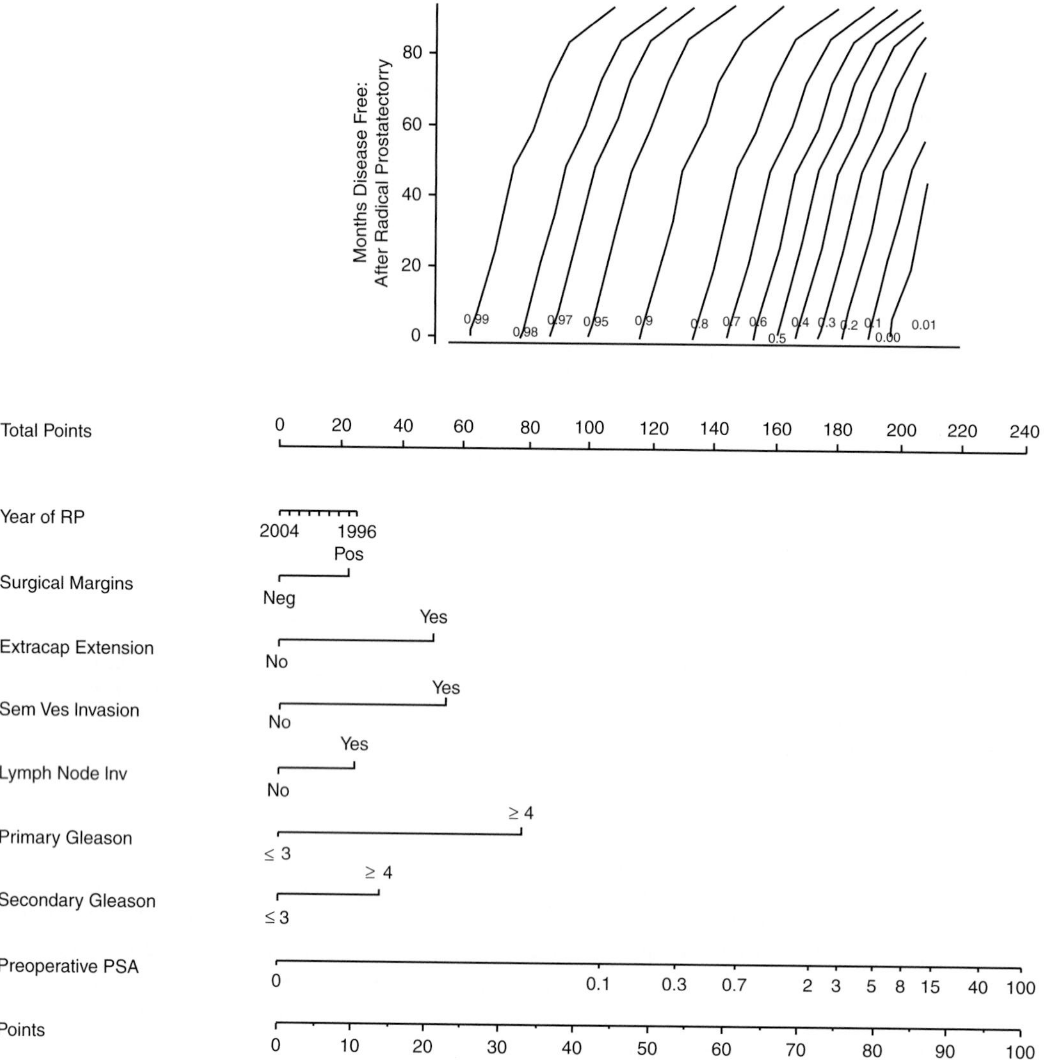

Instructions for physician: Locate patient's surgical margin status on the Surgical Margins axis. Draw a straight line down to the Points axis to determine how many points towards disease recurrence that patient receives for his surgical margin status. Repeat this process for each of the remaining axes. Sum the points for each predicator and locate this sum on the Total Points axis. Draw a line straight up from the Total Points axis unitl it intersects with the horizontal line drawn from the Months Disease-Free After Redical Prostateclomy, corresponding to the number of months the patient has maintained an undetectable PSA (this would equal zero for the immediate postoperative prediction). The slanted vertical line that crosses this intersection point corresponds to the calculated 10-years progression-free probability from the time of radical prostateclomy.

Instruction to patient: "Mr. X. if we had 100 men exactly like you, we would expect <predicated probability from nomogram x 100> to remain free of biochemical progression at 10 years following radical prostateclomy, and progression after 10 years is exceedingly rare.

Fig. 7.5 Postoperative nomogram predicting 10-year freedom from prostate-specific antigen (*PSA*) recurrence based on the pathological features of prostate cancer (primary and secondary pathological Gleason grade, extracapsular extension, seminal vesicle invasion, lymph node invasion, surgical margins) and preoperative PSA level. *RP* radical prostatectomy. (Used with permission from [17])

the same period. The model showed that primary and secondary Gleason grade 4 or 5, SVI, and year of surgery were significant predictors. The *c*-index was noted to be 0.92 with the externally validated cohort.

External-Beam Radiotherapy

To predict the 5-year PFP after treatment with three-dimensional conformal external-beam radiotherapy, Kattan et al. developed a pretreatment nomogram based on clinical stage, biopsy Gleason score, pretreatment PSA level, use of neoadjuvant androgen deprivation therapy, and radiation dose [18]. The model was based on a series of 1042 men treated at MSKCC between 1988 and 1998. The ASTRO criterion was used, which defines PSA failure as three cumulative rises of serum PSA level. The failure date was designated as the midpoint in time between the first rise and the PSA level immediately before this rise. Bootstrap analysis yielded a *c*-index of 0.73 and external validation with a cohort of 912 men treated at the Cleveland Clinic yielded a *c*-index of 0.76, which was significantly superior to the best risk grouping model available [18]. To also include patients treated with intensity-modulated radiotherapy (IMRT), the model was updated and the predictions were extended to 10 years. The biochemical recurrence endpoint was changed to correspond to the Phoenix definition of 2 ng/mL above the nadir PSA level (Fig. 7.6) [19]. The model was based on a cohort of 2253 patients treated with external-beam radiotherapy at MSKCC between 1988 and 2004. Using internal validation methods with bootstrapping, the *c*-index of the model was 0.72. We also developed a model to predict the 5-year metastasis-free probability after conformal external-beam

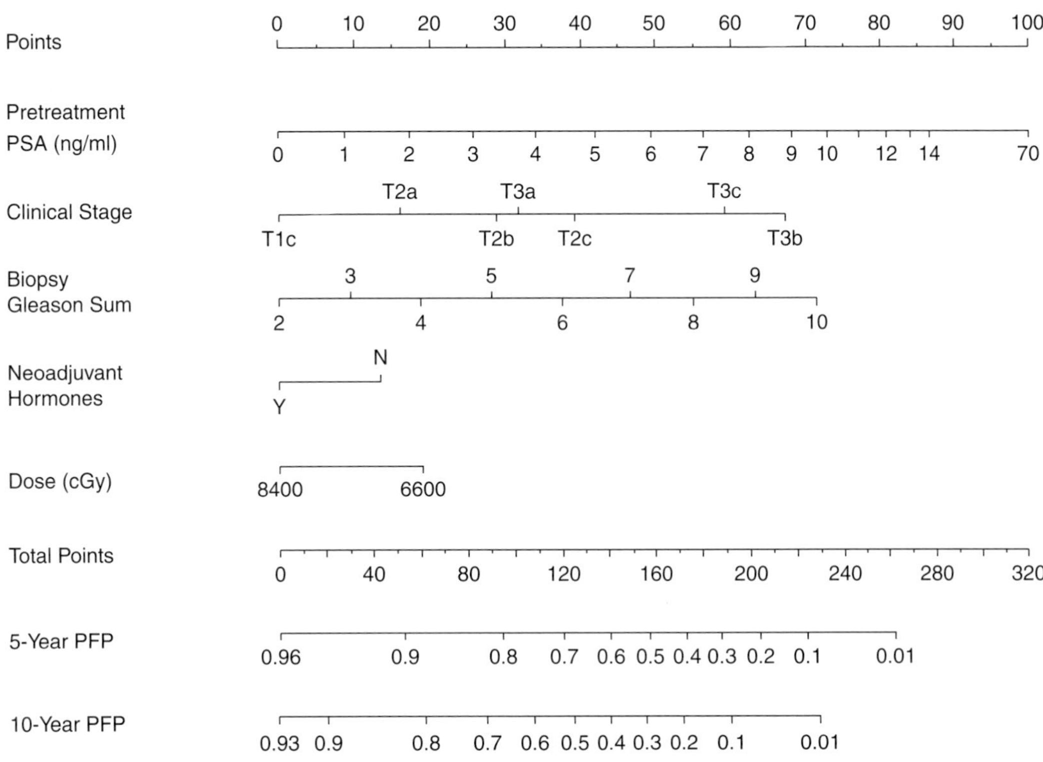

Fig. 7.6 Pretreatment nomogram predicting 5- or 10-year freedom from prostate-specific antigen (*PSA*) recurrence after three-dimensional conformal radiation therapy or intensity modulated radiation therapy based on 2253 patients treated at MSKCC between 1988 and 2004. The parameters used in the nomogram are pretreatment *PSA* level, clinical stage, biopsy Gleason score, use of neoadjuvant androgen deprivation therapy, and radiation dose. *PFP* progression-free probability. (Used with permission from [19])

radiotherapy based on a similar set of predictors [20]. The model was developed on 1677 patients treated at MSKCC between 1988 and 2000 and externally validated on 1626 patients treated at Cleveland Clinic during the same period. The *c*-index of the model was 0.81. Some of the limitations of this nomogram include the short interval to assess for metastatic disease (5 years), the lack of standardized surveillance imaging schedule to detect metastases, and the failure to adjust for the use of androgen deprivation therapy, which may substantially delay the appearance of distant metastasis.

Brachytherapy

Based on pretreatment PSA level, clinical stage, biopsy Gleason score, and the coadministration of external-beam radiotherapy, Kattan et al. developed a pretreatment nomogram that predicts the 5-year PFP after transperineal brachytherapy with ^{125}I seeds in the absence of adjuvant hormonal therapy [21]. The model was based on 920 men treated for T1–2 prostate cancer at MSKCC. Treatment failure was defined by (1) a modified version of the ASTRO criteria, (2) the administration of adjuvant androgen deprivation therapy, (3) clinical evidence of disease progression (local, regional, or distant), or (4) death from prostate cancer. The model was externally validated with a series of 1827 men treated at the Seattle Prostate Institute demonstrating a *c*-index of 0.61. Further validation with 765 men treated at Arizona Oncology Services yielded a *c*-index of 0.64. Potters et al. updated a postpermanent prostate brachytherapy version of this nomogram to also include postimplant dosimetry; disease progression was defined by the Phoenix criteria and the predictions of the model were extended to 9 years (Fig. 7.7) [22]. Clinical information from 5931 patients, who underwent brachytherapy for clinically localized prostate cancer from six centers, was used in the model and the internally validated *c*-index was 0.71. This model should be used as designed, that is, as a posttreatment model. Its predictions should not be used to influence the primary treatment decision of a patient

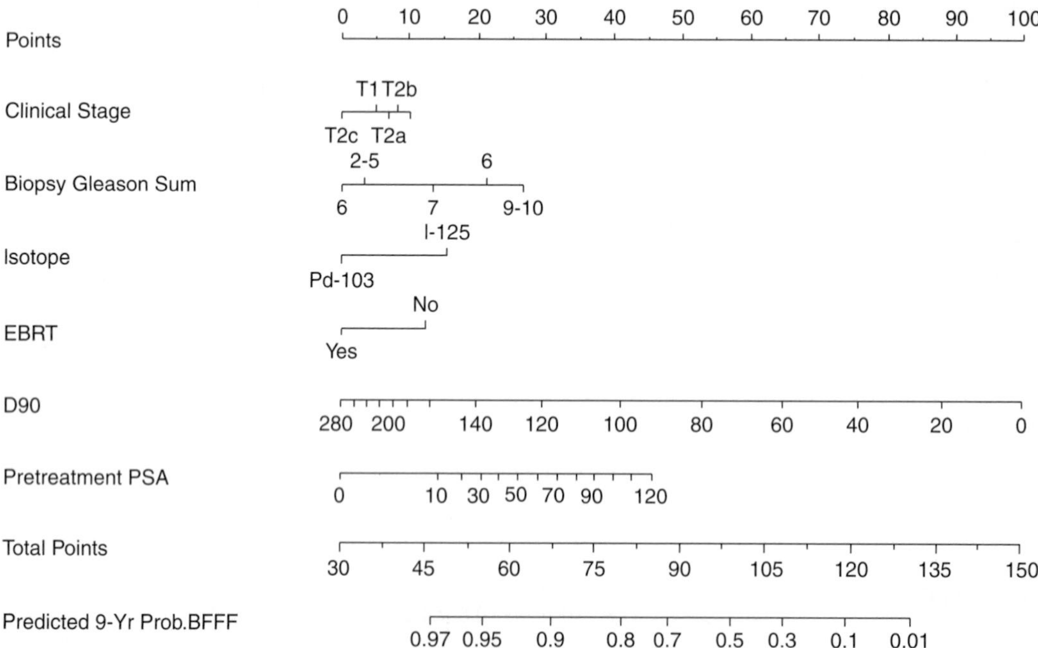

Fig. 7.7 Posttreatment nomogram predicting 9-year freedom from prostate-specific antigen (*PSA*) recurrence after permanent prostate brachytherapy without neoadjuvant androgen ablative therapy based on clinical stage, biopsy Gleason score, pretreatment *PSA* level, radioisotope, and the minimum calculated dose to 90 % of the prostate (D90). *EBRT* external beam radiation therapy, *BFFF* biochemical freedom from failure. (Used with permission from [22])

since the biologic equivalent dose administered is not known prior to treatment.

Active Surveillance or Watchful Waiting

The decision process for men with localized prostate cancer includes choosing to observe or monitoring with no invasive therapy, a decision based on the patient's comfort with placing more value on quality of life over side effects from treatment alternatives. Taking this into consideration, Kattan et al. developed a nomogram for men who did not receive any definitive local therapy with the ability to predict prostate cancer-specific survival at 10 years (Fig. 7.8) [23]. The model was based on a series of 1911 patients who did not receive any form of local therapy within 6 months of diagnosis identified from six cancer registries in England between 1990 and 1996. The patient information including PSA, biopsy Gleason score (centrally reviewed), clinical stage, method of diagnosis (biopsy vs. transurethral resection of the prostate, TURP), percentage of cancer, age, and the use of androgen deprivation therapy within 6 months of diagnosis were used in the modeling. The *c*-index of the model was 0.73, when using a two-thirds/one-third split-sample validation.

For patients wanting assistance with predicting if they have an indolent form of prostate cancer, which may not warrant aggressive treatment, Kattan et al. developed a nomogram to predict the probability of indolent prostate cancer [24]. These cancers were defined as a tumor volume <0.5 cc, pathological Gleason score ≤ 6, and confined to the prostate (Fig. 7.9). It is very unlikely that tumors that meet these criteria would progress to declare themselves with any symptomatology or cause a man's demise over the course of his lifetime in the absence of local therapy.

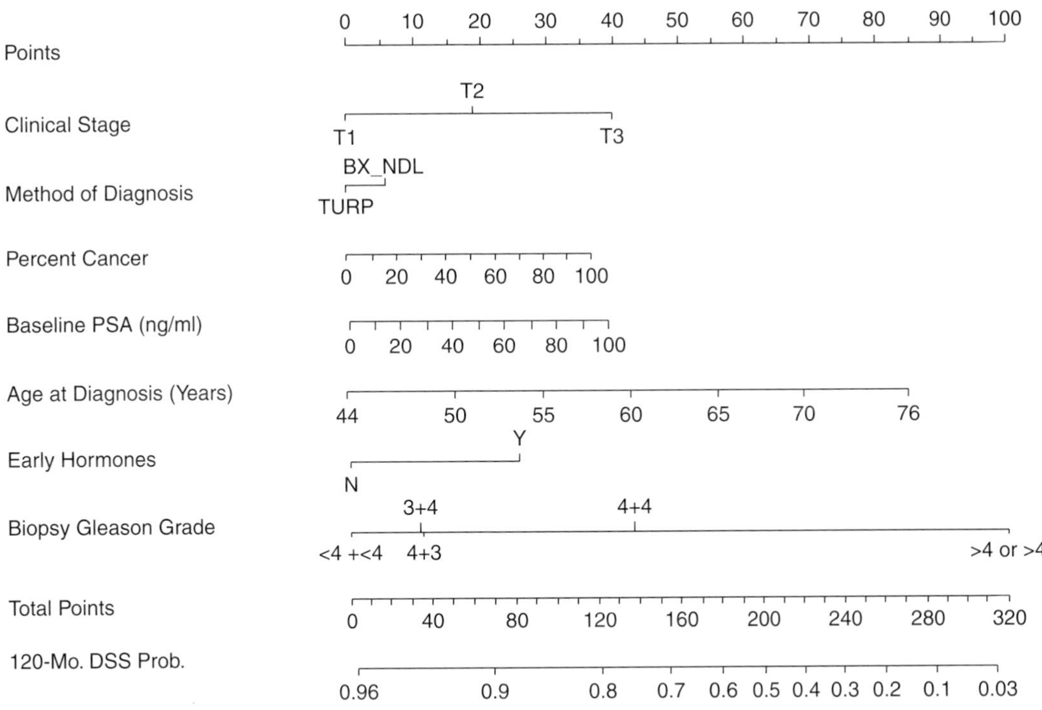

Fig. 7.8 Nomogram for predicting 10-year disease-specific survival for men with localized prostate cancer who are initially managed with a deferred treatment strategy. The parameters included in the nomogram are clinical stage, method of diagnosis (needle biopsy (*BX_NDL*) vs. transurethral resection of the prostate, *TURP*), percentage of cancer in the biopsy specimen, prostate-specific antigen (*PSA*) level at diagnosis, age at diagnosis, the use of early androgen deprivation therapy (within 6 months of diagnosis), and biopsy Gleason score. DSS = Disease Specific Survival (Used with permission from [23])

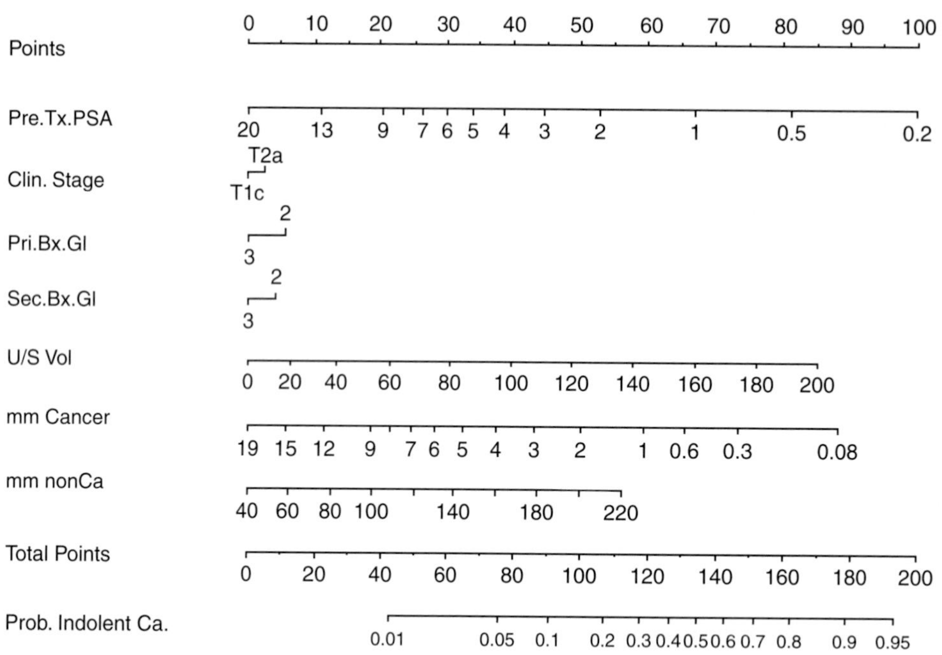

Instructions for Physician: Locate the patient's PSA on the **PreTx PSA** axis. Draw a line straight upwards to the **Points** axis determine how many points towards having an indolent cancer the patient receives for his PSA Repeat this process for the remaining axes, each time drawing straight upward to the **Points** axis. Sum the points achieved for each predictor and locate this sum on the **Total Points** axis Draw a line straight down to find the patient's probability of having indolent cancer.

Instruction to Patient: " Mr. X, if we had 100 men exactly like you, we would excep <predicted probability rom nomogran * 100 > to have indolent cancer."

Fig. 7.9 Nomogram predicting the presence of indolent prostate cancer (pathological Gleason score $\leq 3+3$, cancer volume <0.5 cc, organ confined) based on pretreatment prostate-specific antigen (*PSA*) level (*Pre.Tx.PSA*), clinical stage (*Clin.Stage*), primary (*Pri.Bx.Gl*) and secondary (*Sec.Bx.Gl*) biopsy Gleason grade, prostate volume by ultrasound (*U/S Vol*), length of cancer (mm) in biopsy specimens (*mm Cancer*), and length of noncancer (mm) in biopsy specimens (*mm nonCa*)

Therefore, patients who have been accurately identified based on pretreatment parameters before radical prostatectomy are optimal candidates for surveillance. The model was based on 409 patients with complete information on systematic prostate biopsy results that had low-risk prostate cancer-pretreatment PSA <20, clinical stage T1-T2a, no primary or secondary Gleason grade 4 or 5 cancer in biopsy, $<50\,\%$ positive cores, and <20 mm total cancer in biopsy cores. The nomogram uses PSA, clinical stage, primary and secondary biopsy Gleason grade, prostate volume by ultrasound, and length of cancer and noncancer in biopsy cores. The *c*-index for the internally validated base model was 0.64 and for the full model, which included all the parameters, it was 0.79. When applied to an external cohort of 296 low-risk patients the externally validated *c*-index of the model was 0.77. The external cohort included men treated by radical prostatectomy at Cleveland Clinic between 1999 and 2007 [25].

Prostate Cancer Metagram

In efforts to be most clinically useful, a nomogram addressing each endpoint of interest at each clinical state in the Fig. 7.3 clinical states should be available. To efficiently present the information to the patient, it should be organized in a tabular form with the pros and cons for each management strategy clearly identified, so he may identify those outcomes that are most important to him. To address this need, Nguyen and Kattan

Outcome	Surveillance	Radical Prostatectomy	External-Beam Radiotherapy	Brachytherapy
Biochemical Recurrence		***	***	***
Metastasis		***	***	
Survival	***	***	***	
Life Expectancy	***	***	***	***
Prostate Cancer-Specific Mortality	***	***	***	
Impotence		***		
Incontinence		***		
Bladder Dysfunction				
Bowel Dysfunction				
Convalescence				

Fig. 7.10 Metagram for determining treatment for clinically localized prostate cancer. A blank cell indicates an outcome for a specific treatment for which no validated prediction model exists. Ideally, a probability from a validated nomogram should populate every cell of the table. (Modified with permission from [26])

developed a metagram that considers all the available treatments for localized prostate cancer as well as outcomes relevant to cancer control, survival, and quality of life (Fig. 7.10) [26]. To allow for the patient and physician to make an unbiased and nonarbitrary treatment decision, the data are presented in a simple tabular format, which can provide evidence-based data on the advantages and disadvantages of all treatment options simultaneously. Optimally, every cell of the table should be populated with the probability from a validated nomogram. If one considers that there may be 16 different treatment options with ten important outcomes of interest for patients with localized prostate cancer, then there are potentially 160 treatment/outcome combinations that comprise the metagram for which an outcome prediction tool is needed. At this time, only 31 of the 160 cells of the metagram can be populated with currently available tools.

Nomograms for Other Clinical States

Risk of Prostate Cancer on Biopsy

Thompson et al. developed a nomogram, using data from 5519 men in the placebo arm of the Prostate Cancer Prevention Trial, to predict the risk of any prostate cancer and high-grade cancer based on age, ethnicity, PSA, DRE findings, prior history of biopsy, and use of finasteride [27]. The high-grade cancer was any pathology report with Gleason grade 4 or 5. This model has an advantage over others, as all patients were biopsied to determine the presence or absence of cancer and biopsy specimens were centrally reviewed.

Rising PSA After Radical Prostatectomy

A rising PSA for men after radical prostatectomy can cause anxiety and concern; therefore, Pound et al. [28] and Freedland et al. [29] have developed risk groups to predict the risk of developing distant metastases and PCSM, respectively. Teeter et al. further evaluated the role of postoperative nomograms in predicting PCSM [30]. They evaluated the Duke Prostate Center (DPC) nomogram, the Kattan postoperative nomogram, the Johns Hopkins Hospital (JHH) nomogram, and the joint Center for Prostate Disease Research (CPDR)/Cancer of the Prostate Strategic Urologic Research Endeavor (CaPSURE) nomogram, and noted that each could better predict PCSM than BCR. However, a limitation of these tables is that they do not distinguish between local versus systemic recurrence and thus should not be used to dictate the use of local versus systemic salvage therapy.

To determine which patients would most benefit from salvage radiotherapy after biochemical failure, Stephenson et al. developed a nomogram that predicts the 6-year PFP after salvage

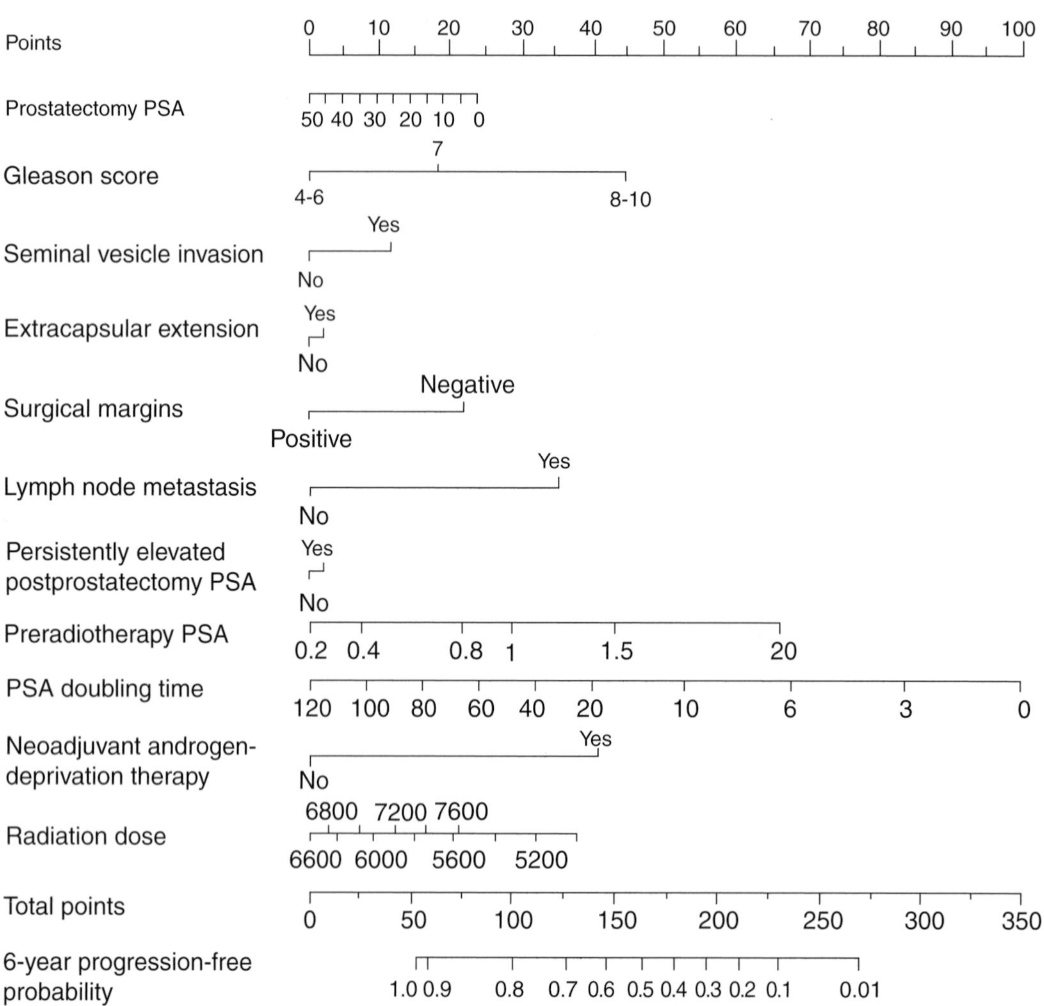

Fig. 7.11 Pretreatment nomogram predicting 6-year freedom from prostate-specific antigen (*PSA*) progression for men with rising *PSA* level after radical prostatectomy (defined as *PSA* ≥0.2 Ngami and rising) who receive salvage radiotherapy with or without neoadjuvant androgen deprivation therapy. (Used with permission from [31])

radiotherapy ± preradiotherapy androgen deprivation therapy (Fig. 7.11) [31]. The model used clinical information from 1545 patients treated with salvage radiotherapy for evidence of biochemical recurrence (defined as rising PSA level >0.2 ng/mL) from 17 institutions. The nomogram uses 11 standard clinical and pathological parameters available before salvage radiotherapy with an internally validated *c*-index of 0.69. The SEARCH database was used to externally validate the model with a *c*-index of 0.65 [32].

Castrate-Resistant Metastatic Prostate Cancer

Over the last few years, new and effective therapies have been introduced for the treatment of metastatic castrate resistant prostate cancer. Therefore, nomograms predicting the overall survival for men in this cohort need to be revalidated [33]. Omlin et al. [34] recently sought to revalidate the nomogram initially developed by Halabi et al. [35], which was modeled to predict overall survival at 1 and 2 years by using the clinical variables including lactate dehydrogenase, PSA, alkaline phosphatase, Gleason sum, Eastern Cooperative Oncology Group performance status, hemoglobin, and the presence of visceral disease. They found improved survival, and determined that participation in phase I, II, and III clinical trials was safe for patients.

Limitations of Nomograms

For the patient and physician, nomograms provide tools to personalize the decision of how to proceed with treatment, yet these models are not perfect and may not fit all men with prostate cancer. This is generally due to the modeling for the nomograms usually being based on patient populations from tertiary, referral, and/or academic centers. The outcomes at these centers may be considerably different than those in the community, including variation to the access and quality of treatment at the patient's home institution and the level of experience by the treating physician. To address this concern, Greene et al. validated the preoperative nomogram to estimate disease recurrence after radical prostatectomy on a cohort of patients treated at both academic and community centers [36]. They observed that the nomogram tended to overestimate the likelihood of cure amongst this patient population (particularly for those with probabilities of recurrence less than 35 %).

The use of PSA in the posttreatment setting should be used with caution. While a rising PSA universally antedates clinical disease recurrence, it has not been validated as a surrogate endpoint for PCSM. Therefore, it is fair to use PSA recurrence as a valuable endpoint for counseling patients regarding the likelihood of treatment success, although the probability of developing clinical recurrence and death from prostate cancer are more meaningful endpoints to predict.

The appropriate nomogram should be selected after the patient has made his decision for treatment, and not to use as a tool to compare the predicted outcome based on radical prostatectomy, external-beam radiotherapy, and brachytherapy. The nomograms do not predict the success of one therapy over another and the interpretation of the freedom from disease recurrence based on PSA should be done with care, as the definition of PSA recurrence varies. When Gretzer et al. [37] applied the ASTRO criteria of recurrence to a cohort of men who underwent a radical prostatectomy it produced an apparent improvement in the 15-year PFP from 68 % (based on a single PSA rise $\geq$0.2 ng/mL) to 90 %. When comparing all three treatment modalities with a similar definition for PSA recurrence, there is a bias for radiotherapy (external-beam and brachytherapy). This occurs because the patient who is treated with radiotherapy needs to reach a PSA nadir, which may take several years. For those treated with a radical prostatectomy, that PSA nadir is achieved within the first few weeks post procedure. Therefore, for patients who have biochemical recurrence after radical prostatectomy, they will fail earlier than those treated with radiotherapy. Biochemical progression is not an equivalent endpoint when comparing radical prostatectomy and external-beam radiotherapy. When evaluating the median interval from biochemical recurrence to metastatic disease (in the absence of salvage androgen-deprivation therapy), for patients undergoing a radical prostatectomy it is 8 years compared to only 3 years after external-beam radiotherapy. This would make it seem like patients who develop biochemical recurrence after external-beam radiotherapy are at a considerably higher risk of early metastatic progression than those men who recur following radical prostatectomy.

For the patient and physician, nomograms provide the most accurate tool for predicting outcomes. The modeling used evaluates variables as continuous, thus allowing to best predict accurate treatment success for the different treatment modalities for localized prostate cancer. The decision of how to manage his localized prostate cancer is a difficult one for the patient. Yet with the appropriate information to determine accurate estimation of the success the patient can make a decision that best fits his lifestyle and beliefs, whether it is radical prostatectomy, external-beam radiotherapy, or brachytherapy. It is important to appreciate the value of nomograms to make predictions, and should be interpreted as such, they are not to make treatment recommendation or serve as proxy for physician–patient interactions.

We are well served by current nomograms as they provide the patient a strong tool in making management decisions. They also provide the patient and physician the opportunity to discuss all the different variables that influence the management of localized prostate cancer. As a field it would behoove us to continue to update and revalidate nomograms that predict the likelihood of long-term urinary and sexual function, along with other outcomes, as patients and physicians explore treatment alternatives, especially to adequately reflect novel treatments and longer series follow-up.

References

1. Albertsen PC, Hanley JA, Fine J. 20-year outcomes following conservative management of clinically localized prostate cancer. JAMA. 2005;293(17):2095–101.
2. Ross PL, Gerigk C, Gonen M, Yossepowitch O, Cagiannos I, Sogani PC, et al. Comparisons of nomograms and urologists' predictions in prostate cancer. Semin Urol Oncol. 2002;20(2):82–8.
3. D'Amico AV, Whittington R, Malkowicz SB, Schultz D, Blank K, Broderick GA, et al. Biochemical outcome after radical prostatectomy, external beam radiation therapy, or interstitial radiation therapy for clinically localized prostate cancer. JAMA. 1998;280(11):969–74.
4. Cooperberg MR, Pasta DJ, Elkin EP, Litwin MS, Latini DM, Du Chane J, et al. The University of California, San Francisco cancer of the prostate risk assessment score: a straightforward and reliable preoperative predictor of disease recurrence after radical prostatectomy. J Urol. 2005;173(6):1938–42.
5. Mitchell JA, Cooperberg MR, Elkin EP, Lubeck DP, Mehta SS, Kane CJ, et al. Ability of 2 pretreatment risk assessment methods to predict prostate cancer recurrence after radical prostatectomy: data from CaPSURE. J Urol. 2005;173(4):1126–31.
6. Partin AW, Kattan MW, Subong EN et al. Combination of prostate-specific antigen, clinical stage, and Gleason score to predict pathological stage of localized prostate cancer. A multi-institutional update. JAMA 1997; 277:1445–51.
7. Chan T, Partin A, Walsh P, Epstein J. Prognostic significance of Gleason score 3+4 versus Gleason score 4+3 tumor at radical prostatectomy. Urology. 2000;56(5):823–7.
8. Kattan MW, Scardino P. Prediction of progression: nomograms of clinical utility. Clin Prostate Cancer. 2002;1(2):90–6.
9. Scher HI, Heller G. Clinical states in prostate cancer: toward a dynamic model of disease progression. Urology. 2000;55(3):323–7.
10. Ross PL, Scardino PT, Kattan MW. A catalog of prostate cancer nomograms. J Urol. 2001;165(5):1562–8.
11. Bianco FJ Jr., Scardino PT, Eastham JA. Radical prostatectomy: long-term cancer control and recovery of sexual and urinary function ("trifecta"). Urology. 2005;66(5 Suppl):83–94.
12. Graefen M, Karakiewicz PI, Cagiannos I, Quinn DI, Henshall SM, Grygiel JJ, et al. International validation of a preoperative nomogram for prostate cancer recurrence after radical prostatectomy. J Clin Oncol. 2002;20(15):3206–12.
13. Bianco FJ Jr., Kattan MW, Scardino PT, Powell IJ, Pontes JE, Wood DP Jr.. Radical prostatectomy nomograms in black American men: accuracy and applicability. J Urol. 2003;170(1):73–6; discussion 6–7.
14. Stephenson AJ, Kattan MW, Eastham JA, Dotan ZA, Bianco FJ Jr., Lilja H, et al. Defining biochemical recurrence of prostate cancer after radical prostatectomy: a proposal for a standardized definition. J Clin Oncol. 2006;24(24):3973–8.
15. Stephenson AJ, Scardino PT, Eastham JA, Bianco FJ Jr., Dotan ZA, Fearn PA, et al. Preoperative nomogram predicting the 10-year probability of prostate cancer recurrence after radical prostatectomy. J Natl Cancer Inst. 2006;98(10):715–7.
16. Stephenson AJ, Kattan MW, Eastham JA, Bianco FJ Jr., Yossepowitch O, Vickers AJ, et al. Prostate cancer-specific mortality after radical prostatectomy for patients treated in the prostate-specific antigen era. J Clin Oncol. 2009;27(26):4300–5.
17. Stephenson AJ, Scardino PT, Eastham JA, Bianco FJ Jr., Dotan ZA, DiBlasio CJ, et al. Postoperative nomogram predicting the 10-year probability of prostate cancer recurrence after radical prostatectomy. J Clin Oncol. 2005;23(28):7005–12.
18. Kattan MW, Zelefsky MJ, Kupelian PA, Scardino PT, Fuks Z, Leibel SA. Pretreatment nomogram for predicting the outcome of three-dimensional conformal radiotherapy in prostate cancer. J Clin Oncol. 2000;18(19):3352–9.
19. Zelefsky MJ, Kattan MW, Fearn P, Fearon BL, Stasi JP, Shippy AM, et al. Pretreatment nomogram predicting ten-year biochemical outcome of three-dimensional conformal radiotherapy and intensity-modulated radiotherapy for prostate cancer. Urology. 2007;70(2):283–7.
20. Kattan MW, Zelefsky MJ, Kupelian PA, Cho D, Scardino PT, Fuks Z, et al. Pretreatment nomogram that predicts 5-year probability of metastasis

following three-dimensional conformal radiation therapy for localized prostate cancer. J Clin Oncol. 2003;21(24):4568–71.
21. Kattan MW, Potters L, Blasko JC, Beyer DC, Fearn P, Cavanagh W, et al. Pretreatment nomogram for predicting freedom from recurrence after permanent prostate brachytherapy in prostate cancer. Urology. 2001;58(3):393–9.
22. Potters L, Roach M 3rd, Davis BJ, Stock RG, Ciezki JP, Zelefsky MJ, et al. Postoperative nomogram predicting the 9-year probability of prostate cancer recurrence after permanent prostate brachytherapy using radiation dose as a prognostic variable. Int J Radiat Oncol Biol Phys. 2010;76(4):1061–5.
23. Kattan MW, Cuzick J, Fisher G, Berney DM, Oliver T, Foster CS, et al. Nomogram incorporating PSA level to predict cancer-specific survival for men with clinically localized prostate cancer managed without curative intent. Cancer. 2008;112(1):69–74.
24. Kattan MW, Eastham JA, Wheeler TM, Maru N, Scardino PT, Erbersdobler A, et al. Counseling men with prostate cancer: a nomogram for predicting the presence of small, moderately differentiated, confined tumors. J Urol. 2003;170(5):1792–7.
25. Dong F, Kattan MW, Steyerberg EW, Jones JS, Stephenson AJ, Schroder FH, et al. Validation of pretreatment nomograms for predicting indolent prostate cancer: efficacy in contemporary urological practice. J Urol. 2008;180(1):150–4; discussion 4.
26. Nguyen CT, Kattan MW. Development of a prostate cancer metagram: a solution to the dilemma of which prediction tool to use in patient counseling. Cancer. 2009;115(13 Suppl):3039–45.
27. Thompson IM, Ankerst DP, Chi C, Goodman PJ, Tangen CM, Lucia MS, et al. Assessing prostate cancer risk: results from the prostate cancer prevention trial. J Natl Cancer Inst. 2006;98(8):529–34.
28. Pound CR, Partin AW, Eisenberger MA, Chan DW, Pearson JD, Walsh PC. Natural history of progression after PSA elevation following radical prostatectomy. JAMA. 1999;281(17):1591–7.
29. Freedland SJ, Humphreys EB, Mangold LA, Eisenberger M, Dorey FJ, Walsh PC, et al. Risk of prostate cancer-specific mortality following biochemical recurrence after radical prostatectomy. JAMA. 2005;294(4):433–9.
30. Teeter AE, Presti JC Jr., Aronson WJ, Terris MK, Kane CJ, Amling CL, et al. Do nomograms designed to predict biochemical recurrence (BCR) do a better job of predicting more clinically relevant prostate cancer outcomes than BCR? A report from the SEARCH database group. Urology. 2013;82(1):53–8.
31. Stephenson AJ, Scardino PT, Kattan MW, Pisansky TM, Slawin KM, Klein EA, et al. Predicting the outcome of salvage radiation therapy for recurrent prostate cancer after radical prostatectomy. J Clin Oncol. 2007;25(15):2035–41.
32. Moreira DM, Jayachandran J, Presti JC Jr., Aronson WJ, Terris MK, Kane CJ, et al. Validation of a nomogram to predict disease progression following salvage radiotherapy after radical prostatectomy: results from the SEARCH database. BJU Int. 2009;104(10):1452–6.
33. Halabi S, Lin CY, Small EJ, Armstrong AJ, Kaplan EB, Petrylak D, et al. Prognostic model predicting metastatic castration-resistant prostate cancer survival in men treated with second-line chemotherapy. J Natl Cancer Inst. 2013;105(22):1729–37.
34. Omlin A, Pezaro C, Mukherji D, Mulick Cassidy A, Sandhu S, Bianchini D, et al. Improved survival in a cohort of trial participants with metastatic castration-resistant prostate cancer demonstrates the need for updated prognostic nomograms. Eur Urol. 2013;64(2):300–6.
35. Halabi S, Small EJ, Kantoff PW, Kattan MW, Kaplan EB, Dawson NA, et al. Prognostic model for predicting survival in men with hormone-refractory metastatic prostate cancer. J Clin Oncol. 2003;21(7):1232–7.
36. Greene KL, Meng MV, Elkin EP, Cooperberg MR, Pasta DJ, Kattan MW, et al. Validation of the Kattan preoperative nomogram for prostate cancer recurrence using a community based cohort: results from cancer of the prostate strategic urological research endeavor (capsure). J Urol. 2004;171(6 Pt 1):2255–9.
37. Gretzer MB, Trock BJ, Han M, Walsh PC. A critical analysis of the interpretation of biochemical failure in surgically treated patients using the American society for therapeutic radiation and oncology criteria. J Urol. 2002;168(4 Pt 1):1419–22.

Genetic Determinants of Familial and Hereditary Prostate Cancer

8

Jesse K. McKenney, Christopher G. Przybycin and Cristina Magi-Galluzzi

Introduction

Prostate carcinoma (PCa) is a multifactorial disease influenced by both environmental and genetic factors. After advancing age and ethnic background, the strongest epidemiological risk factor for PCa is a positive family history. Although genetic factors implicated in the development of PCa are as yet ill defined, over the past 20 years the body of evidence that gene abnormalities may be specifically associated with prostate cancer risk has grown immensely, ranging from familial aggregation and twin studies, to family-based linkage studies, to detection of likely functional genes via mutation screening, to molecular epidemiological studies of both rare and common polymorphisms of candidate genes [1]. Gene–environment interactions play a crucial role in cancer development, particularly when low penetrance genes such as genetic polymorphisms are the major contributor. Strengthening the genetic evidence is a high frequency of prostate cancer in monozygotic as compared to dizygotic twins. Two different analyses have revealed a concordance for prostate cancer diagnosis of 21.1 and 27.1 % for monozygotic versus 6.4 and 7.1 % for dizygotic twins, respectively [2, 3]. Using a model developed to determine the effects of heritable versus environmental factors, heritable factors have been estimated to account for 42 % of prostate cancer risk in one study [2].

For practical purposes, PCa can be divided into three groups: hereditary, familial, and sporadic. Up to 85 % of all prostate cancers are sporadic and only 10–15 % are genetically determined [4]. Hereditary PCa, compatible with Mendelian inheritance criteria, is demonstrated only in 5 % of cases with PCa family history, whereas familial PCa accounts for about 13–25 % of cases. Hereditary prostate cancer has been defined as families that meet at least one of the following three criteria: 1—three or more first-degree relatives (e.g., father, son, brother) affected with PCa in any nuclear family; 2—occurrence of PCa in each of three successive generations in either of the proband's paternal or maternal lineages; or 3—at least two relatives, both affected with PCa diagnosed before age 55 [5]. Familial aggregations of PCa that do not fulfill the previously reported criteria but have at least two affected first-degree relatives are defined as familial forms. Sporadic PCa are likely due to nonhereditary causes. Even if there is more than one case in the family, there is no particular pattern of inheritance.

C. Magi-Galluzzi (✉)
Department of Pathology, Cleveland Clinic, Robert J. Tomsich Pathology and Laboratory Medicine Institute, Cleveland, OH, USA
e-mail: magic@ccf.org

J. K. McKenney
Department of Pathology, Cleveland Clinic, Robert J. Tomsich Pathology and Laboratory Medicine Institute, Cleveland, OH, USA
e-mail: mckennj@ccf.org

C. G. Przybycin
Department of Pathology, Cleveland Clinic, Robert J. Tomsich Pathology and Laboratory Medicine Institute, Cleveland, OH, USA
e-mail: przybyc@ccf.org

C. Magi-Galluzzi, C. G. Przybycin (eds.), *Genitourinary Pathology,* DOI 10.1007/978-1-4939-2044-0_8,

The relative risk of PCa in a man with a brother or father with PCa is 3.4 and 2.2, respectively [6, 7], and increases proportionally to the number of diseased relatives and their decrease in age at diagnosis, so that the risk of developing PCa is assessed 8.5 for men with both first-and second-degree affected relatives [1]. Family history is associated with 2.2-fold risk of PCa before age 65 years and 1.7-fold risk for onset after age 65; in the presence of a family history that includes both PCa and either breast or ovarian cancer, the risk is approximately 5.8, but results differ between studies [8, 9].

No distinct clinicopathologic characteristics or tumor progression attributes have been generally identified for hereditary versus sporadic PCa, except an earlier age at diagnosis (hereditary PCa occurs on average 6 years earlier than the sporadic form) [10, 11].

Apart from *RNaseL*-, *ElaC2*-, *MSR1*-, *HOXB13*- as well as low number of CAG repeats in the androgen receptor (AR) gene, there are no other identified high-risk genetic variants which might be considered responsible for hereditary PCa. These findings suggest that even familial PCa is a genetically heterogeneous disease, related to changes in many gene loci rather than a specific major susceptibility gene. These genetic changes likely interact not only reciprocally, but also with environmental conditions that are generally more strongly associated with sporadic PCa initiation [1].

Strong Candidates for Susceptibility Genes

Recent studies suggest that hereditary prostate cancer is a complex disease, involving multiple susceptibility genes with variable phenotypic expression. Family-based studies have identified three strong candidate susceptibility genes involved in the hereditary form of prostate cancer: the endoribonuclease *RNaseL* gene (*RNaseL/hereditary prostate cancer 1* (*HPC1*)), the 3′ processing endoribonuclease *ELaC2/HPC2* gene, the macrophage scavenger receptor 1 gene (*MSR1*), and *HOXB13* (Table 8.1).

RNaseL/HPC1 (1q24–25)

The identification of genetic susceptibility loci for prostate cancer has been extremely difficult. It was only in 1996 that the first prostate cancer susceptibility locus, *HPC1*, was mapped to chromosome 1q24–25, which was subsequently identified as the RNaseL gene. RNaseL is a uniquely regulated endoribonuclease requiring 5′-triphosphorylated, 2′,5′-linked oligoadenylates (2–5A) for its activity. This enzyme is important in immune response to viral infection, induction of apoptosis, and cell cycle and cell differentiation regulation. The presence of germ-line mutations in RNaseL that segregate with disease within hereditary-prostate-cancer-affected families and the loss of heterozygosity (LOH) in tumor tissues suggest a relationship between innate immunity and tumor suppression.

RNaseL mutations have an autosomal dominant type of inheritance with high penetrance; consequently, carriers of this mutant variant have a high risk of prostate cancer development [4]. The *HPC1* locus is associated with disease that affects younger men (age <66 years) and multiple family members [12]. Men with this predisposition typically have more aggressive cancer (higher Gleason score), often locally advanced or even metastatic. Germ-line mutations in the tumor-suppressor gene *RNaseL* have been reported to track in PCa families, and have been implicated in up to 13 % of all prostate cancer cases [13].

ElaC2/HPC2 (17p11.2)

The *ElaC2/HPC2* gene at 17p11.2 is the first candidate gene identified for human prostate cancer based on linkage analysis and positional cloning [14]. *HPC2* gene encodes ElaC protein 2, a zinc phosphodiesterase located in the nucleus. *ElaC2* displays transfer ribonucleic acid (tRNA) 3′-processing endonuclease activity, inducing tRNA maturation. The *ELaC2/HPC2* gene displayed several sequence variants: missense mutations Ser217Leu, Ala541Thr, and Arg781His and a frame-shift mutation 1641 insG [14]. Two previous studies found an association between

Table 8.1 Genes involved in prostate cancer development

Gene localization	Candidate gene/locus	Gene function	Key features
Strong candidates for susceptibility genes			
1q25.3	*RNaseL/HPC1*	Antiviral and pro-apoptotic role	<65 year old, high GS, advanced disease at diagnosis, strong relationship with PCa in families with >5 affected men
17p11	*ELaC2/HPC2*	Induces tRNA maturation	
8p22–23	*MSR1*	Involved in arterial wall deposition of cholesterol and in endocytosis of low density lipoproteins	Meta analysis failed to reveal correlation between locus for *MSR1* and hereditary risk for PCa
17q21–22	*HOXB13*		5 % of families, predominantly of European descent, more frequent in males diagnosed with PCa with early-onset disease and family history
Weak candidates for susceptibility genes (low-risk alleles)			
Xq27–28	*HPCX*		Gonosomal inheritance, higher risk of PCa in men with affected brother than with affected father; early-onset prostate cancer, responsible for 16 % of hereditary PCa
20q13	*HPC20*		PCa diagnosed at older age
17q21	*BRCA1*	Regulation of cell cycle progression and DNA repair	Germ-line mutations observed in 0.44 % of PCa cases; 9.5 % lifetime risk of PCa by age 65 years
13q12–13	*BRCA2*	DNA recombination and repair	Relative risks estimated as high as fivefold to sevenfold at young age (≤65 years); 20 % lifetime risk of PCa
1q42–43	*PCAP*		Male-to-male transmission, average age at diagnosis <66 years, and ≥5 affected individuals

GS Gleason score, *PCa* prostate cancer, *tRNA* transfer ribonucleic acid

Ser217Leu and Ala541Thr and their combination with PCa [14, 15].

The finding of a nonsense mutation in the *HPC2/ELaC2* gene confirms its potential role in genetic susceptibility to prostate cancer. However, *HPC2/ELaC2* germ-line mutations are rare in hereditary prostate cancer and variants Leu217 and Thr541 do not appear to influence the risk for hereditary prostate cancer, suggesting that alterations within the *HPC2/ELaC2* gene play a limited role in genetic susceptibility to hereditary prostate cancer [16].

MSR1 (8p22–23)

The *MSR1* gene at 8p22–23 has been implicated as a candidate gene for hereditary prostate cancer. *MSR1* encodes membrane glycoproteins, MSR type-I and type-II, involved in the modulation of interaction between foreign cells and macrophages, cell adhesion and phagocytosis, arterial wall deposition of cholesterol during atherogenesis, and endocytosis of low density lipoproteins. The frequencies of deleterious alleles is low, and the penetrance is apparently moderate, suggesting that *MSR1* is not a major susceptibility gene in prostate cancer families [17]. Meta analysis of existing data has failed to show any clear correlation between the *MSR1* locus and the hereditary risk of prostate cancer [18].

HOXB13 (17q21–22)

HOXB13 is a transcription factor gene important in prostate development. *HOXB13* is suppressed in AR negative prostate cancer cells and its overexpression results in significant inhibition of cell growth. In addition, *HOXB13* has been shown to suppress androgen-stimulated AR activity by interacting with the receptor [19].

A recurrent germ-line mutation (G84E) in the *HOXB13* has been recently identified by Ewing et al. in a previously recognized region of linkage at 17q21–22 as harboring an increased risk for familial prostate cancer [20]. Xu et al. have utilized a large sample of prostate cancer-prone families recruited by the International Consortium for Prostate Cancer Genetics (ICPCG) to confirm that the *HOXB13* G84E mutation is rare, but significantly associated with predisposition to PCa. G84E mutation was present in ~5% of prostate cancer families, predominantly of European descent, and was encountered more frequently in males diagnosed with PCa (51%) than in unaffected male family members (30%) [21]. The frequency of the mutation was higher in PCa patients with early-onset disease (age at diagnosis ≤55 years, 2.2%) or with positive family history (2.2%), and most common in patients with both features (3.1%). In a family-based analysis, the proportion of G84E mutation-associated PCa was highest in families from the Nordic countries of Finland (22.4%) and Sweden (8.2%), particularly for early-onset PCa and cases with substantially elevated prostate-specific antigen (PSA) [22]. *HOXB13* G84E variant poses a statistically significant risk of hereditary PCa, while accounting for only a small fraction of all prostate cancers.

Weak Candidates for Susceptibility Genes

An indeterminate number of weak candidate susceptibility loci have been suggested to be involved in hereditary PCa (Table 8.1). However, high-risk PCa alleles, associated with a lifetime penetrance of at least 66%, have a frequency unlikely above 2–3% of the cases, whereas low-risk PCa alleles may have a more frequent impact on sporadic PCa.

HPCX (Xq27–28)

A linkage analysis of 360 families at high risk for PCa identified the q27–28 region on chromosome X as the potential location of a gene, hereditary prostate cancer X-linked (*HPCX*), involved in prostate cancer susceptibility [23]. Results supporting this localization were obtained in another analysis of 153 American families. The most significant evidence of linkage to this locus was found in pedigrees without male-to-male transmission and with early-onset prostate cancer [24]. Studies have revealed a higher relative risk of prostate cancer for men with a brother affected by PCa than for men with an affected father. It is presumed that *HPCX* is responsible for 16% of hereditary PCas [25]. *HPCX* variants seem to be associated with prostate tumor aggressiveness [12].

HPC20 (20q13)

A recent study of hereditary prostate cancer has provided evidence for a prostate cancer-susceptibility locus, *HPC20*, which maps to 20q13. It is speculated that *HPC20* may potentially play a role in men with PCa diagnosed at older age [26].

PCAP (1q42–43)

PCAP (predisposing for cancer prostate) was identified on 1q42.2–43 on a combined analysis of French and German families [27]. PCa tumor antigen-1 (*PCTA-1*), located within the PCa susceptibility locus 1q42.2–43, is not a high-risk PCa gene, but data suggest that it might make a low-risk contribution [28]. *PCTA-1* belongs to the family of galectins. Galectins expression correlates with tumor growth and differentiation, modulates tumor cell adhesion, and mediates cell proliferation, survival, and apoptosis. Linkage studies using microsatellite markers on 144 prostate cancer families found suggestive evidence for linkage to *PCAP* in 21 families that met the criteria of male-to-male transmission, average age at diagnosis <66 years, and ≥5 affected individuals [29]. The role of *PCAP* in prostate cancer warrants further investigation.

8q24

Two independent genome-wide association studies of prostate cancer, using different methodologies, converged on the same chromosomal locus, 8q24 [30, 31]. A 3.8-megabase region of 8q24 has been identified as significantly associated with prostate cancer risk. The region contains nine known genes, including the oncogene *MYC*, commonly gained in PCa. Single nucleotide polymorphisms (SNPs) within three adjacent regions at 8q24 have been recently identified to be connected with familiar PCa risk [32, 33]. In 2009, two additional risk regions were discovered at 8q24 [34]. At least nine SNPs, all independently associated with PCa risk, reside within these five loci. Notably, all 8q24 risk polymorphisms reside in intergenic, noncoding regions of the genome [35]. Chung et al. have recently shown that a critical region at 8q24 is transcribed as a ~13 kb intron-less non-coding RNA (ncRNA), termed *PRNCR1* (prostate cancer ncRNA 1). *PRNCR1* expression was found to be upregulated in some prostate cancer cells as well as the precursor lesion prostatic intraepithelial neoplasia [36].

Variability at 8q24 seems to be associated with high risk of aggressive PCa patterns at diagnosis.

16q23

Prostate cancer linkage to the region of 16q23 has been observed in a SNP-based genome-wide linkage scan on 131 Caucasian prostate cancer families participating in the University of Michigan Prostate Cancer Genetics Project. Linkage to this same region, which contains several strong candidate genes including the known prostate cancer tumor-suppressor genes *ATBF1* and *WWOX*, has also been observed [37].

Prostate Cancer Associated with Other Tumors

Several epidemiological studies have shown a possible, either synchronous or metachronous association of different tumors (e.g., breast, brain, gastrointestinal tumors, and lymphomas) with PCa, thus suggesting common genetic risk factors.

BRCA1 (17q21), *BRCA2* (13q12)

The breast cancer susceptibility genes 1 (*BRCA1*) and 2 (*BRCA2*) are tumor-suppressor genes that are inherited in an autosomal dominant fashion with incomplete penetrance. They are normally expressed in breast, ovary, prostate, and other tissues. Their germ-line mutation is the cause of hereditary breast-ovarian cancer syndromes. Both genders have the same probability of inheriting the trait; however, the phenotype is different in males and females, and the risk of cancer is significantly lower in males. Although the results of some studies are conflicting, it has been clearly shown that male *BRCA* mutation carriers are predisposed to an increased risk of breast, prostate, pancreas, gastric, and hematologic cancers when compared to non-carriers.

Deleterious mutations in both genes have been associated with more aggressive prostate cancer and poor clinical outcome [38].

BRCA1 is on chromosome 17q21 and encodes a protein that has been implicated in the regulation of cell cycle progression, DNA damage response and repair, transcriptional regulation and chromatin modeling. BRCA1 has been associated with an increased risk of sporadic PCa (3.5-fold), even though germ-line mutations in this gene have only been observed in 0.44% of PCa cases [39] (Table 8.1).

BRCA2 is on chromosome 13q12 and its function seems to be limited to DNA recombination and repair processes. There is consistent evidence that germ-line mutations in BRCA2 lead to an increased risk of prostate cancer, with relative risks estimated as high as fivefold to sevenfold, and some evidence suggesting a more important role in prostate cancer presenting at a young age (≤65 years) [38] (Table 8.1).

The lifetime risk of PCa in *BRCA2* mutation carriers has been estimated to be 20 %, while for BRCA1 the risk is 9.5 % by age 65 years [39], similar to that in non-carriers.

Currently, the IMPACT study is evaluating the utility of PSA-based PCa screening in asymptomatic *BRCA1* and *BRCA2* mutation carriers [40].

CAPB (1p35–36)

The *CAPB* (prostate and brain cancer) gene, localized to 1p36 is reportedly linked to a predisposition to both brain and prostate cancer. Strong evidence of linkage to this locus was reported with 12 families showing both hereditary prostate cancer and a history of brain tumors [41]. However, other investigations have reported data that do not support linkage to this locus based on an independent analysis of 13 pedigrees representing the same clinical profile [29].

E-cadherin (16q)

Somatic mutations in the E-cadherin (*CDH1*) gene have frequently been reported in cases with diffuse gastric and lobular breast cancers. Germ-line mutations of the CDH1 gene at 16q have recently been associated with familial gastric cancer. Specifically, diffuse-type gastric cancers (such as signet-ring adenocarcinoma), while relatively uncommon, have a strong genetic association with mutation of the *CDH1* gene. Prostate-specific cancer antigen (PSCA) was demonstrated to be associated with an increased risk of diffuse gastric cancer, but not with intestinal-type gastric cancer [42].

Individual rare mutations and polymorphisms in the *CDH1* gene, such as S270A, may contribute to the onset of PCa. A significant rise in gastric cancer has been shown in pedigrees of PCa patients diagnosed before the age of 55 years; however, no association between PCa and *CDH1* germ-line mutation has been found so far [43].

2q, 16q, 17q

Some hereditary PCa families have a co-occurrence of pancreatic adenocarcinoma. Three chromosomal regions (2q, 16q, 17q) have been noted as harboring potential susceptibility loci, suggesting a linkage between prostate and pancreatic cancer [44].

NBN (8q21)

Nibrin (*NBN*), located on chromosome 8q21, is a gene involved in DNA double-strand break repair that has been implicated in the rare autosomal recessive chromosomal instability syndrome known as Nijmegen Breakage Syndrome (NBS). NBS is characterized by specific physical characteristics (microcephaly and dysmorphic facies), immunodeficiency, and increased risk of malignancy. Individuals who are heterozygous for NBN mutations are clinically asymptomatic, but may display an elevated risk for certain cancers including, but not limited to, ovarian and prostate cancer and various lymphoid malignancies [45].

Androgen Receptor and Steroid Hormone Metabolism-Related Genes' Involvement in Prostate Cancer

Conversion of testosterone to dihydrotestosterone (DHT), its active metabolite on prostatic target cells, is catalyzed in prostatic tissue by the enzyme 5-α-steroid-reductase (srd5α). The two genes *srd5α1* and *srd5α2*, encoding for srd5α isoforms type I and type II, are located on chromosomes 5p15 and 2p23, respectively. It is believed that isoform type II predominates in the prostate. A larger number of dinucleotide thymine-adenine (TA) repeats (≥18) on the last exon of the *srd5α2* gene (locus 2p22–23) is common in African-American men, and seems to confer an increased PCa predisposition [46].

AR is encoded by a gene located on the short arm of chromosome X (Xq11–12). This locus is one of the most conserved regions of the human genome, with only very rare mutations occurring at this site [47]. One of the critical functions of the product of the AR gene is to activate the expression of target genes. This activity resides in the transcriptional N-terminal domain of the protein, which is encoded in exon 1 and contains polymorphic guanine-guanine-cytosine (GGC) and cytosine-adenine-guanine (CAG) repeats. The variability in the *AR* gene length is determined by polymorphisms in the N-terminal region. A smaller number of either GGC (< 16) or CAG (< 18) repeats appears to be associated with a higher level of AR activity, resulting in an increased PCa risk [48]. The number of CAG and GGC base triplet repetition in the first exon of the AR gene is substantially lower in African-American than in Caucasian men [4, 49].

Loss of chromosomal Y segment is the most common chromosomal alteration that may be identified in prostate cancer tissue. Sex-related gene on chromosome Y (*SRY*) is downregulated in PCa. Since *SRY* acts as negative regulator of AR, the loss of chromosome Y results in an increase in prostate cancer growth [50].

Immunohistochemical studies have shown that the percentage of AR-positive cancer cells is higher in hereditary PCa than in sporadic forms, whereas the mean number of estrogen-α-receptor-positive stromal cells is higher in sporadic PCa than in the hereditary form [51].

Gene Mutations Possibly Associated with Prostate Cancer Development and Progression

PTEN (10q23.3)

Phosphatase and tensin homologue deleted on chromosome 10 (*PTEN*), also referred to as mutated in multiple advanced cancers (*MMAC1*) and transforming growth factor-beta (TGF-β) regulated and epithelial cell enriched phosphatase (*TEP1*), was first discovered in 1997 [52, 53]. *PTEN*, mapped to 10q23.3, is frequently inactivated in somatic cancers and is the second most common mutated tumor-suppressor gene after *p53* [54]. It plays a role in various cell processes including apoptosis, cell cycle progression, cell proliferation, angiogenesis, aging, and DNA damage response [55]. *PTEN* encodes a dual specificity phosphatase with the ability to dephosphorylate both lipid and protein substrates. By dephosphorylating PIP3 thereby opposing PI3K activity and resulting in subsequent downregulation of Akt, *PTEN* is the main negative regulator of the PI3K/Akt pathway [55].

PTEN functions may be impaired by mutations and other genetic alterations. *PTEN* inactivation may be due to inappropriate subcellular compartmentalization, altered proteasome degradation, somatic intragenic mutations, and epigenetic inactivation in sporadic tumors [55]. *PTEN* alterations include a variety of possible posttranslational modifications which may alter the phosphatase activity, direct subcellular localization, affect PTEN complexes and influence protein stability. PTEN function can be impaired not only by heterozygous mutations and homozygous losses, but also by other molecular mechanisms, such as transcriptional regression, epigenetic silencing, and microRNAs regulation [56].

Normal cells usually show strong nuclear *PTEN* expression which is lost during transformation to neoplasia. Germ-line mutations of *PTEN* cause the *PTEN* hamartoma tumor syndrome (PHTS), which includes those previously called Cowden, Bannayan-Riley-Ruvalcaba, Proteus, Proteus-like, and Lhermitte-Duclos syndromes [57]. Somatic mutations of *PTEN* have been observed in glioblastoma, prostate cancer, and breast cancer cell lines, to mention only few tissues where the involvement has been proven [52]. A common feature of *PTEN* somatic mutations is the association with advanced stage tumors (mainly glial and prostate cancers) [57].

Monoallelic [58, 59] and biallelic *PTEN* loss has been reported in approximately 42 and 10 % of prostate cancers, respectively [52, 53].

In mice, heterozygous loss (mutations in one allele) of PTEN has been shown to lead to cancers in various organs or systems, such as prostate, thyroid, colon, lymphatic system, breast, and endometrium [60]. There is compelling evidence in mice confirming *PTEN* as a haploinsufficient tumor-suppressor gene [56]: loss of one allele leads to the progression of a lethal polyclonal autoimmune disorder [61]; epithelial cancers, such as prostate cancer, are driven by *PTEN* heterozygosity [62]; cellular levels of *PTEN* protein inversely correlate with the occurrence of invasive prostate cancer [56]. Consequently, functional loss of one *PTEN* allele is critical for the onset of cancer in mice.

KLF 6 (10p15)

The loss-of-function mutation of Krüppel-like factor 6 (*KLF 6*) at chromosome 10p15 is a genetic change that can lead to deregulation of cell proliferation. *KLF 6* is a tumor-suppressor gene inactivated in a significant percentage (up to 55 %) of sporadic prostate cancers [63], however, its role in hereditary PCa has not been confirmed [64, 65]. KLF 6 is a ubiquitously expressed zinc finger transcription factor, which is part of a growing family of KLFs. The KLF family is broadly involved in differentiation and development, growth-related signal transduction, cell proliferation, apoptosis, and angiogenesis [65].

References

1. Alberti C. Hereditary/familial versus sporadic prostate cancer: few indisputable genetic differences and many similar clinicopathological features. Eur Rev Med Pharmacol Sci. 2010;14(1):31–41.
2. Lichtenstein P, Holm NV, Verkasalo PK, Iliadou A, Kaprio J, Koskenvuo M, et al. Environmental and heritable factors in the causation of cancer—analyses of cohorts of twins from Sweden, Denmark, and Finland. N Engl J Med. 2000;343(2):78–85.
3. Page WF, Braun MM, Partin AW, Caporaso N, Walsh P. Heredity and prostate cancer: a study of World War II veteran twins. Prostate. 1997;33(4):240–5.
4. Kral M, Rosinska V, Student V, Grepl M, Hrabec M, Bouchal J. Genetic determinants of prostate cancer: a review. Biomed Pap Med Fac Univ Palacky Olomouc Czech Repub. 2011;155(1):3–9.
5. Carter BS, Bova GS, Beaty TH, Steinberg GD, Childs B, Isaacs WB, et al. Hereditary prostate cancer: epidemiologic and clinical features. J Urol. 1993;150(3):797–802.
6. Bruner DW, Moore D, Parlanti A, Dorgan J, Engstrom P. Relative risk of prostate cancer for men with affected relatives: systematic review and meta-analysis. Int J Cancer. 2003;107(5):797–803.
7. Zeegers MP, Jellema A, Ostrer H. Empiric risk of prostate carcinoma for relatives of patients with prostate carcinoma: a meta-analysis. Cancer. 2003;97(8):1894–903.
8. Chen YC, Page JH, Chen R, Giovannucci E. Family history of prostate and breast cancer and the risk of prostate cancer in the PSA era. Prostate. 2008;68(14):1582–91.
9. Mastalski K, Coups EJ, Ruth K, Raysor S, Giri VN. Substantial family history of prostate cancer in black men recruited for prostate cancer screening: results from the prostate cancer risk assessment program. Cancer. 2008;113(9):2559–64.
10. Gronberg H, Damber L, Tavelin B, Damber JE. No difference in survival between sporadic, familial and hereditary prostate cancer. Br J Urol. 1998;82(4):564–7.
11. Roupret M, Fromont G, Bitker MO, Gattegno B, Vallancien G, Cussenot O. Outcome after radical prostatectomy in young men with or without a family history of prostate cancer. Urology. 2006;67(5):1028–32.
12. Agalliu I, Leanza SM, Smith L, Trent JM, Carpten JD, Bailey-Wilson JE, et al. Contribution of HPC1 (RNASEL) and HPCX variants to prostate cancer in a founder population. Prostate. 2010;70(15):1716–27.
13. Casey G, Neville PJ, Plummer SJ, Xiang Y, Krumroy LM, Klein EA, et al. RNASEL Arg462Gln variant is implicated in up to 13 % of prostate cancer cases. Nat Genet. 2002;32(4):581–3.
14. Tavtigian SV, Simard J, Teng DH, Abtin V, Baumgard M, Beck A, et al. A candidate prostate cancer susceptibility gene at chromosome 17p. Nat Genet. 2001;27(2):172–80.
15. Rebbeck TR, Walker AH, Zeigler-Johnson C, Weisburg S, Martin AM, Nathanson KL, et al. Association of HPC2/ELAC2 genotypes and prostate cancer. Am J Hum Genet. 2000;67(4):1014–9.
16. Wang L, McDonnell SK, Elkins DA, Slager SL, Christensen E, Marks AF, et al. Role of HPC2/ELAC2 in hereditary prostate cancer. Cancer Res. 2001;61(17):6494–9.
17. Maier C, Vesovic Z, Bachmann N, Herkommer K, Braun AK, Surowy HM, et al. Germline mutations of the MSR1 gene in prostate cancer families from Germany. Hum Mutat. 2006;27(1):98–102.
18. Sun J, Hsu FC, Turner AR, Zheng SL, Chang BL, Liu W, et al. Meta-analysis of association of rare mutations and common sequence variants in the MSR1 gene and prostate cancer risk. Prostate. 2006;66(7):728–37.
19. Kim SD, Park RY, Kim YR, Kim IJ, Kang TW, Nam KI, et al. HOXB13 is co-localized with androgen receptor to suppress androgen-stimulated prostate-specific antigen expression. Anat Cell Biol. 2010;43(4):284–93.
20. Ewing CM, Ray AM, Lange EM, Zuhlke KA, Robbins CM, Tembe WD, et al. Germline mutations in HOXB13 and prostate-cancer risk. N Engl J Med. 2012;366(2):141–9.

21. Xu J, Lange EM, Lu L, Zheng SL, Wang Z, Thibodeau SN, et al. HOXB13 is a susceptibility gene for prostate cancer: results from the International Consortium for Prostate Cancer Genetics (ICPCG). Hum Genet. 2013;132(1):5–14.
22. Laitinen VH, Wahlfors T, Saaristo L, Rantapero T, Pelttari LM, Kilpivaara O, et al. HOXB13 G84E mutation in Finland; population-based analysis of prostate, breast and colorectal cancer risk. Cancer Epidemiol Biomarkers Prev. 2013;22(3):452–60.
23. Xu J, Meyers D, Freije D, Isaacs S, Wiley K, Nusskern D, et al. Evidence for a prostate cancer susceptibility locus on the X chromosome. Nat Genet. 1998;20(2):175–9.
24. Lange EM, Chen H, Brierley K, Perrone EE, Bock CH, Gillanders E, et al. Linkage analysis of 153 prostate cancer families over a 30-cM region containing the putative susceptibility locus HPCX. Clin Cancer Res. 1999;5(12):4013–20.
25. Baffoe-Bonnie AB, Smith JR, Stephan DA, Schleutker J, Carpten JD, Kainu T, et al. A major locus for hereditary prostate cancer in Finland: localization by linkage disequilibrium of a haplotype in the HPCX region. Hum Genet. 2005;117(4):307–16.
26. Berry R, Schroeder JJ, French AJ, McDonnell SK, Peterson BJ, Cunningham JM, et al. Evidence for a prostate cancer-susceptibility locus on chromosome 20. Am J Hum Genet. 2000;67(1):82–91.
27. Berthon P, Valeri A, Cohen-Akenine A, Drelon E, Paiss T, Wohr G, et al. Predisposing gene for early-onset prostate cancer, localized on chromosome 1q42.2–43. Am J Hum Genet. 1998;62(6):1416–24.
28. Maier C, Rosch K, Herkommer K, Bochum S, Cancel-Tassin G, Cussenot O, et al. A candidate gene approach within the susceptibility region PCaP on 1q42.2–43 excludes deleterious mutations of the PCTA-1 gene to be responsible for hereditary prostate cancer. Eur Urol. 2002;42(3):301–7.
29. Berry R, Schaid DJ, Smith JR, French AJ, Schroeder JJ, McDonnell SK, et al. Linkage analyses at the chromosome 1 loci 1q24–25 (HPC1), 1q42.2–43 (PCAP), and 1p36 (CAPB) in families with hereditary prostate cancer. Am J Hum Genet. 2000;66(2):539–46.
30. Amundadottir LT, Sulem P, Gudmundsson J, Helgason A, Baker A, Agnarsson BA, et al. A common variant associated with prostate cancer in European and African populations. Nat Genet. 2006;38(6):652–8.
31. Freedman ML, Haiman CA, Patterson N, McDonald GJ, Tandon A, Waliszewska A, et al. Admixture mapping identifies 8q24 as a prostate cancer risk locus in African-American men. Proc Natl Acad Sci U S A. 2006;103(38):14068–73.
32. Cussenot O, Azzouzi AR, Bantsimba-Malanda G, Gaffory C, Mangin P, Cormier L, et al. Effect of genetic variability within 8q24 on aggressiveness patterns at diagnosis and familial status of prostate cancer. Clin Cancer Res. 2008;14(17):5635–9.
33. Sun J, Lange EM, Isaacs SD, Liu W, Wiley KE, Lange L, et al. Chromosome 8q24 risk variants in hereditary and non-hereditary prostate cancer patients. Prostate. 2008;68(5):489–97.
34. Al Olama AA, Kote-Jarai Z, Giles GG, Guy M, Morrison J, Severi G, et al. Multiple loci on 8q24 associated with prostate cancer susceptibility. Nat Genet. 2009;41(10):1058–60.
35. Pomerantz MM, Freedman ML. Genetics of prostate cancer risk. Mt Sinai J Med. 2010;77(6):643–54.
36. Chung S, Nakagawa H, Uemura M, Piao L, Ashikawa K, Hosono N, et al. Association of a novel long non-coding RNA in 8q24 with prostate cancer susceptibility. Cancer Sci. 2011;102(1):245–52.
37. Lange EM, Beebe-Dimmer JL, Ray AM, Zuhlke KA, Ellis J, Wang Y, et al. Genome-wide linkage scan for prostate cancer susceptibility from the University of Michigan prostate cancer genetics project: suggestive evidence for linkage at 16q23. Prostate. 2009;69(4):385–91.
38. Castro E, Eeles R. The role of BRCA1 and BRCA2 in prostate cancer. Asian J Androl. 2012;14(3):409–14.
39. Leongamornlert D, Mahmud N, Tymrakiewicz M, Saunders E, Dadaev T, Castro E, et al. Germline BRCA1 mutations increase prostate cancer risk. Br J Cancer. 2012;106(10):1697–701.
40. Mitra AV, Bancroft EK, Barbachano Y, Page EC, Foster CS, Jameson C, et al. Targeted prostate cancer screening in men with mutations in BRCA1 and BRCA2 detects aggressive prostate cancer: preliminary analysis of the results of the IMPACT study. BJU Int. 2011;107(1):28–39.
41. Gibbs M, Stanford JL, McIndoe RA, Jarvik GP, Kolb S, Goode EL, et al. Evidence for a rare prostate cancer-susceptibility locus at chromosome 1p36. Am J Hum Genet. 1999;64(3):776–87.
42. Lao-Sirieix P, Caldas C, Fitzgerald RC. Genetic predisposition to gastro-oesophageal cancer. Curr Opin Genet Dev. 2010;20(3):210–7.
43. Ikonen T, Matikainen M, Mononen N, Hyytinen ER, Helin HJ, Tommola S, et al. Association of E-cadherin germ-line alterations with prostate cancer. Clin Cancer Res. 2001;7(11):3465–71.
44. Pierce BL, Friedrichsen-Karyadi DM, McIntosh L, Deutsch K, Hood L, Ostrander EA, et al. Genomic scan of 12 hereditary prostate cancer families having an occurrence of pancreas cancer. Prostate. 2007;67(4):410–5.
45. Zuhlke KA, Johnson AM, Okoth LA, Stoffel EM, Robbins CM, Tembe WA, et al. Identification of a novel NBN truncating mutation in a family with hereditary prostate cancer. Fam Cancer. 2012;11(4):595–600.
46. Ntais C, Polycarpou A, Ioannidis JP. SRD5A2 gene polymorphisms and the risk of prostate cancer: a meta-analysis. Cancer Epidemiol Biomarkers Prev. 2003;12(7):618–24.
47. Brooke GN, Bevan CL. The role of androgen receptor mutations in prostate cancer progression. Curr Genomics. 2009;10(1):18–25.
48. Cancel-Tassin G, Cussenot O. Prostate cancer genetics. Minerva Urol Nefrol. 2005;57(4):289–300.

49. Silva Neto B, Koff WJ, Biolchi V, Brenner C, Biolo KD, Spritzer PM, et al. Polymorphic CAG and GGC repeat lengths in the androgen receptor gene and prostate cancer risk: analysis of a Brazilian population. Cancer Invest. 2008;26(1):74–80.
50. Yuan X, Lu ML, Li T, Balk SP. SRY interacts with and negatively regulates androgen receptor transcriptional activity. J Biol Chem. 2001;276(49):46647–54.
51. Fromont G, Yacoub M, Valeri A, Mangin P, Vallancien G, Cancel-Tassin G, et al. Differential expression of genes related to androgen and estrogen metabolism in hereditary versus sporadic prostate cancer. Cancer Epidemiol Biomarkers Prev. 2008;17(6):1505–9.
52. Li J, Yen C, Liaw D, Podsypanina K, Bose S, Wang SI, et al. PTEN, a putative protein tyrosine phosphatase gene mutated in human brain, breast, and prostate cancer. Science. 1997;275(5308):1943–7.
53. Steck PA, Pershouse MA, Jasser SA, Yung WK, Lin H, Ligon AH, et al. Identification of a candidate tumour suppressor gene, MMAC1, at chromosome 10q23.3 that is mutated in multiple advanced cancers. Nat Genet. 1997;15(4):356–62.
54. Georgescu MM. PTEN tumor suppressor network in PI3K-Akt pathway control. Genes Cancer. 2010;1(12):1170–7.
55. Govender D, Chetty R. Gene of the month: PTEN. J Clin Pathol. 2012;65(7):601–3.
56. Salmena L, Carracedo A, Pandolfi PP. Tenets of PTEN tumor suppression. Cell. 2008;133(3):403–14.
57. Romano C, Schepis C. PTEN gene: a model for genetic diseases in dermatology. ScientificWorldJournal. 2012;2012:252457.
58. Feilotter HE, Nagai MA, Boag AH, Eng C, Mulligan LM. Analysis of PTEN and the 10q23 region in primary prostate carcinomas. Oncogene. 1998;16(13):1743–8.
59. Rubin MA, Gerstein A, Reid K, Bostwick DG, Cheng L, Parsons R, et al. 10q23.3 loss of heterozygosity is higher in lymph node-positive (pT2–3,N+) versus lymph node-negative (pT2–3,N0) prostate cancer. Hum Pathol. 2000;31(4):504–8.
60. Podsypanina K, Ellenson LH, Nemes A, Gu J, Tamura M, Yamada KM, et al. Mutation of Pten/Mmac1 in mice causes neoplasia in multiple organ systems. Proc Natl Acad Sci U S A. 1999;96(4):1563–8.
61. Di Cristofano A, Kotsi P, Peng YF, Cordon-Cardo C, Elkon KB, Pandolfi PP. Impaired Fas response and autoimmunity in Pten+/- mice. Science. 1999;285(5436):2122–5.
62. Di Cristofano A, De Acetis M, Koff A, Cordon-Cardo C, Pandolfi PP. Pten and p27KIP1 cooperate in prostate cancer tumor suppression in the mouse. Nat Genet. 2001;27(2):222–4.
63. Narla G, Heath KE, Reeves HL, Li D, Giono LE, Kimmelman AC, et al. KLF6, a candidate tumor suppressor gene mutated in prostate cancer. Science. 2001; 294(5551):2563–6.
64. Koivisto PA, Hyytinen ER, Matikainen M, Tammela TL, Ikonen T, Schleutker J. Kruppel-like factor 6 germ-line mutations are infrequent in Finnish hereditary prostate cancer. J Urol. 2004;172(2):506–7.
65. Narla G, Friedman SL, Martignetti JA. Kruppel cripples prostate cancer: KLF6 progress and prospects. Am J Pathol. 2003;162(4):1047–52.

New Molecular Markers of Diagnosis and Prognosis in Prostate Cancer

9

Rajal B. Shah and Ritu Bhalla

Introduction

Serum prostate-specific antigen (PSA) has remained the mainstay biomarker for the prostate cancer diagnosis and management since its wide spread utilization as a screening tool almost 25 years ago. Although it has led to a dramatic increase in prostate cancer detection, PSA has substantial drawbacks both with sensitivity and specificity. Detection of clinically insignificant disease is another important issue. Together, these drawbacks of PSA emphasize the need for biomarkers that can supplement PSA as a diagnostic test, provide better cancer specificity than currently available tissue-based markers, reduce the number of unnecessary biopsies, and distinguish indolent from clinically significant prostate cancer. New genomic and bioinformatics technologies have allowed the discovery and study of an expanding universe of novel tissue-, urine- or body fluid-based biomarkers due to their higher cancer specificity and their prognostic or predictive utilities. Such efforts have also produced several notable success stories that involve rapidly moving biomarkers from the bench to the clinic. α-Methylacyl-CoA racemase (AMACR), ERG fusion protein, *PTEN*, and *PCA3* are important examples of biomarkers, which have found their way from bench to clinic. This chapter summarizes selected novel promising prostate cancer biomarkers of utility for the diagnosis, biological stratification, and prognosis of prostate cancer. The biomarkers addressed in the chapter are classified based on their diagnostic and prognostic applications as well as their functions as tissue- and urine-based markers (Table 9.1).

R. B. Shah (✉)
Department of Pathology, Division of Urologic Pathology, Miraca Life Sciences, Irving, TX, USA
e-mail: rshah@miracals.com; rajalbshah@gmail.com

R. Bhalla
Department of Pathology, LSU Health Sciences Center, New Orleans, LA, USA
e-mail: rbhall@lsuhsc.edu

Molecular Markers of Diagnosis

Tissue-Based Molecular Markers of Diagnosis

α-Methylacyl-CoA Racemase

Biology

AMACR was discovered as a leading candidate gene by differential display and complementary deoxyribonucleic acid (DNA) subtraction microarray analysis [1, 2]. It is consistently overexpressed in prostate cancer compared to benign prostatic tissue [1, 2]. It encodes a cytoplasmic protein involved in the β-oxidation of branched chain fatty acids. AMACR is not prostate cancer specific; it is also expressed by other cancers most notably, colorectal carcinomas and renal cell carcinomas, papillary type [3].

C. Magi-Galluzzi, C. G. Przybycin (eds.), *Genitourinary Pathology,* DOI 10.1007/978-1-4939-2044-0_9,

Table 9.1 Selected molecular markers of diagnosis and prognosis in prostate cancer

Biomarker	Functional role	Clinical application	Category
AMACR	β-oxidation of branched chain fatty acids	Diagnostic	Tissue
TMPRSS2:ERG gene fusions	Oncogenic transcription factor	Diagnostic, prognostic, predictive	Tissue or urine
GSTP1	Caretaker gene	Diagnostic	Tissue
PCA3	Prostate cancer-specific marker, produces *PCA3* RNA with no resultant protein	Diagnostic, prognostic	Urine
PCA3+ERG fusions	*See* PCA3 and ERG	Diagnostic, prognostic	Urine
PTEN	Tumor-suppressor gene	Prognostic, predictive	Tissue
EZH2	Transcriptional memory	Prognostic	Tissue
SPINK1	Functional role in ETS rearrangement-negative prostate cancer	Prognostic, diagnostic	Tissue, urine

RNA ribonucleic acid, *ETS* E26 transformation-specific

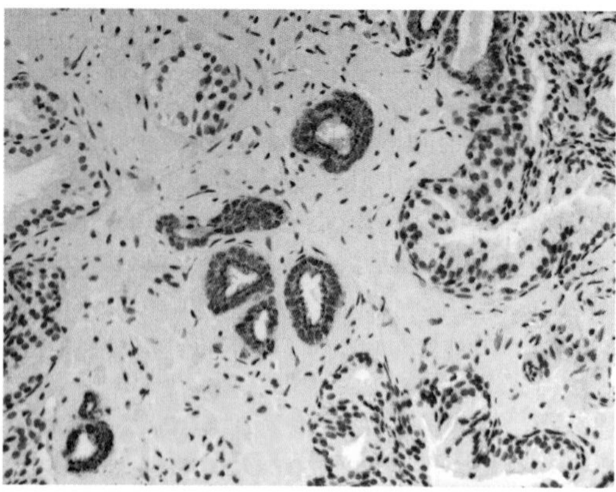

Fig. 9.1 An example of limited prostate carcinoma immunostained with P504S monoclonal antibody to AMACR (×200). Expression of AMACR appears as granular staining predominantly in apical portion of cancer glands. Adjacent benign glands are negative for AMACR

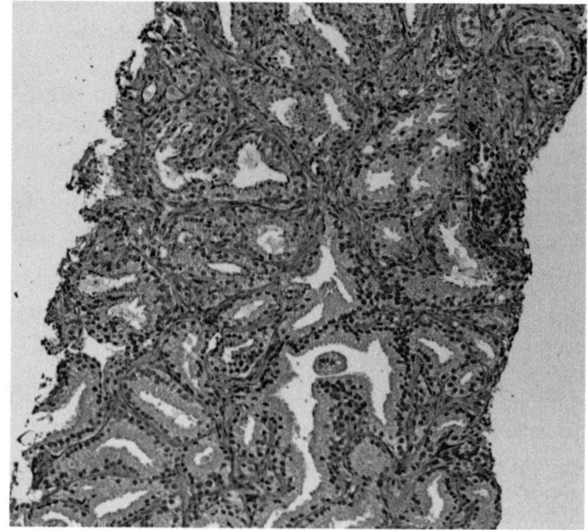

Fig. 9.2 Heterogeneous AMACR staining in cancer glands. The staining is strong in some cancer glands and weak or negative in others. This staining pattern is typical in prostate cancer and accounts for an 80% AMACR positive rate in prostate cancer detected on needle biopsy

Clinical Applications

Both monoclonal and polyclonal antibodies to AMACR have been developed. P504S, commercially available monoclonal antibody to AMACR, is most widely used, clinically. In our experience both monoclonal and polyclonal antibodies demonstrate similar levels of sensitivity and specificity for prostate cancer [4]. AMACR expression is cytoplasmic with granular staining pattern. The staining shows apical predominance (Fig. 9.1) and frequent heterogeneity (Fig. 9.2). Proportion of benign glands may also express AMACR; therefore interpretation of AMACR expression must be evaluated relative to the background staining of benign glands in the same biopsy. If benign glands demonstrate similar intensity of staining compared to atypical glands, then staining should be interpreted as negative.

AMACR in the Diagnosis of Limited Prostate Cancer in Prostate Needle Biopsy

AMACR was the first prostate cancer tissue biomarker identified. Currently, AMACR is more commonly applied to complement basal cell markers in antibody cocktail formats. The cocktails are now routinely utilized to resolve the diagnosis of "atypical glands" or to confirm the diagnosis of small volume cancer in needle biopsies (Fig. 9.1) [5]. Average sensitivity for the detection of limited prostate carcinoma in needle biopsies is in the range of 70–80% with lower sensitivity reported in certain morphologic variants including foamy, pseudohyperplastic, and atrophic variants of usual acinar prostate adenocarcinoma [6, 7]. AMACR is expressed in ~90% of irradiated prostate carcinomas; its expression is reduced in hormone-deprived cancers [8].

Positive AMACR staining supports a diagnosis of cancer in morphologically suspicious atypical glands. A diagnosis of cancer should not be reversed if AMACR and basal cell markers are negative and the morphology of the atypical glands is suspicious for carcinoma as a small proportion of prostate cancer lacks AMACR expression.

Utility of AMACR in Resolving an "Atypical Glands Suspicious for Prostate Cancer" Diagnosis

One of the challenges encountered during biopsy evaluation is the diagnosis of atypical glands suspicious for cancer (ATYP), which typically require immunohistochemistry (IHC) for further diagnostic work up. Two studies have demonstrated that in a subset of ATYP cases, positive AMACR may convert an ATYP to cancer diagnosis where morphology is suspicious for but not diagnostic of cancer and basal cell markers are negative [6, 9]. Caution should be exercised, however, before making a cancer diagnosis based on AMACR positivity alone as AMACR has significant limitations with prostate cancer specificity. The diagnosis of high-grade prostatic intraepithelial neoplasia (HGPIN), partial atrophy, adenosis (atypical adenomatous hyperplasia) and nephrogenic adenoma must be ruled out on morphological grounds before making a diagnosis of limited prostate cancer based on AMACR positivity.

Pitfalls

AMACR is not entirely specific for prostate cancer detection. The majority of HGPIN, nephrogenic adenomas, a subset of partial atrophy lesions, adenosis, and even benign glands may demonstrate AMACR expression [6, 10–12]. A summary of biology, clinical applications, and pitfalls of AMACR biomarker is summarized in Table 9.2.

TMPRSS2:ERG Gene Fusions

Biology of ETS Gene Fusions in Prostate Cancer

Recurrent chromosomal rearrangements in prostate carcinoma were discovered through

Table 9.2 α-Methylacyl-CoA racemase (AMACR, P504S)

Types of antibodies
Monoclonal (P504S) and polyclonal, both with comparable sensitivity and specificity
Staining pattern in prostate cancer
Granular cytoplasmic staining in apical distribution pattern
Diagnostic utility
1. Positive AMACR staining in atypical glands morphologically suspicious for cancer supports a cancer diagnosis
2. Positive AMACR may convert an ATYP to cancer diagnosis where morphology is suspicious but not diagnostic of cancer and basal cell markers are negative
Pitfalls
Staining intensity often heterogeneous in cancer glands
~20% of prostate carcinomas diagnosed on needle biopsy lack AMACR expression
Lower positive rate in several histologic variants (foamy gland, atrophic, and pseudohyperplastic) of prostate carcinoma
Positive in >90% HGPIN, 20% adenosis, majority of nephrogenic adenomas; frequently positive in partial atrophy and morphologically benign glands
Expressed in nonprostatic tumors (urothelial carcinoma, colon cancer, renal cell carcinoma, clear cell adenocarcinoma)

AMACR α-methylacyl-CoA racemase, *ATYP* atypical glands suspicious for cancer, *HGPIN* high-grade prostatic intraepithelial neoplasia

an unconventional bioinformatics approach termed as the "Cancer Outlier Profile Analysis" (COPA) algorithm used to analyze DNA microarray studies. Using the results of COPA analysis of many prostate cancer profiling studies, in 2005 Tomlins et al. discovered recurrent chromosomal rearrangements in prostate cancer demonstrating fusion of the 5′ untranslated region of the androgen-regulated gene *TMPRSS2* with *ERG* or *ETV1*, two members of the *E26 transformation-specific* (*ETS*) transcription factor family genes [13]. Many subsequent studies have validated *ETS* gene fusions in the majority (~50 %) of PSA-screened prostate cancer surgical cohorts [14–17]. Fusions between *TMPRSS2* and *ERG* represent the most common molecular subtype accounting for ~90 % of all *ETS* gene fusions [13, 14, 16, 17]. In addition to the most common *TMPRSS2:ERG* rearrangements, several other novel 5′ promoter or other upstream sequences of androgen-inducible genes (*HERV_K22q11.23, SLC45A3, C15orf21, HNRPA2B1, KLK2, CANT1*) and 3′ *ETS* transcription factors genes (*ETV4, ETV5, and ELK4*) have also been identified, which comprise about 5–10 % of all gene fusions in prostate cancers [17–19]. Rearrangements of *ERG* at the chromosomal level are highly specific to prostate cancer and are an early molecular event seen in ~18 % of HGPIN lesions immediately adjacent to cancer demonstrating identical gene fusions [15, 20]. HGPIN lesions expressing *TMPRSS2:ETS* rearrangements are invariably associated with invasive cancer, suggesting that they are a subset of true neoplastic precursors for *TMPRSS2:ETS*-positive cancers [15, 17, 20]. Clinically localized prostate cancer is typically a multifocal disease, with heterogeneous rearrangement for *TMPRSS2:ETS* fusions between different tumor foci [21]. In this schema of multifocal disease, a primary focus rearranged for *TMPRSS2:ETS* may progress and become capable of dissemination and give rise to metastatic disease. All metastatic disease foci retain similar *TMPRSS2:ETS* rearrangement like the primary focus, indicating that *ETS* rearrangement occurs before progression to metastatic disease and that the metastatic disease arises through the clonal expansion of a single focus of primary cancer capable of dissemination [22]. In summary, *ETS* gene fusions have been implicated to play a critical role in prostate carcinogenesis. *ERG* gene fusions have yet not been demonstrated in benign prostate tissue, isolated HGPIN, or benign cancer mimics [23–25]. Taken together, *ERG* gene fusions are the best prostate cancer-specific biomarker yet identified and define a specific molecular subtype of prostate cancer with important implications in diagnosis and management.

Anti-ERG Antibody as a Surrogate for *ERG* Gene Fusions in Prostate Cancer

TMPRSS2:ERG gene fusions result in the overexpression of chimeric fusion transcripts that encode a truncated ERG protein product. Park et al. characterized a rabbit anti-ERG monoclonal antibody [26]. A positive immunostain with this antibody highly correlated with the *ERG* gene rearrangement status determined by fluorescent in situ hybridization (FISH), with 96 % sensitivity and specificity for determining *ERG* rearrangement in prostate cancer. Several subsequent studies have validated this observation and demonstrated that ERG immunohistochemical expression has a high accuracy for defining the *TMPRSS2:ERG* fusion status in prostate cancer [27–31]. Table 9.3 summarizes the published studies highlighting the type of ERG antibody utilized, frequency of expression in prostate cancer, and its sensitivity and specificity for the detection of *ERG* gene fusions in prostate carcinoma. In summary, ERG oncoprotein detection in prostate cancer is highly concordant with *ERG* gene fusion status and can be reliably utilized as a surrogate of *ERG* gene fusions in prostate cancer diagnosis and management.

Clinical Applications of ERG IHC

Two monoclonal antibodies to C-terminus (clone EPR3864) and N-terminus (9FY) have been developed and are now commercially available. A recent study demonstrated similar levels of sensitivity and specificity for detecting the *ERG* gene fusions for the two monoclonal antibodies [30]. Overall, C-terminus antibody clone EPR3864 has been the most widely utilized ERG antibody in published studies (Table 9.3). The vascular

Table 9.3 Published studies demonstrating the frequency of ERG positivity and sensitivity and specificity of the detection of underlying *ERG* gene fusions in prostate carcinoma for two classes of ERG antibody

Type of antibody	Source of ERG antibody	Frequency of ERG positivity (%)	Detection of underlying ERG fusions		Study
			Sensitivity (%)	Specificity (%)	
C-terminus (clone EPR3864)	Epitomics	44	96	97	Park et al.
N-terminus (CPDR ERG-MAb)	Noncommercial[a]	Concordance rate of 82.8 %[b]			Furusato et al.
C-terminus (clone EPR3864)	Epitomics	45	86	89	Chaux et al.
C-terminus (clone EPR3864)	Epitomics	61	100	85	Leenders et al.
C-terminus (clone EPR3864)	Epitomics	33	96	99	Falzarano et al.
C-terminus (clone EPR3864)	Epitomics	45	96	99	Braun M et al.
N-terminus (clone 9FY)	Biocare	45	98	98	Braun M et al.

[a] The center for Prostatic Disease Research of Walter Reed Army Medical Center and Uniformed Services University (Rockville, MD)

[b] Correlation between mRNA levels of *TMPRSS2:ERG* type A transcript and ERG protein (35 cases)

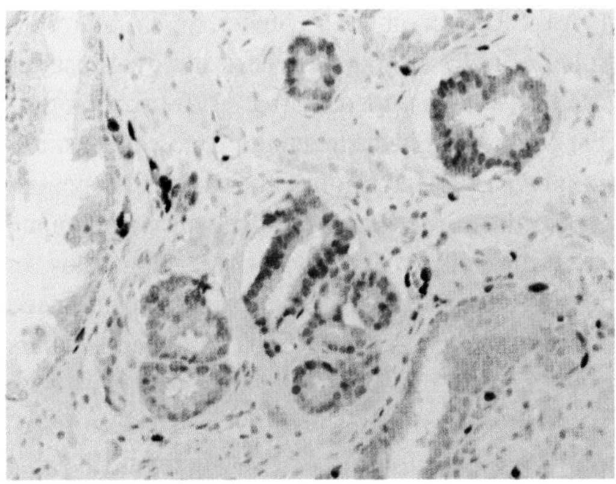

Fig. 9.3 An example of limited prostate carcinoma immunostained with ERG antibody (×200). The vascular endothelial cells (*asterisk*) that are present ubiquitously in prostate biopsy demonstrate strong nuclear staining and are utilized as an internal control. Cancerous glands demonstrate uniform strong nuclear ERG (*arrow*) reactivity. Adjacent benign glands are negative for ERG

endothelial cells present ubiquitously in prostate biopsy are utilized as internal positive control (Fig. 9.3). ERG expression in cancer cell nuclei is typically diffuse and strong (Fig. 9.3) [23–25]. Heterogeneous staining within the same cancer focus is relatively uncommon but heterogeneity of staining between different tumor foci of multifocal cancer is frequently reported [21, 25].

ERG in the Diagnosis of Limited PCa in Prostate Needle Biopsy

Basal cell markers including high-molecular weight cytokeratin and p63, and prostate cancer marker AMACR (P504S), individually or as a part of PIN-4 cocktail, are currently the most commonly utilized IHC markers in clinical practice [32, 33]. AMACR is preferentially overexpressed in approximately 80 % of prostate cancer detected in prostate biopsies [5, 6, 32, 33]. However, its expression is also found in most cases of HGPIN, in a significant proportion of adenosis, nephrogenic adenoma and partial atrophy, and occasionally even in morphologically benign prostatic glands [6, 10–12]. Therefore, a tumor marker that demonstrates better specificity for prostate cancer and is not expressed in noncancerous lesions may complement basal cell markers and AMACR and will greatly facilitate the identification of limited cancer in prostate biopsies.

Several studies have analyzed the utility of ERG immunostain in the work up of limited prostate cancer and have consistently found high specificity of ERG for prostate cancer detection. The reported frequency of ERG expression in limited cancer ranges from 40 to 60 % [23–25, 27, 29, 34, 35]. ERG expression has been observed in a small proportion of HGPIN or benign glands, invariably associated with adjacent prostate cancer [23–25, 34]. Benign lesions distant from cancerous glands, including simple and partial atrophy, are typically negative for ERG. Overall, ERG has much higher specificity for prostate cancer than AMACR; hence, ERG staining in an atypical focus (where HGPIN or atypical glands adjacent to HGPIN can be excluded) supports a diagnosis of cancer, irrespective of AMACR staining. A representative example of limited prostate cancer stained with ERG antibody is represented in Fig. 9.3.

Utility of ERG in Resolving an "Atypical Glands Suspicious for Prostate Cancer" Diagnosis

Only a few studies have examined the significance of ERG in the setting of ATYP [23, 24]. We studied 84 ATYP cases using multiplex ERG/AMACR/high molecular weight cytokeratin/p63 IHC to determine clinical utility of ERG in resolving an ATYP diagnosis [23]. A final diagnosis of benign, ATYP and cancer was rendered following review of morphology and all markers in 3, 30, and 51 cases, respectively. Of 51 cancer diagnoses, 45 and 94 % were positive for ERG and AMACR, respectively. Of 30 atypical diagnoses, 10 and 67 % were positive for ERG and AMACR, respectively. Of three benign diagnoses, none and 83 % were positive for ERG and AMACR, respectively. All three ERG-positive atypical cases were classified as "HGPIN with adjacent ATYP." ERG was expressed in adjacent noncancer glands of 20 % of prostate cancers, while AMACR was expressed in noncancer glands in all diagnostic categories in 40 % of cases. In ERG-positive ATYP focus, the expression was predominantly uniform within the focus with minimal staining heterogeneity. Overall, ERG has a low sensitivity but high specificity for prostate cancer detection. Therefore, ERG positivity in small atypical glands where the diagnosis of HGPIN is excluded can be utilized to establish a definitive cancer diagnosis in the majority of ATYP cases.

Utility of ERG in Resolving an ATYP Diagnosis Beyond that Provided by Traditional AMACR and Basal Cell Markers

An important clinical question remains: is a positive ERG staining used merely to confirm a malignant diagnosis that could otherwise be established based on routine hematoxylin and eosin (H&E) histology and traditionally utilized PIN-4 cocktail antibodies composed of AMACR and basal cell markers? Alternatively, could a positive ERG staining be used to convert an atypical diagnosis to cancer in cases that otherwise would not be diagnostic of prostate cancer based on histology and traditionally utilized AMACR and basal cell markers? In our experience addressed in the earlier section of utility of ERG in resolving an "ATYP" diagnosis, traditionally utilized AMACR and basal markers were adequate to resolve ATYP diagnosis in the vast majority of cases [23]. However, owing to the high specificity of ERG for prostate cancer, ERG positivity in small atypical glands where the diagnosis of HGPIN was excluded helped establish a definitive cancer diagnosis in small proportion of additional ATYP cases where either morphology and/or traditional markers were not deemed adequate enough to offer a definitive cancer diagnosis. In this series, 12/48 (28 %) atypical diagnoses based on morphology, AMACR, and basal cell markers were changed to cancer after incorporating a positive ERG staining. These cases were morphologically suspicious for cancer and in all cases AMACR was expressed but a definitive diagnosis of cancer could not be rendered due to either quantitatively or qualitatively less than optimal morphology or inconclusive basal cell IHC. A positive AMACR staining was not sufficient in these cases to make a definitive cancer diagnosis as AMACR is also known to be expressed in a significant proportion of benign prostate cancer mimics. In this study, 67 % of lesions which were classified as atypical and 40 % of noncancer glands in all diagnostic categories demonstrated AMACR expression, indicating that AMACR expression is not cancer specific and by itself is not sufficient to convert an atypical diagnosis to cancer. On the contrary, ERG expression in small proportion of benign or HGPIN glands has been

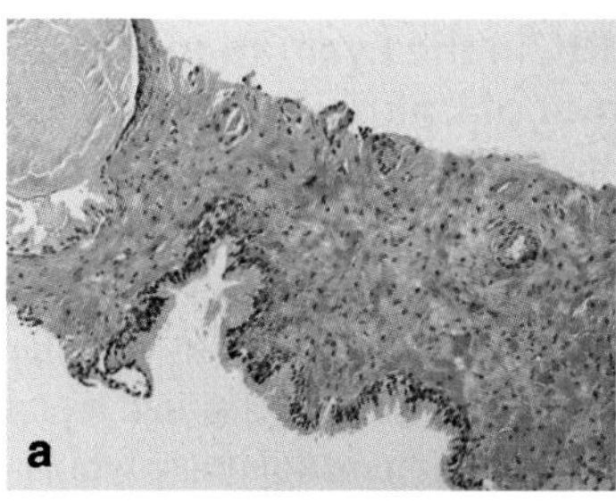
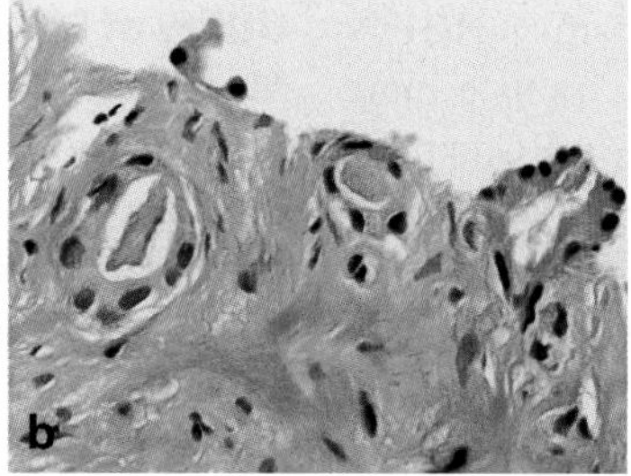
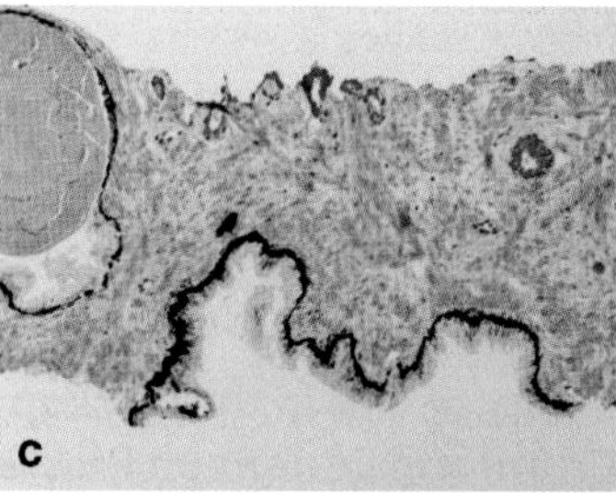

Fig. 9.4 An example of "atypical glands suspicious for cancer" (diagnosis based on morphology, AMACR, and basal cell markers) due to qualitatively less than optimal morphological features converted to cancer after incorporating positive ERG staining. The atypical glands are partially atrophic, lack obvious infiltrative architecture (**a**, ×200) and prominent atypia at higher magnification (**b**, ×400) required to render a definitive cancer diagnosis despite lack of basal cell staining and AMACR expression. The presence of strong diffuse nuclear ERG staining in atypical glands as demonstrated by PIN4-ERG multiplex stains supports the cancer diagnosis.

predominantly reported in the setting of adjacent cancer, therefore ERG positivity in small atypical glands, where the diagnosis of PINATYP or HGPIN is excluded, is virtually diagnostic of cancer [23, 24]. An example of "ATYP" (diagnosis based on morphology, AMACR, and basal cell markers) due to qualitatively less than optimal morphological features converted to cancer after incorporating positive ERG staining is represented in Fig. 9.4a–c.

ERG Expressing HGPIN and ATYP Lesions as a Predictive Biomarker of Prostate Cancer Risk Stratification in Subsequent Prostate Biopsy

Previous FISH-based evaluations of the genomic rearrangements associated with prostate cancer development have consistently revealed that about 20 % of HGPIN lesions in proximity to cancer are also positive for *ERG* rearrangement with identical *ERG* gene fusions. Evaluation of ERG oncoprotein expression in whole mount sections using clone 9FY has revealed a strong concordance between focally ERG-positive HGPIN and homogenously ERG-positive prostate cancer in 96.5 % of cases [31]. These findings indicate a clonal relationship between gene fusion-positive HGPIN and cancer and thus potential implications for utilization of ERG as a marker for prostate cancer risk stratification in patients with HGPIN diagnosis. Two studies examined the significance of ERG-positive HGPIN for future cancer risk stratification and came to contrasting conclusions. Gao et al. found that the presence of *ERG* rearrangement in HGPIN lesions detected on initial biopsy warrants repeat biopsy [36]. He et al., however, did not find the utility of ERG to stratify cancer risk associated with HGPIN [37]. Patients with initial HGPIN in biopsies and at least one follow-up prostate biopsy were included and were immunostained for ERG. The cancer detection rate was not significantly different between ERG-positive and ERG-negative HGPIN cases. The authors concluded that ERG expression is distinctly uncommon in isolated HGPIN (5.3 %) and positive ERG expression is not associated with increased cancer detection in subsequent repeat biopsies [37].

A repeat prostate biopsy after 3–6 months is recommended for patients with ATYP diagnosis due to its high predictive value for cancer detection in repeat biopsy. In a study of follow-up biopsies from 103 patients with a preliminary diagnosis of ATYP, ERG expression was detected in 16 cases (15.5 %). Of these 16 ERG-positive cases, the atypical glands were positive for ERG in nine [34]. Five of these patients (55.6 %) had cancer on repeat biopsies, compared with 42 of the 87 (48.3 %) with ERG-negative preliminary biopsies. The authors concluded that ERG expression is unlikely to help identify patients suitable for subsequent biopsies. Of note, in the study the repeat biopsies were not directed to the ERG-positive ATYP sites. Overall, additional biopsy studies assessing ERG-positive HGPIN and ATYP lesions are needed to evaluate more thoroughly the utility of measuring ERG expression as prostate cancer risk stratification in subsequent biopsies in patients with HGPIN or ATYP.

Utility of ERG in the Workup of Atypical Cribriform Lesions on Prostate Needle Biopsy

Atypical cribriform lesions of the prostate gland are defined as cribriform or rarely solid prostate glands populated by cytologically malignant cells with preservation of basal cells. It may represent cribriform HGPIN or intraductal carcinoma of the prostate (IDC-P) [38]. IDC-P is almost always associated with high-grade and high-volume invasive carcinoma. On the other hand, cribriform HGPIN is a putative neoplastic precursor lesion; recent studies have shown that the significance of HGPIN as a predictive marker of cancer has reduced significantly in the range of 25 % [39, 40]. The diagnosis of focal HGPIN, defined by <2 cores involvement, currently does not mandate a repeat biopsy within the first year of diagnosis [39]. In contrast, prostate cancer with associated IDC-P component has a significantly worse prognosis than cancer without IDC-P [40]. Therefore, the distinction of cribriform PIN from IDC-P is of paramount importance due to its widely differing clinical significance. In a study evaluating *ERG* gene fusions in a subset of cribriform HGPIN (noncancer-associated atypical cribriform lesions) and IDC-P lesions (cancer-associated atypical cribriform lesions) in totally embedded radical prostatectomy specimens, isolated cribriform HGPIN lesions consistently lacked *ERG* gene rearrangements, while IDC-P lesions regardless of their morphologic spectrum were highly enriched in these gene fusions [38]. *ERG* gene rearrangements were observed in up to 75 % of IDC-P. Therefore, all cancer-associated atypical cribriform lesions essentially represent an intraductal spread of prostate cancer, and ERG IHC has potential utility in stratification of an atypical cribriform lesion encountered in prostate biopsy. Essentially all ERG expressing atypical cribriform lesions, especially when associated with adjacent prostate cancer represent examples of IDC-P.

Utility of ERG IHC in the Evaluation of Metastatic Tumor of Unknown Origin

ERG is known to be expressed in endothelial cells, and oncogenic *ERG* gene fusions occur in subsets of prostatic carcinoma, acute myeloid leukemia, and Ewing sarcoma [41, 42]. In vascular tumors, ERG oncoprotein is expressed in a broad range of tumors including hemangiomas, lymphangiomas, angiosarcomas, epithelioid hemangioendotheliomas, and Kaposi sarcomas. Among nonvascular mesenchymal tumors, Ewing sarcoma and blastic extramedullary myeloid tumors express ERG. Among epithelial tumors, diffuse ERG expression is largely restricted to prostatic adenocarcinomas. Rare other carcinomas and epithelial tumors that may demonstrate focal ERG expression include large cell undifferentiated pulmonary carcinomas, mesotheliomas, thymomas, squamous cell carcinomas of the skin and lung, carcinosarcomas of the uterus, gastrointestinal stromal tumors, hepatocellular carcinomas, teratomas of the testis, anaplastic carcinomas of the thyroid, giant cell tumors of the tendon sheath, and benign fibrous histiocytomas of the skin [43]. Overall, ERG has a very narrow biological role in highly selected tissues and among epithelial tumors in appropriate clinical setting, strong and diffuse ERG expression would essentially support the diagnosis of prostate carcinoma [25]. Similarly, in the setting of small cell carcinoma of unknown origin, ERG positivity would support the prostatic origin of small cell carcinoma [44, 45].

Limitations of ERG IHC as Diagnostic Biomarker

Despite several promising clinical applications, ERG has several important limitations as a diagnostic prostate cancer biomarker that needs to be addressed. While positive ERG establishes a diagnosis of prostate cancer in the majority of cases, negative ERG expression offers no value in the work up of atypical cases as ERG overall has a low sensitivity for prostate cancer detection [23]. In addition, ERG expression should be interpreted with caution if the small atypical glands are either intermingled or closely associated with HGPIN glands (PINATYP) [23, 24]. As ERG is

Table 9.4 ERG protein

Genetics
ERG is a member of the *ETS* gene family, which is commonly (~50%) involved by chromosomal translocation in prostate cancer
Fusions between *TMRSS2* and *ERG* represent the most common molecular subtype accounting for ~90% of *ETS* gene fusions
Staining pattern
Nuclear staining
ERG immunostaining correlates highly with *ERG* gene alteration
Endothelial cells are strongly positive for ERG and serve as the positive internal control
Clinical utility
In small atypical glands where the diagnosis of HGPIN is ruled out, positive staining supports the cancer diagnosis
In small proportion of cases, positive ERG may help convert an ATYP diagnosis to cancer
ERG expression in atypical cribriform lesion (containing basal cells) supports the diagnosis of intraductal carcinoma of the prostate, specifically when associated with adjacent invasive carcinoma
Diffuse ERG expression in metastatic carcinoma of unknown origin supports the prostatic origin of carcinoma
Measurement of ERG overexpression in conjunction with *PTEN* loss may improve prostate cancer risk stratification
Pitfalls
Low sensitivity for prostate cancer detection; positive in 40–50% of prostate carcinomas
Positive in 20% of HGPIN that intermingles with prostate carcinoma
ERG expression may demonstrate frequent inter-focal tumor heterogeneity

HGPIN high-grade prostatic intraepithelial neoplasia, *ATYP* atypical glands suspicious for cancer

expressed in small proportion of HGPIN glands, a diagnosis of HGPIN or PINATYP cannot be ruled out with certainty in such cases. Whether ERG protein expression in such situations is a marker of unsampled adjacent cancer still remains to be addressed. Similarly, inter-focal tumor heterogeneity for ERG expression observed within multifocal prostate cancer may also potentially affect the utilization of ERG as a diagnostic, prognostic, or predictive prostate cancer biomarker.

A summary of biology, clinical applications, and pitfalls of ERG oncoprotein is summarized in Table 9.4.

Glutathione s-Transferase π 1

Biology

Glutathione s-transferase π 1 (*GSTP1*) gene methylation is the most common epigenetic change in prostate cancer [46]. Methylation silences the gene depriving normal cells of protection against damage by oxidation and electrophilic substances and subsequent malignant transformation [46]. *GSTP1* expression is rarely detected in prostate cancers. Methylation of the *GSTP1* gene is present in PIN and cancer but not in benign glands.

Clinical Applications

Using methylation-specific polymerase chain reaction (PCR) assay, detection of the methylated *GSTP1* promoter region is utilized as a tissue-based diagnostic marker to differentiate PIN and cancer from benign prostate tissue including BPH. Absent or decreased GSTP1 activity in cancerous tissue has been suggested as a potential prognostic marker [47].

Urine-Based Molecular Markers of Diagnosis

Prostate Cancer Antigen-3

Biology

First identified in 1999, initially known as *DD3* gene and later called *prostate cancer antigen-3* (*PCA3*), is overexpressed in more than 95% of all prostate cancers with high prostate specificity. The *PCA3* gene is located at 9q21–22, and encodes a nontranslational transcript [48–50]. *PCA3* assays have been developed using ribonucleic acid (RNA) detection methods since no protein products have been detected from *PCA3* RNA.

Clinical Applications

Urinary test, to detect *PCA3*, is performed following thorough digital rectal examination (with three strokes on each lobe). In the first voided urine sample, *PCA3* and *PSA* RNAs are selected, amplified by transcription-mediated amplification and detected by hybridization protection assay. *PCA3* score is calculated as *PCA3/PSA* ratio multiplied by 1000. The test is considered positive when the *PCA3/PSA* ratio is equal to or greater than 35. Clinical studies have demonstrated the sensitivity of the PCA3 test (range: 54–82 %) to be less than serum PSA, whereas the specificity of PCA3 (66–89 %) to be better. The positive predictive values (48–75 %) and negative predictive values (74–90 %) for PCA3 are also better than for PSA. The accuracy of the urinary PCA3 test ranges from 66 to 84 % [51]. Patient's age, inflammation, trauma, 5 α-reductase inhibitor use, or prostate volume do not significantly influence the test [52].

PCA3 test has been FDA approved for its ability to predict cancer in patients with increased PSA and negative biopsy (Fig. 9.5). Additionally, it has also shown utility in refining prostate cancer risk in men undergoing initial prostate biopsy (most commonly due to elevated serum PSA) [53].

Patients with atypical small acinar proliferation and high-grade prostatic intraepithelial neoplasm have a higher mean PCA3 score as compared to patients with noncancerous prostate. The mean score, however, is significantly lower than for patients with a definitive diagnosis of prostate cancer [51].

There have been conflicting reports regarding the usefulness of PCA3 in active surveillance of prostate cancer and is undergoing further evaluation. A recent study incorporated PCA3 in the management of prostate cancer. PCA3 score combined with traditional tools may aid in identifying men with clinically insignificant disease who would be candidates for active surveillance. A low PCA3 score (of 20) may have the highest utility for selecting men with clinically insignificant prostate cancer in whom active surveillance may be appropriate; a higher PCA3 score (of 50) may be useful to identify men at higher risk of harboring significant prostate cancer who would be candidates for radical prostatectomy [53].

Pitfalls

Issues arise in regard to the cutoff of PCA3 score used to determine a positive test since specificity decreases with a lower PCA3 score. A low

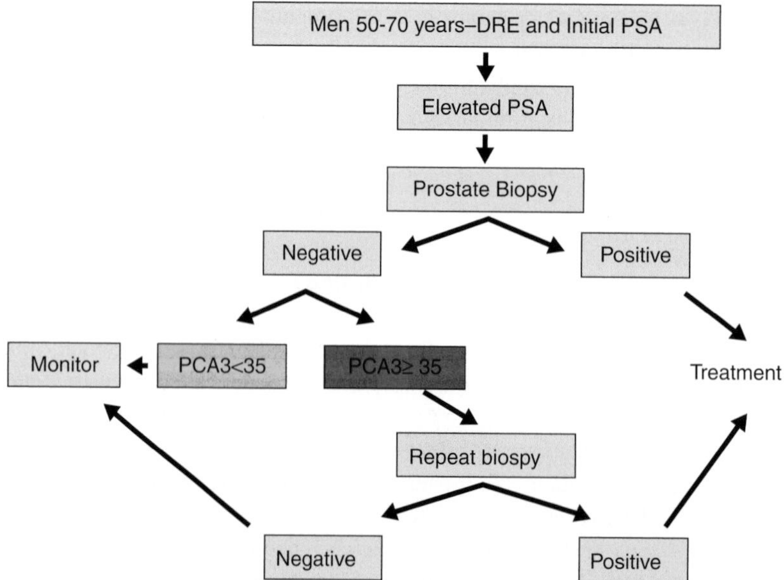

Fig. 9.5 Flow chart demonstrating current clinical applications of urine PCA3 test. *PSA* prostate-specific antigen, *DRE Digital rectal examination*

Table 9.5 PCA3

Genetics
PCA3 gene is located on 9q21–22
Overexpressed in >95 % prostate cancers
Encodes nontranslational transcript, hence assays developed using RNA detection methods
Assay: urinary test
Performed on first voided urine sample following thorough digital rectal examination (three strokes on each lobe)
PCA3 and PSA RNAs are selected, amplified by transcription-mediated amplification, and detected by hybridization protection assay
PCA3 score = *PCA3*/PSA × 1000
Positive score ≥35
Clinical utility
FDA approved for its utility in patients with increased PSA and negative biopsy
Patients with atypical acinar proliferation and high-grade prostatic intraepithelial neoplasm have higher *PCA3* score as compared to patients with noncancerous prostate
PCA3 in combination with clinical tools may identify patients with clinically insignificant disease, who could be active surveillance candidates. A low *PCA3* score may identify men with clinically insignificant disease; while a high *PCA3* score may identify patients with significant prostate cancer
Pitfalls
A low *PCA3* score does not rule out prostate cancer
Issues arise in the cutoff of *PCA3* score, specificity decreases with a lower *PCA3* score

PSA prostate-specific antigen

PCA3 test does not exclude a cancer diagnosis [52]. PCA3 test by itself may ignore the heterogeneity of prostate cancer development; hence, the preferred approach may be the use of a panel of biomarkers [54]. PCA3 represents a promising screening biomarker that may require to be used with other biomarkers for screening, given that a low PCA3 score does not exclude cancer [52].

A summary of biology, clinical applications, and pitfalls of PCA3 is summarized in Table 9.5.

Measurement of *PCA3* Multiplexed with *TMPRSS2:ERG* Fusion Genes Transcript (T2-ERG + PCA3)

Biology

Recurrent gene fusions involving the E26 transformation-specific (*ETS*) family of transcription factors *ERG, ETV1, ETV4, and ETV5,* fused to androgen-regulated *TMPRSS2* and other 5′ partner genes, have been identified in approximately 50 % of prostate cancers [13, 18, 19, 55–59]. *TMPRSS2-ERG* gene fusions represent the most specific prostate cancer biomarker reported, with FISH- and IHC-based studies reporting more than 99.99 % specificity for prostate cancer [31, 60, 61]. Similar to *PCA3*, *TMPRSS2-ERG* fusion gene transcripts can be detected in urine after digital rectal examination [62]. Addition of *TMPRSS2-ERG* fusion transcripts in PCA3 assay improves the overall accuracy of the test [63, 64].

Clinical Applications

TMPRSS2-ERG expression in urine has been quantified using reverse transcriptase PCR and transcription-mediated amplification assays [54, 63, 64]. Detection of *TMPRRS2-ERG* in urine has greater than 90 % specificity and 94 % positive predictive value for prostate cancer detection [63]. A negative biopsy with a positive *TMPRSS2-ERG* test would indicate an unsampled cancer in the patient, since *ETS* gene rearrangements have not been reported in benign prostate tissue [20, 60, 65]. Such a scenario highlights the possible utility of *TMPRSS2-ERG* fusion status in identifying a subgroup of patients that need to be followed up more closely for possible repeat biopsy, despite their negative prostate biopsy result [54, 65]. *TMPRSS2-ERG* score in urine is associated with the presence of cancer, tumor volume and clinically significant cancer in prostatectomy, and biopsy specimens [66]. *ERG* fusion status also may help predict the outcome of hormone therapy. Recent study demonstrated

ERG fusion-positive patients to be more receptive to adjuvant androgen-deprivation therapy [67]. Given the high specificity for prostate cancer, in the future, specific therapeutic solutions for *TMPRSS2-ERG*-positive men may be expected [66]. Hence, urinary ERG test would help in identifying the subgroup of *ERG*-positive men who would benefit from such therapy.

There are issues related to urine *TMPRSS2-ERG* test including the lower frequency of fusion in some populations, lowering screening sensitivity, and the identification of a cut-off that is applicable to all patient populations [52]. The reported sensitivity is 23.5 % [54]. Multiple studies have attempted to combine *TMPRSS2-ERG* gene fusions with *PCA3* for early detection of prostate cancer [54, 63, 64]. Combining *TPRSS2-ERG* with *PCA3* has a reported sensitivity of 73 % [63]. The addition of *TMPRSS2-ERG* to *PCA3* would add significant value in the prediction of biopsy Gleason score, clinical tumor stage, and extraprostatic extension in radical prostatectomy specimen [66]. The combination of both these markers could be of value for men who have persistently elevated serum PSA and a history of negative prostate biopsies. Furthermore, both tests combined could give a better indication to which patient would need to be re-biopsied and as such, could aid the diagnosis of prostate cancer as a reflex test to serum PSA [51].

Multiplex *T2-ERG* + *PCA3* + SPINK1 + GOLPH2

GOLPH2 is a Golgi apparatus-associated protein coded by the gene *GOLM1* on chromosome 9q21.33. It was originally cloned from a library derived from liver tissue of a patient with adult giant cell hepatitis. The function and the mechanisms of GOLPH2 regulation in normal and neoplastic tissues are still unclear. It can be generally assumed that it is either involved in posttranslational protein modification, transport of secretory proteins, cell signaling regulation, or simply maintenance of Golgi apparatus functions. More recently, GOLPH2 was found in the serum of patients with hepatocellular carcinoma, compared with normal individuals. Furthermore, it was found to be strongly expressed in adenocarcinoma of colorectum, breast, and prostate [68].

Laxman et al. recently explored a multiplexed qPCR urine-based diagnostic assay for prostate cancer utilizing GOLPH2, serine peptidase inhibitor, Kazal type 1 (SPINK1), *TMPRSS2-ERG*, and *PCA3* and determined that multiplexing biomarkers for cancer detection improves testing characteristics over single biomarker. This technique advances the sensitivity of urine-based tests, without sacrificing specificity. In the study, transcript expression levels of GOLPH2, SPINK1, PCA3, and *TMPRSS2-ERG* gene fusion significantly predicted prostate cancer. Sensitivity and specificity of the four-marker model for prostate cancer was 65.9 and 76.0 %, respectively. Positive and negative predictive values were 79.8 and 60.8 % respectively. *SPINK1* expression in urine samples was higher in *TMPRSS2-ERG*-negative compared with *TMPRSS2-ERG*-positive samples, corresponding with the mutual exclusivity of *SPINK1* expression and *ETS* fusions. Multiplexed urine assay, for patients presenting for prostate biopsy or prostatectomy, outperformed serum PSA or PCA3 alone [69].

Molecular Markers of Prognosis in Prostate Cancer

Biology of PTEN Deletion

PTEN (phosphatase and tensin homolog) on chromosome 10q23 is a key tumor-suppressor gene that is often deleted or inactivated in prostate cancer [70]. *PTEN* is a caretaker gene that is involved in the regulation of DNA repair, genomic instability, stem cell self-renewal, cellular senescence, and cell migration. Loss of *PTEN* function results in increased PIP3 (phosphatidylinositol (3,4,5)-triphosphate) levels and subsequent AKT phosphorylation and modulation of its downstream molecular oncogenic processes. Work over the last decade has firmly established that loss of *PTEN* is one of the most common somatic genetic aberrations in prostate cancer and is frequently associated with high-risk prostate cancer disease [70–78]. A series of in vivo studies

a

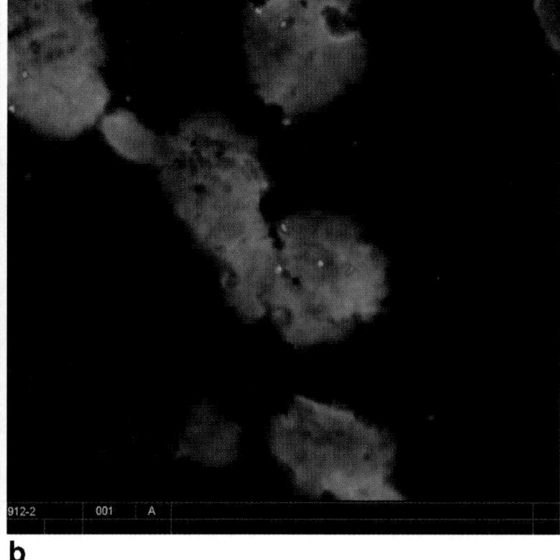

b

Fig. 9.6 **a** and **b** Prostate cancer cells demonstrate homozygous *PTEN* deletion with loss of both *PTEN* signals (*red*). *Green* signal indicates retained chromosome ten control probe (**a**). Adjacent benign prostatic tissue from same patient demonstrates retention of both copies of *PTEN* signal (*red*) and two copies of chromosome ten control probe (*green*, **b**). (**b**: Courtesy of Nallasivam Palanisamy, PhD, Michigan Center for Translational Pathology, University of Michigan)

have also demonstrated critical role of *PTEN* in prostate carcinogenesis.

Genomic deletions are the most common method for *PTEN* inactivation. Heterozygous (loss of one allele) deletions far outnumber homozygous (loss of both alleles) deletions (Fig. 9.6 a, b). Clinically, deletion or mutation of at least one *PTEN* allele was reported to occur in 20–40 % of localized cancers and up to 60 % of metastases [70]. Other uncommon and less characterized mechanisms of *PTEN* inactivation include mutation and epigenetic modifications such as methylation [79]. To date, the relative frequency of *PTEN* inactivation by mechanisms other than genomic deletion in clinical prostate cancer specimens remain unclear.

Measurement of Loss of PTEN by IHC

Recent studies have suggested that alternative mechanisms of *PTEN* inactivation or posttranscriptional down regulation may also play an important role in prostate cancer [72, 79]. Therefore, it is likely that *PTEN* FISH analysis may fail to detect some cases of prostate cancer with *PTEN* inactivation and an additional or alternative assay such as analysis of *PTEN* loss by IHC could detect additional cases where *PTEN* inactivation occurs by mechanisms other than genomic deletions. Lotan et al. utilized a rabbit monoclonal antibody and found that the antibody performed much more reliably than older clones or polyclonal antibodies [72]. They found that PTEN IHC is highly sensitive for the detection of *PTEN* genomic loss, detecting nearly 80 % of cases with loss by FISH and more than 80 % of cases with loss by high-resolution single nucleotide polymorphism (SNP) array [72]. Interestingly, 45 and 37 % of tumors with PTEN protein loss did not show genomic deletions detected by FISH or high-resolution SNP microarray, respectively. We reported a detection of 52 % of cases with *PTEN* loss by FISH using IHC if only cases with 0+ immunostaining were considered to be true negative. In this study, 35 % of their PTEN protein-negative cases did not show genomic deletions by FISH [70].

These results suggest that PTEN evaluation by IHC may provide additional benefit or supplement genomic analysis by picking up more cases of *PTEN* inactivation, which may be missed by FISH-only assay. An example of PCa showing loss of PTEN is represented in Fig. 9.7.

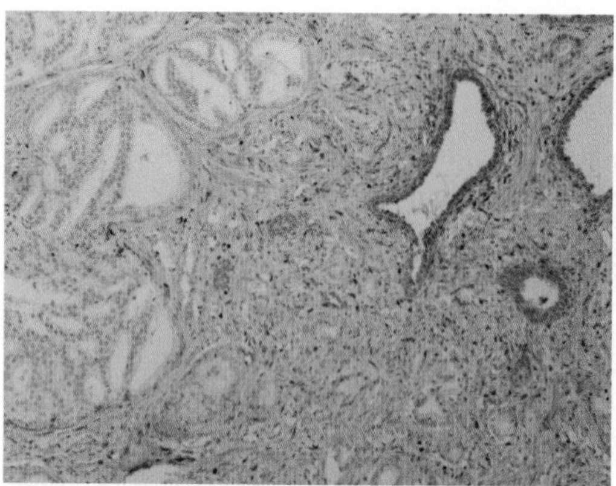

Fig. 9.7 An example of prostate cancer demonstrating loss of PTEN immunostaining in cancer cells. Adjacent benign glands and stromal cells demonstrate strong cytoplasmic staining, serving as internal positive control

Loss of PTEN and Prostate Cancer Outcomes

The majority of studies utilizing FISH or immunohistochemical methods have demonstrated that *PTEN* genomic deletion and absence of PTEN expression are frequently associated with unfavorable clinical outcome measures. Several studies have demonstrated that *PTEN* inactivation is an independent prognostic variable at multivariable analysis that is associated with a variety of different adverse pathologic outcomes including metastasis and disease-specific death [77, 79–81]. Both heterozygous (loss of one allele) and homozygous (loss of both alleles) *PTEN* deletions have been variably associated with poor prostate cancer outcomes; however, the association is strongest and consistent for homozygous *PTEN* loss. Other studies have demonstrated an association between decreased PTEN protein expression and higher Gleason grade and advanced tumor stage [74]. Recent studies also showed that *PTEN* inactivation plays an important role in prostate cancer during progression to androgen independence and development of metastasis [75, 82].

TMPRSS2:ERG Gene Fusions as a Prognostic PCa Biomarker

The prognostic association of *ERG* alterations remains uncertain in prostate cancer. Numerous genomic studies have examined the association of *ERG* and prostate cancer outcomes and have found variable results. Several studies have found independent association with poor outcomes including cancer-specific death [16, 83–85], while some studies have found no association [86], and paradoxically one study has shown association of *ERG* gene fusions and favorable outcomes [87]. Certain mechanisms of *ERG* rearrangement have shown to be more consistently associated with poor outcomes. We reported deletion as an exclusive mechanism of *ERG* rearrangement in patients who died of hormone refractory metastatic prostate cancer [22]. Deletion of the intermediate region between *TMPRSS2* and *ERG* combined with duplication of the *TMPRSS2:ERG* fusion sequences are predictive of poor cancer-specific survival, an observation supported by several studies [22, 83].

The studies analyzing ERG oncoprotein and prostate cancer outcomes have also not found consistent evidence of prognostic association [88–90]. It is important to note, however, that to study prognostic associations in prostate cancer, use of ERG antibody may not be an optimal approach, as ERG expression does not stratify underlying mechanisms of *ERG* rearrangements in prostate cancer. Notably, as explained in the earlier section, several studies have demonstrated poor outcomes when *ERG* rearrangements occur through deletion or deleted and amplified (EDel2+) mechanisms.

Combined Measurement of PTEN Loss and ERG Overexpression as Prognostic Biomarker

PTEN loss and *ETS* gene rearrangements are the most common molecular events in prostate carcinogenesis and are proposed to be critically important. In particular, there is a strong relationship between the two events in clinical and mouse models demonstrating cooperation [70]. *PTEN* deletion appears to be a late genetic event in human prostate cancer, presumably a “second hit” after *ERG* rearrangement. Several studies have analyzed the effect of *PTEN* loss on prostate cancer survival and its relationship to the

Table 9.6 PTEN

Genetics
PTEN (phosphatase and tensin homolog) on chromosome 10q23 is a key tumor-suppressor gene that is often deleted or inactivated in prostate cancer. *PTEN* is a caretaker gene that is involved in the regulation of DNA repair, genomic instability, stem cell self-renewal, cellular senescence, and cell migration
Clinically, deletion or mutation of at least one *PTEN* allele occurs in 20–40% of localized cancers and up to 60% of metastases
Staining pattern
Cytoplasmic staining in prostate cancer cells is considered intact PTEN; complete or partial loss of PTEN staining is considered loss of PTEN
Loss of PTEN staining in prostate cancer cells correlates with *PTEN* inactivation or deletion as measured by FISH and SNP array
Adjacent benign glands and stromal cells staining serve as the positive internal control
Clinical utility
Several studies have demonstrated that *PTEN* inactivation or *PTEN* loss is an independent prognostic variable at multivariable analysis that is associated with variety of different adverse pathologic outcomes including Gleason grade, pathologic stage, metastasis, and disease-specific death
PTEN loss in atypical cribriform lesion (containing basal cells) supports the diagnosis of intraductal carcinoma of the prostate over high grade prostatic intraepithelial neoplasia (HGPIN)
Pitfalls
Measurement of PTEN loss may be affected by both inter and intra-focal tumor heterogeneity

DNA deoxyribonucleic acid, *FISH* fluorescent in situ hybridization, *SNP* single nucleotide polymorphism

ETS rearrangements. Reid et al. identified three molecular prognostic groups. *PTEN* gene loss with no *ERG/ETV1* rearrangement identified a poor prognosis group [91]. In this cohort, 21% of patients had Gleason score <7, supporting that molecular reclassification of prostate cancer may be relevant. *ERG/ETV1* gene rearranged tumors with and without *PTEN* loss formed two intermediate prognostic groups. No *ERG/ETV1* gene rearrangement and no *PTEN* loss identified a good prognosis group. Yoshimoto et al. also proposed three molecular groups: poor genomic grade for prostate cancer with both *PTEN* deletion and *ERG* fusion, intermediate grade when either *PTEN* deletion or *ERG* fusion, and favorable grade when neither rearrangements present [81].

In conclusion, characterization of *PTEN, ERG,* and *ETV1* gene status might be used in future to determine the risk of prostate cancer death. This has implications both for potentially deciding which patients should be conservatively or aggressively treated and also for risk stratification of patients in clinical trials. A summary of biology, significance, clinical applications, and pitfalls of determination of *PTEN* loss in prostate cancer is summarized in Table 9.6.

SPINK1

Biology

ETS gene fusions are present in only ~50% of the cases, leaving nearly 50% of the remaining cases where the driving genetic aberration is largely unknown. Recently identified, SPINK1 is overexpressed in a subset of prostate cancers (10%) that are *ETS*-rearrangement negative [92]. *SPINK1* mRNA is normally found in pancreas as well as in a number of cancers [93–99]. It encodes a peptide that protects pancreas from auto digestion, by preventing premature activation of pancreatic proteases [100]. Prostate gland, like pancreas, also secretes a number of proteases, notably the kallikrien enzyme PSA, but also the trypsin, the expression of which is increased in prostate cancer [101]. SPINK1 expression may have a role in modulating the activity of cancer-related proteases.

Clinical Applications

Expression of SPINK1 has been correlated with aggressive disease [92]. In a subsequent study, it was reported that SPINK1 mediates its neoplastic effects in part through interactions with the epidermal growth factor receptor (EGFR).

Antibodies to both EGFR and SPINK1 block the growth of SPINK1+/ETS− tumors more than either antibody alone and do not affect ETS− tumors, thus suggesting a potential therapeutic avenue for a subset of prostate cancers with SPINK1 overexpression [102]. The identification of SPINK1 in prostate cancer may, hence, have dual function in detecting patients with more aggressive outcome and in identifying patients who may benefit from emerging therapeutics. SPINK1 can be detected in tissue samples by IHC as well as quantitative PCR and similarly in urine by quantitative PCR following RNA amplification [92]. SPINK1 has been used as one of the markers in multiplexing study to detect prostate cancer [69]. Urine being easily available and noninvasive would be a simple way to recognize patients with aggressive cancer and direct them towards targeted therapy.

Enhancer of Zeste Homolog 2

Biology

Enhancer of zeste homolog 2 (EZH2) is a component of polycomb repressive complex 2 (PRC2) along with embryonic ectoderm development (EED) and suppressor of zeste 12 (SUZ12). PRC2 complex is postulated to control gene expression during proliferation of normal cells. Dysregulation of components of the PRC2 complex, such as EZH2, has a significant impact on the expression of cell-cycle regulatory genes [103, 104]. MicroRNA 101 negatively regulates EZH2 expression and concurrently attenuates the invasion ability of prostate cancer cells, which can be rescued by ectopically expressed EZH2. Deletions of microRNA 101 have been described in prostate cancer, thus providing a mechanism for EZH2 overexpression. Restoring microRNA 101 may, hence, be an effective approach for treatment [105, 106].

Clinical Applications

EZH2 may be a potential biomarker which could provide valuable prognostic information. Polycomb group protein enhancer of zeste homolog 2 (EZH2) is overexpressed in hormone-refractory, metastatic prostate cancer and other aggressive cancers. Its expression status is predictive of disease progression, poor prognosis, and treatment outcome [107]. Similarly, it has been proposed that development of EZH2 inhibitors may be antiangiogenic and antimetastatic [108].

Summary

New genomic and bioinformatics technologies have enabled us to discover and study an expanding universe of novel tissue-, urine-, or body fluid-based biomarkers. Despite great promise and extensive research, very few biomarkers have come into routine clinical practice. Lack of vigorous prospective-blinded studies to validate biomarkers is one of the important reasons for poor clinical acceptance. In addition, biomarkers development and validation are affected by many compounding factors, including specimen collection and assay platforms. A summary of potential clinical applications of proposed biomarkers in clinical practice is summarized in Fig. 9.8.

Acknowledgments We acknowledge Nallasivam Palanisamy, PhD, Michigan Center for Translational Pathology, University of Michigan for providing Fig. 9.6b; M. Carmen Frias-Kletecka, MD, LSU, for critical reading of the chapter; and Monica Brynes, graphics manager, LSU, for assistance with the images.

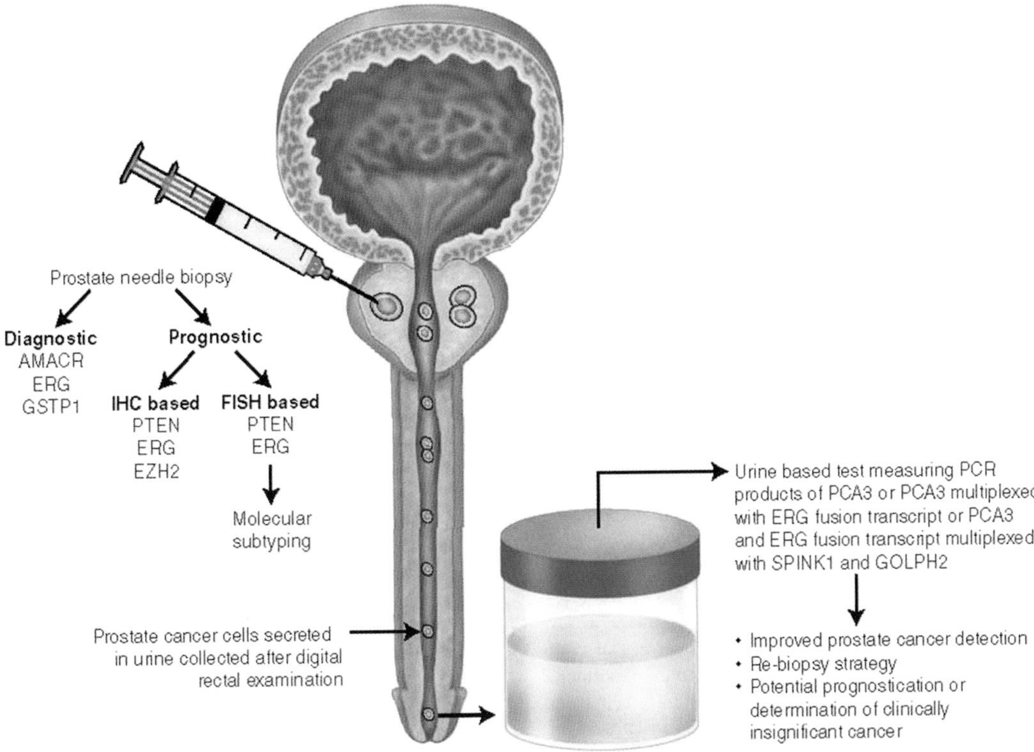

Fig. 9.8 Summary of potential diagnostic and prognostic applications of selected tissue- and urine-based biomarkers in prostate cancer. *IHC* immunohistochemistry, *FISH* fluorescent in situ hybridization, *PCR* polymerase chain reaction

References

1. Rubin MA, Zhou M, Dhanasekaran SM, Varambally S, Barrette TR, Sanda MG, et al. Alpha-Methylacyl coenzyme A racemase as a tissue biomarker for prostate cancer. JAMA. 2002;287(13):1662–70.
2. Luo J, Zha S, Gage WR, Dunn TA, Hicks JL, Bennett CJ, et al. Alpha-methylacyl-CoA racemase: a new molecular marker for prostate cancer. Cancer Res. 2002;62(8):2220–6.
3. Zhou M, Chinnaiyan AM, Kleer CG, Lucas PC, Rubin MA. Alpha-Methylacyl-CoA racemase: a novel tumor marker over-expressed in several human cancers and their precursor lesions. Am J Surg Pathol. 2002;26(7):926–31.
4. Kunju LP, Chinnaiyan AM, Shah RB. Comparison of monoclonal antibody (P504S) and polyclonal antibody to alpha methylacyl-CoA racemase (AMACR) in the work-up of prostate cancer. Histopathology. 2005;47(6):587–96.
5. Paner GP, Luthringer DJ, Amin MB. Best practice in diagnostic immunohistochemistry: prostate carcinoma and its mimics in needle core biopsies. Arch Pathol Lab Med. 2008;132(9):1388–96.
6. Kunju LP, Rubin MA, Chinnaiyan AM, Shah RB. Diagnostic usefulness of monoclonal antibody P504S in the workup of atypical prostatic glandular proliferations. Am J Clin Pathol. 2003;120(5):737–45.
7. Zhou M, Jiang Z, Epstein JI. Expression and diagnostic utility of alpha-methylacyl-CoA-racemase (P504S) in foamy gland and pseudohyperplastic prostate cancer. Am J Surg Pathol. 2003;27(6):772–8.
8. Yang XJ, Laven B, Tretiakova M, Blute RD Jr., Woda BA, Steinberg GD, et al. Detection of alpha-methylacyl-coenzyme A racemase in postradiation prostatic adenocarcinoma. Urology. 2003;62(2):282–6.
9. Zhou M, Aydin H, Kanane H, Epstein JI. How often does alpha-methylacyl-CoA-racemase contribute to resolving an atypical diagnosis on prostate needle biopsy beyond that provided by basal cell markers? Am J Surg Pathol. 2004;28(2):239–43.
10. Przybycin CG, Kunju LP, Wu AJ, Shah RB. Partial atrophy in prostate needle biopsies: a detailed analysis of its morphology, immunophenotype, and cellular kinetics. Am J Surg Pathol. 2008;32(1):58–64.
11. Skinnider BF, Oliva E, Young RH, Amin MB. Expression of alpha-methylacyl-CoA racemase (P504S) in nephrogenic adenoma: a significant immunohistochemical pitfall compounding the differential diagnosis with prostatic adenocarcinoma. Am J Surg Pathol. 2004;28(6):701–5.

12. Yang XJ, Wu CL, Woda BA, Dresser K, Tretiakova M, Fanger GR, et al. Expression of alpha-Methylacyl-CoA racemase (P504S) in atypical adenomatous hyperplasia of the prostate. Am J Surg Pathol. 2002;26(7):921–5.
13. Tomlins SA, Rhodes DR, Perner S, Dhanasekaran SM, Mehra R, Sun XW, et al. Recurrent fusion of TMPRSS2 and ETS transcription factor genes in prostate cancer. Science. 2005;310(5748):644–8.
14. Mehra R, Tomlins SA, Shen R, Nadeem O, Wang L, Wei JT, et al. Comprehensive assessment of TMPRSS2 and ETS family gene aberrations in clinically localized prostate cancer. Mod Pathol. 2007;20(5):538–44.
15. Mosquera JM, Mehra R, Regan MM, Perner S, Genega EM, Bueti G, et al. Prevalence of TMPRSS2-ERG fusion prostate cancer among men undergoing prostate biopsy in the United States. Clin Cancer Res. 2009;15(14):4706–11.
16. Perner S, Demichelis F, Beroukhim R, Schmidt FH, Mosquera JM, Setlur S, et al. TMPRSS2:ERG fusion-associated deletions provide insight into the heterogeneity of prostate cancer. Cancer Res. 2006;66(17):8337–41.
17. Shah RB, Chinnaiyan AM. The discovery of common recurrent transmembrane protease serine 2 (TMPRSS2)-erythroblastosis virus E26 transforming sequence (ETS) gene fusions in prostate cancer: significance and clinical implications. Adv Anat Pathol. 2009;16(3):145–53.
18. Han B, Mehra R, Dhanasekaran SM, Yu J, Menon A, Lonigro RJ, et al. A fluorescence in situ hybridization screen for E26 transformation-specific aberrations: identification of DDX5-ETV4 fusion protein in prostate cancer. Cancer Res. 2008;68(18):7629–37.
19. Helgeson BE, Tomlins SA, Shah N, Laxman B, Cao Q, Prensner JR, et al. Characterization of TMPRSS2:ETV5 and SLC45A3:ETV5 gene fusions in prostate cancer. Cancer Res. 2008;68(1):73–80.
20. Perner S, Mosquera JM, Demichelis F, Hofer MD, Paris PL, Simko J, et al. TMPRSS2-ERG fusion prostate cancer: an early molecular event associated with invasion. Am J Surg Pathol. 2007;31(6):882–8.
21. Mehra R, Han B, Tomlins SA, Wang L, Menon A, Wasco MJ, et al. Heterogeneity of TMPRSS2 gene rearrangements in multifocal prostate adenocarcinoma: molecular evidence for an independent group of diseases. Cancer Res. 2007;67(17):7991–5.
22. Mehra R, Tomlins SA, Yu J, Cao X, Wang L, Menon A, et al. Characterization of TMPRSS2-ETS gene aberrations in androgen-independent metastatic prostate cancer. Cancer Res. 2008;68(10):3584–90.
23. Shah RB, Tadros Y, Brummell B, Zhou M. The diagnostic use of ERG in resolving an "atypical glands suspicious for cancer" diagnosis in prostate biopsies beyond that provided by basal cell and alpha-methylacyl-CoA-racemase markers. Hum Pathol. 2013;44(5):786–94.
24. Tomlins SA, Palanisamy N, Siddiqui J, Chinnaiyan AM, Kunju LP. Antibody-based detection of ERG rearrangements in prostate core biopsies, including diagnostically challenging cases: ERG staining in prostate core biopsies. Arch Pathol Lab Med. 2012;136(8):935–46.
25. Shah RB. Clinical applications of novel ERG immunohistochemistry in prostate cancer diagnosis and management. Adv Anat Pathol. 2013;20(2):117–24.
26. Park K, Tomlins SA, Mudaliar KM, Chiu YL, Esgueva R, Mehra R, et al. Antibody-based detection of ERG rearrangement-positive prostate cancer. Neoplasia. 2010;12(7):590–8.
27. Chaux A, Albadine R, Toubaji A, Hicks J, Meeker A, Platz EA, et al. Immunohistochemistry for ERG expression as a surrogate for TMPRSS2-ERG fusion detection in prostatic adenocarcinomas. Am J Surg Pathol. 2011;35(7):1014–20.
28. Falzarano SM, Zhou M, Carver P, Tsuzuki T, Simmerman K, He H, et al. ERG gene rearrangement status in prostate cancer detected by immunohistochemistry. Virchows Arch. 2011;459(4):441–7.
29. van Leenders GJ, Boormans JL, Vissers CJ, Hoogland AM, Bressers AA, Furusato B, et al. Antibody EPR3864 is specific for ERG genomic fusions in prostate cancer: implications for pathological practice. Mod Pathol. 2011;24(8):1128–38.
30. Braun M, Goltz D, Shaikhibrahim Z, Vogel W, Bohm D, Scheble V, et al. ERG protein expression and genomic rearrangement status in primary and metastatic prostate cancer—a comparative study of two monoclonal antibodies. Prostate Cancer Prostatic Dis. 2012;15(2):165–9.
31. Furusato B, Tan SH, Young D, Dobi A, Sun C, Mohamed AA, et al. ERG oncoprotein expression in prostate cancer: clonal progression of ERG-positive tumor cells and potential for ERG-based stratification. Prostate Cancer Prostatic Dis. 2010;13(3):228–37.
32. Hameed O, Humphrey PA. Immunohistochemistry in diagnostic surgical pathology of the prostate. Semin Diagn Pathol. 2005;22(1):88–104.
33. Varma M, Jasani B. Diagnostic utility of immunohistochemistry in morphologically difficult prostate cancer: review of current literature. Histopathology. 2005;47(1):1–16.
34. He H, Magi-Galluzzi C, Li J, Carver P, Falzarano S, Smith K, et al. The diagnostic utility of novel immunohistochemical marker ERG in the workup of prostate biopsies with "atypical glands suspicious for cancer". Am J Surg Pathol. 2011;35(4):608–14.
35. Yaskiv O, Zhang X, Simmerman K, Daly T, He H, Falzarano S, et al. The utility of ERG/P63 double immunohistochemical staining in the diagnosis of limited cancer in prostate needle biopsies. Am J Surg Pathol. 2011;35(7):1062–8.
36. Gao X, Li LY, Zhou FJ, Xie KJ, Shao CK, Su ZL, et al. ERG rearrangement for predicting subsequent cancer diagnosis in high-grade prostatic intraepithelial neoplasia and lymph node metastasis. Clin Cancer Res. 2012;18(15):4163–72.

37. He H, Osunkoya AO, Carver P, Falzarano S, Klein E, Magi-Galluzzi C, et al. Expression of ERG protein, a prostate cancer specific marker, in high grade prostatic intraepithelial neoplasia (HGPIN): lack of utility to stratify cancer risks associated with HGPIN. BJU Int. 2012;110(11 Pt B):E751–5.
38. Shah RB, Zhou M. Atypical cribriform lesions of the prostate: clinical significance, differential diagnosis and current concept of intraductal carcinoma of the prostate. Adv Anat Pathol. 2012;19(4):270–8.
39. Epstein JI, Herawi M. Prostate needle biopsies containing prostatic intraepithelial neoplasia or atypical foci suspicious for carcinoma: implications for patient care. J Urol. 2006; 175(3 Pt 1):820–34.
40. Shah RB, Magi-Galluzzi C, Han B, Zhou M. Atypical cribriform lesions of the prostate: relationship to prostatic carcinoma and implication for diagnosis in prostate biopsies. Am J Surg Pathol. 2010;34(4):470–7.
41. Miettinen M, Wang ZF, Paetau A, Tan SH, Dobi A, Srivastava S, et al. ERG transcription factor as an immunohistochemical marker for vascular endothelial tumors and prostatic carcinoma. Am J Surg Pathol. 2011;35(3):432–41.
42. Wang WL, Patel NR, Caragea M, Hogendoorn PC, Lopez-Terrada D, Hornick JL, et al. Expression of ERG, an ETS family transcription factor, identifies ERG-rearranged Ewing sarcoma. Mod Pathol. 2012;25(10):1378–83.
43. Minner S, Luebke AM, Kluth M, Bokemeyer C, Janicke F, Izbicki J, et al. High level of ETS-related gene expression has high specificity for prostate cancer: a tissue microarray study of 11 483 cancers. Histopathology. 2012;61(3):445–53.
44. Guo CC, Dancer JY, Wang Y, Aparicio A, Navone NM, Troncoso P, et al. TMPRSS2-ERG gene fusion in small cell carcinoma of the prostate. Hum Pathol. 2011;42(1):11–7.
45. Han B, Mehra R, Suleman K, Tomlins SA, Wang L, Singhal N, et al. Characterization of ETS gene aberrations in select histologic variants of prostate carcinoma. Mod Pathol. 2009;22(9):1176–85.
46. Meiers I, Shanks JH, Bostwick DG. Glutathione S-transferase pi (GSTP1) hypermethylation in prostate cancer: review 2007. Pathology. 2007;39(3):299–304.
47. Ellinger J, Bastian PJ, Jurgan T, Biermann K, Kahl P, Heukamp LC, et al. CpG island hypermethylation at multiple gene sites in diagnosis and prognosis of prostate cancer. Urology. 2008;71(1):161–7.
48. Bussemakers MJ, van Bokhoven A, Verhaegh GW, Smit FP, Karthaus HF, Schalken JA, et al. DD3: a new prostate-specific gene, highly overexpressed in prostate cancer. Cancer Res. [Research Support, Non-U.S. Gov't]. 1999;59(23):5975–9.
49. de Kok JB, Verhaegh GW, Roelofs RW, Hessels D, Kiemeney LA, Aalders TW, et al. DD3(PCA3), a very sensitive and specific marker to detect prostate tumors. Cancer Res. 2002;62(9):2695–8.
50. Hessels D, Klein Gunnewiek JM, van Oort I, Karthaus HF, van Leenders GJ, van Balken B, et al. DD3(PCA3)-based molecular urine analysis for the diagnosis of prostate cancer. Eur Urol. [Comparative Study]. 2003;44(1):8–15; discussion 6.
51. Vlaeminck-Guillem V, Ruffion A, Andre J, Devonec M, Paparel P. Urinary prostate cancer 3 test: toward the age of reason? Urology. [Review]. 2010;75(2):447–53.
52. Truong M, Yang B, Jarrard DF. Toward the detection of prostate cancer in urine: a critical analysis. J Urol. 2013;189(2):422–9.
53. van Poppel H, Haese A, Graefen M, de la Taille A, Irani J, de Reijke T, et al. The relationship between prostate cancer gene 3 (PCA3) and prostate cancer significance. BJU Int. [Meta-Analysis]. 2012;109(3):360–6.
54. Leyten GH, Hessels D, Jannink SA, Smit FP, de Jong H, Cornel EB, et al. Prospective multicentre evaluation of PCA3 and TMPRSS2-ERG gene fusions as diagnostic and prognostic urinary biomarkers for prostate cancer. Eur Urol. 2014;65(3):534–42.
55. Tomlins SA, Mehra R, Rhodes DR, Smith LR, Roulston D, Helgeson BE, et al. TMPRSS2:ETV4 gene fusions define a third molecular subtype of prostate cancer. Cancer Res. 2006;66(7):3396–400.
56. Hermans KG, Bressers AA, van der Korput HA, Dits NF, Jenster G, Trapman J. Two unique novel prostate-specific and androgen-regulated fusion partners of ETV4 in prostate cancer. Cancer Res. 2008;68(9):3094–8.
57. Attard G, Clark J, Ambroisine L, Mills IG, Fisher G, Flohr P, et al. Heterogeneity and clinical significance of ETV1 translocations in human prostate cancer. Br J Cancer. [Research Support, N.I.H., ExtramuralResearch Support, Non-U.S. Gov't]. 2008;99(2):314–20.
58. Tomlins SA, Laxman B, Dhanasekaran SM, Helgeson BE, Cao X, Morris DS, et al. Distinct classes of chromosomal rearrangements create oncogenic ETS gene fusions in prostate cancer. Nature. 2007;448(7153):595–9.
59. Kumar-Sinha C, Tomlins SA, Chinnaiyan AM. Recurrent gene fusions in prostate cancer. Nat Rev Cancer. 2008;8(7):497–511.
60. Tomlins SA, Bjartell A, Chinnaiyan AM, Jenster G, Nam RK, Rubin MA, et al. ETS gene fusions in prostate cancer: from discovery to daily clinical practice. Eur Urol. 2009;56(2):275–86.
61. Young A, Palanisamy N, Siddiqui J, Wood DP, Wei JT, Chinnaiyan AM, et al. Correlation of urine TMPRSS2:ERG and PCA3 to ERG+ and total prostate cancer burden. Am J Clin Pathol. [Research Support, N.I.H., Extramural Research Support, Non-U.S. Gov't]. 2012;138(5):685–96.
62. Laxman B, Tomlins SA, Mehra R, Morris DS, Wang L, Helgeson BE, et al. Noninvasive detection of TMPRSS2:ERG fusion transcripts in the urine of men with prostate cancer. Neoplasia. 2006;8(10):885–8.
63. Hessels D, Smit FP, Verhaegh GW, Witjes JA, Cornel EB, Schalken JA. Detection of TMPRSS2-ERG fusion transcripts and prostate cancer antigen 3 in urinary sediments may improve

diagnosis of prostate cancer. Clin Cancer Res. 2007;13(17):5103–8.

64. Tomlins SA, Aubin SM, Siddiqui J, Lonigro RJ, Sefton-Miller L, Miick S, et al. Urine TMPRSS2:ERG fusion transcript stratifies prostate cancer risk in men with elevated serum PSA. Sci Transl Med. [Research Support, N.I.H., Extramural Research Support, Non-U.S. Gov't]. 2011;3(94):94ra72.
65. Salami SS, Schmidt F, Laxman B, Regan MM, Rickman DS, Scherr D, et al. Combining urinary detection of TMPRSS2:ERG and PCA3 with serum PSA to predict diagnosis of prostate cancer. Urol Oncol. 2013;31(5):566–71.
66. Salagierski M, Schalken JA. Molecular diagnosis of prostate cancer: PCA3 and TMPRSS2:ERG gene fusion. J Urol. [Research Support, Non-U.S. Gov't Review]. 2012;187(3):795–801.
67. Karnes RJ, Cheville JC, Ida CM, Sebo TJ, Nair AA, Tang H, et al. The ability of biomarkers to predict systemic progression in men with high-risk prostate cancer treated surgically is dependent on ERG status. Cancer Res. [Research Support, N.I.H., Extramural Research Support, Non-U.S. Gov't]. 2010;70(22):8994–9002.
68. Kristiansen G, Fritzsche FR, Wassermann K, Jager C, Tolls A, Lein M, et al. GOLPH2 protein expression as a novel tissue biomarker for prostate cancer: implications for tissue-based diagnostics. Br J Cancer. 2008;99(6):939–48.
69. Laxman B, Morris DS, Yu J, Siddiqui J, Cao J, Mehra R, et al. A first-generation multiplex biomarker analysis of urine for the early detection of prostate cancer. Cancer Res. 2008;68(3):645–9.
70. Han B, Mehra R, Lonigro RJ, Wang L, Suleman K, Menon A, et al. Fluorescence in situ hybridization study shows association of PTEN deletion with ERG rearrangement during prostate cancer progression. Mod Pathol. 2009;22(8):1083–93.
71. Halvorsen OJ, Haukaas SA, Akslen LA. Combined loss of PTEN and p27 expression is associated with tumor cell proliferation by Ki-67 and increased risk of recurrent disease in localized prostate cancer. Clin Cancer Res. 2003;9(4):1474–9.
72. Lotan TL, Gurel B, Sutcliffe S, Esopi D, Liu W, Xu J, et al. PTEN protein loss by immunostaining: analytic validation and prognostic indicator for a high risk surgical cohort of prostate cancer patients. Clin Cancer Res. 2011;17(20):6563–73.
73. McCall P, Witton CJ, Grimsley S, Nielsen KV, Edwards J. Is PTEN loss associated with clinical outcome measures in human prostate cancer? Br J Cancer. 2008;99(8):1296–301.
74. McMenamin ME, Soung P, Perera S, Kaplan I, Loda M, Sellers WR. Loss of PTEN expression in paraffin-embedded primary prostate cancer correlates .with high Gleason score and advanced stage. Cancer Res. 1999;59(17):4291–6.
75. Schmitz M, Grignard G, Margue C, Dippel W, Capesius C, Mossong J, et al. Complete loss of PTEN expression as a possible early prognostic marker for prostate cancer metastasis. Int J Cancer. 2007;120(6):1284–92.
76. Whang YE, Wu X, Suzuki H, Reiter RE, Tran C, Vessella RL, et al. Inactivation of the tumor suppressor PTEN/MMAC1 in advanced human prostate cancer through loss of expression. Proc Natl Acad Sci U S A. 1998;95(9):5246–50.
77. Yoshimoto M, Cunha IW, Coudry RA, Fonseca FP, Torres CH, Soares FA, et al. FISH analysis of 107 prostate cancers shows that PTEN genomic deletion is associated with poor clinical outcome. Br J Cancer. 2007;97(5):678–85.
78. Yoshimoto M, Cutz JC, Nuin PA, Joshua AM, Bayani J, Evans AJ, et al. Interphase FISH analysis of PTEN in histologic sections shows genomic deletions in 68 % of primary prostate cancer and 23 % of high-grade prostatic intra-epithelial neoplasias. Cancer Genet Cytogenet. 2006;169(2):128–37.
79. Chaux A, Peskoe SB, Gonzalez-Roibon N, Schultz L, Albadine R, Hicks J, et al. Loss of PTEN expression is associated with increased risk of recurrence after prostatectomy for clinically localized prostate cancer. Mod Pathol. 2012;25(11):1543–9.
80. Krohn A, Diedler T, Burkhardt L, Mayer PS, De Silva C, Meyer-Kornblum M, et al. Genomic deletion of PTEN is associated with tumor progression and early PSA recurrence in ERG fusion-positive and fusion-negative prostate cancer. Am J Pathol. 2012;181(2):401–12.
81. Yoshimoto M, Joshua AM, Cunha IW, Coudry RA, Fonseca FP, Ludkovski O, et al. Absence of TMPRSS2:ERG fusions and PTEN losses in prostate cancer is associated with a favorable outcome. Mod Pathol. 2008;21(12):1451–60.
82. Bertram J, Peacock JW, Fazli L, Mui AL, Chung SW, Cox ME, et al. Loss of PTEN is associated with progression to androgen independence. Prostate. 2006;66(9):895–902.
83. Attard G, Clark J, Ambroisine L, Fisher G, Kovacs G, Flohr P, et al. Duplication of the fusion of TMPRSS2 to ERG sequences identifies fatal human prostate cancer. Oncogene. 2008;27(3):253–63.
84. Demichelis F, Fall K, Perner S, Andren O, Schmidt F, Setlur SR, et al. TMPRSS2:ERG gene fusion associated with lethal prostate cancer in a watchful waiting cohort. Oncogene. 2007;26(31):4596–9.
85. Nam RK, Sugar L, Wang Z, Yang W, Kitching R, Klotz LH, et al. Expression of TMPRSS2:ERG gene fusion in prostate cancer cells is an important prognostic factor for cancer progression. Cancer Biol Ther. 2007;6(1):40–5.
86. Gopalan A, Leversha MA, Satagopan JM, Zhou Q, Al-Ahmadie HA, Fine SW, et al. TMPRSS2-ERG gene fusion is not associated with outcome in patients treated by prostatectomy. Cancer Res. 2009;69(4):1400–6.
87. Hermans KG, Boormans JL, Gasi D, van Leenders GJ, Jenster G, Verhagen PC, et al. Overexpression of prostate-specific TMPRSS2(exon 0)-ERG fusion transcripts corresponds with favorable

prognosis of prostate cancer. Clin Cancer Res. 2009;15(20):6398–403.

88. Hoogland AM, Jenster G, van Weerden WM, Trapman J, van der Kwast T, Roobol MJ, et al. ERG immunohistochemistry is not predictive for PSA recurrence, local recurrence or overall survival after radical prostatectomy for prostate cancer. Mod Pathol. 2012;25(3):471–9.
89. Minner S, Enodien M, Sirma H, Luebke AM, Krohn A, Mayer PS, et al. ERG status is unrelated to PSA recurrence in radically operated prostate cancer in the absence of antihormonal therapy. Clin Cancer Res. 2011;17(18):5878–88.
90. Pettersson A, Graff RE, Bauer SR, Pitt MJ, Lis RT, Stack EC, et al. The TMPRSS2:ERG rearrangement, ERG expression, and prostate cancer outcomes: a cohort study and meta-analysis. Cancer Epidemiol Biomarkers Prev. 2012;21(9):1497–509.
91. Reid AH, Attard G, Ambroisine L, Fisher G, Kovacs G, Brewer D, et al. Molecular characterisation of ERG, ETV1 and PTEN gene loci identifies patients at low and high risk of death from prostate cancer. Br J Cancer. 2010;102(4):678–84.
92. Tomlins SA, Rhodes DR, Yu J, Varambally S, Mehra R, Perner S, et al. The role of SPINK1 in ETS rearrangement-negative prostate cancers. Cancer Cell. 2008;13(6):519–28.
93. Lukkonen A, Lintula S, von Boguslawski K, Carpen O, Ljungberg B, Landberg G, et al. Tumor-associated trypsin inhibitor in normal and malignant renal tissue and in serum of renal-cell carcinoma patients. Int J Cancer. [Research Support, Non-U.S. Gov't]. 1999;83(4):486–90.
94. Kelloniemi E, Rintala E, Finne P, Stenman UH, Finnbladder G. Tumor-associated trypsin inhibitor as a prognostic factor during follow-up of bladder cancer. Urology. 2003;62(2):249–53.
95. Haglund C, Huhtala ML, Halila H, Nordling S, Roberts PJ, Scheinin TM, et al. Tumour-associated trypsin inhibitor, TATI, in patients with pancreatic cancer, pancreatitis and benign biliary diseases. Br J Cancer. [Research Support, Non-U.S. Gov't]. 1986;54(2):297–303.
96. Higashiyama M, Monden T, Tomita N, Murotani M, Kawasaki Y, Morimoto H, et al. Expression of pancreatic secretory trypsin inhibitor (PSTI) in colorectal cancer. Br J Cancer. [Research Support, Non-U.S. Gov't]. 1990;62(6):954–8.
97. Huhtala ML, Kahanpaa K, Seppala M, Halila H, Stenman UH. Excretion of a tumor-associated trypsin inhibitor (TATI) in urine of patients with gynecological malignancy. Int J Cancer. [Comparative Study Research Support, Non-U.S. Gov't]. 1983;31(6):711–4.
98. Paju A, Vartiainen J, Haglund C, Itkonen O, von Boguslawski K, Leminen A, et al. Expression of trypsinogen-1, trypsinogen-2, and tumor-associated trypsin inhibitor in ovarian cancer: prognostic study on tissue and serum. Clin Cancer Res. [Research Support, Non-U.S. Gov't]. 2004;10(14):4761–8.
99. Ohmachi Y, Murata A, Matsuura N, Yasuda T, Yasuda T, Monden M, et al. Specific expression of the pancreatic-secretory-trypsin-inhibitor (PSTI) gene in hepatocellular carcinoma. Int J Cancer. 1993;55(5):728–34.
100. Kazal LA, Spicer DS, Brahinsky RA. Isolation of a crystalline trypsin inhibitor-anticoagulant protein from pancreas. J Am Chem Soc. 1948;70(9):3034–40.
101. Bjartell A, Paju A, Zhang WM, Gadaleanu V, Hansson J, Landberg G, et al. Expression of tumor-associated trypsinogens (TAT-1 and TAT-2) in prostate cancer. Prostate. [In Vitro Research Support, Non-U.S. Gov't]. 2005;64(1):29–39.
102. Ateeq B, Tomlins SA, Laxman B, Asangani IA, Cao Q, Cao X, et al. Therapeutic targeting of SPINK1-positive prostate cancer. Sci Transl Med. [Research Support, N.I.H., Extramural Research Support, Non-U.S. Gov't Research Support, U.S. Gov't, Non-P.H.S.]. 2011;3(72):72ra17.
103. Bracken AP, Pasini D, Capra M, Prosperini E, Colli E, Helin K. EZH2 is downstream of the pRB-E2F pathway, essential for proliferation and amplified in cancer. EMBO J. [Research Support, Non-U.S. Gov't]. 2003;22(20):5323–35.
104. Pasini D, Bracken AP, Helin K. Polycomb group proteins in cell cycle progression and cancer. Cell Cycle. [Research Support, Non-U.S. Gov't]. 2004;3(4):396–400.
105. Varambally S, Cao Q, Mani RS, Shankar S, Wang X, Ateeq B, et al. Genomic loss of microRNA-101 leads to overexpression of histone methyltransferase EZH2 in cancer. Science. [Research Support, N.I.H., Extramural Research Support, Non-U.S. Gov't Research Support, U.S. Gov't, Non-P.H.S.]. 2008;322(5908):1695–9.
106. Cao P, Deng Z, Wan M, Huang W, Cramer SD, Xu J, et al. MicroRNA-101 negatively regulates Ezh2 and its expression is modulated by androgen receptor and HIF-1alpha/HIF-1beta. Mol Cancer. [Research Support, N.I.H., Extramural Research Support, Non-U.S. Gov't]. 2010;9:108.
107. Varambally S, Dhanasekaran SM, Zhou M, Barrette TR, Kumar-Sinha C, Sanda MG, et al. The polycomb group protein EZH2 is involved in progression of prostate cancer. Nature. [Clinical Trial Research Support, Non-U.S. Gov't Research Support, U.S. Gov't, P.H.S.]. 2002;419(6907):624–9.
108. Crea F, Fornaro L, Bocci G, Sun L, Farrar WL, Falcone A, et al. EZH2 inhibition: targeting the crossroad of tumor invasion and angiogenesis. Cancer Metastasis Rev. [Research Support, Non-U.S. Gov't]. 2012;31(3–4):753–61.

Intraoperative Consultation for Prostate Tumors: Challenges and Implications for Treatment

10

Hiroshi Miyamoto and Steven S. Shen

Introduction

The widespread use of prostate-specific antigen (PSA) testing and screening has led to a marked increase in the diagnosis and treatment of early localized prostate cancer. Clinically organ-confined disease can be treated by external beam radiotherapy, brachytherapy, or radical prostatectomy (conventional open or robot-assisted laparoscopic surgery). Long-term outcomes for these treatment modalities are comparable, and the choice of treatment is dependent on a variety of clinical and pathologic factors as well as patient preference. Patients to whom radical prostatectomy, mostly nerve-sparing surgery, either unilateral or bilateral, are offered should be carefully selected to ensure complete surgical resection of tumor and minimize postoperative urine incontinence and erectile dysfunction.

Due to the advancement of surgical and imaging techniques over the last few decades, anatomical planes of dissection are predictable during radical prostatectomy, and their alteration prompts suspicion of extra-prostatic disease. However, obtaining a negative apical margin remains challenging for the surgeon because: (1) there is no clear tissue plane that defines the apex and benign prostatic tissue, which is often admixed with skeletal muscle bundles; and (2) the apical area is anatomically compact so that good surgical technique is needed to completely resect prostatic tissue while preserving adequate sphincter function and minimizing the risk of postsurgical incontinence.

S. S. Shen (✉)
Department of Pathology and Genomic Medicine, Houston Methodist Hospital, Houston, TX, USA
e-mail: stevenshen@houstonmethodist.org

H. Miyamoto
Departments of Pathology and Urology, The Johns Hopkins Medical Institutions, Baltimore, MD, USA
e-mail: hmiyamo1@jhmi.edu

Common Indications for Intraoperative Consultation

- The status of surgical margins at the apex, bladder neck, and lateral area/neurovascular bundle during radical prostatectomy
- Histopathologic diagnosis of lymph nodes during radical prostatectomy

Assessment of Surgical Margins During Radical Prostatectomy

The goal of radical prostatectomy is to resect the entire cancerous prostate with clear surgical margins. Careful clinical staging and application of recently developed preoperative nomograms [1] can predict the final pathologic stage fairly well. Most of prostatectomies for organ-confined disease can thus be performed without recourse to intraoperative assessment of surgical margins. However, positive surgical margins are not uncommonly (e.g., 11–38 % [2, 3]) seen in radical prostatectomy specimens, mainly due to unexpected extension of the tumor.

C. Magi-Galluzzi, C. G. Przybycin (eds.), *Genitourinary Pathology,* DOI 10.1007/978-1-4939-2044-0_10,

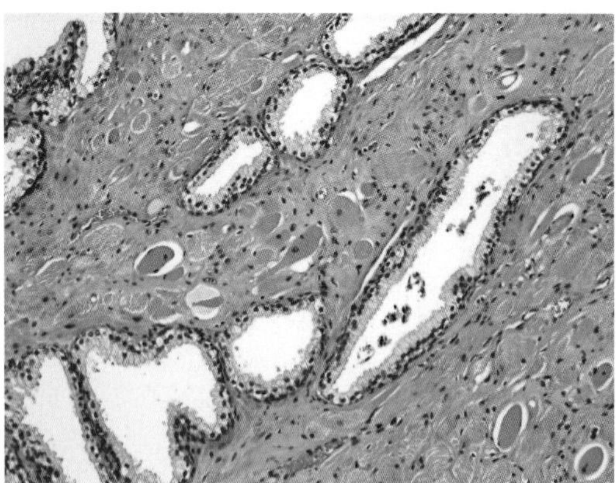

Fig. 10.1 Benign glands "infiltrating" skeletal muscle at the apex. Original magnification ×100

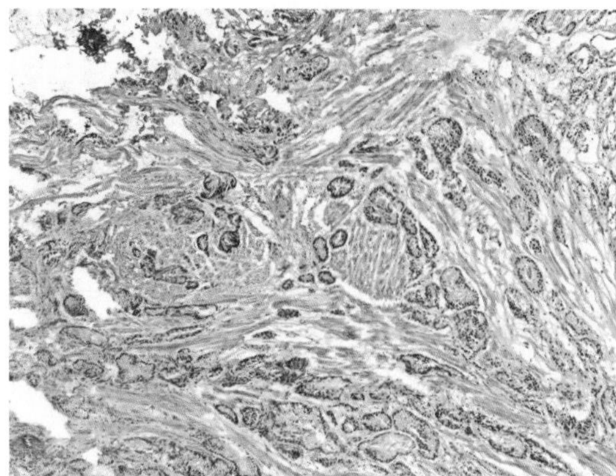

Fig. 10.2 Frozen section of bladder neck tissue showing small malignant glands dissecting smooth muscle bundles in a haphazard infiltrative fashion, although the cytologic details are obscured by cautery and frozen artifacts. Original magnification ×40

Various studies have evaluated the utility of intraoperative frozen section assessment (FSA) of surgical margins during radical prostatectomy [4]. In a recent study by one of the authors comparing cases with (n=1128) versus without (n=1480) intraoperative consultation, use of FSA did not dramatically change the overall surgical margin status of radical prostatectomy (final surgical margin positivity 9.7 vs. 11.0%, P=0.264) [3]. However, it was noteworthy that FSA during prostatectomy was useful in a select group of patients (biopsy Gleason score of 7 or higher; 10.1 vs. 15.3%, P=0.012) and at a specific site (distal urethra/apex; 7.5 vs. 11.0%, P=0.035).

With the current approaches to radical prostatectomy, virtually all the specimens submitted for FSA are small biopsies, and the pathologist is rarely summoned to sample margins from the entire prostatectomy specimen. The biopsied specimens are usually unoriented and should be embedded in its entirety. The presence of carcinoma anywhere in the specimen should be considered a positive margin. The three most common sites for FSA are:

- Apex: If carcinoma is identified in the specimen, additional apical tissue will be excised until a negative FSA is obtained. One of the pitfalls in the diagnosis of apical biopsies is that benign prostatic glands are intimately associated with skeletal muscle fibers in this location, and the mere presence of the glands "infiltrating" skeletal muscle should not be mistaken for carcinoma (Fig. 10.1).

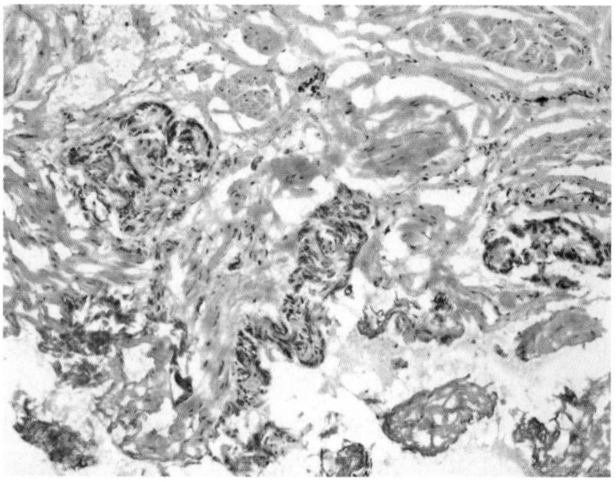

Fig. 10.3 Frozen section of a surgical margin showing fibromuscular tissue with small atypical glands highly suspicious for prostatic carcinoma. Original magnification ×100

- Bladder neck: The specimen submitted for FSA is usually larger than biopsies from other locations, often in excess of 1 cm. It should be sectioned, if necessary, and submitted entirely for FSA. These biopsies usually consist of more prominent smooth muscle fibers, occasionally with benign prostatic epithelium, and their diagnosis is often straightforward (Figs. 10.2 and 10.3).
- Lateral area: When a nerve-sparing procedure is planned, the surgeon may submit a biopsy from the area of the neurovascular bundle. The presence of carcinoma in the

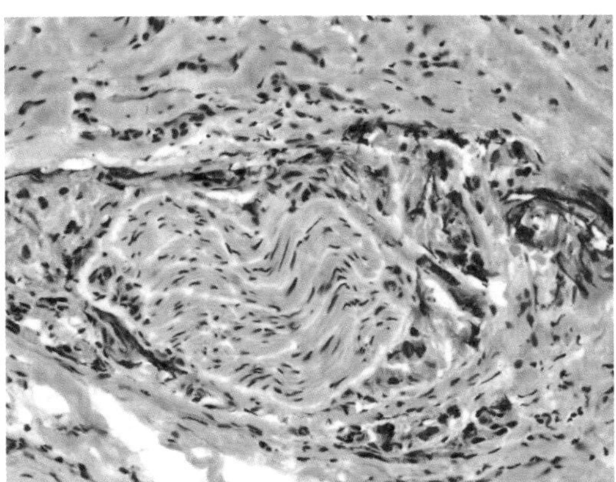

Fig. 10.4 Frozen section showing a focus of circumferential perineural invasion by prostatic carcinoma. Marked cautery and frozen artifacts are seen. Original magnification ×200

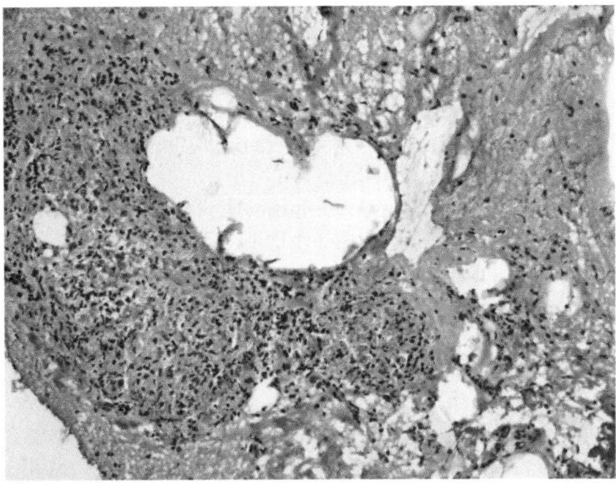

Fig. 10.5 Frozen section of ganglion tissue showing a well circumscribed nest of loosely cohesive cells and occasional large cells with abundant amphophilic cytoplasm and large nucleus, mimicking high-grade prostatic carcinoma. Original magnification ×100

biopsy will result in abandonment of nerve sparing on that side. The biopsy is usually quite small and multiple levels should be prepared because cautery artifact may complicate the interpretation (Fig. 10.4). An additional pitfall is that cauterized nests of nerve and ganglion cells that may have prominent nucleoli similar to those seen in prostate cancer cells should not be mistaken for carcinoma with perineural invasion (Fig. 10.5).

Assessment of Pelvic Lymph Nodes During Radical Prostatectomy

Lymph node dissection is potentially therapeutic when performed with prostatectomy, while nodal metastasis implies disseminated carcinoma and is classically a contraindication for radical surgery. However, an apparent stage migration has been reported in recent years resulting in a significant decrease in the rate of nodal metastasis in men undergoing radical prostatectomy [5]. A number of nomograms that combine preoperative variables, including serum PSA level, clinical tumor stage, biopsy findings (e.g., Gleason score, number of positive cores, percentage of cancer in positive cores), and others (e.g., age, digital rectal examination finding, prostate volume) have been developed to predict pathologic stage and/or the risk of lymph node metastasis [1]. Because the chance of nodal metastasis is minimal in patients with a low or intermediate risk [6], routine FSA of the lymph nodes during radical prostatectomy may be unnecessary. In contrast, nodal dissection is often performed in high-risk patients. When FSA of lymph node is requested, it is critical to avoid false positive diagnosis because positive nodal metastasis identified by FSA may be used by surgeon in making the decision of aborting the radical prostatectomy procedure [7].

The choice of FSA versus macroscopic examination only can be best determined cooperatively by the surgeon and pathologist. All lymph nodes should be identified from the submitted specimen and carefully examined with serial sectioning in 3–4 mm intervals. In patients with clinically low-risk of nodal metastasis, macroscopic examination may suffice. However, any areas grossly suspicious for metastatic carcinoma should be submitted for FSA. In high-risk patients, all the lymph nodes grossly identified may need to be submitted for FSA.

It is relatively easy to diagnose metastatic high-grade carcinoma on FSA. However, well-differentiated tumors often lack prominent desmoplastic stroma and the tumor cells show bland cytologic features. A small focus of metastasis, particularly when it is subjected to freezing

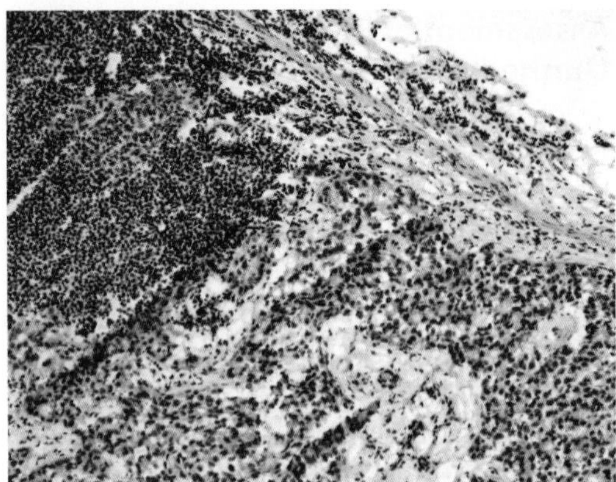

Fig. 10.6 Frozen section of a pelvic lymph node showing metastatic carcinoma. Prostatic carcinoma usually shows minimal pleomorphism and does not induce prominent desmoplasia; it can be difficult to recognize it on gross or microscopic examination due to frozen artifact. Original magnification ×100

artifact, can easily be overlooked (Fig. 10.6). Rarely, false positive FSA result has been reported in patients following hip joint replacement that may predispose them to have pelvic lymph node histiocytosis simulating metastatic foamy gland prostate cancer cells (Fig. 10.7). Awareness of these pitfalls and review of the previous biopsy material prior to FSA are very helpful for adequate interpretation of the specimens.

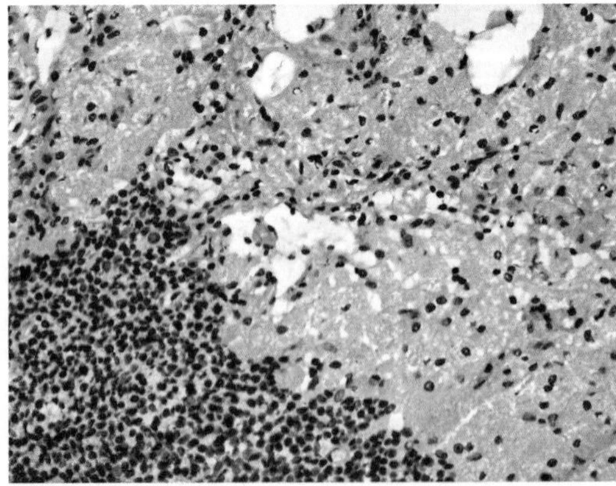

Fig. 10.7 Frozen section of a pelvic lymph node showing prominent sinus histiocytes that may be mistaken for metastatic high-grade or foamy gland prostatic carcinoma. Original magnification ×200

References

1. Lughezzani G, Briganti A, Karakiewicz PI, Kattan MW, Montorsi F, Shariat SF, Vickers AJ. Predictive and prognostic models in radical prostatectomy candidates: a critical analysis of the literature. Eur Urol. 2010;58(5):687–700.
2. Yossepowitch O, Bjartell A, Eastham JA, Graefen M, Guillonneau BD, Karakiewicz PI, Montironi R, Montorsi F. Positive surgical margins in radical prostatectomy: outlining the problem and its long-term consequences. Eur Urol. 2009;55(1):87–99.
3. Kakiuchi Y, Choy B, Gordetsky J, Izumi K, Wu G, Rashid H, Joseph JV, Miyamoto H. Role of frozen section analysis of surgical margins during robot-assisted laparoscopic radical prostatectomy: a 2608-case experience. Hum Pathol. 2013;44(8):1556–62.
4. Ramírez-Backhaus M, Rabenalt R, Jain S, Do M, Liatsikos E, Ganzer R, Horn LC, Burchardt M, Jiménez-Cruz F, Stolzenburg JU. Value of frozen section biopsies during radical prostatectomy: significance of the histological results. World J Urol. 2009;27(2):227–34.
5. Ploussard G, Briganti A, de la Taille A, Haese A, Heidenreich A, Menon M, Sulser T, Tewari AK, Eastham JA. Pelvic lymph node dissection during robot-assisted radical prostatectomy: Efficacy, limitations, and complications—A systematic review of the literature. Eur Urol. 2014;65(1):7–16.
6. Kakehi Y, Kamoto T, Okuno H, Terai A, Terachi T, Ogawa O. Per-operative frozen section examination of pelvic nodes is unnecessary for the majority of clinically localized prostate cancers in the prostate-specific antigen era. Int J Urol. 2000;7(8):281–6.
7. Beissner RS, Stricker JB, Speights VO, Coffield KS, Spiekerman AM, Riggs M. Frozen section diagnosis of metastatic prostate adenocarcinoma in pelvic lymphadenectomy compared with nomogram prediction of metastasis. Urology. 2002;59(5):721–5.

Genomics and Epigenomics of Prostate Cancer

11

Juan Miguel Mosquera, Pei-Chun Lin and Mark A. Rubin

Introduction

Prostate cancer is a clinically heterogeneous disease. Over 900,000 cases of prostate cancer are diagnosed worldwide annually [1]. Many of these men will have aggressive disease with progression, metastasis, and death from prostate cancer, remaining as the second most common cause of cancer death worldwide. However, many others will have indolent disease that will not threaten health during their natural lifespan. Overtreatment of low-risk disease with radical therapy imports significant morbidity and compromise to quality of life. The emergence and application of new technology has allowed a rapid expansion of our understanding of the molecular basis of prostate cancer, and has revealed a remarkable genetic heterogeneity that may underlie the clinically variable behavior of the disease [2–7].

M. A. Rubin (✉) · J. M. Mosquera
Department of Pathology and Laboratory Medicine, Institute for Precision Medicine, Weill Medical College of Cornell University, New York, NY, USA
e-mail: rubinma@med.cornell.edu

J. M. Mosquera
e-mail: Jmm9018@med.cornell.edu

P.-C. Lin
Innovative Genomics Initiative, University of California, Berkeley, CA, USA
e-mail: Peichun.lin@berkeley.edu

Genomic Alterations

Somatic Mutations

Alterations in tumor cells but not in the germline DNA are referred to as somatic mutations. The term mutation includes point mutations, copy number alterations (i.e., copy gain and loss), and genomic rearrangements. Recent high throughput studies have nominated a number of recurrent somatic mutations that may represent gain of function oncogenes and loss of function of tumor suppressor genes.

Phosphoinositide 3-Kinase (PI3K) Pathway

The phosphoinositide 3-kinase (PI3K) pathway is among the most commonly altered signaling pathways in human cancer. This pathway is activated by lesions in several different signaling components, and affects cell proliferation, survival, and invasion. The PI3K pathway is altered in approximately 25–70% of prostate cancers, with metastatic tumors having significantly higher incidence.

Phosphatase and tensin homologue (*PTEN*), located on chromosome 10q23, is among the most frequently mutated tumor suppressors in human cancer. *PTEN* acts to dephosphorylate lipid-signaling intermediates, thereby deactivating PI3K-dependent signaling. Heterozygous and less commonly homozygous deletions at the *PTEN* locus occur in about 40% of primary

C. Magi-Galluzzi, C. G. Przybycin (eds.), *Genitourinary Pathology,* DOI 10.1007/978-1-4939-2044-0_11,

prostate cancers and inactivating mutations in another 5–10% [2, 3, 8]. Inactivating lesions are more common in advanced disease [2, 3, 6, 9, 10]. Multiple functional studies in cell lines, xenografts, and mouse models support the role of *PTEN* as a critical tumor suppressor in prostate cancer [11–13].

Gene amplification and gain of function point mutations of *PIK3CA*, encoding a catalytic subunit of PI3K, result in overactivation of the pathway. Amplification of *PIK3CA* has been reported in about 25% of prostate cancers and recent sequencing studies have revealed activating point mutations in about 5% of cases [2, 14]. Activating lesions in *PIK3CA* and inactivation of *PTEN* are often, but not completely, mutually exclusive, supporting similar endpoints in driving downstream signaling. However, *PTEN* inactivation seems to be the dominant mechanism of altering the pathway.

Like *PTEN*, the *PHLPP1* gene (PH domain and leucine-rich repeat protein) located at 18q21, is recurrently deleted in a number of cancers, including prostate cancer, and acts to dephosphorylate components of the PI3K pathway (specifically the protein kinase Akt) [6]. Interestingly, deletion of PHLPP appears to have its most potent effects in cells with *PTEN* inactivation, suggesting that PHLPP plays a redundant role in cells with intact PTEN signaling [12]. As additional data emerge, rarer events affecting the PI3K pathway are also being discovered. These include rearrangement of *MAGI2*, encoding a PTEN scaffolding protein, point mutations and genomic deletions of *CDKN1B*, a tumor suppressor that functions as an inhibitor of cell cycle progression downstream of Akt signaling, and mutations in *GSK3B*, another regulatory kinase downstream of PI3K [2, 6, 7, 15]. In total, these recurrent lesions in multiple nodes of the PI3K pathway reinforce its central importance in the pathogenesis of prostate cancer and confirm interest in its potential for targeted therapy.

Ras/Raf/MAPK Pathway

The mitogen-activated protein kinase (MAPK) pathway plays a critical role in many cancers (including lung, ovary, melanoma, pancreas, and GI tract); however, its role in prostate cancer is less well established. MAPK signaling is activated in response to upstream signals such as growth factors, cytokines, and adhesion molecules. Other signaling intermediates commonly activated in cancer, such as Ras and Raf, activate MAPK signaling and may enhance transcriptional activity of the androgen receptor (AR) [16]. Up-regulation of MAPK pathway components and upstream intermediates are common and enriched in prostate cancer metastases; however, mutations in these components are relatively rare [2, 3, 6]. In addition, rare fusion genes involving *KRAS*, *RAF1*, and *BRAF* may confer pathway activation in advanced prostate cancers [17, 18].

p53

The tumor suppressor p53 (*TP53*) is the most commonly mutated gene in human cancer. In response to cell stress, the p53 protein acts as a sequence-specific transcription factor, activating the transcription of genes involved in cell cycle arrest, DNA repair, and apoptosis. Recent data show deletions at the *TP53* locus in about 25–40% of prostate cancer samples, with point mutations in 5–40% of cases [2, 3, 6, 9, 10, 19].

Rb

The retinoblastoma protein Rb, is a classic tumor suppressor that acts to check cell cycle progression, and is deleted or mutated in a number of human cancers. *RB1*, located at 13q14, is only rarely deleted in clinically localized prostate cancer; however, *RB1* is commonly inactivated in castration-resistant prostate cancer (CRPC), in up to 45% of cases [3, 6, 9]. Recent data suggest that Rb modulates AR signaling and inhibits progression to castration resistance [20].

Myc

MYC encodes a transcription factor (c-Myc) with multiple downstream target genes, leading to cell cycle progression, cell survival, and tumorigenesis. Mutations, amplification, overexpression, rearrangements, and translocations involving *MYC* are common in epithelial and hematopoietic malignancies, making it one of the most commonly activated oncogenes in human cancer. *MYC*, at chromosome 8q24, is commonly amplified in prostate cancer [2, 3, 6, 9]; however, this often involves amplification of this entire arm of chromosome 8, leading to the possibility of other oncogenes in the region.

Mutations Affecting Androgen Signaling

Since the discovery that castration of men with advanced prostate cancer resulted in disease regression, androgen signaling has been a central axis in the pathogenesis of prostate cancer. Genomic data confirming recurrent lesions in components of androgen signaling serves to reinforce its cardinal importance to the development and progression of prostate cancer. These include alterations in the *AR* gene itself, as well as in interacting proteins that can modulate the activity of the AR and its downstream target genes.

The AR is a ligand-dependent nuclear transcription factor. The *AR* gene undergoes multiple alterations leading to increased activity in prostate cancer, including gene amplification, point mutations, and alteration in splicing leading to constitutively active variants [21–24]. However, these alterations take place largely, if not exclusively, in metastatic, CRPC [25–27]. Recent studies reported amplification of *AR* in 23/50 (46%) and point mutations in an additional 5/50 (10%) of treated, metastatic tumors, but these lesions were absent in over 100 clinically localized prostate cancers [2, 3]. This is consistent with analysis by Taylor et al., with *AR* amplification in 40% and mutation in an additional 10% of metastatic prostate cancers (largely CRPC), but completely absent in primary tumors [6]. These findings support the hypothesis that lesions in the *AR* gene itself do not play a role in the pathogenesis of prostate cancer, but instead emerge during treatment as a mechanism of resistance to therapies targeting the androgen axis. Even in advanced cancers that no longer respond to androgen deprivation therapy, accumulating evidence has shown that AR signaling remains active and plays a critical role in disease progression; this has led to the abandonment of the term "androgen independent" in favor of "castration resistant" for this disease state [28].

Alterations have also been found in genes encoding proteins that interact with and modulate AR activity. These include transcriptional coactivators (*NCOA2*, *EP300*), transcriptional corepressors (*NCOR2*), interacting transcription factors, and chromatin regulatory elements [2, 3, 6, 19]. Interestingly, mutations or other means of deregulation of these genes are present in primary as well as metastatic tumors, indicating that although *AR* itself may not be altered in clinically localized disease, other elements of the signaling pathway may be recurrently altered.

The forkhead-box family of transcription factors is involved in cell growth and differentiation. Forkhead box A1 (*FOXA1*) interacts with the AR and modulates its transcriptional activity in the prostate. Recurrent point mutations in *FOXA1* have been found in both primary tumors and metastatic lesions [2, 3]. These likely represent activating mutations as *FOXA1* is overexpressed in metastatic and CRPC, and observed *FOXA1* mutants increase proliferation in the presence of androgen [3, 29]. Interestingly, other members of the forkhead-box family have also been implicated in prostate cancer pathogenesis; *FOXP1 at* 3p14, *FOXO1 at* 13q14, and *FOXO3 at* 6q21 are in areas recurrently deleted, suggesting a possible role as tumor suppressors [2, 6, 30].

The *NCOA2* gene encodes nuclear receptor coactivator 2 (also known as steroid receptor coactivator 2, SRC2), a transcriptional coactivator that modulates gene expression by a number of hormone receptors, including AR. Taylor et al. identified 6.2% of prostate cancers with amplification of the *NCOA2* gene (on chromosome 8q, in an amplicon previously attributed to the *MYC* gene) with significant correlation between amplification and elevated *NCOA2* mRNA, as well as rare somatic mutations of *NCOA2* (2/91 prostate cancers; 2.2%) [6]. Functionally, increased *NCOA2* levels amplified AR pathway transcriptional output.

In addition, genes encoding multiple other AR-interacting proteins are mutated or otherwise dysregulated in prostate cancer. These include transcriptional corepressors such as *NCOR2* and coactivators such as *NRIP1* and *EP300* [3, 6]. Furthermore, there is extensive interaction between AR signaling and other oncogenic signaling pathways. For instance, the PI3K/Akt signaling pathway has been shown to inhibit AR signaling, and by reciprocal negative feedback, AR inhibition activates Akt signaling [31]. This type of complex interplay between the AR components that modulate its transcriptional activity, and other pathways may help explain the eventual failure of androgen deprivation therapy, and further investigation to map out these interactions may nominate key therapeutic targets.

A distinct and intriguing role for androgen signaling in driving prostate carcinogenesis has been proposed based on recent findings. The importance of genomic rearrangements in prostate cancer is well established; rearrangements may occur when the genomic loci are brought into close physical proximity to each other. Interestingly, rearrangement breakpoints are significantly more likely to occur near AR-bound sites in the genome than predicted by chance [7]. This raises the possibility that AR complexes mediate the formation of "transcriptional hubs" that bring together distant genomic loci, and predispose to genomic rearrangements through transcriptional stress. In support of this concept, androgen stimulation can bring the *TMPRSS2* and *ERG* loci into proximity and induce fusion of these genes *de novo* [32]. More recently, whole genome sequencing in a German cohort suggested a high incidence of androgen-driven structural rearrangements, especially in early onset prostate cancer [33]. Essentially, this suggests that androgen-mediated transcriptional activity could act as the initial driver of many genomic rearrangements in prostate cancer. Overall, these findings reinforce androgen signaling as potentially the most impactful pathway in both primary and advanced prostate cancer.

ETS Gene Fusions

A major advance toward the understanding of the molecular nature of prostate cancer came with the identification of recurrent gene fusions consisting of androgen-regulated genes and members of the ETS family of oncogenic transcription factors in a majority of prostate cancers [34–36]. These most commonly occur as fusion of the *TMPRSS2* gene and the transcription factor *ERG*. Over ten androgen-regulated genes have been identified as 5′ fusion partners; other members of the ETS family that serve as 3′ partners include *ETV1*, *ETV4*, and *ETV5* [36]. The prevalence of ETS rearrangements ranges from 27 to 79% in radical prostatectomy and biopsy samples; these generally represent prostate-specific antigen (PSA)-screened patients (reviewed in [36]) (Fig. 11.1a–d). Prostate-specific expression of ETS family members in mice results in the development of prostatic intraepithelial neoplasia (PIN), and combination with other lesions such as *AR* overexpression or *PTEN* loss leads to invasive adenocarcinoma [11, 37, 38]. Overall, these findings and the high frequency of recurrent *ETS* gene fusions in prostate cancer support dysregulation of the ETS signaling axis as an important factor in prostate tumorigenesis.

SPOP Mutations

Mutations in *SPOP* in prostate cancer have been recently discovered in systematic sequencing studies [2, 7, 19, 39]. These represent the most common point mutations in primary prostate cancer, with recurrent mutations in *SPOP* in 6–13% of multiple independent cohorts. The *SPOP* gene encodes for the substrate-recognition component of a Cullin3-based E3-ubiquitin ligase; missense mutations are found exclusively in the structurally defined substrate-binding cleft of SPOP, indicating that prostate cancer-derived mutations will alter substrate binding [2, 39] (Fig. 11.2a, b).

Mutations Affecting Gene Expression and Chromatin Regulation

Regulation of chromatin remodeling, the process of modifying DNA architecture through histone modifications and other restructuring processes, has emerged as a major mechanism for alterations across the spectrum of human cancers. Alteration in proteins involved in chromatin regulation can have far reaching cellular effects, affecting

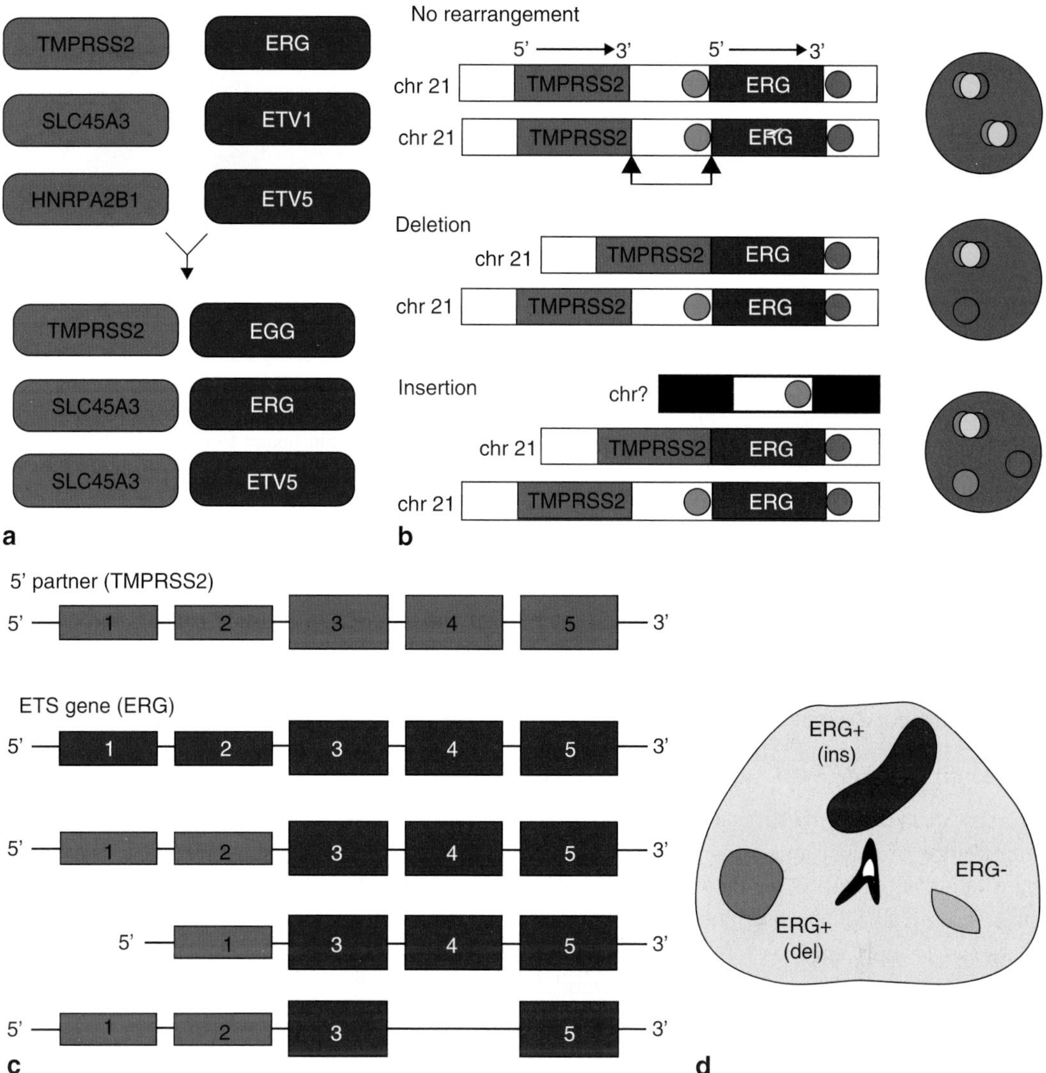

Fig. 11.1 Complexity of *ETS* gene fusions in prostate cancer. **a** Multiple 50 partners (*red*) and *ETS* genes (*blue*) have been identified. **b** Two genomic mechanisms of *TMPRSS2:ERG* gene fusions have been identified. The prostate-specific androgen-induced transmembrane protease serine 2 gene, *TMRPSS2*, and the v-ets erythroblastosis virus E26 oncogene homolog gene, *ERG*, are located approximately 3 megabases (Mb) apart on chromosome 21, and fusion can occur either through deletion of the intervening genomic region (*arrows*) or insertion of the intervening region to another chromosome. Stylized results obtained by fluorescence in situ hybridization (FISH) using probes located 50 (*green*) and 30 (*red*) to ERG are shown to the right of the structural diagrams, with colocalization of 50/30 ERG probes indicated in *yellow*. **c** Multiple fusion transcript isoforms have been characterized. Stylized structures for *TMPRSS2* (*red*) and *ERG* (*blue*) are shown. Noncoding and coding exons are shown in small and large boxes, respectively. Transcripts differ in the location of the junction between the 50 partners and the *ETS* gene, as well as the included exons. **d** Localized prostate cancer is commonly multifocal, with several distinct appearing foci of cancer. A single prostate can contain foci without *ETS* gene rearrangements, foci with *TMPRSS2:ERG* fusion through deletion (*del*), or foci with *TMRPSS2:ERG* fusion through insertion (*ins*). (Used with permission from [36])

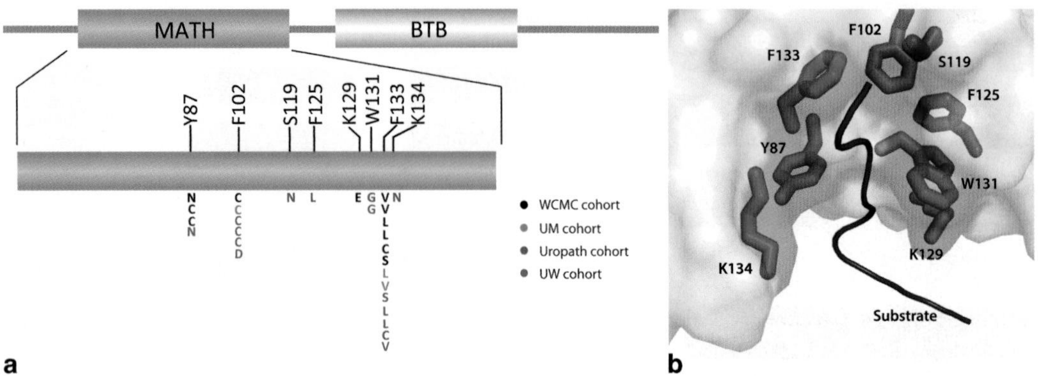

Fig. 11.2 Structural studies of recurrent *SPOP* alterations in prostate cancer. **a** Positional distribution of somatic alterations in *SPOP* across the Weill Cornell Medical College (*WCMC*), University of Michigan (*UM*), Uropath, and University of Washington (*UW*) prostate tumor cohorts. **b** Mutated residues in the crystal structure of the SPOP MATH domain bound to substrate (PDB 3IVV). *MATH* meprin and TRAF homology domain, *BTB* broad complex, tramtrack and bric-a-brac domain. (Used with permission from [2])

genome-wide control of gene expression and playing key roles in DNA repair and genome maintenance. Mutations in a number of genes involved in histone modifications have been identified in prostate cancer. These include *KDM6A/UTX, MLL2, and MLL3* [2, 3, 6, 19]. Interestingly, proteins encoded by these genes all act to alter methylation of the histone variant H3, known to be a key component of regulation of chromatin states and involved in transcriptional control.

CHD1 at 5q21 encodes a chromodomain helicase DNA-binding protein that acts to remodel chromatin states (partly by acting as a chaperone of H3.3), and is involved in transcriptional control across the genome. The *CHD1* locus is recurrently deleted in prostate cancer, at roughly 10–25 % frequency in both primary and metastatic tumors; rearrangements and point mutations have also been identified [2, 3, 6, 7]. Furthermore, prostate tumors with CHD1 deletion have a significant increase in genomic rearrangements [40]. Future studies will elucidate the role of this putative tumor suppressor in the pathogenesis of prostate cancer.

Enhancer of zeste homolog 2 (*EZH2*) acts as a histone methyltransferase (HMT) to silence gene expression and plays a critical role in chromatin regulation. Dysregulation of *EZH2* occurs in a variety of human cancers, through mutation, overexpression, and other mechanisms. *EZH2* is overexpressed in prostate cancer, and overexpression is associated with aggressive and metastatic disease [41] (Fig. 11.3a, b). Interestingly, recent data show that the role of EZH2 in prostate cancer may be independent of its function in silencing gene expression, but instead it acts as an activator of the AR and other transcription factors [42]. These discoveries raise the possibility that therapeutic targeting of EZH2 activity may be a potential strategy for advanced prostate cancer (see below in epigenetics section).

Prognostic Significance of Genetic Changes

Although we have begun to catalogue the alterations in prostate cancer, the prognostic significance of the majority of these changes remains unclear. The long natural history of prostate cancer complicates establishing predictive relationships, and raises the possibility that many mutations that drive tumorigenesis in the prostate are not associated with disease progression or mortality. Instead, lesions that initiate cancer may occur decades before the disease becomes clinically relevant, and may have no effect on prognosis. Furthermore, long follow-up on large well-annotated cohorts are necessary to establish effects on prognosis.

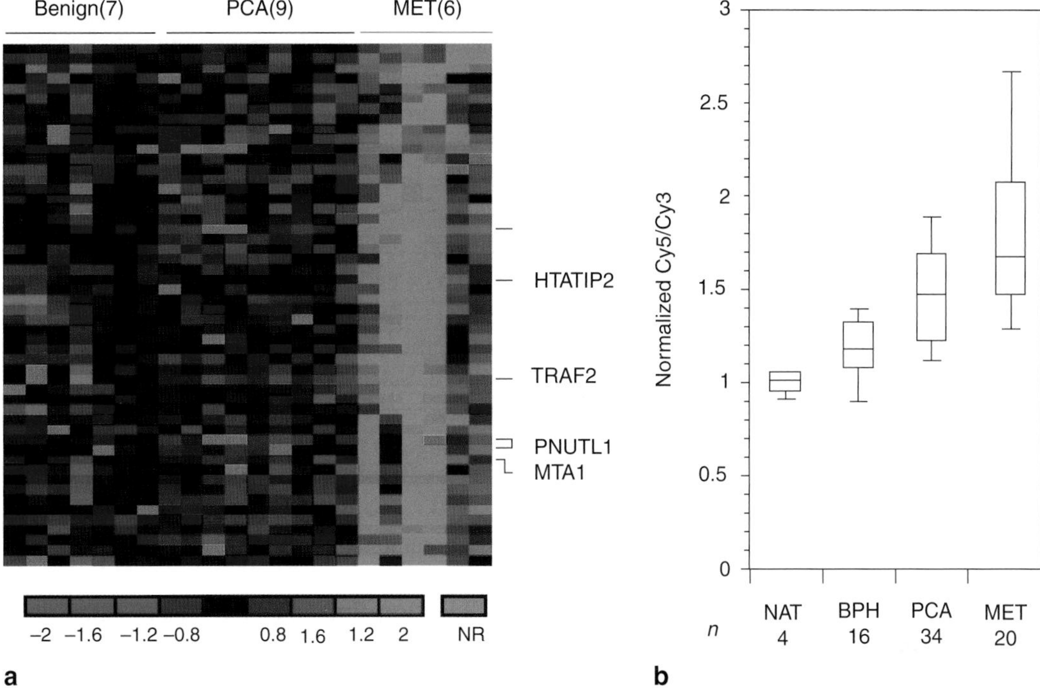

Fig. 11.3 Overexpression of *EZH2* in metastatic hormone-refractory prostate cancer (*MET*). **a** Cluster diagram depicting genes that distinguish MET from clinically localized prostate cancer (*PCA*). Genes upregulated in METs relative to prostate cancer are shown. *Red* and *green* represent upregulation and downregulation, respectively, relative to the median of the reference pool. *Grey* represents technically inadequate or missing data, and *black* represents equal expression relative to the reference sample. **b** DNA microarray analysis of prostate cancer shows upregulation of EZH2 in METs. *BPH* benign prostatic hyperplasia, *NAT* normal adjacent prostate tissue. (Used with permission from [41])

PTEN

Dysregulation of PTEN is the lesion most consistently associated with poor prognosis in prostate cancer. A preponderance of evidence shows that deletion of PTEN is associated with advanced localized or metastatic disease, higher Gleason grade, and higher risk of progression, recurrence after therapy, and death from disease [8, 43–47].

TMPRSS2-ERG

As the most common event in prostate cancer, numerous studies have investigated the effect of TMPRSS2-ERG fusion on prognosis. Data are conflicting; ETS fusions have been reported as associated with both more aggressive and more indolent disease, likely representing heterogeneity of study cohorts and management, the impact of sampling, multifocality and intraprostate molecular heterogeneity, and the variability of measured outcomes. Here we will discuss briefly what Tomlins et al. have reviewed in details [36]. Population-based studies focused on non-PSA screened populations with prostate cancer diagnosed by transurethral resection of the prostate (TURP) and conservatively managed (watchful waiting) have shown a significant association between *ERG* rearrangement and adverse clinicopathologic predictors, metastases, or disease-specific death [48, 49]. Studies investigating the impact of ETS fusions on aggressive features or outcome following radical prostatectomy have produced conflicting results, with several showing association between ETS fusion status and features of aggressive prostate cancer (including increased Gleason grade, stage, or biochemical recurrence [BCR]), while others have found no such associations, or even the opposite (association with lower Gleason grade or increased recurrence-free survival). In summary, population-based studies of watchful waiting cohorts have shown ETS fusions associated with poor prognosis, while retrospective radical prostatectomy series have conflicting results regarding aggressiveness and prognosis of ETS fusion-positive cancers; variation in techniques to detect ERG rearrangement also confounds interpretation across studies.

Somatic Copy Number Alterations (SCNAs) and Gene Expression

In addition to the effect of specific genomic events on the prognosis of prostate cancer, the implications of genome-wide or transcriptome-wide changes have also been investigated. Multiple authors have shown that the overall number of SCNAs correlates with Gleason grade, tumor stage, and other poor prognostic features [6, 15, 50]. This may reflect the impact of the overall degree of genomic instability in these tumors, or may represent the accumulation of driving events, with prognosis worsening as the tumor accumulates additional "hits." Studies investigating gene expression have been also attempted to define patterns associated with aggressive disease; many studies have reported gene expression signatures predictive of disease progression or aggressiveness, but limited value has been demonstrated across cohorts and transition to the clinical setting remains elusive.

Tumor Heterogeneity and Potential Targets

The heterogeneity of prostate cancer complicates risk stratification and selection of management strategies. However, molecular classification holds the promise of identifying specific subclasses of prostate cancer associated with distinct patterns of genomic abnormalities. Genomic and transcriptomic analyses reveal that prostate tumors can be subclassified based on gene expression and SCNA signatures, with some success in predicting aggressive features of disease or impact on prognosis [6, 15, 50, 51]. Systematic sequencing studies continue to add data allowing the definition of molecular subclasses based on mutations and copy number aberrations. These discoveries raise the possibility that prostate cancer might soon transition from a poorly understood, clinically heterogeneous disease to a collection of homogenous subtypes identifiable by molecular criteria, associated with specific genetic abnormalities, with distinct effects on patient prognosis, amenable to specific management strategies, and perhaps vulnerable to specific targeted therapies. As these subclasses emerge, selection of model systems based on genetic context becomes critical; for instance, studying *SPOP* mutations in a cell line that has *TMPRSS2-ERG* fusion or *TP53* mutations may be futile, since these events are mutually exclusive in tumors.

ETS Fusion-Positive Tumors

Due to the approximately 50% prevalence of ETS fusions, attempts to molecularly characterize prostate often begin with division into ETS-positive and ETS-negative subclasses. It is likely that the different *ETS* fusions genes have similar functional consequences to the cancer cell. Although prostate tumors have been reported with more than one type of ETS fusion, in general only a single ETS fusion is present in a given tumor, consistent with functional redundancy [52]. Multiple studies have defined distinct gene expression profiles in ETS fusion-positive and ETS fusion-negative prostate cancers [36, 51, 53]. In addition, tumors with *ERG* rearrangement have distinct SCNA profiles and increased lesions in *TP53* and *PTEN*, suggesting that they represent a biologically distinct entity [2, 6, 54].

The high prevalence and simple identification of prostate cancers with ETS rearrangement led to interest in potential therapeutic targeting. Although successful targeted therapy against oncogenic transcription factors has proven notoriously difficult, Brenner et al. identified the enzyme poly (ADP-ribose) polymerase 1 (PARP1) as an ERG-interacting protein critical for the oncogenic action of ETS proteins in prostate cancer cells, and demonstrated that inhibition of PARP resulted in decreased growth of ETS fusion-positive, but not ETS-negative prostate cancer xenografts [55]. These findings suggest that PARP inhibitors, currently under clinical investigation in a number of cancers, including breast and ovarian, represent a potential therapeutic avenue specifically for ETS-positive prostate cancers.

SPOP Mutations Define a Distinct Molecular Class of Prostate Cancer

Mutations in *SPOP* occur in up to 15% of prostate cancers; importantly, *SPOP* mutations are mutually exclusive with *TMPRSS-ERG* fusion and other ETS rearrangements, and SPOP-mutant tumors generally lack lesions in the PI3K pathway [2, 3, 19] (Fig. 11.4). Moreover, SPOP mutations are also mutually exclusive with deletions and mutations in the *TP53* tumor suppressor [2, 19]. Finally, SPOP-mutant tumors show a distinct pattern of genomic aberrations; specifically, deletions of *CHD1 at* 5q21.1 and deletion in the 6q21 region are significantly associated with *SPOP* mutations [2]. Taken together, these findings support SPOP mutations as a driver lesion that underlies a distinct molecular subclass of prostate cancer.

SPINK1

As studies have characterized the molecular nature of prostate cancer, additional potential subtypes have emerged. The serine peptidase inhibitor, Kazal type 1 (*SPINK1*) is a secreted protein overexpressed specifically in a subset of ETS-negative cancers [56–58]. *SPINK1* overexpression is associated with decreased BCR-free survival, and monoclonal antibodies to SPINK1 attenuate the growth and invasion of SPINK1-positive cells in prostate cancer models. Furthermore, EGFR, through interaction with SPINK1, may in part mediate the oncogenic effects of SPINK1, and inhibition of EGFR signaling with already clinically established agents may be another route of targeted therapy for this specific subclass of

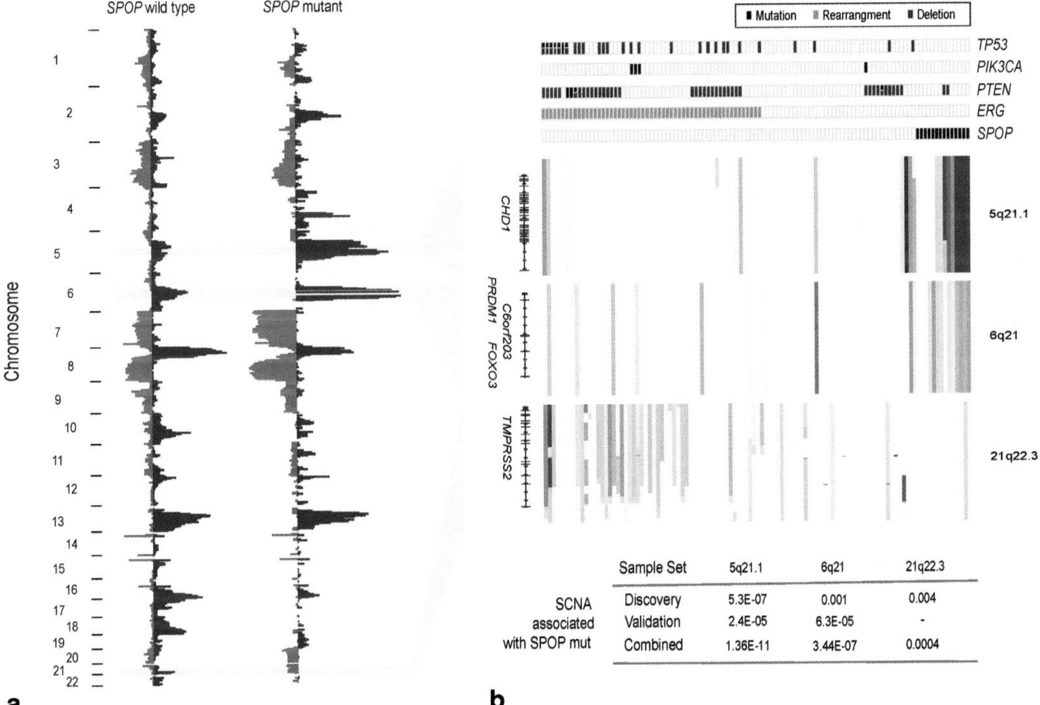

	Sample Set	5q21.1	6q21	21q22.3
SCNA associated with SPOP mut	Discovery	5.3E-07	0.001	0.004
	Validation	2.4E-05	6.3E-05	-
	Combined	1.36E-11	3.44E-07	0.0004

Fig. 11.4 *SPOP* mutation defines a distinct genetic subclass of prostate cancer. **a** Heat map showing selected recurrent somatic copy-number aberrations (SCNAs). **b** Each column represents a single prostate cancer sample. Samples are annotated for mutations in *SPOP*, *PTEN*, *PIK3CA* and *TP53*, deletions of *PTEN,* and *ERG* rearrangements. Deletions positively correlated (5q21.1, 6q21) or inversely correlated (21q22.3) with *SPOP* mutation are shown. *P* values of peak association with *SPOP* mutation in both discovery and validation cohorts are given below (Fisher's exact test). (Used with permission from [2])

prostate cancer [59]. These studies on ETS fusion and SPINK1-positive prostate cancer subclasses can serve as a model for how further classification efforts can benefit patients; identifying molecular subclasses with specific underlying genetic abnormalities, finding effects on patient prognosis, defining the signaling pathways associated with these lesions that may drive prostate tumorigenesis, and identifying potential targets for therapy.

IL-6 and Cytokine Signaling

Accumulating evidence also implicates cytokine signaling as a targetable axis in prostate cancer. Interleukin-6 (IL-6) is an inflammatory cytokine that is overexpressed in prostate cancer; it regulates proliferation, apoptosis, and angiogenesis through activation of multiple downstream pathways, including MAPKs and Akt. While no specific mutations in elements of IL-6 signaling have been reported, preclinical studies in multiple prostate tumor models reveal the potential of the anti-IL-6 antibody siltuximab, and clinical trials have been initiated [60]. Endogenous inhibitors of cytokine signaling are also relevant in prostate cancer; Suppressor of Cytokine Signaling 3 (*SOCS3*) inhibits apoptosis in AR-negative models [61]. IL-6 has pleomorphic effects that are cell-context dependent, complicating the search for biomarkers and design of trials [62].

Rare Lesions and Opportunities for Precision Medicine

The high incidence of prostate cancer and the diverse and heterogeneous pattern of alterations in the disease imply that even alterations only impacting a few percent of patients may have clinical utility; this is the paradigm of personalized medicine. Highlighting this are recent studies identifying rare fusion genes involving the Ras/Raf kinase pathways. Rearrangements of the *BRAF* or *RAF1* genes have been reported in 1–2 % of prostate cancers [9, 17] (Fig. 11.5a–d), while

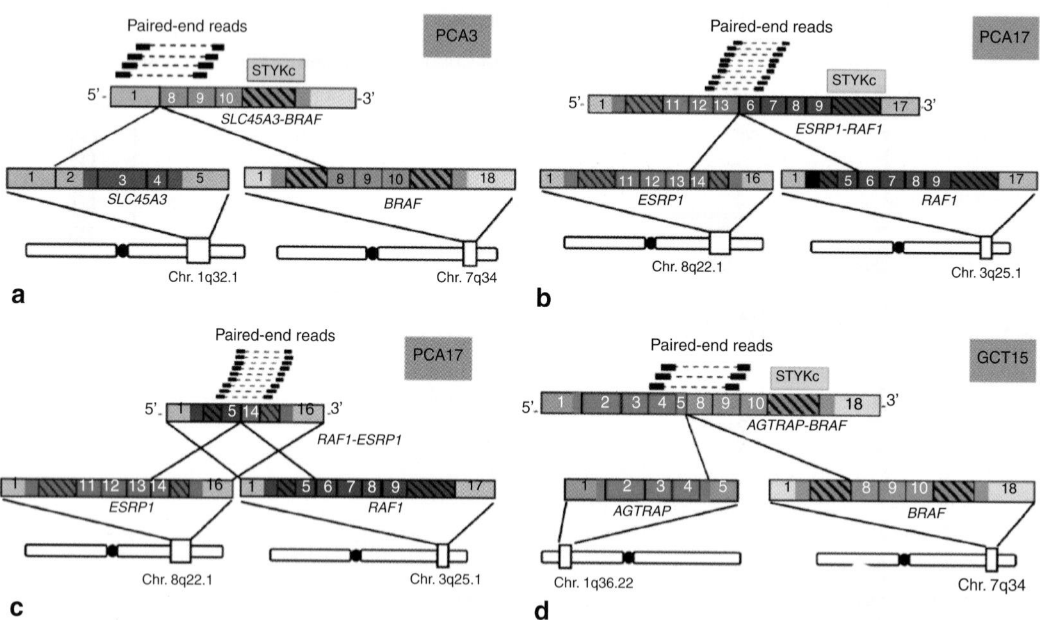

Fig. 11.5 Discovery of the *SLC45A3-BRAF* and *ESRP1-RAF1* gene fusions in prostate cancer by paired-end transcriptome sequencing. **a** Schematic representation of reliable paired-end reads supporting the interchromosomal gene fusion between *SLC45A3* (*purple*) and *BRAF* (*orange*). The protein kinase domain in the *BRAF* gene (*yellow*) remains intact following the fusion event. Respective exons are numbered. **b**, **c** As in **a**, except showing the fusions between *ESRP1* (*red*) and *RAF1* (*blue*), resulting in reciprocal fusion genes *ESRP1-RAF1* and *RAF1-ESRP1*. **d** As in **a**, except showing the fusion between *AGTRAP* (*red*) and *BRAF* (*orange*). (Used with permission from [17])

KRAS rearrangement has also been discovered in advanced prostate cancer [18]. Importantly, activating events in these pathways are considered targetable by existing Raf kinase inhibitors. These studies suggest that while uncommon, such events may define a model where evaluation of the molecular profile of an individual's prostate cancer could reveal rare but actionable alterations that can be treated with existing pharmacologic agents.

A subtype of prostate cancer that can rarely arise de novo, neuroendocrine prostate cancer (NEPC), is a lethal subtype that most commonly develops after hormonal therapy for the disease [63]. It is estimated that up to 30 % of late stage prostate cancers harbor a predominance of neuroendocrine differentiation. NEPC does not secrete PSA or express AR, and should be suspected in patients with rapid disease progression especially metastases to visceral organs, low or modestly elevated serum PSA level and elevated serum markers of neuroendocrine differentiation (i.e., chromogranin A or neuronspecific enolase). Recent transcriptome sequencing and assessment of DNA copy number changes of both prostate cancer and NEPC has brought new insight into NEPC pathogenesis [9]. Despite clonal origin of NEPC from adenocarcinoma cells, there exist dramatic gene expression differences with nearly 1000 genes showing differential expression. In addition, the genome of NEPC is widely aberrant with frequent amplifications and deletions. There are subpopulations of prostate cancer patients that demonstrate mixed molecular features and may be at high risk for progression to NEPC. For instance, co-amplification of the genes encoding the oncogenes Aurora kinase A *(AURKA)* and N-myc (*MYCN*) are frequently found in primary tumors of patients that later develop treatment-related NEPC, and are infrequent in other primary prostate adenocarcinomas [64]. Therefore, *AURKA* and *MYCN* amplifications may predict patients at high risk for the development of treatment-related NEPC.

Temporal Relationships Among Genomic Events

Establishing the temporal sequence of genomic events in prostate cancer—which lesions occur early and likely initiate cancer, versus those that come later and are associated with disease progression—is critical for defining prostate cancer progression and aggressiveness at the molecular level. A molecular definition of progression may be invaluable for patients on active surveillance or for risk-stratification of intermediate-risk patients. *ERG* rearrangement has been shown in both isolated high-grade prostatic intraepithelial neoplasia (HGPIN) and in HGPIN adjacent to invasive prostate cancer [36, 65]. *SPOP* mutations have also been identified in HGPIN, and are only observed in ETS-negative tumors, suggesting that *SPOP* mutation and ETS rearrangements are mutually exclusive early events in the natural history of prostate cancer [2]. In contrast, lesions in *PTEN*, *RB1*, *TP53*, and *AR* are more commonly reported in advanced tumors. Whole genome sequencing has provided additional insight in this endeavor. Analysis of the clonality of genomic events (in essence, the percentage of cells in a tumor with a specific lesion) allows investigators to extrapolate the hierarchy of these events in a tumor's natural history. Using this approach, Baca et al. have reported *ERG* rearrangement, *NKX3-1* deletion, and mutations in *SPOP* and *FOXA1* as clonal, early events in the history of prostate cancer. These are followed by lesions in *CDKN1B* and *TP53*, and finally by inactivation of *PTEN* [40] (Fig. 11.6). Findings such as these establish a framework for defining the sequence of molecular events in the natural history of prostate cancer, from disease initiation to progression, metastases, emergence of treatment resistance, and death.

Section Summary

Major advances have been made in cataloguing the genomic alterations in prostate cancer, understanding the molecular mechanisms underlying the disease, and using this information to

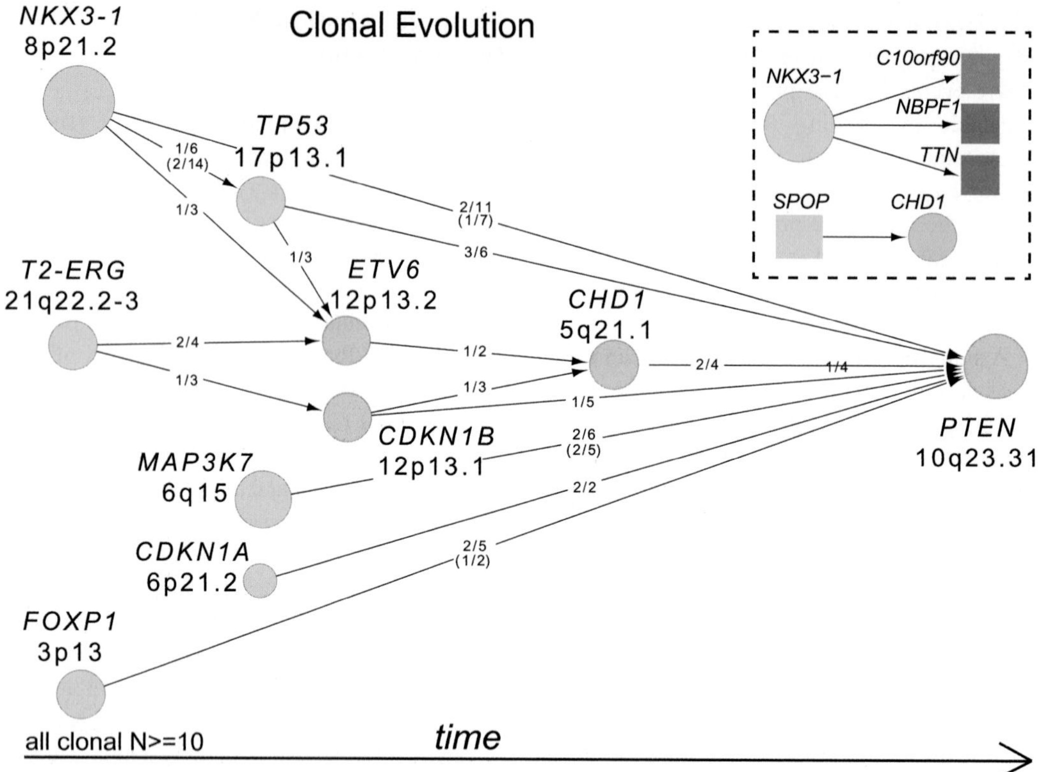

Fig. 11.6 Clonality and evolution of prostate cancer. Patterns of tumor evolution were inferred on the basis of clonality estimates. *Arrows* indicate the direction of clonal–subclonal hierarchy between genes that are deleted in the same sample in multiple cases. Deleted genes are represented by *circles* with size and color intensity reflecting the frequency of overall deletions and subclonal deletions, respectively. Ratios along the *arrows* indicate the number of samples demonstrating directionality of the hierarchy out of samples with deletion of both genes. (Used with permission from [40])

subclassify tumors. These findings raise the possibility that prostate cancer could soon transition from a poorly understood, heterogeneous disease with a variable clinical course to a collection of homogenous subtypes, identifiable by molecular criteria, associated with distinct risk profiles, and perhaps amenable to specific management strategies or targeted therapies [66] (Fig. 11.7).

Epigenetic Alterations in Prostate Cancer

Epigenetic alterations occur more frequently than somatic mutations. They arise early and associate with prostate cancer and disease progression, including DNA methylation, histone modifications, and microRNA (miRNA) regulation. These heritable alterations affect gene expression without changing the DNA sequences during the development of prostate cancer. As epigenetic alterations can be reversed, inhibitors blocking the processes are being tested for their effectiveness in treating prostate cancer. In addition, there appear to be many opportunities for biomarker development based on epigenetic alterations as these changes can be robustly measured.

DNA Methylation

GSTP1

The best-known gene-specific hypermethylation in prostate cancer is *Glutathione-S-*

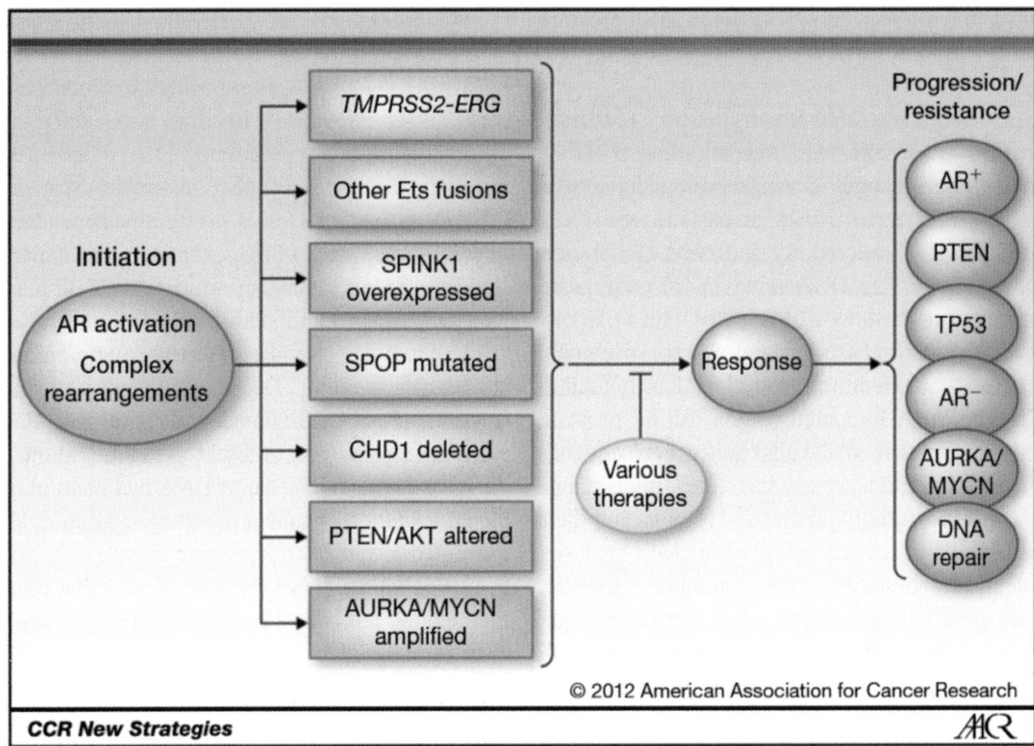

Fig. 11.7 Molecular subclassification of prostate cancer. Disease initiation occurs through activation of androgen signaling, complex rearrangements, or other proposed mechanisms, leading to prostate tumor—wide clinical heterogeneity and distinct molecular subtypes. Disease progression and resistance to therapy lead to acquisition of new and potentially overlapping molecular alterations. (Used with permission from [66] Copyright © American Association for Cancer Research.)

transferase P1 (*GSTP1*) [67]. Loss of expression of *GSTP1* is frequently found in prostate cancer, as well as in HGPIN, and its silencing is a result of promoter hypermethylation. These observations support that promoter hypermethylation is an early event in tumorigenesis. *GSTP1* is involved in oxidative damage response and can protect cells from DNA damage and cancer initiation. Lack of *GSPT1* expression might enable cells to tolerate DNA damage and mutations. Hypermethylation at the *GSTP1* promoter in prostate cancer is well characterized and documented. Since it can be detected in tumor tissues and body fluids (urine and blood), extensive work has been done in an attempt to make *GSTP1* a useful biomarker. When screening for *GSTP1* promoter hypermethylation, it shows high specificity, but various sensitivities in urine and serum/plasma. The discrepancies among different studies reflect the differences in methodologies and patient cohorts. Detecting *GSTP1*-promoter hypermethylation has been suggested as biomarker for diagnosis, prognosis, and treatment response. For example, serum *GSTP1* promoter hypermethylation has been suggested as a predictor of BCR in patients with localized disease at radical prostatectomy. Still, some prostate cancer cases do not have *GSTP1* promoter hypermethylation, and examination of panels of multiple genes has been proposed to balance this scenario. Combination of multiple genes has greatly enhanced the detection while maintaining high specificity; gene selection is critical and should be carefully evaluated. In a recent large-scale study, the panel of *GSTP1*, *HIF3A*, *HAAO*, and *RARβ* provided high sensitivity and high specificity to distinguish prostate cancer from benign prostate tissues [68].

Genome-Wide DNA Methylation Profiling

In the last decade, our understanding of DNA methylation changes in prostate cancer have been greatly improved, thanks in part to new technologies (e.g., microarray and Next Generation Sequencing). The DNA methylation patterns in prostate cancer show global losses with a particular enrichment at CpG island promoter regions. Regions with medium to low CpG density tend to develop DNA hypomethylation during prostate cancer initiation. While next generation sequencing allows for deeper coverage, new understanding of differentially methylated regions and their associated genes are being identified. Analyses integrating mutations, copy number variation, and gene expression data can further provide relevant information to the cancer genome. Different from candidate gene-based approaches, genome-wide site-specific DNA methylation events can now be studied and previously unknown differential methylation regions can be identified to provide a more complete map of DNA methylation changes.

Methylation profiling with microarray technology is limited by defined probes; however, several studies have uncovered biomarkers for predicting BCR [69], associated with prostate cancer progression [70, 71] (Fig. 11.8a–c), and the combination of methylation and copy number changes has shown that in CRPC copy number loss and promoter hypermethylation occur together for tumor suppressor genes (e.g., RB) in the same tumor [72]. These results suggest that multiple mechanisms are utilized simultaneously by cancer cells to gain growth advantages.

Large-scale DNA methylation profiling between prostate cancer and normal prostate tissue has also been carried out to identify diagnostic and prognostic DNA methylation alterations [68, 73]. Deep sequencing enables investigators to study CpG sites outside of gene promoters or CpG islands, including repetitive sequences, and allows the evaluation of methylation states at specific alleles. The challenge is how to distinguish the "drivers" and "passengers" of DNA methylation alterations. Differential methylation is observed in repeat elements (e.g., LINE-1) between *ERG* gene fusion-positive and negative cancer [74]. Moreover, bisulfite sequencing of chromatin immunoprecipitated DNA (BisChIP-seq) has demonstrated that in prostate cancer cells DNA methylation is not totally dependent of H3K27me3 marks [75], expanding our understanding from a previous finding that EZH2 may lead DNA methyltransferases (DNMTs) to specific genomic loci and connect the two epigenetic modes together. Deep sequencing has also revealed most CpG dinucleotide sites and has provided a clear look of total CpG methylation.

To understand the role of DNA methylation in clonal evolution of cancer metastases, Aryee et al. examined a metastatic prostate cancer autopsy cohort of 13 patients [76]. They found that total methylation patterns are preserved among metastases from the same individual, but heterogeneous among men. Functional consequences from the gene expression patterns suggest that hypomethylation is likely to promote genetic instability instead of affecting gene expression. Hypermethylation at promoters is generally correlated with downregulated gene expression, particularly at methylated regions showing significant variation. These inheritable marks may be highly enriched for driver alterations. New forms of DNA methylation have recently been discovered, including 5-hydroxymethylcytosine, 5-formylcytosine, and 5-carboxylcytosine [77]; however, their importance in prostate cancer remains to be determined. Taken together, DNA methylation alterations warrant further investigations for biomarker development and therapeutic strategies.

Histone Modifications

Histone modifications refer to the changes of basic amino acid residues (i.e., lysine, arginine, and serine) on histone tails, including acetylation, phosphorylation, methylation, ubiquitylation, sumoylation, citrullination, and ADP-ribosylation. These modifications affect histone tails' affinity to DNA, change chromatin structure (open or closed chromatin conformation),

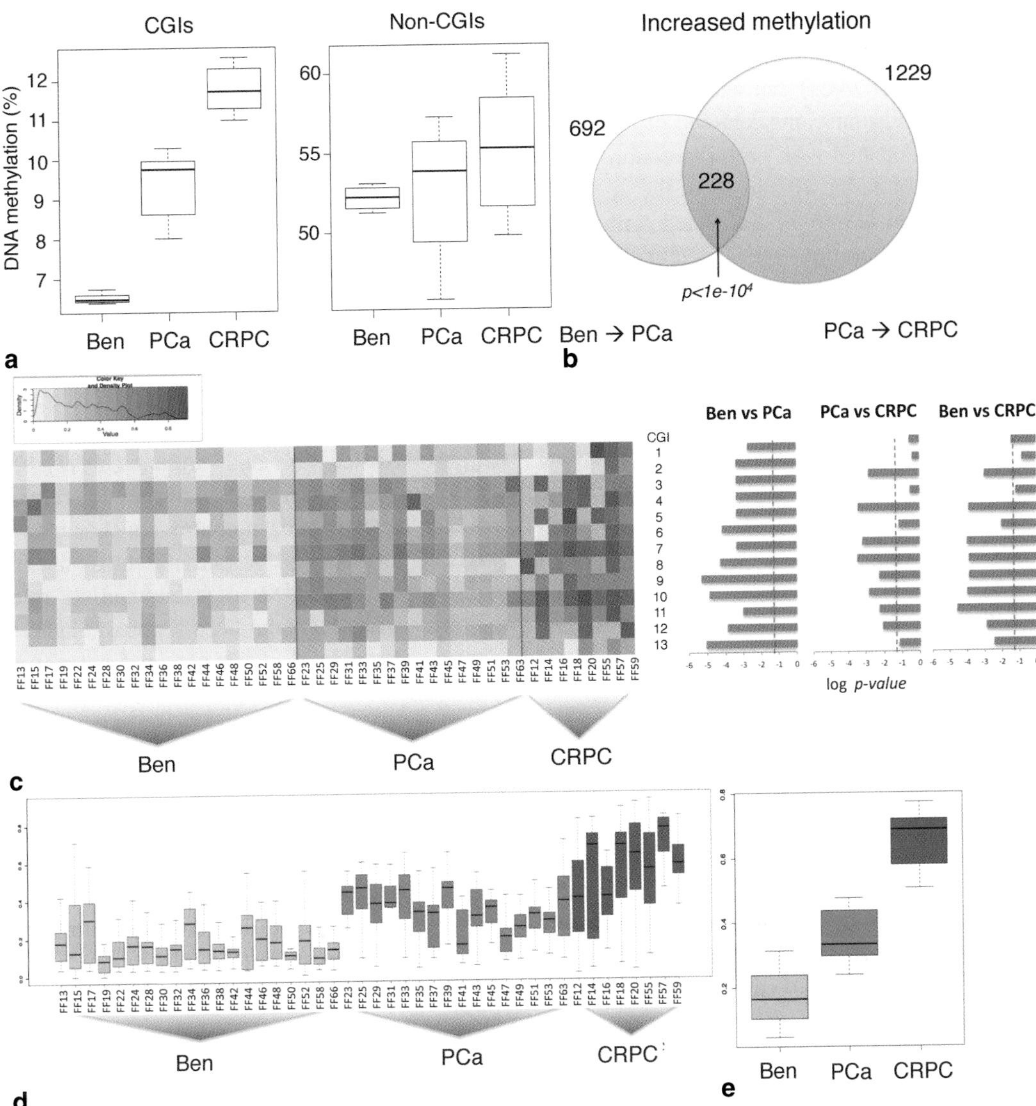

Fig. 11.8 DNA methylation increases with and may predict disease severity. **a** *Left*: Heat map of DNA methylation levels of the panel of 13 CpG islands (*CGIs*) in the three groups, 20 benign prostate tissues and 16 PCa and 8 CRPC samples (value range, 0–1). *Right*: Comparison between the three groups with adjusted log *P* values (Benjamini-Hochberg correction false discovery rate (FDR) controlled at 0.05). **b** Boxplots of the average DNA methylation levels of the panel for individual samples. **c** Boxplots of the average DNA methylation levels of the panel for the three groups. The AUC, sensitivity, and specificity for the comparison of benign and PCa are 0.9375, 100, and 75 %, and those for the comparison of PCa and CRPC are 0.975, 95, and 95 %. The boxplots at the bottom show average DNA methylation levels in individual samples (**d**) and in the three groups (**e**). (Used with permission of [71])

and consequently impact gene expression. The malleability of histone modifications allows temporal and spatial changes in gene expression that are needed for cellular homeostasis. The complexities of histone modifications present a big challenge to study them in prostate cancer disease progression. For example, addition of methyl groups (mono-, di-, or tri-methylation) by HMTs to H3, H4 lysine, and arginine residues can lead to gene activation or repression, depending on the location of target residues. Histone acetyltransferases (HATs) and histone deacetylases (HDACs) can change the acetylation state of histones, and removal of the acetyl groups is associated with gene repression. Phosphorylation of serine 10 and 28 of the histone 3 (H3S10ph, H3S28ph) is associated with chromosomal condensation; on the other hand, the combination of H3S10ph and H3K14Ac would suggest active transcription. Few studies have demonstrated patterns of histone modifications by using immunohistochemistry, suggesting that global histone modifications can provide prognostic information for prostate cancer. Histone modifiers as mentioned above possess enzymatic activities and have gained tremendous interests for their potentials in therapeutic interventions to treat cancer patients. Here, we discuss the ones pertinent to prostate cancer.

EZH2

The HMT, the enhancer of zeste homolog 2 (EZH2), is responsible for H3K27 trimethylation (H3K27me3) and gene silencing. It physically interacts with DNMTs and helps their binding to EZH2 target promoters. Overexpression of EZH2 and the group of its repressed genes have been associated with aggressive prostate cancer and disease progression. Downregulation of miR-101 or miR-26 is proposed to cause EZH2 elevation during prostate cancer progression. However, most studies have only explored for detected expression levels of EZH2 without showing global levels of H3K27me1, me2, or me3. One study systematically evaluated global H3K27 mono-, di-, and trimethylation in different disease states using immunohistochemistry [78]. It showed that global H3K27 methylation levels were increased in metastatic prostate cancer and CRPC, implying that the detection in bodily fluids with an ELISA-based assay could be beneficial. It remains to be determined if the levels of H3K27 methylation provide relevant information for prostate cancer prognosis. Additional molecular mechanisms have been proposed for EZH2's oncogenic functions. The histone methyltransferase multiple myeloma SET domain (MMSET) was upregulated in prostate cancer cell lines, which results in the activation of TWIST1, a critical gene in regulating epithelial-mesenchymal transition (EMT) and promoting cell migration and invasion [79]. MMSET is responsible for H3K36 dimethylation (H3K36me2) and gene activation. The expression of MMSET is highly correlated with EZH2 in prostate cancer. It acts downstream of EZH2, necessary for mediating EZH2's oncogenic functions [80]. The regulatory link between EZH2 and MMSET suggests that EZH2's oncogenic functions are not limited to transcriptional repression of tumor suppressors (e.g., p16INK4α, WNT pathway, and *CDH1*), but also to oncogene activation. However, the role or EZH2 in cancer has been controversial as it also exerts tumor suppressive activity; thus, further investigation is needed to understand its role. Inhibitors of EZH2 have been reported, such as 3-deazaneplanocin A (DZNep), an S-adenosylhomocysteine hydrolase inhibitor, and the small molecules GKS126 and EPZ00687, but to date none have been approved by the FDA. DZNep has been shown to globally inhibit histone methylation, both active and repressive marks. Its effects on cancer cells are not specific to EZH2. A major concern in the development of inhibitors for epigenetic modifications is cytotoxicity. Therapeutic approaches to totally block EZH2 activity might cause undesired consequences and targeting its downstream effectors, like MMSET, might provide more specific outcomes.

LSD1

Lysine-specific demehtylase 1 (LSD1), can function as a corepressor and a coactivator. When in corepressor complexes, it functions by demethylating mono- and dimethylated H3K4; when in coactivator complexes, it functions as a coactivator through association with AR and other nuclear factors to demethylate repressive mono- and dimethylated H3K9. LSD1 can form complexes with AR and recognize repressor elements of genes that negatively regulate AR signaling and cellular proliferation. In CRPC, low levels of androgen are not sufficient to recruit LSD1 and AR, and therefore, it increases the expression of AR and of multiple genes that contribute to increased androgen synthesis, DNA replication, and proliferation. Overexpression of LSD1 in prostate cancer is associated with aggressiveness and high risk of relapse.

Histone Acetylation

Extensive studies have characterized AR transcriptional coregulators, several of which, including p300/CBP, p/CAF, TIP60, class I and class II HDACs, and p160/SRC proteins, have histone acetylase/deacetylase activity. HDACs inhibitors can be subdivided into the following groups: hydroxamic acids (e.g., trichostatin A, vorinostat/SAHA), cyclic tetrapeptides (e.g., trapoxin B)/depsipeptides, electrophilic ketones, short-chain fatty acids, and benzamides; the former two groups have been clinically tested in prostate cancer. These compounds act on the zinc-containing catalytic domains of the HDACs, thus, blocking substrate recognition. Combination of HDAC inhibitors and conventional chemotherapeutic drugs (suberoylanilide hydroxamic acid [SAHA] and doxorubicin or panobinostat and docetaxel) has been tested in prostate cancer patients, but only partial responses have been observed. Significant cytotoxicity and limited antitumor effects were observed in a phase II clinical trial of cyclic tetrapeptide romidepsin. More recently, a phase II trial for recurrent or CRPC has started with SB939, a new hydroxamic acid-based HDAC inhibitor.

MicroRNAs (miRNAs)

miRNAs are small noncoding RNAs that can simultaneously regulate the expression of multiple genes by deteriorating mRNA stability or interrupting translation. They govern a big variety of cellular functions and their aberrant expression can contribute to tumorigenesis by targeting oncogenes or tumor suppressor genes or affecting important signaling pathways [81, 82]. Therefore, altered expression of miRNAs may play an important role in prostate cancer development and disease progression. Over the past few years, accumulating evidence have implicated miRNA dysregulation in prostate cancer [82, 83]. As many miRNAs are related to prostate cancer growth, disease progression, and responses to treatment, they have potential clinical implications as biomarkers for prostate cancer surveillance. It is worth exploiting their potentials on enhancing PSA-based screening test, improving the accuracy of recurrence predictors, and assisting the prediction of the efficacies of hormone therapy and chemotherapy.

Table 11.1 Altered miRNAs in prostate cancer with validated targets

microRNA	Validated targets
let-7a	CCND2, E2F2, MYC, RAS
miR-15a/miR-16	BCL2, CCND1, FGF-2, FGFR1, WNT3A
miR-101	EZH2
miR-106b-25-93	E2F1, p21/WAF1
miR-125b	ERBB2, ERBB3
miR-143/145	AIF, BNIP3, ERK5, MYO6
miR-146	CXCR4, EGFR, ROCK1
miR-148	MSK1
miR-21	BTG2, PDCD4, PTEN, RECK, SPRY2, TIMP3, TPM1
miR-22	PTEN
miR-23	MYC
miR-203	BMI1, RUNX2, ZEB2
miR-205	AR, BCL2L, E2F6, PRKCE, ZEB1, ZEB2
miR-221/222	p27/kip1
miR-31	AR, BCL2L, E2F1, E2F2, E2F6, MCM2, EXO1, FOXM1
miR-32	BIM, BTG2
miR-34	AKT, BCL2, CD44, E2F3, MYC, TP53, SIRT1
miR-330	E2F1
miR-449	CCND1, HDAC1
miR-99	SMARCA5, SMARD1

Many altered miRNAs affect prostate cancer growth by regulating cell cycle and apoptosis. Table 11.1 lists altered miRNAs in prostate cancer with validated targets [82, 84–90]. In addition, several cellular mechanisms are mediated by miRNAs in prostate cancer bone metastasis. EMT is a key step of establishing cancer metastasis. Downregulation of miR-143, miR-145, or miR-205 in prostate cancer is associated with

EMT. miR-146 targets ROCK1 and results in ROCK1 downregulation, which causes the activation of the ROCK-medicated signaling and promotes metastasis. Downregulation of miR-203 also promotes bone metastasis through ZEB2 and RUNX2, which are an EMT factor and a transcription regulator for bone homing and osteoblast proliferation, respectively. miR-101 targets EZH2, whose increased expression is related to invasion by repressing E-cadherin. Genomic loss and downregulation of miR-101 may increase the invasiveness by upregulating EZH2. Genomic loss of miR-15 and miR-16.2 in cancer-associated fibroblasts promotes prostate cancer development and progression by enhancing expression of *FGF-2* and *FGFR1*.

Treatment with abiraterone acetate and enzalutamide (MDV3100) in CRPC patients underlines the importance of AR-signaling in prostate cancer disease progression. Several miRNAs are implicated in regulating AR signaling and their dysregulation may uphold AR activity during androgen deprivation therapy. Let-7c inhibits AR transcription through targeting c-MYC, while miR-31 and miR-488* directly target AR mRNA. Using a miRNA library, additional miRNAs that target AR 3′UTR are identified, including miR-135b, miR-185, miR-299-3p, miR-34a/c, miR-371-3p, miR-421, miR-449a/b, miR-634, miR-654-5p, and miR-9. MiR-31 also indirectly represses AR by downregulating E2F1 and CDK1. MiR-130a, miR-203, and miR-205 repress AR coactivators, CDK1, PSAP, PSMC3IP, and PARK7, and inhibit the MAPK signaling pathway, which facilitates ligand-independent AR activation. On the other hand, AR regulates miRNAs at the transcriptional level, inducing the expression of miR-125b-2, miR-21, and miR-32, and suppressing the expression of miR-31. Overexpressing miR-21 supports androgen-independent growth in vitro and in vivo.

Malfunction of the miRNA machinery may also contribute to prostate cancer. Dicer, an essential RNase III endonuclease for the cleavage of 70–100 nucleotides long pre-miRNA in the cytoplasm, is frequently upregulated in prostate cancer, and its expression levels are correlated with clinical status, lymph node status, and Gleason score [83]. Dicer and several components of the miRNA machinery, XPO5, EIF2C2, EIF2C1, HSPCA, MOV10, and TNRC6B, have shown increased expression in metastatic prostate cancer and have been associated with aggressiveness. Immunohistochemical analysis shows that in normal prostate tissues, Dicer is only detected in the basal cells; during tumorigenesis, Dicer expression in neoplastic luminal cells arises and continues to increase during disease progression. The appearance of Dicer may potentiate malignant transition and promote aggressiveness by mediating expression of miRNAs with oncogene features. As miRNAs are involved in various cellular functions, dysregulation of Dicer may provide growth advantages to prostate cancer at all stages.

MiRNAs are believed to be more stable than mRNA in serum, urine, archived formalin-fixed paraffin-embedded (FFPE) or frozen tissues, making them ideal for biomarker development. Epigenetic changes also affect miRNA expression in prostate cancer. We recently found that miR-31 is frequently downregulated due to promoter DNA hypermethylation [91]. Downregulation of miR-31 and DNA hypermethylation at the miR-31 promoter are associated with prostate cancer disease progression. The frequent hypermethylation of the *miR-31* promoter in prostate cancer suggests that epigenetic drugs, such as DNA demethylating agents, could complement existing therapeutic strategies. Such combinatorial treatment might decrease the emergence of CRPC, which represents a major cause of progression and mortality in prostate cancer patients.

Section Summary

The enthusiasm for using DNA methylation alterations as biomarkers or as the base for therapeutic intervention has attenuated, in part due to the uncertainty whether DNA methylation or other epigenetic marks are stable to drive prostate cancer tumorigenesis and disease progression. Aryee et al. recently showed that like copy number alterations, total DNA methylation can be maintained in different metastases [76]. The critical issue here is to separate and distinguish between "driver" and "passenger" epigenetic alterations.

References

1. Siegel R, Naishadham D, Jemal A. Cancer statistics, 2012. CA Cancer J Clin. 2012;62(1):10–29.
2. Barbieri CE, Baca SC, Lawrence MS, Demichelis F, Blattner M, Theurillat JP, et al. Exome sequencing identifies recurrent SPOP, FOXA1 and MED12 mutations in prostate cancer. Nat Genet. 2012;44(6):685–9.
3. Grasso CS, Wu YM, Robinson DR, Cao X, Dhanasekaran SM, Khan AP, et al. The mutational landscape of lethal castration-resistant prostate cancer. Nature. 2012;487(7406):239–43.
4. Lindberg J, Klevebring D, Liu W, Neiman M, Xu J, Wiklund P, et al. Exome sequencing of prostate cancer supports the hypothesis of independent tumour origins. Eur Urol. 2013;63(2):347–53.
5. Kumar A, White TA, MacKenzie AP, Clegg N, Lee C, Dumpit RF, et al. Exome sequencing identifies a spectrum of mutation frequencies in advanced and lethal prostate cancers. Proc Natl Acad Sci U S A. 2011;108(41):17087–92.
6. Taylor BS, Schultz N, Hieronymus H, Gopalan A, Xiao Y, Carver BS, et al. Integrative genomic profiling of human prostate cancer. Cancer Cell. 2010;18(1):11–22.
7. Berger MF, Lawrence MS, Demichelis F, Drier Y, Cibulskis K, Sivachenko AY, et al. The genomic complexity of primary human prostate cancer. Nature. 2011;470(7333):214–20.
8. Cairns P, Okami K, Halachmi S, Halachmi N, Esteller M, Herman JG, et al. Frequent inactivation of PTEN/MMAC1 in primary prostate cancer. Cancer Res. 1997;57(22):4997–5000.
9. Beltran H, Yelensky R, Frampton GM, Park K, Downing SR, Macdonald TY, et al. Targeted next-generation sequencing of advanced prostate cancer identifies potential therapeutic targets and disease heterogeneity. Eur Urol. 2013;63(5):920–6.
10. Kumar A, White TA, MacKenzie AP, Clegg N, Lee C, Dumpit RF, et al. Exome sequencing identifies a spectrum of mutation frequencies in advanced and lethal prostate cancers. Proc Natl Acad Sci U S A. 2011;108(41):17087–92.
11. Carver BS, Tran J, Gopalan A, Chen Z, Shaikh S, Carracedo A, et al. Aberrant ERG expression cooperates with loss of PTEN to promote cancer progression in the prostate. Nat Genet. 2009;41(5):619–24.
12. Chen M, Pratt CP, Zeeman ME, Schultz N, Taylor BS, O'Neill A, et al. Identification of PHLPP1 as a tumor suppressor reveals the role of feedback activation in PTEN-mutant prostate cancer progression. Cancer Cell. 2011;20(2):173–86.
13. Trotman LC, Niki M, Dotan ZA, Koutcher JA, Di Cristofano A, Xiao A, et al. Pten dose dictates cancer progression in the prostate. PLoS Biol. 2003;1(3):E59.
14. Sun X, Huang J, Homma T, Kita D, Klocker H, Schafer G, et al. Genetic alterations in the PI3K pathway in prostate cancer. Anticancer Res. 2009;29(5):1739–43.
15. Lapointe J, Li C, Giacomini CP, Salari K, Huang S, Wang P, et al. Genomic profiling reveals alternative genetic pathways of prostate tumorigenesis. Cancer Res. 2007;67(18):8504–10.
16. Bakin RE, Gioeli D, Sikes RA, Bissonette EA, Weber MJ. Constitutive activation of the Ras/mitogen-activated protein kinase signaling pathway promotes androgen hypersensitivity in LNCaP prostate cancer cells. Cancer Res. 2003;63(8):1981–9.
17. Palanisamy N, Ateeq B, Kalyana-Sundaram S, Pflueger D, Ramnarayanan K, Shankar S, et al. Rearrangements of the RAF kinase pathway in prostate cancer, gastric cancer and melanoma. Nat Med. 2010;16(7):793–8.
18. Wang XS, Shankar S, Dhanasekaran SM, Ateeq B, Sasaki AT, Jing X, et al. Characterization of KRAS rearrangements in metastatic prostate cancer. Cancer Discov. 2011;1(1):35–43.
19. Lindberg J, Mills IG, Klevebring D, Liu W, Neiman M, Xu J, et al. The mitochondrial and autosomal mutation landscapes of prostate cancer. Eur Urol. 2013;63(4):702–8.
20. Aparicio A, Den RB, Knudsen KE. Time to stratify? The retinoblastoma protein in castrate-resistant prostate cancer. Nat Rev Urol. 2011;8(10):562–8.
21. Linja MJ, Visakorpi T. Alterations of androgen receptor in prostate cancer. J Steroid Biochem Mol Biol. 2004;92(4):255–64.
22. Visakorpi T, Hyytinen E, Koivisto P, Tanner M, Keinanen R, Palmberg C, et al. In vivo amplification of the androgen receptor gene and progression of human prostate cancer. Nat Genet. 1995;9(4):401–6.
23. Hu R, Lu C, Mostaghel EA, Yegnasubramanian S, Gurel M, Tannahill C, et al. Distinct transcriptional programs mediated by the ligand-dependent full-length androgen receptor and its splice variants in castration-resistant prostate cancer. Cancer Res. 2012;72(14):3457–62.
24. Hu R, Dunn TA, Wei S, Isharwal S, Veltri RW, Humphreys E, et al. Ligand-independent androgen receptor variants derived from splicing of cryptic exons signify hormone-refractory prostate cancer. Cancer Res. 2009;69(1):16–22.
25. Visakorpi T, Hyytinen E, Koivisto P, Tanner M, Keinanen R, Palmberg C, et al. In vivo amplification of the androgen receptor gene and progression of human prostate cancer. Nat Genet. 1995;9(4):401–6.
26. Linja MJ, Visakorpi T. Alterations of androgen receptor in prostate cancer. J Steroid Biochem Mol Biol. 2004;92(4):255–64.

27. Koivisto P, Kononen J, Palmberg C, Tammela T, Hyytinen E, Isola J, et al. Androgen receptor gene amplification: a possible molecular mechanism for androgen deprivation therapy failure in prostate cancer. Cancer Res. 1997;57(2):314–9.
28. Waltering KK, Urbanucci A, Visakorpi T. Androgen receptor (AR) aberrations in castration-resistant prostate cancer. Mol Cell Endocrinol. 2012;360(1–2):38–43.
29. Zhang C, Wang L, Wu D, Chen H, Chen Z, Thomas-Ahner JM, et al. Definition of a FoxA1 Cistrome that is crucial for G1 to S-phase cell-cycle transit in castration-resistant prostate cancer. Cancer Res. 2011;71(21):6738–48.
30. Lapointe J, Li C, Giacomini CP, Salari K, Huang S, Wang P, et al. Genomic profiling reveals alternative genetic pathways of prostate tumorigenesis. Cancer Res. 2007;67(18):8504–10.
31. Carver BS, Chapinski C, Wongvipat J, Hieronymus H, Chen Y, Chandarlapaty S, et al. Reciprocal feedback regulation of PI3K and androgen receptor signaling in PTEN-deficient prostate cancer. Cancer Cell. 2011;19(5):575–86.
32. Haffner MC, Aryee MJ, Toubaji A, Esopi DM, Albadine R, Gurel B, et al. Androgen-induced TOP2B-mediated double-strand breaks and prostate cancer gene rearrangements. Nat Genet. 2010;42(8):668–75.
33. Weischenfeldt J, Simon R, Feuerbach L, Schlangen K, Weichenhan D, Minner S, et al. Integrative genomic analyses reveal an androgen-driven somatic alteration landscape in early-onset prostate cancer. Cancer Cell. 2013;23(2):159–70.
34. Tomlins SA, Rhodes DR, Perner S, Dhanasekaran SM, Mehra R, Sun XW, et al. Recurrent fusion of TMPRSS2 and ETS transcription factor genes in prostate cancer. Science. 2005;310(5748):644–8.
35. Tomlins SA, Laxman B, Dhanasekaran SM, Helgeson BE, Cao X, Morris DS, et al. Distinct classes of chromosomal rearrangements create oncogenic ETS gene fusions in prostate cancer. Nature. 2007;448(7153):595–9.
36. Tomlins SA, Bjartell A, Chinnaiyan AM, Jenster G, Nam RK, Rubin MA, et al. ETS gene fusions in prostate cancer: from discovery to daily clinical practice. Eur Urol. 2009;56(2):275–86.
37. Klezovitch O, Risk M, Coleman I, Lucas JM, Null M, True LD, et al. A causal role for ERG in neoplastic transformation of prostate epithelium. Proc Natl Acad Sci U S A. 2008;105(6):2105–10.
38. King JC, Xu J, Wongvipat J, Hieronymus H, Carver BS, Leung DH, et al. Cooperativity of TMPRSS2-ERG with PI3-kinase pathway activation in prostate oncogenesis. Nat Genet. 2009;41(5):524–6.
39. Lindberg J, Klevebring D, Liu W, Neiman M, Xu J, Wiklund P, et al. Exome sequencing of prostate cancer supports the hypothesis of independent tumour origins. Eur Urol. 2013;63(2):347–53.
40. Baca SC, Prandi D, Lawrence MS, Mosquera JM, Romanel A, Drier Y, et al. Punctuated evolution of prostate cancer genomes. Cell. 2013;153(3):666–77.
41. Varambally S, Dhanasekaran SM, Zhou M, Barrette TR, Kumar-Sinha C, Sanda MG, et al. The polycomb group protein EZH2 is involved in progression of prostate cancer. Nature. 2002;419(6907):624–9.
42. Xu K, Wu ZJ, Groner AC, He HH, Cai C, Lis RT, et al. EZH2 oncogenic activity in castration-resistant prostate cancer cells is Polycomb-independent. Science. 2012;338(6113):1465–9.
43. Attard G, Swennenhuis JF, Olmos D, Reid AH, Vickers E, A'Hern R, et al. Characterization of ERG, AR and PTEN gene status in circulating tumor cells from patients with castration-resistant prostate cancer. Cancer Res. 2009;69(7):2912–8.
44. Cairns P, Evron E, Okami K, Halachmi N, Esteller M, Herman JG, et al. Point mutation and homozygous deletion of PTEN/MMAC1 in primary bladder cancers. Oncogene. 1998;16(24):3215–8.
45. Choucair K, Ejdelman J, Brimo F, Aprikian A, Chevalier S, Lapointe J. PTEN genomic deletion predicts prostate cancer recurrence and is associated with low AR expression and transcriptional activity. BMC Cancer. 2012;12:543.
46. McMenamin ME, Soung P, Perera S, Kaplan I, Loda M, Sellers WR. Loss of PTEN expression in paraffin-embedded primary prostate cancer correlates with high Gleason score and advanced stage. Cancer Res. 1999;59(17):4291–6.
47. Reid AH, Attard G, Ambroisine L, Fisher G, Kovacs G, Brewer D, et al. Molecular characterisation of ERG, ETV1 and PTEN gene loci identifies patients at low and high risk of death from prostate cancer. Br J Cancer. 2010;102(4):678–84.
48. Attard G, de Bono JS, Clark J, Cooper CS. Studies of TMPRSS2-ERG gene fusions in diagnostic trans-rectal prostate biopsies. Clin Cancer Res. 2010;16(4):1340. Author reply.
49. Demichelis F, Fall K, Perner S, Andren O, Schmidt F, Setlur SR, et al. TMPRSS2:ERG gene fusion associated with lethal prostate cancer in a watchful waiting cohort. Oncogene. 2007;26(31):4596–9.
50. Lapointe J, Li C, Higgins JP, van de Rijn M, Bair E, Montgomery K, et al. Gene expression profiling identifies clinically relevant subtypes of prostate cancer. Proc Natl Acad Sci U S A. 2004;101(3):811–6.
51. Setlur SR, Mertz KD, Hoshida Y, Demichelis F, Lupien M, Perner S, et al. Estrogen-dependent signaling in a molecularly distinct subclass of aggressive prostate cancer. J Natl Cancer Inst. 2008;100(11):815–25.
52. Svensson MA, LaFargue CJ, MacDonald TY, Pflueger D, Kitabayashi N, Santa-Cruz AM, et al. Testing mutual exclusivity of ETS rearranged prostate cancer. Lab Invest. 2011;91(3):404–12.
53. Tomlins SA, Mehra R, Rhodes DR, Cao X, Wang L, Dhanasekaran SM, et al. Integrative molecular concept modeling of prostate cancer progression. Nat Genet. 2007;39(1):41–51.
54. Demichelis F, Setlur SR, Beroukhim R, Perner S, Korbel JO, Lafargue CJ, et al. Distinct genomic aberrations associated with ERG rearranged

prostate cancer. Genes Chromosomes Cancer. 2009;48(4):366–80.
55. Brenner JC, Ateeq B, Li Y, Yocum AK, Cao Q, Asangani IA, et al. Mechanistic rationale for inhibition of poly(ADP-ribose) polymerase in ETS gene fusion-positive prostate cancer. Cancer Cell. 2011;19(5):664–78.
56. Tomlins SA, Rhodes DR, Yu J, Varambally S, Mehra R, Perner S, et al. The role of SPINK1 in ETS rearrangement-negative prostate cancers. Cancer Cell. 2008;13(6):519–28.
57. Paju A, Hotakainen K, Cao Y, Laurila T, Gadaleanu V, Hemminki A, et al. Increased expression of tumor-associated trypsin inhibitor, TATI, in prostate cancer and in androgen-independent 22Rv1 cells. Eur Urol. 2007;52(6):1670–9.
58. Lippolis G, Edsjo A, Stenman UH, Bjartell A. A high-density tissue microarray from patients with clinically localized prostate cancer reveals ERG and TATI exclusivity in tumor cells. Prostate Cancer Prostatic Dis. 2013;16(2):145–50.
59. Ateeq B, Tomlins SA, Laxman B, Asangani IA, Cao Q, Cao X, et al. Therapeutic targeting of SPINK1-positive prostate cancer. Sci Transl Med. 2011;3(72):72ra17.
60. Karkera J, Steiner H, Li W, Skradski V, Moser PL, Riethdorf S, et al. The anti-interleukin-6 antibody siltuximab down-regulates genes implicated in tumorigenesis in prostate cancer patients from a phase I study. Prostate. 2011;71(13):1455–65.
61. Puhr M, Santer FR, Neuwirt H, Susani M, Nemeth JA, Hobisch A, et al. Down-regulation of suppressor of cytokine signaling-3 causes prostate cancer cell death through activation of the extrinsic and intrinsic apoptosis pathways. Cancer Res. 2009;69(18):7375–84.
62. Malinowska K, Neuwirt H, Cavarretta IT, Bektic J, Steiner H, Dietrich H, et al. Interleukin-6 stimulation of growth of prostate cancer in vitro and in vivo through activation of the androgen receptor. Endocr Relat Cancer. 2009;16(1):155–69.
63. Flechon A, Pouessel D, Ferlay C, Perol D, Beuzeboc P, Gravis G, et al. Phase II study of carboplatin and etoposide in patients with anaplastic progressive metastatic castration-resistant prostate cancer (mCRPC) with or without neuroendocrine differentiation: results of the French Genito-Urinary Tumor Group (GETUG) P01 trial. Ann Oncol. 2011;22(11):2476–81.
64. Mosquera JM, Beltran H, Park K, MacDonald TY, Robinson BD, Tagawa ST, et al. Concurrent AURKA and MYCN gene amplifications are harbingers of lethal treatment-related neuroendocrine prostate cancer. Neoplasia. 2013;15(1):1–10.
65. Mosquera JM, Perner S, Genega EM, Sanda M, Hofer MD, Mertz KD, et al. Characterization of TMPRSS2-ERG fusion high-grade prostatic intraepithelial neoplasia and potential clinical implications. Clin Cancer Res. 2008;14(11):3380–5.
66. Beltran H, Rubin MA. New strategies in prostate cancer: translating genomics into the clinic. Clin Cancer Res. 2013;19(3):517–23.
67. Chiam K, Ricciardelli C, Bianco-Miotto T. Epigenetic biomarkers in prostate cancer: Current and future uses. Cancer Lett. 2014;342(2):248–56.
68. Mahapatra S, Klee EW, Young CY, Sun Z, Jimenez RE, Klee GG, et al. Global methylation profiling for risk prediction of prostate cancer. Clin Cancer Res. 2012;18(10):2882–95.
69. Cottrell S, Jung K, Kristiansen G, Eltze E, Semjonow A, Ittmann M, et al. Discovery and validation of 3 novel DNA methylation markers of prostate cancer prognosis. J Urol. 2007;177(5):1753–8.
70. Kron K, Pethe V, Briollais L, Sadikovic B, Ozcelik H, Sunderji A, et al. Discovery of novel hypermethylated genes in prostate cancer using genomic CpG island microarrays. PLoS One. 2009;4(3):e4830.
71. Lin PC, Giannopoulou EG, Park K, Mosquera JM, Sboner A, Tewari AK, et al. Epigenomic alterations in localized and advanced prostate cancer. Neoplasia. 2013;15(4):373–83.
72. Friedlander TW, Roy R, Tomlins SA, Ngo VT, Kobayashi Y, Azameera A, et al. Common structural and epigenetic changes in the genome of castration-resistant prostate cancer. Cancer Res. 2012;72(3):616–25.
73. Kobayashi Y, Absher DM, Gulzar ZG, Young SR, McKenney JK, Peehl DM, et al. DNA methylation profiling reveals novel biomarkers and important roles for DNA methyltransferases in prostate cancer. Genome Res. 2011;21(7):1017–27.
74. Kim JH, Dhanasekaran SM, Prensner JR, Cao X, Robinson D, Kalyana-Sundaram S, et al. Deep sequencing reveals distinct patterns of DNA methylation in prostate cancer. Genome Res. 2011;21(7):1028–41.
75. Statham AL, Robinson MD, Song JZ, Coolen MW, Stirzaker C, Clark SJ. Bisulfite sequencing of chromatin immunoprecipitated DNA (BisChIP-seq) directly informs methylation status of histone-modified DNA. Genome Res. 2012;22(6):1120–7.
76. Aryee MJ, Liu W, Engelmann JC, Nuhn P, Gurel M, Haffner MC, et al. DNA methylation alterations exhibit intraindividual stability and interindividual heterogeneity in prostate cancer metastases. Sci Transl Med. 2013;5(169):169ra10.
77. Ito S, Shen L, Dai Q, Wu SC, Collins LB, Swenberg JA, et al. Tet proteins can convert 5-methylcytosine to 5-formylcytosine and 5-carboxylcytosine. Science. 2011;333(6047):1300–3.
78. Ellinger J, Kahl P, von der Gathen J, Heukamp LC, Gutgemann I, Walter B, et al. Global histone H3K27 methylation levels are different in localized and metastatic prostate cancer. Cancer Invest. 2012;30(2):92–7.
79. Ezponda T, Popovic R, Shah MY, Martinez-Garcia E, Zheng Y, Min DJ, et al. The histone methyltransferase MMSET/WHSC1 activates TWIST1 to

promote an epithelial-mesenchymal transition and invasive properties of prostate cancer. Oncogene. 2013;32(23):2882–90.

80. Asangani IA, Ateeq B, Cao Q, Dodson L, Pandhi M, Kunju LP, et al. Characterization of the EZH2-MMSET Histone Methyltransferase regulatory axis in cancer. Mol Cell. 2013;49(1):80–93.
81. Iorio MV, Croce CM. MicroRNA dysregulation in cancer: diagnostics, monitoring and therapeutics. A comprehensive review. EMBO Mol Med. 2012;4(3):143–59.
82. Maugeri-Sacca M, Coppola V, Bonci D, De Maria R. MicroRNAs and prostate cancer: from preclinical research to translational oncology. Cancer J. 2012;18(3):253–61.
83. Chiosea S, Jelezcova E, Chandran U, Acquafondata M, McHale T, Sobol RW, et al. Up-regulation of dicer, a component of the MicroRNA machinery, in prostate adenocarcinoma. Am J Pathol. 2006;169(5):1812–20.
84. Benassi B, Flavin R, Marchionni L, Zanata S, Pan Y, Chowdhury D, et al. MYC is activated by USP2a-mediated modulation of microRNAs in prostate cancer. Cancer Discov. 2012;2(3):236–47.
85. Coppola V, De Maria R, Bonci D. MicroRNAs and prostate cancer. Endocr Relat Cancer. 2010;17(1):F1–17.
86. Coppola V, Musumeci M, Patrizii M, Cannistraci A, Addario A, Maugeri-Sacca M, et al. BTG2 loss and miR-21 upregulation contribute to prostate cell transformation by inducing luminal markers expression and epithelial-mesenchymal transition. Oncogene. 2013;32(14):1843–53.
87. Hagman Z, Haflidadottir BS, Ceder JA, Larne O, Bjartell A, Lilja H, et al. miR-205 negatively regulates the androgen receptor and is associated with adverse outcome of prostate cancer patients. Br J Cancer. 2013;108(8):1668–76.
88. Lin PC, Chiu YL, Banerjee S, Park K, Mosquera JM, Giannopoulou E, et al. Epigenetic repression of miR-31 disrupts androgen receptor homeostasis and contributes to prostate cancer progression. Cancer Res. 2013;73(3):1232–44.
89. Majid S, Dar AA, Saini S, Shahryari V, Arora S, Zaman MS, et al. miRNA-34b inhibits prostate cancer through demethylation, active chromatin modifications, and AKT pathways. Clin Cancer Res. 2013;19(1):73–84.
90. Tucci P, Agostini M, Grespi F, Markert EK, Terrinoni A, Vousden KH, et al. Loss of p63 and its microRNA-205 target results in enhanced cell migration and metastasis in prostate cancer. Proc Natl Acad Sci U S A. 2012;109(38):15312–7.
91. Lin PC, Chiu YL, Banerjee S, Park K, Mosquera JM, Giannopoulou E, et al. Epigenetic repression of miR-31 disrupts androgen receptor homeostasis and contributes to prostate cancer progression. Cancer Res. 2013;73(3):1232–44.

Part II

Update on Bladder Tumor Pathology

Anatomy of the Urinary Bladder Revisited: Implications for Diagnosis and Staging of Bladder Cancer

12

Victor E. Reuter

Introduction

The most important risk factor in predicting disease progression in primary urothelial carcinoma of the bladder is pathological stage. As such, understanding the microscopic anatomy of this organ is crucial. While the urinary bladder appears to be an anatomically simple organ, it is not. Benign surface epithelium can invaginate in the underlying connective tissue, mimicking invasive disease. The lamina propria and muscularis propria can be of variable thickness and may contain variable anatomic elements in different portions of the bladder. We are commonly asked to evaluate bladder specimens in areas of prior intervention, where biopsy site changes mask normal anatomic landmarks. To add to this complexity, invasive urothelial carcinoma may be associated with an intense stromal reaction and we are often asked to evaluate transurethral biopsies and resections in patients who have undergone prior excisions, both of which distort the anatomy of the organ. What follows is a review of the gross and microscopic anatomy of the bladder, highlighting the implications for the diagnosis and staging of bladder cancer and illustrating anatomic features that may cause problems in staging tumors properly. More detailed descriptions of the embryology and normal anatomy of the bladder are available in other publications [1, 2].

Embryology and Gross Anatomy

The urinary bladder is an epithelial-lined organ, a component of the lower urinary tract. The lining epithelium, called urothelium, is surrounded by a lamina propria and muscularis propria, which in turn is surrounded by pelvic soft tissue (Fig. 12.1). The urinary bladder is a hollow viscus with the ability to distend and accommodate up to 500 mL of urine without a change in luminal pressure. Its outer layer is composed of smooth muscle, the muscularis propria, which has the ability to voluntarily initiate and maintain a contraction until the organ is empty of urine. Interestingly, micturition may be initiated or inhibited voluntarily despite the involuntary nature of the organ. The ureters transport the urine from the kidneys and these enter the bladder at the trigone. The bladder neck is the most distal portion of the urinary bladder and opens into the urethra.

The bladder urothelium is of endodermal origin, derived from the cranial portion of the urogenital sinus in continuity with the allantois. The lamina propria, the muscularis propria, and the adventitia develop from the adjacent splanchnic mesenchyme. While the mesonephric ducts contribute initially to the formation of the mucosa of the trigone, this is subsequently entirely replaced by endodermal epithelium of the urogenital sinus. During embryologic development, the

V. E. Reuter (✉)
Department of Pathology, Memorial Sloan Kettering Cancer Center, New York, NY, USA
e-mail: reuterv@mskcc.org

C. Magi-Galluzzi, C. G. Przybycin (eds.), *Genitourinary Pathology,* DOI 10.1007/978-1-4939-2044-0_12,

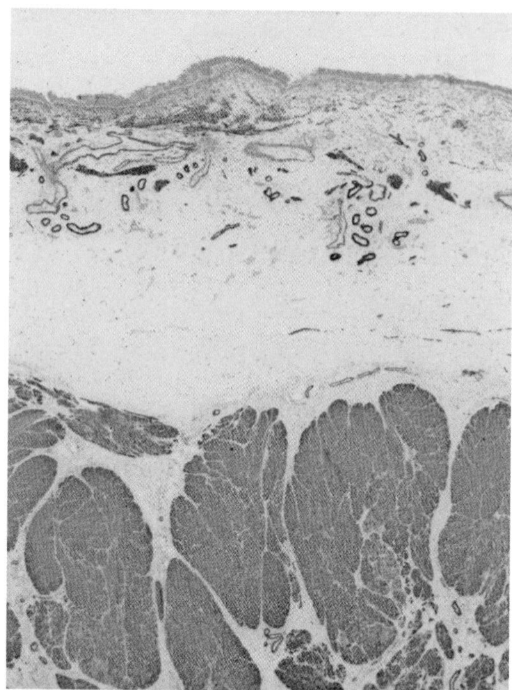

Fig. 12.1 Normal microscopic anatomy of the bladder (actin immunohistochemical stain). The urothelium rests on a lamina propria composed of connective tissue, vessels, and nerves. A few small wisps of smooth muscle are present within, near medium caliber vessels. The underlying muscularis propria is composed of thick, compact smooth muscle bundles

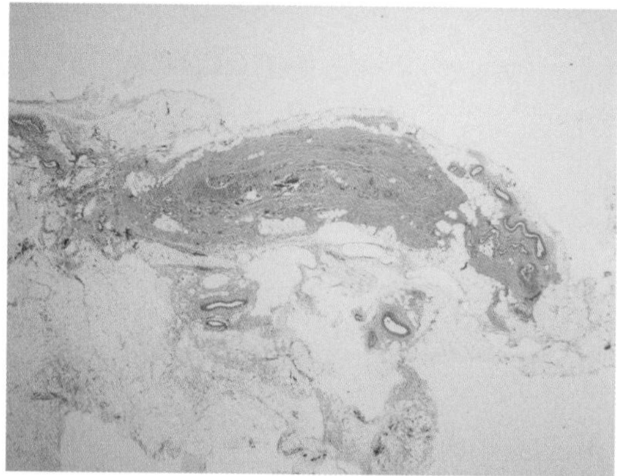

Fig. 12.2 Median umbilical ligament composed of dense fibro-connective tissue. At the time of prosecting, close examination of the bladder dome and anterior wall is required to visualize this remnant

allantois regresses completely, forming the urachus, an epithelial-lined tube which extends from the umbilicus to the apex (dome) of the bladder [3]. Before or shortly after birth, the urachus involutes, becoming a fibrous cord which is called the median umbilical ligament (Fig. 12.2); the term urachal remnant should be limited to those instances when remnants of epithelium persist within the median umbilical ligament. The epithelial lining of the urachus is urothelium, similar to that of the urinary bladder and ureter, but it frequently undergoes metaplastic change, mostly glandular.

In adults, the empty urinary bladder lies within the anteroinferior portion of the pelvis minor, inferior to the peritoneum, while in infants and children it is located partially within the abdomen, even when empty [4]. In adults, as the bladder fills it will distend and may extend into the abdomen. The bladder lies relatively free within the fibrofatty tissues of the pelvis except in the area of the bladder neck where it is firmly secured by the pubovesical ligaments in the female and the puboprostatic ligaments in the male [4, 5]. The relative freedom of the rest of the bladder allows for expansion superiorly as the organ fills with urine.

The empty bladder in an adult has the shape of a four-sided inverted pyramid and is enveloped by the vesical fascia [4]. The superior surface faces superiorly and is covered by the pelvic parietal peritoneum. The posterior surface, also known as the base of the bladder, faces posteriorly and inferiorly. It is separated from the rectum by the uterine cervix and the proximal portions of the vagina in females and by the seminal vesicles and the ampulla of the vasa deferentia in males. These posterior anatomic relationships are very important clinically. Since many bladder neoplasms arise in the posterior wall adjacent to the ureteral orifices, invasive tumor may extend into adjacent soft tissue and organs. The close anatomic relationship of organs explains why hysterectomy and partial anterior vaginectomy are commonly performed at the time of radial cystectomy in women. Similarly, perivesical soft tissue and seminal vesicle involvement is a bad prognostic marker in bladder carcinoma in males [6–8], a reflection of high pathologic stage. The latter is a rare occurrence but these patients do not appear to have a similarly bad prognosis unless prostatic stromal invasion is present. The two inferolateral surfaces of the bladder face laterally, inferiorly, and anteriorly and are in contact with the fascia of the levator ani muscles. The most anterosuperior point of the bladder is known as the apex or dome and it is located at the point of contact of the superior surfaces and the two inferolateral surfaces. It marks the point of insertion of the median umbilical ligament and consequently is the area where urachal carcinomas are located. Sometimes the insertion of the medial umbilical ligament is more towards the anterior apex.

The trigone is a complex anatomic structure located at the base of the bladder and extending to the posterior bladder neck. In the proximal and lateral aspects of the trigone, the ureters enter into the bladder (ureteral orifices) obliquely. The muscle underlying the mucosa in this region is a combination of smooth muscle of the longitudinal layer of the intramural ureter and detrusor muscle [9–13]. The intramural ureter is surrounded by a fibromuscular sheath (Waldeyer's sheath), which is fused into the ureteral muscle (Fig. 12.3). This fibromuscular tissue fans out in the area of the trigone and mixes with the detrusor muscle, thus fixing the intramural ureter to the bladder. As the bladder distends, the surrounding musculature exerts pressure on the obliquely oriented intramural ureter, producing closure of the ureteral lumen and thus avoiding reflux of urine. During micturition, there is contraction of the bladder musculature which also closes the intramural ureter. The bladder neck is the most distal portion of the bladder. It is the area where the posterior and the infero-lateral walls converge and open into the urethra (Fig. 12.4). The bladder neck is formed with contributions from the trigonal musculature (inner longitudinal ureteral muscle and Waldeyer's sheath), the detrusor musculature, and the urethral musculature [9–14]. The internal sphincter is located in this general area, with major contributions from the middle circular layer of the detrusor muscle. In the male, the bladder neck merges with the prostate gland and one may occasionally observe several prostatic ducts present in this area (Fig. 12.4).

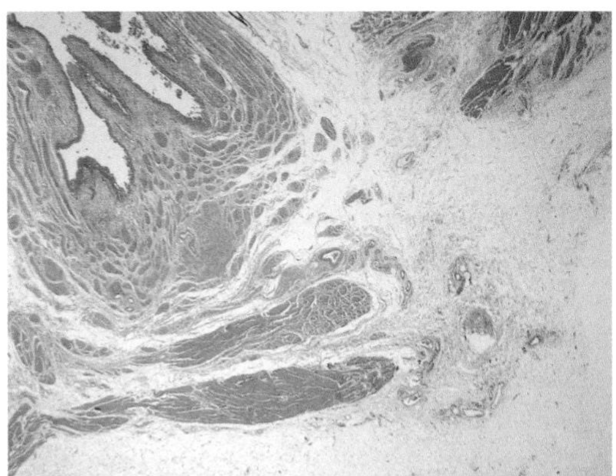

Fig. 12.3 Intramural ureter. At this site, the ureter exhibits a variable amount of lamina propria and longitudinal fibers of its own muscularis propria, which intermingle with the muscularis propria of the bladder

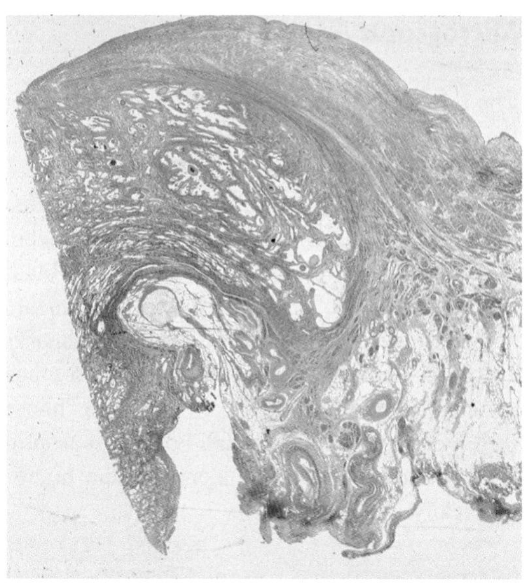

Fig. 12.4 Bladder neck. Notice displacement of muscle fibers of the muscularis propria towards the lumen of the bladder, compressing the lamina propria. There is intermingling of muscle fibers of the muscularis propria and the musculature of the prostate

The bladder bed (structures on which the bladder neck rests) is formed posteriorly by the rectum in males and vagina in females. Anteriorly and laterally it is formed by the internal obturator and levator ani muscles as well as the pubic bones. These structures may be involved in advanced tumors occupying the anterior, lateral, or bladder neck regions and render the patient inoperable except in a salvage setting, in order to relieve local symptoms.

Microscopic Anatomy

The urinary bladder, ureter, and renal pelvis for the most part have a similar anatomic composition, the innermost layer being an epithelial lining and, extending outwards, a lamina propria, smooth muscle (muscularis propria), and adventitia (Fig. 12.1). The superior surface of the bladder comes in contact with parietal peritoneum and hence has a serosa. The anatomic landmarks are used clinically and pathologically to stage patients with urothelial cancer in order to choose therapy and estimate survival. For this reason, it is important to accurately identify them microscopically.

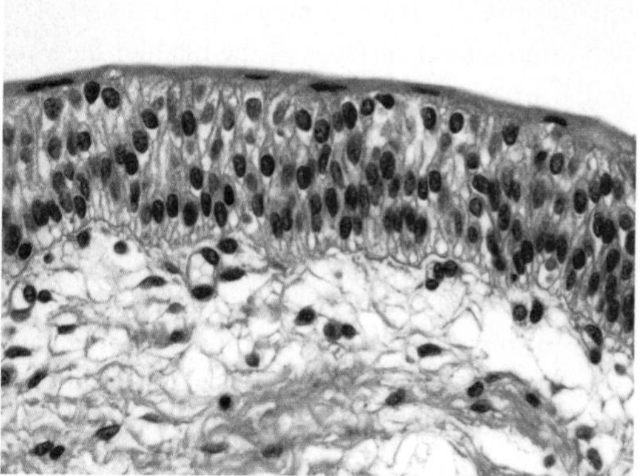

Fig. 12.5 Normal urothelium. The superficial (umbrella) cells span the luminal surface. The intermediate cell layer exhibits cells arranged perpendicular to the basement membrane, with regular nuclear contours, fine chromatin, and absent or minute nucleoli. In this section, the basal cell layer is inconspicuous but a very thin basement membrane is evident, as well as small capillaries

Urothelium

The urinary bladder is lined by urothelium, formerly referred to as "transitional mucosa." The thickness of the urothelium will vary according to the degree of distension and anatomical location; in the contracted bladder, it is usually six to seven cells thick. One can identify three regions: the superficial or "umbrella" cells which are in contact with the urinary space, the intermediate cells, and the basal cells which lie on a basement membrane [15, 16] (Fig. 12.5). In practice, the thickness of the urothelium is dependent not only on the degree of distension but also on the plane on which the tissue is cut. If the cut is tangential to the basement membrane, it is possible to generate an artificially thick mucosa. For these and other reasons, we feel that urothelial thickness is at best of marginal utility in the evaluation of urothelial neoplasms. For the most part, the diagnosis of in situ urothelial carcinoma should be based of the degree of cytologic atypia and disorder.

Superficial (umbrella) cells are large, elliptical cells which lie umbrella-like over the smaller intermediate cells [15–18]. They may be binucleated and have abundant eosinophilic cytoplasm. In a setting of chronic inflammation or intravesical therapy they can be quite atypical and hyperplastic, although the abundant eosinophilic cytoplasm remains. In the distended bladder, they become flattened and barely discernible. While the presence of these cells is taken as a sign of normalcy of the urothelium, one must be aware that they may become detached due to superficial erosion, during instrumentation or tissue processing in the prosecting area. It is possible to see umbrella cells overlying frank carcinoma so their presence or absence cannot be used as a determining factor of malignancy. Ultrastructural studies have shown the superficial urothelial cells to be quite unique, exhibiting what has been known as the "asymmetric unit membrane" (AUM) [17–21], which contains frequent invaginations. When the bladder distends, this unique feature allows for an increase in the surface area and maintenance of the structural integrity of the urothelium.

The intermediate cell layer may be up to five cells thick in the contracted bladder, where they are oriented with the long axis perpendicular to the basement membrane. The nuclei are oval and have finely stippled chromatin with absent or minute nucleoli. Longitudinal nuclear grooves are commonly present. These grooves are rarely, if ever, seen in urothelial carcinoma and certainly not in high-grade disease. Intermediate cells have ample cytoplasm which may be vacuolated. The cytoplasmic membranes are distinct and these cells are attached to each other by desmosomes. In the distended state or near an area of superficial erosion, this layer may be inconspicuous, only one cell thick and flattened. The basal layer is composed of cuboidal cells which are best seen in the contracted bladder. They lie on a thin but continuous basement membrane [22]. All normal urothelial cells may contain glycogen but only the superficial cells are occasional mucicarminophilic.

Table 12.1 Proliferative changes in the urothelium and the tumors they mimic

Benign variants	Carcinoma variants
Brunn nests	Nested variant of urothelial carcinoma
Cystitis cystica	Microcystic carcinoma
Nephrogenic adenoma	Adenocarcinoma
Cystitis glandularis with intestinal metaplasia	Enteric-type adenocarcinoma
Inverted papilloma	Urothelial carcinoma with an inverted pattern of growth

Urothelial Variants and Benign Urothelial Proliferations

While we have described the microscopic features of normal urothelium, we know there are many benign morphologic variants. Koss et al. studied 100 grossly normal bladders obtained at postmortem [23]. Of these, 93 % had either Brunn nests, cystitis cystica, or squamous metaplasia. It is important to understand this morphologic "plasticity" seen in benign urothelium since they can mimic variants of urothelial carcinoma (Table 12.1).

The most common benign urothelial variant is the formation of Brunn nests, which represent invaginations of the surface urothelium into the underlying lamina propria (Fig. 12.6a, b). In some cases, these solid nests of benign-appearing urothelium may lose continuity with the surface. If the proliferation of Brunn nests is profound, it can mimic a large nested variant of urothelial carcinoma. Brunn nests can become cystic due to accumulation of cellular debris or mucin and the term cystitis cystica has been coined to describe this phenomenon (Fig. 12.6a). The lining epithelium of these small cysts is composed of one or several layers of flattened urothelial or cuboidal epithelium. In can mimic microcystic urothelial carcinoma (Fig. 12.6b). In some cases, the epithelial lining undergoes glandular metaplasia, giving rise to what is called cystitis glandularis. The cells become cuboidal or columnar and mucin secreting; some are transformed into intestinal-type goblet cells (cystitis glandularis with intestinal metaplasia) (Fig. 12.7), and may be associated with extravasated mucin. Extreme examples can mimic mucinous adenocarcinoma. Brunn nests, cystitis cystica, and cystitis

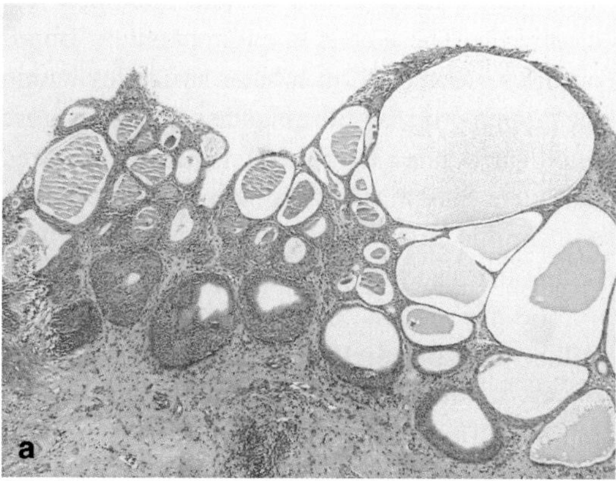

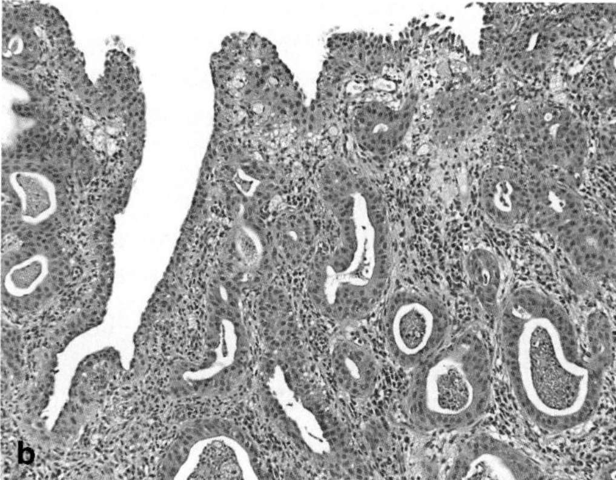

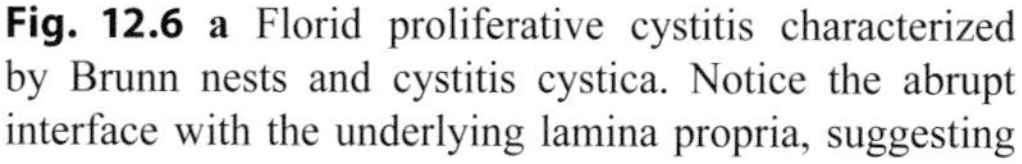

Fig. 12.6 **a** Florid proliferative cystitis characterized by Brunn nests and cystitis cystica. Notice the abrupt interface with the underlying lamina propria, suggesting circumscription. **b** Microcystic carcinoma. The nests of tumor are variable in size and shape and exhibit an infiltrative pattern

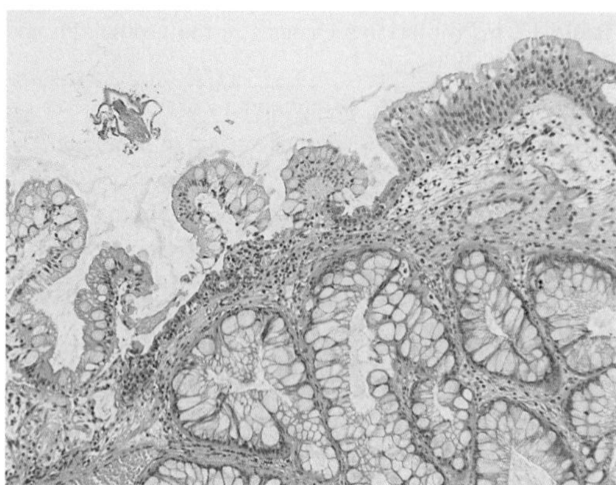

Fig. 12.7 Florid cystitis glandularis with intestinal metaplasia. Notice the transition from normal urothelium with prominent, sometimes vacuolated superficial umbrella cells to intestinal metaplasia of the surface urothelium containing cytologically banal goblet-type cells

glandularis represent a continuum of proliferative or reactive changes and it is common to see all three in the same tissue sample. Most investigators believe that they occur as a result of local inflammatory insult [23–25]. Nevertheless, these proliferative changes are seen in the urothelium of patients with no evidence of local inflammation, so that it is possible that they also represent either normal histologic variants or the residual effects of old inflammatory processes [26, 27]. The high incidence of these proliferative changes in normal bladder suggests that they are not likely to be premalignant changes and that there is no cause-and-effect relationship between their presence and the appearance of bladder cancer. It is true that one or all of these changes are commonly present in biopsy specimens containing bladder cancer, but the coexistence may be coincidental or the cancer itself may be producing the local inflammatory insult that causes them. The fact that exceptional cases may occur in which carcinoma clearly arises within the epithelium of these reactive lesions does not alter this argument [28, 29].

Metaplasia refers to a change in morphology of one cell type into another which is considered aberrant for that location. Urothelium frequently undergoes either squamous or glandular metaplasia, presumably as a response to chronic inflammatory stimuli such as urinary tract infection, calculi, diverticula, or frequent catheterization [24, 27].

Squamous epithelium in the area of the trigone is a common finding in women. It is characterized by abundant intracytoplasmic glycogen and lack of keratinization, making it histologically similar to vaginal or cervical squamous epithelium. In this particular setting, most of us believe that squamous epithelium should be regarded as a variant of urothelium rather than metaplasia. Squamous metaplasia may occur at other sites and at times may undergo keratinization and even exhibit parakeratosis and a granular layer. Squamous metaplasia is not preneoplastic per se but patients with keratinizing squamous metaplasia must be monitored closely since some may progress to squamous carcinoma [30].

Cystitis glandularis is commonly encountered in a setting of chronic inflammation or irritation and also in cases of bladder exstrophy [31, 32]. The epithelium is composed of tall columnar cells with mucin-secreting goblet cells, strikingly similar to colonic or small intestinal epithelium in which one might identify even Paneth cells. As with squamous metaplasia, glandular metaplasia is not of itself a precancerous lesion but may eventually undergo neoplastic transformation in exceptional cases [32]. Patients should be monitored accordingly.

So-called nephrogenic adenoma is a distinct lesion characterized by aggregates of cuboidal or hobnail cells with clear or eosinophilic cytoplasm and small discrete nuclei without prominent nucleoli [33]. These cells line thin papillary fronds on the surface or form tubular structures within the lamina propria of the bladder. The tubules are often surrounded by a thickened and hyalinized basement membrane. Variable numbers of acute and chronic inflammatory cells are commonplace within the bladder wall.

The histogenesis of nephrogenic adenoma is still being debated. Some believe it develops secondary to an inflammatory insult or local injury [33–37]. It was originally described in the trigone and given its name because it was thought to arise from mesonephric rests. We now know that nephrogenic adenoma may occur anywhere in the urothelial tract, although it is most common in the bladder. It is important in that it may present as an exophytic mass mimicking carcinoma grossly and suggesting adenocarcinoma microscopically. The benign histologic appearance of the cells arranged in characteristic tubules surrounded by a prominent basement membrane should provide the correct diagnosis. A very interesting publication described nephrogenic adenomas of the bladder in patients that underwent renal transplantation [38]. The authors demonstrated the nephrogenic adenomatous lesions and the donor kidneys were clonal, suggestion that they developed through a process of shedding of donor renal tubule cells followed by implantation and proliferation within the bladder. Additional support for this hypothesis is postulated by other authors who have shown immunoreactivity for Pax-2, an antigen expressed in renal tubules [39, 40]. While this is interesting, it is unlikely to be the sole mechanism by which nephrogenic adenoma develops. The true specificity of Pax expression in this setting remains to be determined since it may very well be due to differentiation rather than histogenesis.

Inverted papillomas are relatively rare lesions that may occur anywhere along the urothelial tract and may be confused clinically and pathologically with urothelial carcinoma, specifically urothelial carcinoma with an inverted pattern of growth [41, 42]. In order of decreasing frequency, they occur in the bladder, renal pelvis, ureter, urethra, and renal pelvis [43–49]. Patients usually present with hematuria. Cystoscopically, the lesions are polypoid and either sessile or pedunculated. The mucosal surface is smooth or nodular without villous or papillary fronds. Microscopically, the surface transitional epithelium is compressed but otherwise unremarkable. It is undermined by invaginated cords and nests of transitional epithelium, which occupy the lamina propria. The accumulation of these endophytic growths gives the lesion its characteristic polypoid gross appearance. The urothelial cells forming the cords are benign, exhibiting normal maturation and few mitoses. They are similar to the cells of bladder papillomas, differing only in that the epithelial cords are endophytic and consequently more closely packed. Frequently, the cells are oval or spindle shaped. Epithelial nests may become centrally cystic, dilated, and even lined by cuboidal epithelium.

These cords of transitional epithelium in the lamina propria represent invaginations, not invasion. As such, there are no fibrous reactive changes within the stroma. Although mitotic figures can be seen, they are rare, regular, and located at or near the basal layer of the epithelium. Inverted papillomas are discrete lesions and do not exhibit an infiltrative border [43, 44]. One must be careful not to confuse a nested type of urothelial carcinoma infiltrating lamina propria with an inverted papilloma.

The etiology of inverted papilloma is unclear. Most investigators feel that, similar to other proliferative lesions such as Brunn nests and cystitis cystica, they are a reactive, proliferative process secondary to a noxious insult. They are not premalignant, although in exceptional cases they have been associated with carcinoma [45–47]. Given the rarity of this association, we consider it incidental.

Lamina Propria

The lamina propria lies between the mucosal basement membrane and the muscularis propria (Fig. 12.1). It is composed of dense connective tissue containing a rich vascular network, lymphatic channels, sensory nerve endings, and a few elastic fibers [15, 19, 50]. In the deeper aspects of the lamina propria of the urinary bladder and ureter, the connective tissue is loose, allowing for the formation of thick mucosal folds when the viscus is contracted. Its thickness varies, not only with the degree of distention but also with the anatomic location. It is generally thinner in the areas of the trigone and bladder neck and thicker in the dome [51]. In fact, in patients with urinary outflow obstruction (i.e., prostatic hyperplasia) the bladder neck may contain muscularis propria directly beneath the mucosa with the lamina propria being virtually indiscernible (Fig. 12.4). Within the lamina propria lie intermediate-sized arteries and veins. Their exact location within the lamina propria may

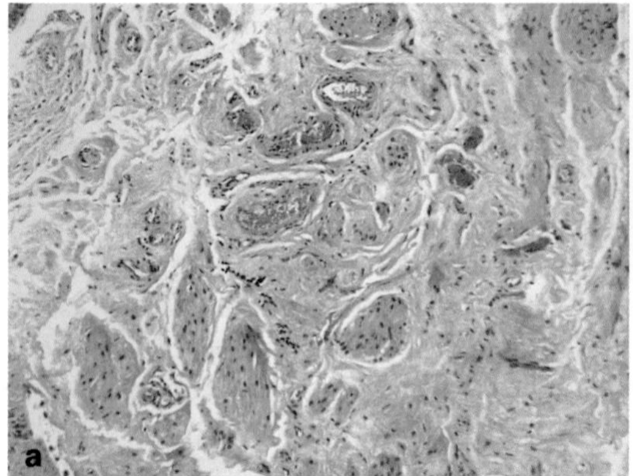

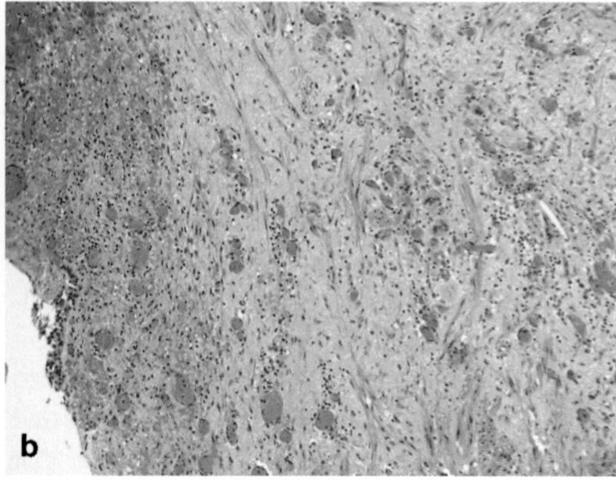

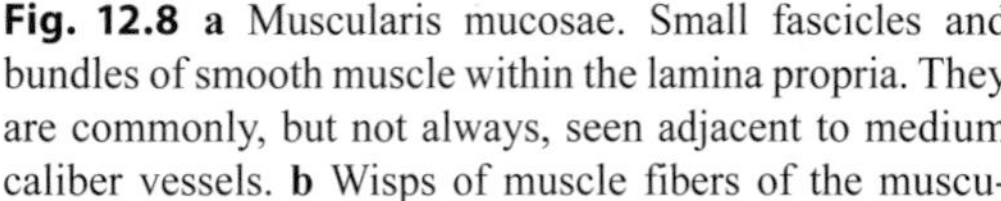

Fig. 12.8 **a** Muscularis mucosae. Small fascicles and bundles of smooth muscle within the lamina propria. They are commonly, but not always, seen adjacent to medium caliber vessels. **b** Wisps of muscle fibers of the muscularis mucosae haphazardly arranged in an area of prior biopsy. Notice how close these fibers reach to the ulcerated surface

vary but they are usually roughly in the middle. Wisps and isolated fibers of smooth muscle are commonly found in the lamina propria, usually adjacent these vessels, and have been referred to as the muscularis mucosae (Fig. 12.8a) [52, 53]. These fascicles of smooth muscle are not connected to the muscularis propria and appear as isolated muscle fibers but may form a discontinuous thin layer of muscle. Uncommonly, these muscle fibers may present as a continuous layer of muscle within the lamina propria, thus forming a true muscularis mucosae [53]. Because the clinical management of tumors that involve the muscularis propria compared to those that invade only the lamina propria is so different, a pathologist must make every effort to make this distinction on biopsies and transurethral dissections (Fig. 12.8b). In cystectomy specimens, it is also important since it places the patient into a different prognostic category. Recent studies have described "hyperplastic" muscularis mucosae, defined as muscle bundles within the lamina propria that are more than four layers in thickness, thus mimicking muscularis propria (Fig. 12.9). These bundles may be arranged haphazardly in which individual fascicles are oriented in different directions or may have a compact arrangement with smooth outlines. When markedly thickened (hyperplastic), this pattern can easily be confused with muscularis propria (Fig. 12.10) [51, 54].

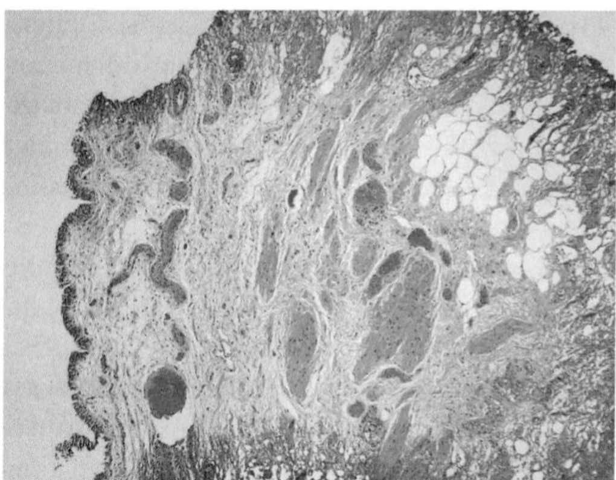

Fig. 12.9 "Hyperplastic" muscularis mucosae. The muscle fascicles and small bundles are four or more layers (fibers) in thickness. Their haphazard orientation and absence of large compact bundles allow us to identify it as muscularis mucosae

The anatomic relationship of these fibers to the overlying urothelium can be severely disrupted by inflammation, tumor-related desmoplasia, or prior therapeutic intervention, when they may be seen immediately beneath the basement membrane (Fig. 12.8b). Once again, every effort should be made to distinguish these muscle fibers of the muscularis mucosae from muscularis propria since a failure to do so will lead to errors in tumor staging and treatment. It goes without saying that a pathologist should not sign out a biopsy as "urothelial carcinoma invading muscle"

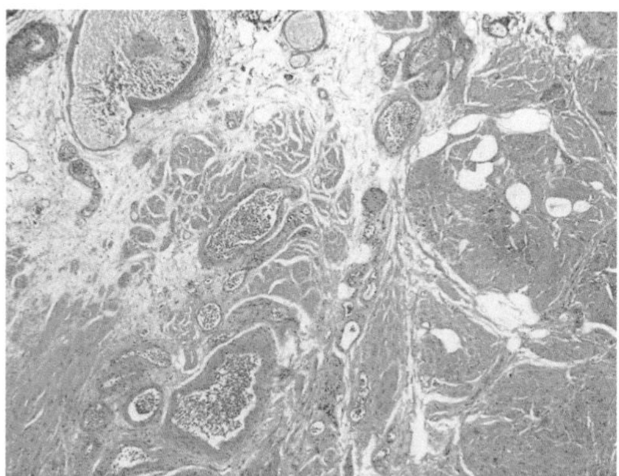

Fig. 12.10 Interface between "hyperplastic" muscularis mucosae and muscularis propria. Notice the large compact bundles that characterize the muscularis propria *(right)*, compared to the haphazard arrangement seen in the muscularis mucosae *(left)*

because this phrase lacks critical information as to the depth of invasion, specifically what level of the bladder wall is involved by tumor.

Recent reports have evaluated the ability of an antibody directed to smoothelin, a smooth muscle-specific contractile protein, in differentiating smooth muscle of the lamina propria from muscularis propria. In theory, this protein is expressed in contractile smooth muscle (muscularis propria) but not the fascicles of the muscularis mucosae. At this point, its utility remains controversial since some authors find it to be very useful while others do not [55, 56]. Occasionally, one may encounter fat within the lamina propria and muscularis [51, 57]. Its presence on a biopsy or transurethral resection should not be interpreted by pathologists as evidence of perivesical fat.

Pathologists are surprised to learn that, in terms of prognosis and treatment, urologists and urologic oncologists in the recent past grouped noninvasive (Ta) and superficially invasive (T1) tumors into a single category. It is our opinion that this is due greatly to the fact that we as pathologists had trouble agreeing as to what constitutes lamina propria invasion. There are many cases of pT1 disease which are unequivocal but there is an equal number of cases in which invasion is, at best, questionable. Pathologist's interpretation in the latter group has been inconsistent and not

Table 12.2 Useful criteria to determine the presence of superficial invasion of the lamina propria

Morphologic feature	Explanation
Arrangement of neoplastic cells	Isolated cells or nests of tumor cells that are variable in size and shape
Absence of capillaries along the basement membrane	No visible capillaries surround the invasive tumor nests
Stromal reaction	A stromal reaction (inflammatory, fibrous, or myxoid) different than what is seen in areas of the lamina propria where there is no suggestion of invasion
Presence of retraction artifact	Cells retract from adjacent stroma, mimicking vascular invasion, or micropapillary carcinoma
Paradoxical differentiation	Tumor cells appear to have more voluminous cytoplasm than the adjacent, noninvasive component

Not all features may be present in any given case. The greater number of features present, the greater the confidence in establishing a diagnosis of superficial invasion

reproducible. While this confusion is partly due to the lack of orientation of transurethral biopsy specimens and disruption of the normal histologic architecture by tumor or prior therapy, it is clear that better parameters are needed to make this distinction. In general, there are five histologic criteria that we have found to be of utility in identifying superficially invasive disease (Table 12.2) [2]. These include the arrangement of the neoplastic cells, the presence of capillaries surrounding the tumor cells, assessment of a stromal reaction, and the presence of retraction artifact and paradoxical differentiation.

There has been great interest in histologic substaging of the lamina propria (superficial and deep) in order to better stratify patient into more precise clinical risk groups [58–61]. I have no doubt that in the future this will be the case but at this moment there is no agreement on how to do it in a reproducible manner and substaging of the lamina propria is not advocated by the present AJCC-UICC classification of bladder cancer nor the College of American Pathologists, although pathologists are encouraged to mention whether lamina propria invasion is "superficial" or "deep" [62, 63]. Some investigators have suggested measuring the distance from the nearest intact basement membrane to the deepest point of invasion whereas others have suggested using the medium caliber vessels of the muscularis mucosae present within the lamina propria as accurate ways to substage these tumors. Some studies have shown a good correlation with disease recurrence and progression. However, none of these studies have been validated across multiple institutions. Given the lack of orientation of cystoscopic samples and the host of confounding factors mentioned above, arriving at consensus on the issue will remain a challenge for some time.

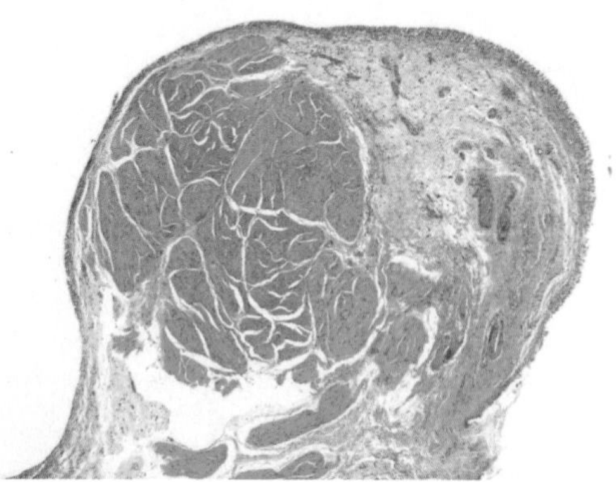

Fig. 12.11 Cold cup biopsy of the bladder containing muscularis propria. The large and compact nature of the smooth muscle bundle defines it as muscularis propria rather than hyperplastic muscularis mucosae

Muscularis Propria

The muscularis propria is said to be composed of three smooth muscle coats, inner and outer longitudinal layers, and a central circular layer. In fact, these layers can only be identified consistently in the area of the bladder neck. In other areas, the longitudinal and circular layers mix freely and have no definite orientation. In the contracted bladder, the muscle fibers are arranged in relatively coarse bundles, which are separated from each other by moderate to abundant connective tissue containing blood vessels, lymphatics, and nerves. Mature adipose tissue may also be present. Muscularis propria may be present even in small cold cup biopsy specimens, and can be identified by the size of the muscle bundle and its compact appearance (Fig. 12.11). Similar to other layers, the thickness of the muscularis propria will vary from patient to patient. Jequier et al. [64] performed sonographic measurements of the bladder wall thickness in 410 urologically normal children and 10 adults. They found that the bladder wall thickness varied mostly with the state of bladder filling and only minimally with age and gender. The bladder wall had a mean thickness of 2.76 mm when empty and 1.55 mm when distended.

For staging purposes, the muscularis propria has been divided into two segments, superficial and deep (T2a and T2b, respectively) [62]. No anatomical landmarks can be used to make this distinction so that it must be done by direct visualization on the light microscope of the full thickness of the bladder. Substaging of the muscularis propria can only be done at the time of cystectomy, never on transurethral resection or biopsy. Importantly, prior transurethral resection will alter the anatomy of the site and mask normal landmarks, making proper staging difficult, if not impossible (Fig. 12.12a, b). In addition, some invasive urothelial carcinomas are associated with extensive stromal desmoplasia in which case establishing the depth of invasion is equally difficult.

Perivesical soft tissue involvement is considered pathologic stage pT3 and is defined as perivesical fat invasion beyond the level of muscularis propria. As previously mentioned, this can only be established at the time of cystectomy. Although this categorization seems to be straightforward, it is anything but simple (Fig. 12.13). The boundary between the muscularis propria and perivesical tissue may be poorly defined due to inherent and anatomic reasons or may exhibit post therapy (biopsy, radiation therapy of chemotherapy) changes, tumor-related stromal desmoplasia, and inflammation. A study by Ananthanarayanan et al. [65] demonstrated a significant level of interobserver variability

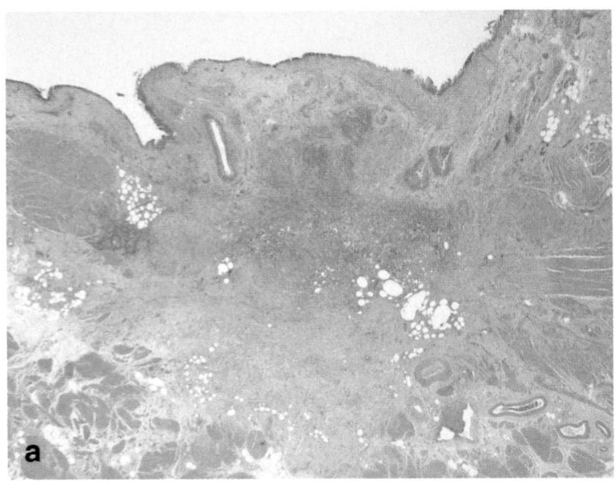

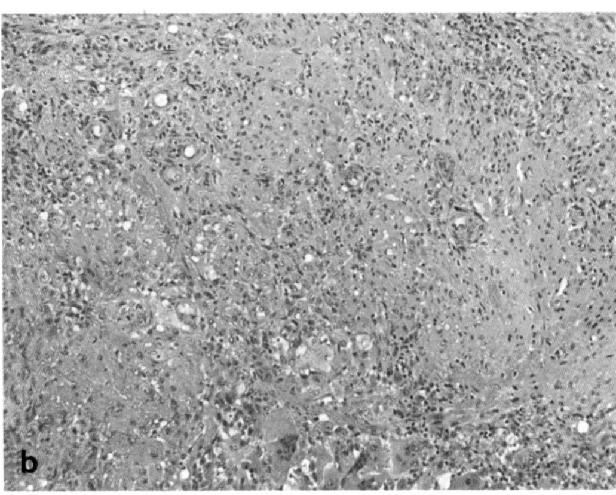

Fig. 12.12 **a** Biopsy site change seen at the time of cystectomy. Notice that the area of fibrosis goes beyond the superficial layer of the muscularis propria with intact muscularis propria seen lateral and deep to the biopsy site where the anatomic landmarks are entirely obscured. **b** Higher-power view of the biopsy site compose of fibrosis, inflammation, and foreign body reaction. If tumor cells were seen within this area, it would be impossible to establish the depth of invasion

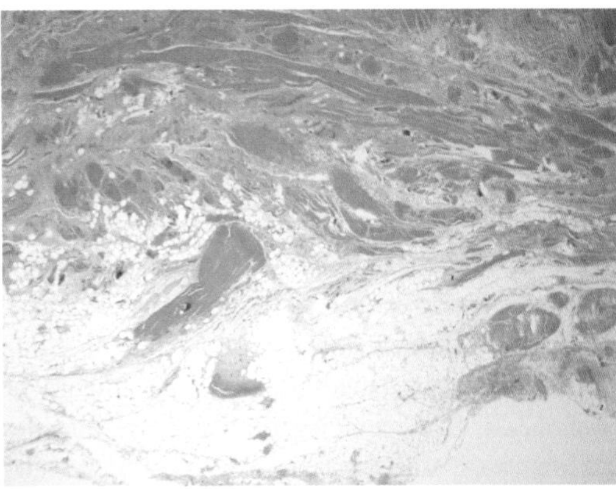

Fig. 12.13 Interface between muscularis propria and perivesical soft tissue. Notice the irregular contour of this interface which makes establishing early pT3 invasion challenging

among expert urologic pathologists in assessing perivesical involvement by tumor in equivocal cases. The study also highlighted the fact that tumor emboli within lymphovascular spaces should not be used to establish the presence of muscularis propria or perivesical soft tissue involvement.

Invasion into adjacent organs is considered pT4 [66]. Examples include extension into prostatic stroma, uterine or vaginal wall, bowel, and pubic bone. Involvement of the surface urothelium of the urethra or ureter does not constitute pT4 disease although it places the patient at a higher risk of recurrence.

Bladder Diverticula

Bladder diverticula are relatively common, yet their etiology remains controversial. Most investigators agree that they develop secondary to increased intravesical pressure as a result of obstruction distal to the diverticulum [67–69]. The obstruction brings about compensatory muscle hypertrophy and eventual mucosal herniation in areas of weakness. Others feel that at least some diverticula are a consequence of congenital defects in the bladder musculature, citing as evidence cases of diverticula in young patients without evidence of obstruction [69, 70]. The most common sites of diverticula are (a) adjacent to the ureteral orifices, (b) the bladder dome, and (c) the region of the internal urethral orifice. Grossly, one sees distortion of the external surface of the bladder. The diverticula may be widely patent but are usually narrow in symptomatic patients. The mucosa adjoining the diverticulum is usually hyperemic or ulcerated. There may be epithelial

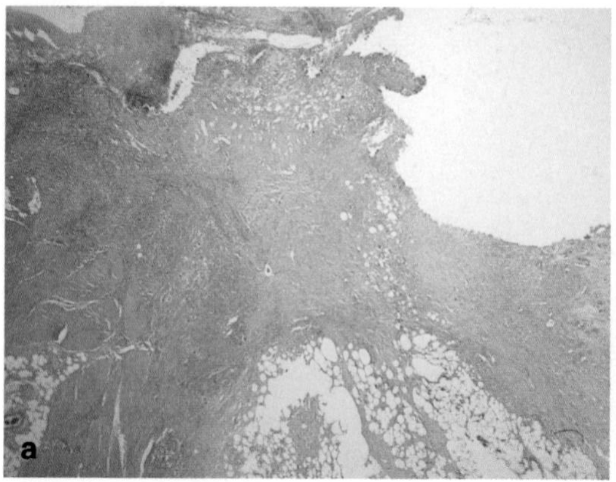

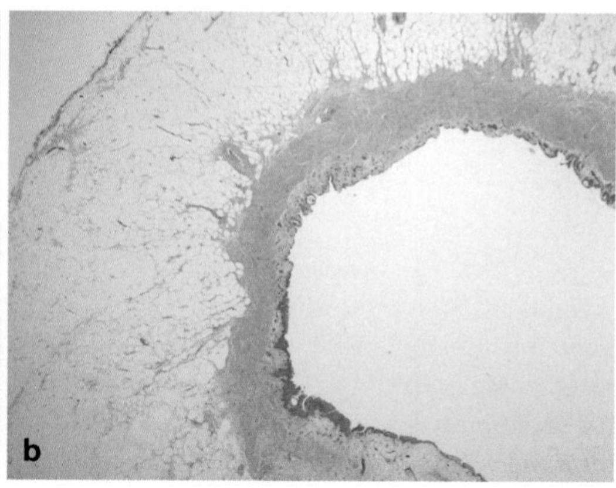

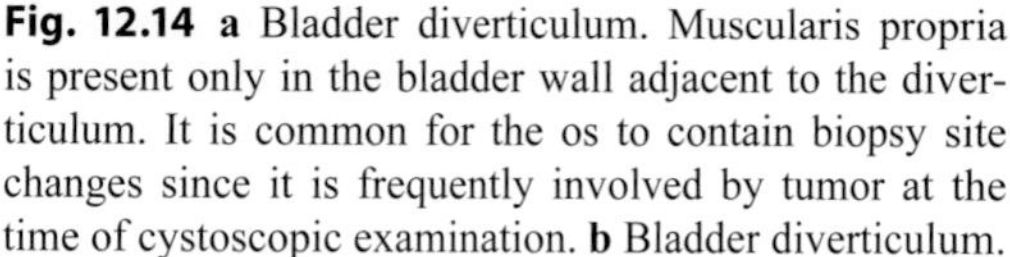

Fig. 12.14 **a** Bladder diverticulum. Muscularis propria is present only in the bladder wall adjacent to the diverticulum. It is common for the os to contain biopsy site changes since it is frequently involved by tumor at the time of cystoscopic examination. **b** Bladder diverticulum. The wall is composed of lamina propria containing a hyperplastic, longitudinally arranged muscularis mucosae, surrounded by peridiverticular soft tissue. No muscularis propria is present

hyperplasia. Very commonly, there is inflammation involving the lamina propria. The wall of the diverticulum itself consists of urothelium and underlying connective tissue, specifically lamina propria. By definition, there is no muscularis propria in an acquired bladder diverticulum although muscularis propria of the bladder is present immediately adjacent to the os (Fig. 12.14a). The lamina propria may contain muscularis mucosae that is commonly thickened and hyperplastic (Fig. 12.14b). It rarely forms tight muscle bundles but rather appears as longitudinally arranged smooth muscle fascicles. This fact has direct implications on the staging of tumors arising in diverticula. Tumors can be either noninvasive (pTa or CIS), pT3 or pT4; there is no such thing as pT2 disease unless the tumor invades the muscularis propria of the bladder wall adjacent to the diverticulum (Fig. 12.14a). The rarely encountered true "congenital" diverticulum contains a thinned outer muscle layer.

Urachal Remnant

The anatomy of a urachal remnant will depend on its location. Since the median umbilical ligament stretches from the umbilicus to the bladder dome, urachal remnants can be encountered along its entire length. The epithelial remnant will be surrounded be a fibrous wall, the composition of the median umbilical ligament (Fig. 12.2). If the urachal remnant is within the bladder wall, this fibrous covering will be surrounded by either lamina propria or muscularis propria. If the remnant is in the apical perivesical soft tissue, it will be surrounded by fibroadipose tissue while if it arises more proximally, it will be surrounded by soft tissue of the anterior abdominal wall (Fig. 12.15a, b). It goes without saying that pathologic staging of tumors arising within a urachal remnant must be staged according to its specific anatomical location [71–73].

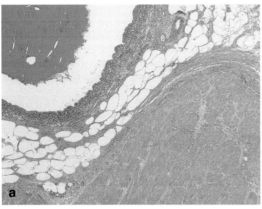

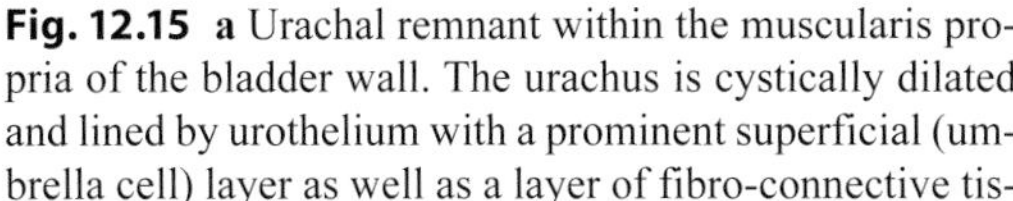

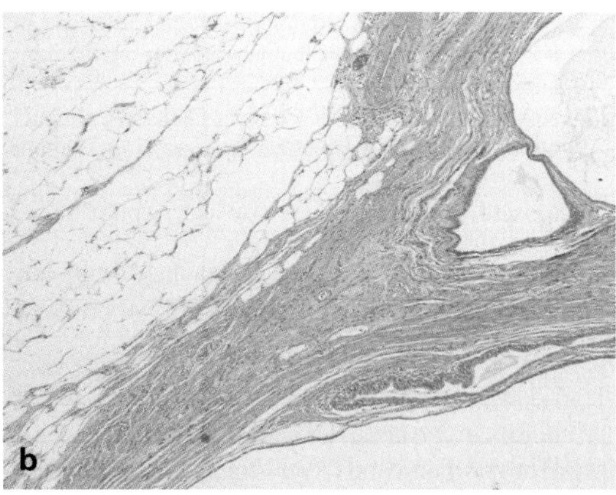

Fig. 12.15 **a** Urachal remnant within the muscularis propria of the bladder wall. The urachus is cystically dilated and lined by urothelium with a prominent superficial (umbrella cell) layer as well as a layer of fibro-connective tissue, the latter being a component of the medial umbilical ligament. **b** Extravesical urachal remnant. Epithelial remnants are present within the medial umbilical ligament, surrounded by perivesical fat

References

1. Reuter VE. Histology for pathologists. 2nd ed. Sternberg SS, editor. New York: Raven Press; 1998. pp. 835–47.
2. Reuter VE. The urothelial tract: renal pelvis, ureter, urinary bladder, and urethra. In: Reuter VE, editor. Sternberg's diagnostic surgical pathology. 2. 4th ed. Philadelphia: Lippincott Williams & Wilkins; 2004. pp. 2035–81.
3. Moore K. The urinary system. In: Moore K, editor. The developing human. 3rd ed. Philadelphia: WB Saunders; 1982. pp. 267–8.
4. Moore KL. The pelvis and perineum. In: Moore KL, editor. Clinically oriented anatomy. 2nd ed. Baltimore: Williams & Wilkens; 1985. pp. 362–5.
5. Tanagho E. Campbell's urology. In: Walsh PC RA, Stamey TA, editors. Anatomy of the lower urinary tract. 6 ed. Philadelphia: WB Saunders; 1992. pp. 49–54.
6. Mahadevia PS, Koss LG, Tar IJ. Prostatic involvement in bladder cancer. Prostate mapping in 20 cystoprostatectomy specimens. Cancer. 1986;58(9):2096–102.
7. Utz DC, Farrow GM, Rife CC, Segura JW, Zincke H. Carcinoma in situ of the bladder. Cancer. 1980;45(7 Suppl):1842–8.
8. Ro JY, Ayala AG, el-Naggar A, Wishnow KI. Seminal vesicle involvement by in situ and invasive transitional cell carcinoma of the bladder. Am J Surg Pathol. 1987;11(12):951–8.
9. Tanagho EA, Smith DR, Meyers FH. The trigone: anatomical and physiological considerations. 2. In relation to the bladder neck. J Urol. 1968;100(5): 633–9.
10. Tanagho EA, Meyers FH, Smith DR. The trigone: anatomical and physiological considerations. I. In relation to the ureterovesical junction. J Urol. 1968;100(5):623–32.
11. Shehata R. A comparative study of the urinary bladder and the intramural portion of the ureter. Acta Anat (Basel). 1977;98(4):380–95.
12. Politano VA. Ureterovesical junction. J Urol. 1972;107(2):239–42.
13. Elbadawi A. Anatomy and function of the ureteral sheath. J Urol. 1972;107(2):224–9.
14. Tanagho EA, Smith DR. The anatomy and function of the bladder neck. Br J Urol. 1966;38(1):54–71.
15. Koss LG. Tumors of the urinary bladder. Fascicle 11. Washington, DC: Armed Forces Institute of Pathology; 1975. pp. 99–102.
16. Fawcett DW. Bloom and Fawcett: a textbook of histology. 11th ed. Philadelphia: WB Saunders; 1986. pp. 787–90.
17. Hicks RM. The function of the golgi complex in transitional epithelium. Synthesis of the thick cell membrane. J Cell Biol. 1966;30(3):623–43.
18. Battifora H, Eisenstein R, McDonald JH. The human urinary bladder mucosa. An electron microscopic study. Invest Urol. 1964;12:354–61.
19. Fawcett DW, Bloom W, Raviola E. A textbook of histology. 12th ed. New York: Chapman & Hall; 1994. pp. xx, 964.
20. Koss LG. The asymmetric unit membranes of the epithelium of the urinary bladder of the rat. An electron microscopic study of a mechanism of epithelial maturation and function. Lab Invest. 1969;21(2):154–68.
21. Newman J, Antonakopoulos GN. The fine structure of the human fetal urinary bladder. Development and maturation. A light, transmission and scanning electron microscopic study. J Anat. 1989;166:135–50.

22. Alroy J, Gould VE. Epithelial-stromal interface in normal and neoplastic human bladder epithelium. Ultrastruct Pathol. 1980;1(2):201–10.
23. Koss LG. Mapping of the urinary bladder: its impact on the concepts of bladder cancer. Hum Pathol. 1979;10(5):533–48.
24. Mostofi FK. Potentialities of bladder epithelium. J Urol. 1954;71:705–14.
25. Morse HD. The etiology and pathology of pyelitis cystica, ureteritis cystica and cystitis cystica. Am J Pathol. 1928;4:33–50.
26. Goldstein AM, Fauer RB, Chinn M, Kaempf MJ. New concepts on formation of Brunn's nests and cysts in urinary tract mucosa. Urology. 1978;11(5):513–7.
27. Wiener DP, Koss LG, Sablay B, Freed SZ. The prevalence and significance of Brunn's nests, cystitis cystica and squamous metaplasia in normal bladders. J Urol. 1979;122(3):317–21.
28. Edwards PD, Hurm RA, Jaeschke WH. Conversion of cystitis glandularis to adenocarcinoma. J Urol. 1972;108(4):568–70.
29. Lin JI, Yong HS, Tseng CH, Marsidi PS, Choy C, Pilloff B. Diffuse cystitis glandularis. Associated with adenocarcinomatous change. Urology. 1980;15(4):411–5.
30. Tannenbaum M. Inflammatory proliferative lesion of urinary bladder: squamous metaplasia. Urology. 1976;7(4):428–9.
31. Engel RM, Wilkinson HA. Bladder exstrophy. J Urol. 1970;104(5):699–704.
32. Nielsen K, Nielsen KK. Adenocarcinoma in exstrophy of the bladder—the last case in Scandinavia? A case report and review of literature. J Urol. 1983;130(6):1180–2.
33. Bhagavan BS, Tiamson EM, Wenk RE, Berger BW, Hamamoto G, Eggleston JC. Nephrogenic adenoma of the urinary bladder and urethra. Hum Pathol. 1981;12(10):907–16.
34. Navarre RJ Jr, Loening SA, Platz C, Narayana A, Culp DA. Nephrogenic adenoma: a report of 9 cases and review of the literature. J Urol. 1982;127(4):775–9.
35. Molland EA, Trott PA, Paris AM, Blandy JP. Nephrogenic adenoma: a form of adenomatous metaplasia of the bladder. A clinical and electron microscopical study. Br J Urol. 1976;48(6):453–62.
36. Ford TF, Watson GM, Cameron KM. Adenomatous metaplasia (nephrogenic adenoma) of urothelium. An analysis of 70 cases. Br J Urol. 1985;57(4):427–33.
37. Satodate R, Koike H, Sasou S, Ohori T, Nagane Y. Nephrogenic adenoma of the ureter. J Urol. 1984;131(2):332–4.
38. Mazal PR, Schaufler R, Altenhuber-Muller R, Haitel A, Watschinger B, Kratzik C, et al. Derivation of nephrogenic adenomas from renal tubular cells in kidney-transplant recipients. N Engl J Med. 2002;347(9):653–9.
39. Fromont G, Barcat L, Gaudin J, Irani J. Revisiting the immunophenotype of nephrogenic adenoma. Am J Surg Pathol. 2009;33(11):1654–8.
40. Tong GX, Melamed J, Mansukhani M, Memeo L, Hernandez O, Deng FM, et al. PAX2: a reliable marker for nephrogenic adenoma. Mod Pathol. 2006;19(3):356–63.
41. DeMeester LJ, Farrow GM, Utz DC. Inverted papillomas of the urinary bladder. Cancer. 1975;36(2):505–13.
42. Henderson DW, Allen PW, Bourne AJ. Inverted urinary papilloma: report of five cases and review of the literature. Virchows Arch A Pathol Anat Histol. 1975;366(3):177–86.
43. Caro DJ, Tessler A. Inverted papilloma of the bladder: a distinct urological lesion. Cancer. 1978;42(2):708–13.
44. Anderstrom C, Johansson S, Pettersson S. Inverted papilloma of the urinary tract. J Urol. 1982;127(6):1132–4.
45. Lazarevic B, Garret R. Inverted papilloma and papillary transitional cell carcinoma of urinary bladder: report of four cases of inverted papilloma, one showing papillary malignant transformation and review of the literature. Cancer. 1978;42(4):1904–11.
46. Whitesel JA. Inverted papilloma of the urinary tract: malignant potential. J Urol. 1982;127(3):539–40.
47. Stein BS, Rosen S, Kendall AR. The association of inverted papilloma and transitional cell carcinoma of the urothelium. J Urol. 1984;131(4):751–2.
48. Assor D. Inverted papilloma of the renal pelvis. J Urol. 1976;116(5):654.
49. Lausten GS, Anagnostaki L, Thomsen OF. Inverted papilloma of the upper urinary tract. Eur Urol. 1984;10(1):67–70.
50. Weiss L. Cell and tissue biology: a textbook of histology. 6th ed. Baltimore: Urban & Schwarzenberg; 1988. pp. xii, 1158, [16] of plates p.
51. Paner GP, Ro JY, Wojcik EM, Venkataraman G, Datta MW, Amin MB. Further characterization of the muscle layers and lamina propria of the urinary bladder by systematic histologic mapping: implications for pathologic staging of invasive urothelial carcinoma. Am J Surg Pathol. 2007;31(9):1420–9.
52. Dixon JS, Gosling JA. Histology and fine structure of the muscularis mucosae of the human urinary bladder. J Anat. 1983;136(2):265–71.
53. Ro JY, Ayala AG, el-Naggar A. Muscularis mucosa of urinary bladder. Importance for staging and treatment. Am J Surg Pathol. 1987;11(9):668–73.
54. Vakar-Lopez F, Shen SS, Zhang S, Tamboli P, Ayala AG, Ro JY. Muscularis mucosae of the urinary bladder revisited with emphasis on its hyperplastic patterns: a study of a large series of cystectomy specimens. Ann Diagn Pathol. 2007;11(6):395–401.
55. Paner GP, Shen SS, Lapetino S, Venkataraman G, Barkan GA, Quek ML, et al. Diagnostic utility of antibody to smoothelin in the distinction of muscularis propria from muscularis mucosae of the urinary bladder: a potential ancillary tool in the pathologic staging of invasive urothelial carcinoma. Am J Surg Pathol. 2009;33(1):91–8.

56. Miyamoto H, Sharma RB, Illei PB, Epstein JI. Pitfalls in the use of smoothelin to identify muscularis propria invasion by urothelial carcinoma. Am J Surg Pathol. 2010;34(3):418–22.
57. Philip AT, Amin MB, Tamboli P, Lee TJ, Hill CE, Ro JY. Intravesical adipose tissue: a quantitative study of its presence and location with implications for therapy and prognosis. Am J Surg Pathol. 2000;24(9):1286–90.
58. Hasui Y, Osada Y, Kitada S, Nishi S. Significance of invasion to the muscularis mucosae on the progression of superficial bladder cancer. Urology. 1994;43(6):782–6.
59. Angulo JC, Lopez JI, Grignon DJ, Sanchez-Chapado M. Muscularis mucosa differentiates two populations with different prognosis in stage T1 bladder cancer. Urology. 1995;45(1):47–53.
60. Nishiyama N, Kitamura H, Maeda T, Takahashi S, Masumori N, Hasegawa T, et al. Clinicopathological analysis of patients with non-muscle-invasive bladder cancer: prognostic value and clinical reliability of the 2004 WHO classification system. Jpn J Clin Oncol. 2013;43(11):1124–31.
61. Hu Z, Mudaliar K, Quek ML, Paner GP, Barkan GA. Measuring the dimension of invasive component in pT1 urothelial carcinoma in transurethral resection specimens can predict time to recurrence. Ann Diagn Pathol 2014;18(2):49–52.
62. Al-Hussain T, Carter HB, Epstein JI. Significance of prostate adenocarcinoma perineural invasion on biopsy in patients who are otherwise candidates for active surveillance. J Urol. 2011;186(2):470–3.
63. Eble JN, Sauter G, Epstein J, Sesterhenn I, editors. Pathology and genetics of tumours of the urinary system and male genital organs. Lyon: IARC press; 2004.
64. Jequier S, Rousseau O. Sonographic measurements of the normal bladder wall in children. AJR Am J Roentgenol. 1987;149(3):563–6.
65. Ananthanarayanan V, Pan Y, Tretiakova M, Amin MB, Cheng L, Epstein JI, et al. Influence of histologic criteria and confounding factors in staging equivocal cases for microscopic perivesical tissue invasion (pT3a): an interobserver study among genitourinary pathologists. Am J Surg Pathol. 2014;38(2):167–75.
66. Edge SB, Compton CC. The American joint committee on cancer: the 7th edition of the AJCC cancer staging manual and the future of TNM. Ann Surg Oncol. 2010;17(6):1471–4.
67. Miller A. The aetiology and treatment of diverticulum of the bladder. Br J Urol. 1958;30:43–56.
68. Kertsschmer HL. Diverticula of the urinary bladder: a clinical study of 236 cases. Surg Gynecol Obstet. 1940;71:491–503.
69. Fox M, Power RF, Bruce AW. Diverticulum of the bladder: presentation and evaluation of treatment of 115 cases. Br J Urol. 1962;34:286–98.
70. Barrett DM, Malek RS, Kelalis PP. Observations on vesical diverticulum in childhood. J Urol. 1976;116(2):234–6.
71. Sheldon CA, Clayman RV, Gonzalez R, Williams RD, Fraley EE. Malignant urachal lesions. J Urol. 1984;131(1):1–8.
72. Gopalan A, Sharp DS, Fine SW, Tickoo SK, Herr HW, Reuter VE, et al. Urachal carcinoma: a clinicopathologic analysis of 24 cases with outcome correlation. Am J Surg Pathol. 2009;33(5):659–68.
73. Kong MX, Zhao X, Kheterpal E, Lee P, Taneja S, Lepor H, et al. Histopathologic and clinical features of vesical diverticula. Urology. 2013;82(1):142–7.

Classification and Histologic Grading of Urothelial Neoplasms by the WHO 2004 (ISUP 1998) Criteria

13

Jesse K. McKenney

Introduction

Numerous histologic grading or classification systems have been applied to urothelial neoplasms, but the World Health Organization (WHO) 2004/ International Society of Urological Pathology (ISUP) system [1] is now widely accepted by pathologists and by both the American Urological Association and the American Joint Committee on Cancer [2]. This system was originally proposed in 1998 by the ISUP consensus committee [3] and subsequently adopted by the WHO in 2004 [1]. It replaced the WHO 1973 classification system [4], which was the most widely utilized system prior to 1998. This chapter addresses the current WHO/ISUP histologic criteria for the grading/classification of both papillary urothelial neoplasia and flat urothelial lesions with atypia.

Flat Urothelial Lesions with Atypia

Reactive Urothelial Atypia

Reactive urothelial atypia most often occurs in a background of acute and chronic inflammation associated with infection, urinary calculi, indwelling catheters, or prior intravesical therapy. The associated inflammatory cells are commonly intraurothelial, but may also involve the lamina propria. Typically, the individual urothelial cells have uniform nucleomegaly with evenly distributed, fine nuclear chromatin (Fig. 13.1a, b). The nuclear enlargement is typically less than three times the size of a lymphocyte, and the nuclei maintain a rather monomorphic appearance with regard to size and shape. Prominent pinpoint nucleoli, or multiple small nucleoli, are also common. The cytoplasm of the reactive cells may have a slightly more basophilic appearance than seen in normal urothelium. Mitotic activity may be easily identified, and may extend into the upper layers of the urothelium; however, atypical mitotic figures are not seen. Reactive atypia is typically most severe in the setting of an indwelling catheter or acute calculi. Distinguishing features for benign reactive changes and urothelial carcinoma in situ are summarized in Table 13.1.

Urothelial Atypia of Uncertain Significance

Atypia of uncertain significance is a descriptive diagnostic term that is utilized for flat urothelial atypias that are difficult to classify as definitively reactive or neoplastic. Most commonly, this diagnosis is made when the "severity of the atypia appears out of proportion to the extent of inflammation such that dysplasia cannot be confidently excluded" [1]. The general recommendation for patients diagnosed with urothelial atypias of this indeterminate type is close clinical follow-up care, typically with at least continued urine cytology screening.

J. K. McKenney (✉)
Department of Pathology, Cleveland Clinic, Robert J. Tomsich Pathology and Laboratory Medicine Institute, Cleveland, OH, USA
e-mail: mckennj@ccf.org

C. Magi-Galluzzi, C. G. Przybycin (eds.), *Genitourinary Pathology,* DOI 10.1007/978-1-4939-2044-0_13,

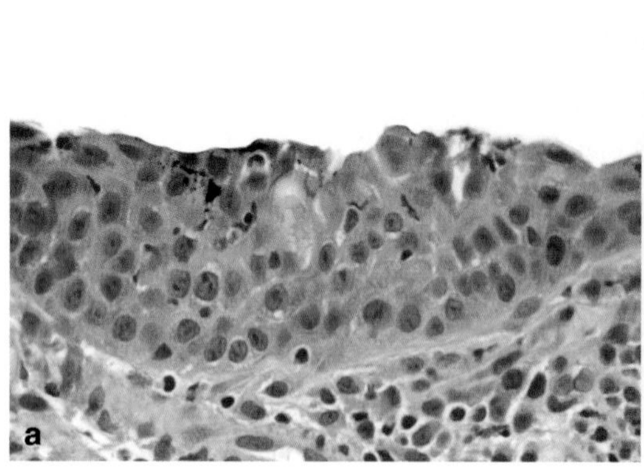

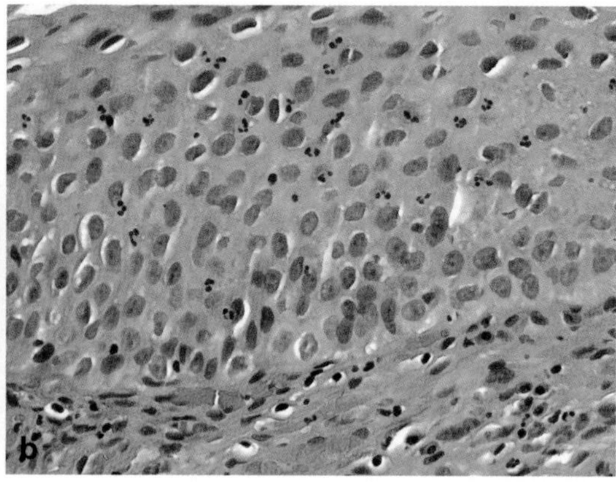

Fig. 13.1 Reactive urothelial atypia (H&E). **a** and **b** Reactive urothelial atypia is characterized by mild nuclear enlargement with fine, evenly distributed nuclear chromatin and small pinpoint nucleoli. Intraurothelial inflammatory cells are common

Table 13.1 Distinguishing features for benign reactive changes and urothelial carcinoma in situ

Histologic features	Reactive atypia	CIS
Nucleomegaly	Typically less than 3 × size of lymphocyte	Often greater than 4 × size of lymphocyte
Nucleoli	Often prominent, but small (pinpoint)	Variable
Chromatin	Fine, evenly distributed	Variable clumping, coarseness
Nuclear membrane	Smooth, round	Irregular
Apoptotic debris	Not typical	May be prominent
Mitotic activity	May be increased (not atypical)	May be increased (with atypical forms)
Cytoplasm	Often basophilic	Often eosinophilic
Nuclear crowding	Not typical	Often present
Intraurothelial inflammation	Typical	Not common

Urothelial Dysplasia (Low-Grade Intraurothelial Neoplasia)

Urothelial dysplasia has been a controversial category because of a lack of easily reproducible criteria for diagnosis [5, 6]. The original ISUP 1998 criteria defined urothelial dysplasia as urothelium with "appreciable cytologic and architectural changes felt to be preneoplastic, yet falling short of the diagnostic threshold for transitional cell carcinoma in situ" [3]. Lesions diagnosed as dysplasia often show a degree of nuclear enlargement that overlaps with reactive atypia, but the loss of cellular polarity is typically more prominent. In addition, although mild, the nuclear chromatin is more hyperchromatic (Fig. 13.2). Nuclear pleomorphism and/or brisk mitotic activity would suggest the diagnosis of urothelial carcinoma in situ over dysplasia. The potential for the over-diagnosis of urothelial dysplasia is significant due to the degree of histologic overlap with benign nonneoplastic urothelial atypias; therefore, the diagnosis of de novo urothelial dysplasia (i.e., with no prior history of urothelial carcinoma) should be made only with great caution.

The clinical significance of urothelial dysplasia is not fully known, mainly due to problems with varying diagnostic thresholds being utilized in different studies. Because of these problems, some genitourinary pathologists combine the groups of urothelial dysplasia and urothelial atypia of uncertain significance for reporting purposes. Using this diagnostic approach that combines the two categories, the flat atypias would be reported as urothelial atypia of uncertain significance with a comment regarding the inability to exclude a neoplastic process and a

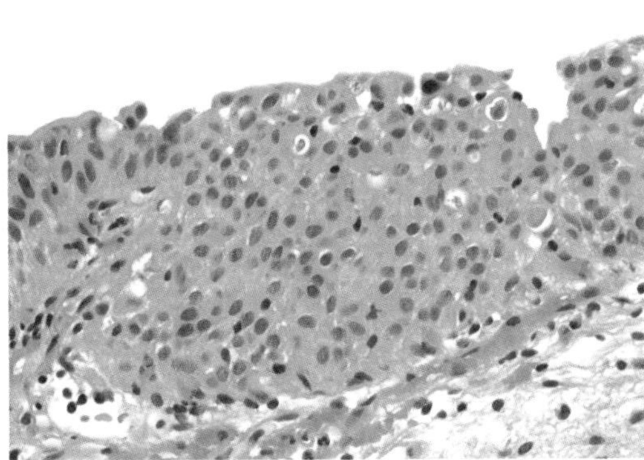

Fig. 13.2 Urothelial dysplasia (H&E). This urothelium shows marked architectural disorder of the urothelial cells with some mild nuclear enlargement. The cytologic features are not sufficient for diagnosis as carcinoma in situ. This lesion might be classified as urothelial dysplasia (or atypia of uncertain significance cannot exclude flat urothelial neoplasia/dysplasia)

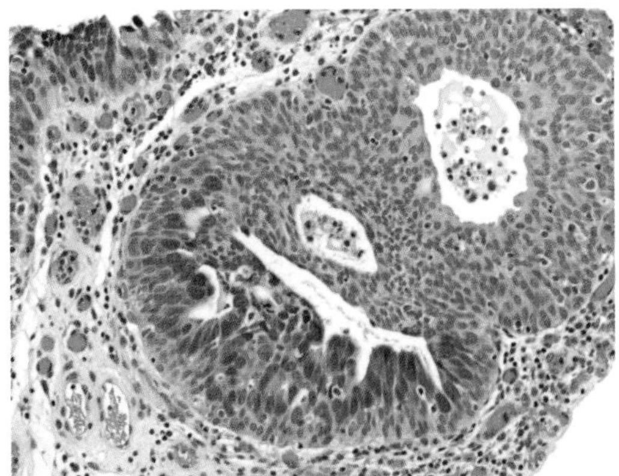

Fig. 13.3 Urothelial carcinoma in situ (H&E). Urothelial carcinoma in situ colonizes a von Brunn nest in the *lower left* and lines the surface in the *upper left* of this photomicrograph. The carcinoma in situ cells are markedly enlarged compared to adjacent normal urothelium, and the chromatin is irregular and dark

recommendation for continued follow-up, which is the general clinical management strategy for either diagnostic category.

Urothelial Carcinoma In-Situ (CIS)

Urothelial CIS is a neoplastic process that has the potential to progress to invasive urothelial carcinoma. The spectrum of cytologic atypia and the patterns of architectural growth seen in CIS are broad; however, nuclear enlargement is a common feature that is often used as an initial histologic screening evaluation. The nuclei of the neoplastic cells in CIS are often four times or more the size of a lymphocyte. These nuclei may be extremely anaplastic at one end of the spectrum, but have a range to include rather monomorphic nuclear atypia in other examples (Fig. 13.3). The nuclei may be more rounded, and cellular crowding and loss of cellular polarity are common. There may also be nuclear membrane irregularity and the nuclear chromatin in all cases is typically irregularly condensed. Macronucleoli may rarely be present, but this feature is not necessary for diagnosis. It is important to realize that the nuclear to cytoplasmic ratio is not always increased, as many examples of CIS have abundant eosinophilic cytoplasm. In contrast to prior classification systems that followed a paradigm similar to cervical dysplasia, the ISUP 1998 criteria also clearly stated that CIS "may be present in the entire thickness of the epithelium or only part of it." Therefore, the presence of any high-grade neoplastic cells, regardless of extent, warrants a diagnosis as CIS. Finally, mitotic figures are commonly identified in CIS, including atypical forms.

A number of varying architectural patterns are also described and include pleomorphic, monomorphic, "small" cell, pagetoid, clinging, and undermining (Fig. 13.4a–f) [7]. The pleomorphic pattern of CIS is the prototypical and most easily recognizable type due to its marked nuclear anaplasia. Some examples have more monomorphic nuclei, and the diagnosis is based on more subtle nuclear features such as more homogeneous nucleomegaly, nuclear hyperchromasia, and irregular nuclear contours. "Small" cell CIS has a very high nuclear to cytoplasmic ratio due to the presence of minimal cytoplasm; this descriptive term does not imply neuroendocrine differentiation. Pagetoid CIS may be histologically subtle because the neoplastic cells may be few in number. The presence of scattered round cells, which often have a rim of eosinophilic cytoplasm and are histologically distinct from the surrounding urothelium, should alert one to this possibility.

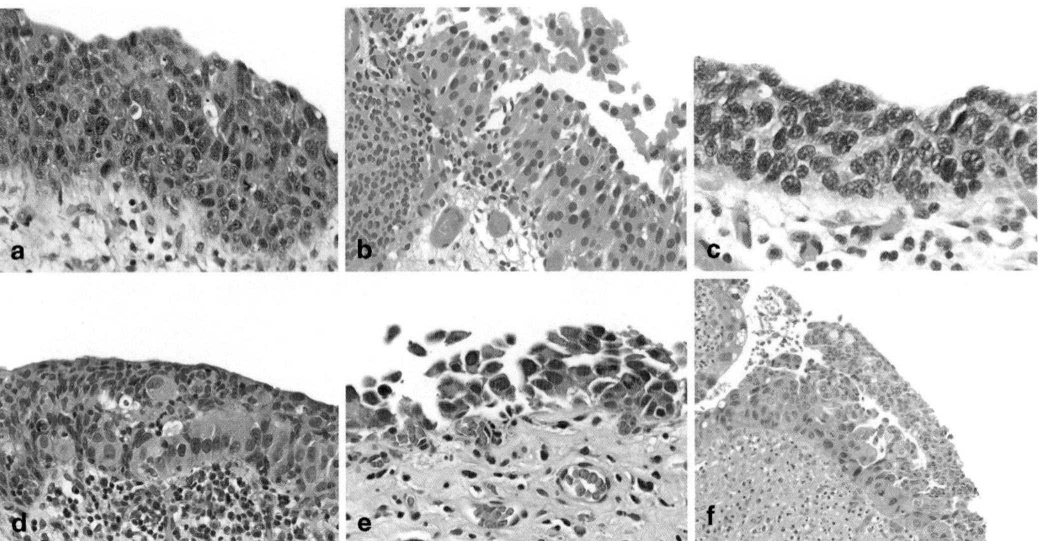

Fig. 13.4 Urothelial carcinoma in situ: architectural patterns. **a** Pleomorphic. **b** Nonpleomorphic. **c** "Small" cell. **d** Pagetoid. **e** Clinging/denuding. **f** Undermining

Denudation of the urothelium is also common in CIS; therefore, a single layer of "clinging" residual CIS cells may be the only remaining neoplastic component. These clinging CIS cells are markedly enlarged compared to normal basal cells and cytologic atypia may be obvious. Finally, CIS may extend into adjacent urothelium along the basement membrane, lifting up the residual normal urothelial cells in an undermining pattern. To date, there is no known clinical implication for these varying architectural patterns of CIS, and we do not report these individual patterns; however, knowledge of this heterogeneity is useful for diagnostic recognition.

Immunophenotypic Analysis of Flat Lesions with Atypia

Multiple studies have addressed possible immunophenotypic differences between these types of urothelial atypia [6, 8–17]. Cytokeratin 20 (CK20), CD44 (standard isoform), and p53 are the most frequently utilized immunohistochemical markers in routine practice (Fig. 13.5a–c). In normal urothelium, the umbrella cells express CK 20, while the basal cell layer may express CD44 to a variable extent. P53 expression typically has significant variation between different laboratories because the antibody seems to be

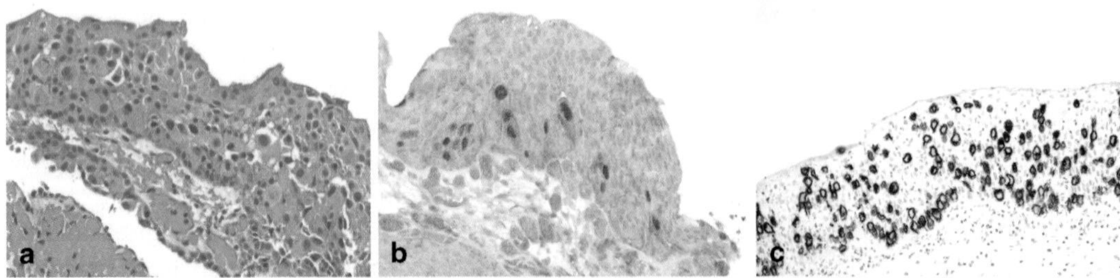

Fig. 13.5 Immunohistochemistry in flat lesions with atypia. **a** H&E: urothelial carcinoma in situ, pagetoid. **b** CK20/CD44/p53 cocktail: cytoplasmic CK20 and nuclear p53 reactivity is seen in the pagetoid CIS cell population (both *brown* chromogen), while cytoplasmic/membranous CD44 is seen in the residual nonneoplastic urothelial cells. **c** CK20: strong and diffuse CK20 immunoreactivity is present in the CIS cells

susceptible to subtle changes in staining conditions. Despite this variation, benign urothelium should not show diffuse and intense nuclear reactivity. Reactive atypia has similar CK 20 and p53 staining to normal urothelium, but CD44 often shows more diffuse membranous expression in the majority of the urothelial cells and this staining extends into the upper cell layers. CIS, in contrast, shows a loss of CD44 immunoreactivity and full thickness expression of CK 20 in the neoplastic cell population. P53 may show diffuse and intense nuclear relativity in a subset of CIS cases. Other markers that have been suggested as having utility in the classification of flat urothelial lesions include Ki-67, cytokeratin 5/6, and p16.

The main problem with these immunophenotypic data is that they are based on morphologic classification and are, therefore, often studied only in cases that are easily diagnosed by routine histology. The clinical prognostic significance of specific immunophenotypes in urothelial atypias has not been adequately addressed in the literature. In addition, we anecdotally see cases, typically in an external re-review or consult setting, in which the immunophenotype does not fit the histologic diagnosis. Until more studies address these issues, the classification of flat urothelial lesions with atypia should remain based primarily on routine histologic evaluation.

Diagnostic Comments for Flat Lesions with Atypia

Urothelium may show gradual histologic changes across a broad continuum that includes normal urothelium at one extreme and carcinoma in situ with marked nuclear pleomorphism at the other. The evaluation and classification of flat urothelial atypias across this continuum is one of the most difficult tasks in genitourinary pathology. For clinical management, the most important role of the surgical pathologist is to set a minimum diagnostic threshold for urothelial carcinoma in situ based on nuclear size, chromatin irregularity, nuclear membrane irregularity, and cellular polarity. This threshold should include the monomorphic forms of urothelial carcinoma in situ, which were classified as varying levels of "dysplasia" or "atypia" in previous classification systems. To maintain an appropriate distinction from florid examples of reactive atypia, it is recommended as a general rule that the diagnosis of CIS be very carefully re-considered if the individual nuclei of the lesional cells are less than or equal to the size of three to four lymphocytes.

Papillary Urothelial Neoplasia

Urothelial Papilloma

Under the WHO 2004 classification, very restrictive criteria are employed for the diagnosis of urothelial papilloma [1, 18–20]. "Urothelial papilloma" without qualifiers refers to the exophytic variant of papilloma, defined as a discrete papillary growth with a central fibrovascular core lined by urothelium of normal thickness and normal cytology. The low-power papillary architecture is a relatively simple branching pattern without irregular fusion between adjacent papillae (Fig. 13.6a–c). The umbrella cell layer is often prominent and may show prominent vacuolization, nuclear enlargement, or cytoplasmic eosinophilia. Some unusual features that have been reported in urothelial papillomas include dilation of lymphatic spaces within the papillae, gland-in-gland patterns, and foamy histiocytes within the papillae. This is a rare, benign condition typically occurring as a small, isolated growth that is commonly, but not exclusively seen in younger patients.

Papillary Urothelial Neoplasm of Low Malignant Potential

These tumors resemble urothelial papillomas, but generally have a markedly thickened (hyperplastic) urothelial lining (Fig. 13.7a, b). By definition, the nuclei may be slightly enlarged, but there is minimal to absent cytologic atypia. There is also normal polarity of the urothelial cells with an orderly, predominantly linear arrangement

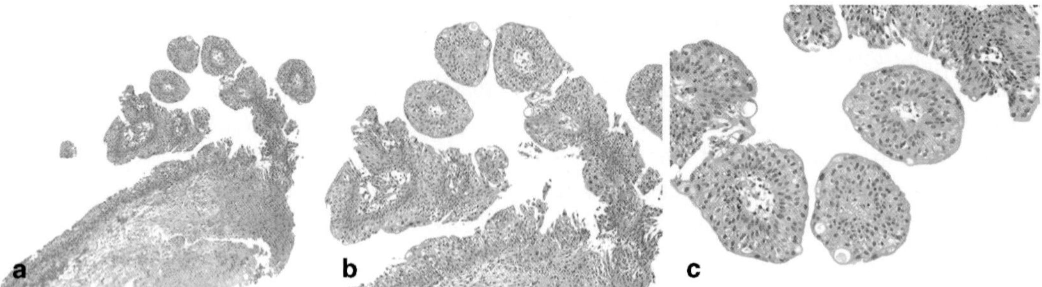

Fig. 13.6 Urothelial papilloma (H&E). **a** Urothelial papilloma typically has a very simple papillary architecture with significant anastomosis between papillae. **b** The urothelium should be evaluated in foci that are not cut tangentially. The urothelium appears relatively normal with retained polarity of the cells perpendicular to the basement membrane. **c** On high-power magnification, the cytology of the urothelial cells is normal. A prominent umbrella cell layer with some vacuolization is also a common feature of papilloma

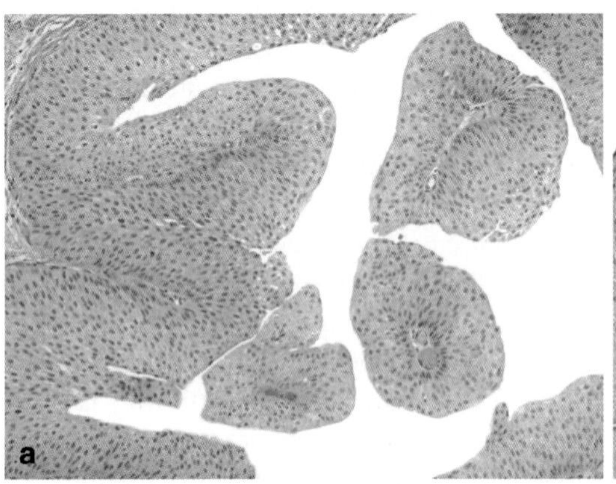

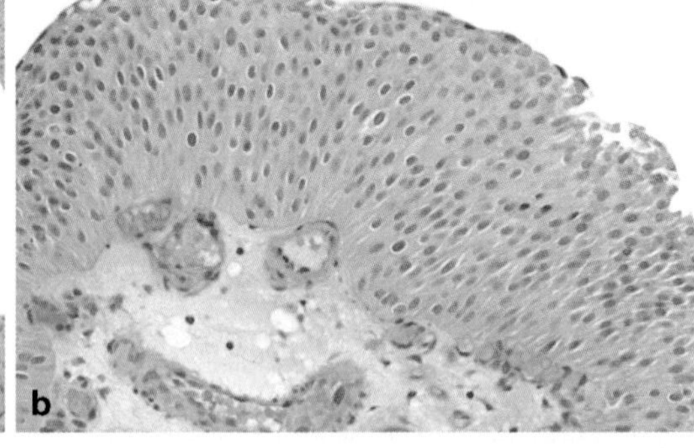

Fig. 13.7 Papillary urothelial neoplasm of low malignant potential (PUNLMP) (H&E). **a** As in papilloma, the papillary architecture of PUNLMP is usually simple, but a greater degree of complexity may be seen. **b** The cytologic features of PUNLMP appear normal, but the urothelium is hyperplastic/thickened compared to papilloma

perpendicular to the basement membrane. Mitotic figures are infrequent in papillary urothelial neoplasms of low malignant potential, and usually limited to the basal layer. The umbrella cell layer is frequently maintained. Like papillomas, the papillae of PUNLMP generally have a simple branching pattern with discrete, slender papillae, but more anastomosis between papillae may be seen. These patients, compared to those with papilloma, are at an increased risk of developing recurrent or new papillary lesions that occasionally are of higher grade and may progress. The diagnosis of PUNLMP should be carefully reconsidered in the presence of stromal invasion because that finding would be highly unusual.

Papillary Carcinoma, Low Grade

Low-grade papillary urothelial carcinomas are characterized by an overall orderly appearance but with easily recognizable variation of architectural and/or cytologic features seen at scanning magnification. Variation in cellular polarity (loss of the perpendicular arrangement of the urothelial cells to the basement membrane) and nuclear size, shape, and chromatin texture comprise the minimal criteria for the diagnosis of low-grade carcinoma (Fig. 13.8a, b). Mitotic figures are infrequent and usually seen in the lower half; but may be seen at any level of the urothelium. Tangential sections near the base of the urothelium

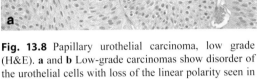

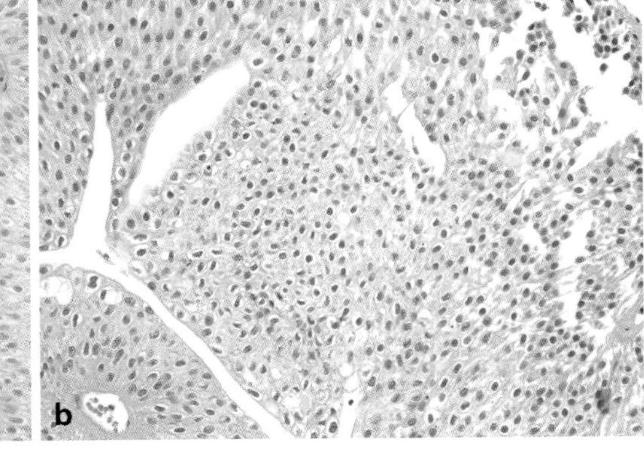

Fig. 13.8 Papillary urothelial carcinoma, low grade (H&E). **a** and **b** Low-grade carcinomas show disorder of the urothelial cells with loss of the linear polarity seen in papilloma and PUNLMP; however, the cytologic features do not reach the threshold of high-grade carcinoma

may be misleading and result in sheets of immature urothelium with frequent mitotic activity. A spectrum of cytologic and architectural abnormalities may exist within a single lesion, stressing the importance of examining the entire lesion and noting the highest grade of abnormality.

Papillary Carcinoma, High Grade

High-grade carcinomas are characterized by a complex, disordered architecture and moderate to marked cytologic atypia. Although the low-power papillary architecture is frequently complex with obvious anastomosis of adjacent papillae creating fused, confluent formations, the definitional feature for a diagnosis of high-grade carcinoma is the cytology of the neoplastic cells (Fig. 13.9a–c). Cytologically, there is a spectrum of pleomorphism ranging from moderate to marked, but obvious nuclear membrane irregularity and irregular, clumped chromatin represent the minimal diagnostic criteria. The individual neoplastic cells are often more rounded than in lower-grade lesions and have a loss of polarity in relation to the basement membrane (random, nonperpendicular arrangement within the urothelium). Mitotic figures, including atypical forms, and apoptotic debris are frequently seen. In tumors with variable histology, the tumor should be graded according to the highest grade. High-grade papillary urothelial carcinomas have a much higher risk of progression than low-grade lesions. These tumors also have a high risk of

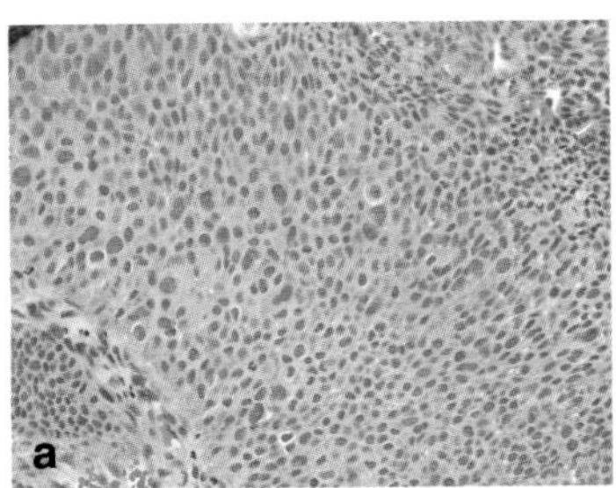

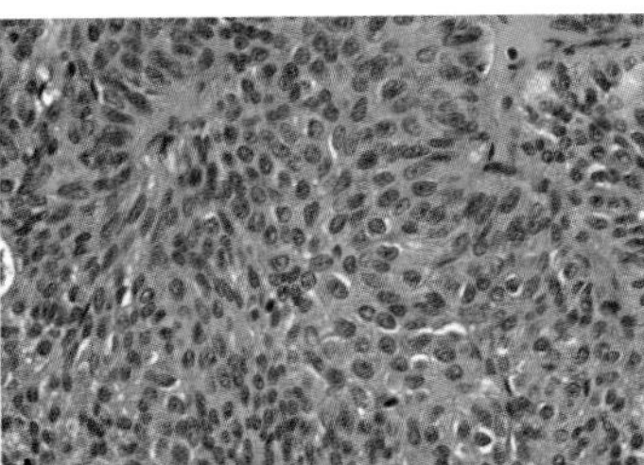

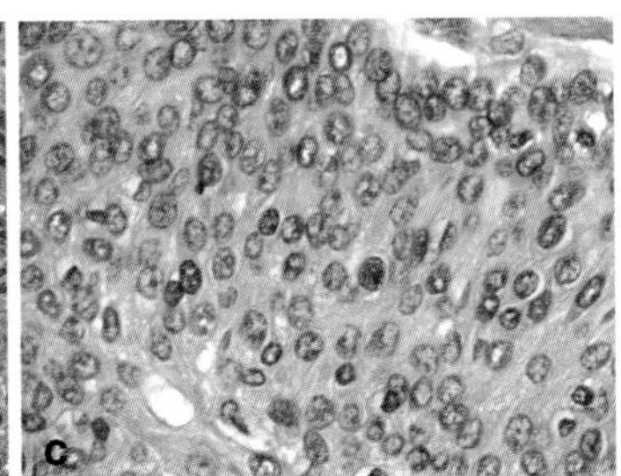

Fig. 13.9 Papillary urothelial carcinoma, high grade (H&E). **a** This degree of nuclear pleomorphism is designated as high grade. **b** and **c** Some high-grade carcinomas are more monomorphic, but have nucleomegaly and nuclear chromatin abnormalities beyond the WHO 2004 threshold for low grade. Such cases would have been classified as grade 2 under the 1973 classification system, but are now regarded as high grade

association with invasive disease at the time of diagnosis. Paralleling the high-grade cytologic atypia within these lesions, the surrounding flat urothelial mucosa may also demonstrate urothelial CIS.

Diagnostic Comments for Papillary Urothelial Neoplasia

As with flat lesions, the most important histologic distinction is the separation of high-grade papillary urothelial carcinoma from the other types because this represents the clinical threshold for intravesical therapy. The threshold for designation as high grade is lower than in the 1973 classification system. This change was based on data showing that "1973 Grade 2 carcinomas" could be divided into two groups, and that those with more nuclear atypia had a lower survival rate [21]. Therefore, cases that were previously classified as grade 2 are now divided into either high grade or low grade [1]. The result is that high-grade carcinoma is now more histologically heterogeneous with varying levels of cytologic atypia, which allows a larger number of patients at higher risk of recurrence/progression to receive intravesical therapy [22, 23]. When papillary urothelial neoplasms have a mixture of both high-grade and low-grade foci, it is generally recommended to assign the highest grade. Further study is needed to assess the prognostic impact of only focal high-grade features. Adjunctive immunohistochemistry has also been suggested as a surrogate for histologic grade, but this has not been adopted into standard practice [24–29].

The distinction of papilloma and PUNLMP from low-grade carcinoma also requires very strict criteria. Superficial umbrella cells are ignored for classification; therefore, any degree of architectural disorder, nuclear variation, or nuclear hyperchromasia should warrant a low-grade carcinoma designation. Also, significant levels of mitotic activity should exclude a case as papilloma or PUNLMP.

Finally, a subset of biopsies shows very early papillary change or undulation that may be early papillary neoplasia. In the absence of any epithelial abnormality, this was originally called papillary hyperplasia; however, this category was not included in the WHO 2004 edition as it was considered to be PUNLMP by many consensus participants. As with flat and papillary lesions, the main point of clinical relevance is the identification of any high-grade cytologic features, which should be regarded as high-grade papillary carcinoma. In some cases with high-grade cytology that are difficult to classify as either flat or papillary, we render a diagnosis of "urothelial carcinoma in situ with early papillary formation." Alternatively, one may simply defer to the clinical cystoscopic impression of a flat or papillary lesion. Similarly, in cases with cytologic atypia falling short of carcinoma in situ and questionable early tufting/papillae, we utilize the descriptive diagnostic term "papillary hyperplasia with dysplasia."

Endophytic Urothelial Neoplasia

Inverted (Urothelial) Papilloma

Inverted (urothelial) papillomas typically consist of complex inter-anastomosing cords of urothelium within the lamina propria of the urinary tract [30–32]. The amount of intervening stroma is variable. There is usually a well-circumscribed border at the base, and there is often a characteristic palisading of basaloid cells at the periphery of the nests/cords (Fig. 13.10a–c). Centrally within the nests/cords, the neoplastic cells may have a spindled appearance or rarely, show nonkeratinizing squamous metaplasia. Mitotic figures are rare or absent. Rarely, cases are hybrid with different areas of the lesion resembling exophytic urothelial papilloma and inverted urothelial papilloma; these lesions are generally classified as papillomas with both exophytic and inverted features. By definition, inverted papillomas lack nuclear pleomorphism,

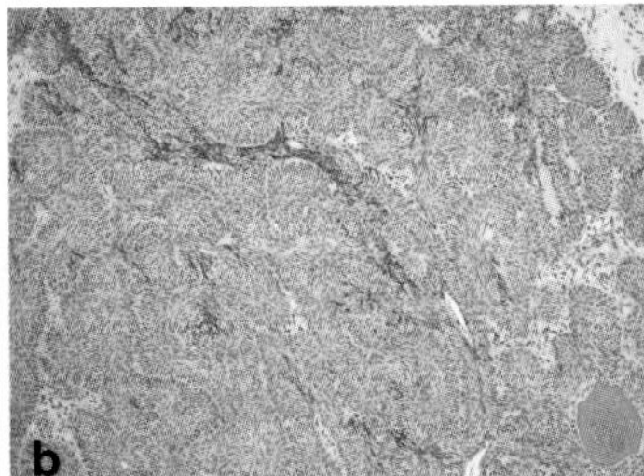

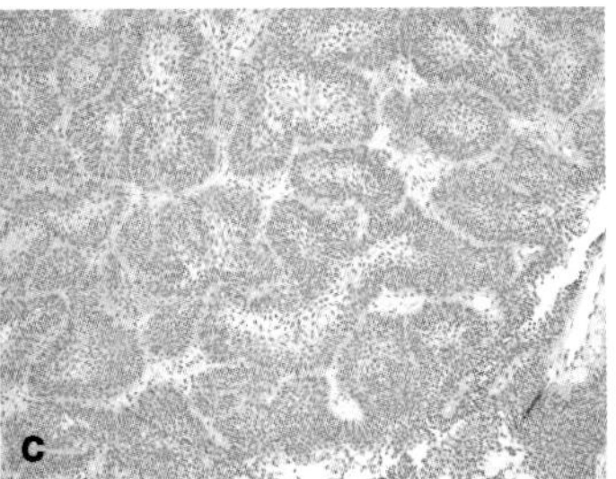

Fig. 13.10 Inverted papilloma (H&E). **a** Anastomosing cord-like growth is the characteristic architecture of inverted papilloma. **b** The cords may be arranged back-to-back, which may mimic solid growth. **c** Urothelial papilloma often has palisading of the peripheral nuclei in the cords and nests and the central region may be spindled with a "stellate reticulum-like" appearance

nuclear hyperchromasia, or significant mitotic activity; however, scattered cells with multinucleation or degenerative-type atypia have been described and do not seem to alter the benign clinical course [33]. In addition, foamy or vacuolated cells are occasionally seen [31]. Central cystic change (cystitis cystica-like or colloid cyst pattern) has also been described [30]. When prominent, this cystitis cystica-like pattern of inverted papilloma may have a glandular appearance at low-power magnification.

When diagnosed by these strict criteria and completely excised, inverted papillomas have a very low risk of recurrence (less than 1 %). The controversy and conflicting reports in the literature regarding the prognosis of inverted papillomas and their association with carcinoma is likely due to endophytic patterns of urothelial carcinoma being classified as inverted papilloma in the older literature.

Inverted/Endophytic Urothelial Neoplasms Other than Papilloma

Endophytic patterns of urothelial carcinoma may also closely resemble inverted papillomas, but the invaginated cords are typically broader with greater variation in size including transition to solid areas. In addition, they may have cytologic atypia beyond what is allowed in urothelial papilloma (Fig. 13.11a–d) [34, 35]. Carcinomas typically have a greater degree of cytologic atypia, do not demonstrate the homogeneous basaloid appearance of inverted papillomas, and may have a prominent exophytic component that does not resemble urothelial papilloma. Any true stromal invasion would warrant classification as carcinoma.

Endophytic growth, on its own merit, should not be regarded as stromal invasion in urothelial carcinomas despite the invagination into the lamina propria. In contrast to irregular small nests and clusters of urothelium in invasion, endophytic growth is characterized by inter-anastomosing cords of urothelium with a relatively smooth, pushing border. Overlying papillary urothelial neoplasms are not uncommon.

This pattern of urothelial neoplasia has been addressed in the literature only rarely. It should be emphasized that the entire spectrum of urothelial neoplasia can grow in this endophytic pattern. We recommend a diagnostic approach identical to that used for papillary neoplasms. Cases may be classified as urothelial neoplasm of low malignant potential, low-grade carcinoma, or high-grade carcinoma based on the same cytologic and architectural criteria utilized for papillary lesions. These endophytic neoplasms should also be staged as otherwise typical urothelial carcinoma. Invasion is typically characterized by the presence of irregular nests of tumor cells, often with more eosinophilic cytoplasm.

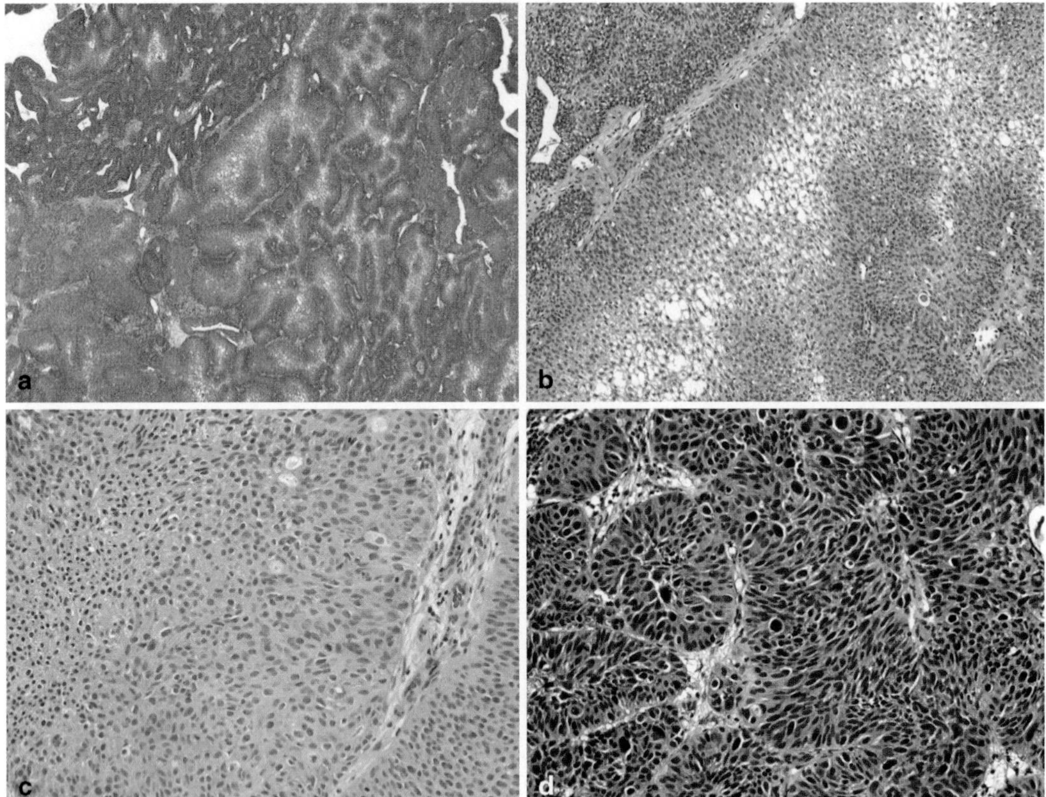

Fig. 13.11 Noninvasive inverted/endophytic carcinoma. **a** The presence of endophytic cords that are expanded and create areas with a more confluent solid appearance are not compatible with inverted papilloma. **b** On higher-power magnification, this neoplasm is cytologically bland and maintains polarity. It would be classified as inverted urothelial neoplasm of low malignant potential due to this architectural expansion. **c** This degree of disorder and cytologic atypia is characteristic of a low-grade carcinoma. **d** This noninvasive endophytic urothelial carcinoma has sufficient nuclear atypia for designation as high grade

References

1. Sauter G, Algaba F, Amin MB, et al. Non-invasive urothelial tumors. In: Eble JN, Sauter G, Epstein JI, Sesterhenn IA, editors. World health organization classification of tumors pathology and genetics of tumours of the urinary system and male genital organs. Lyon: IARC Press; 2004. pp. 110–23.
2. Edge SB, Byrd DR, Compton CC, Fritz AG, Greene FL, Trotti III A, editors. AJCC cancer staging manual. 7th ed. New York: Springer; 2010.
3. Epstein JI, Amin MB, Reuter VR, Mostofi FK. The world health organization/international society of urological pathology consensus classification of urothelial (transitional cell) neoplasms of the urinary bladder. Bladder consensus conference committee. Am J Surg Pathol. 1998;22:1435–48.
4. Mostofi FK, Sobin LH, Torloni H. Histological typing of urinary bladder tumours. Geneva: World Health Organization; 1973.
5. Amin MB, Grignon DJ, Eble JN. Intraepithelial lesions of the urothelium: an interobserver reproducibility study with a proposed terminology and histologic criteria. Mod Pathol. 1997;10:69.
6. Murata S, Iseki M, Kinjo M, et al. Molecular and immunohistologic analyses cannot reliably solve diagnostic variation of flat intraepithelial lesions of the urinary bladder. Am J Clin Path. 2010;134:862–72.
7. McKenney JK, Gomez JA, Desai S, Lee MW, Amin MB. Morphologic expressions of urothelial carcinoma in situ: a detailed evaluation of its histologic patterns with emphasis on carcinoma in situ with microinvasion. Am J Surg Pathol. 2001;25:356–62.
8. McKenney JK, Desai S, Cohen C, Amin MB. Discriminatory immunohistochemical staining of urothelial carcinoma in situ and non-neoplastic urothelium: an analysis of cytokeratin 20, p53, and CD44 antigens. Am J Surg Pathol. 2001;25:1074–8.
9. Edgecombe A, Nguyen BN, Djordjevic B, Belanger EC, Mai KT. Utility of cytokeratin 5/6, cytokeratin 20, and p16 in the diagnosis of reactive urothe-

lial atypia and noninvasive component of urothelial neoplasia. Appl Immunohistochem Mol Morphol. 2012;20:264–71.
10. Harnden P, Eardley I, Joyce AD, Southgate J. Cytokeratin 20 as an objective marker of urothelial dysplasia. B J Urol. 1996;78:870–5.
11. Kunju LP, Lee CT, Montie J, Shah RB. Utility of cytokeratin 20 and Ki-67 as markers of urothelial dysplasia. Pathol Int. 2005;55:248–54.
12. Mallofre C, Castillo M, Morente V, Sole M. Immunohistochemical expression of CK20, p53, and Ki-67 as objective markers of urothelial dysplasia. Mod Pathol. 2003;16:187–91.
13. Oliva E, Pinheiro NF, Heney NM, et al. Immunohistochemistry as an adjunct in the differential diagnosis of radiation-induced atypia versus urothelial carcinoma in situ of the bladder: a study of 45 cases. Hum Pathol. 2013;44:860–6.
14. Yin H, He Q, Li T, Leong AS. Cytokeratin 20 and Ki-67 to distinguish carcinoma in situ from flat nonneoplastic urothelium. Appl Immunohistochem Mol Morphol. 2006;14:260–5.
15. Stepan A, Simionescu C, Margaritescu C, Ciurea R. P16, c-erbB2 and Ki67 immunoexpression in urothelial carcinomas of the bladder. Rom J Morphol Embryol. 2011;52:653–8.
16. Sun W, Zhang PL, Herrera GA. p53 protein and Ki-67 overexpression in urothelial dysplasia of bladder. Appl Immunohistochem Mol Morphol. 2002;10:327–31.
17. Yin M, Bastacky S, Parwani AV, McHale T, Dhir R. p16ink4 immunoreactivity is a reliable marker for urothelial carcinoma in situ. Hum Pathol. 2008;39:527–35.
18. Cheng L, Darson M, Cheville JC, et al. Urothelial papilloma of the bladder. Clinical and biologic implications. Cancer. 1999;86:2098–101.
19. Magi-Galluzzi C, Epstein JI. Urothelial papilloma of the bladder: a review of 34 de novo cases. Am J Surg Pathol. 2004;28:1615–20.
20. McKenney JK, Amin MB, Young RH. Urothelial (transitional cell) papilloma of the urinary bladder: a clinicopathologic study of 26 cases. Mod Pathol. 2003;16:623–9.
21. Malmstrom PU, Busch C, Norlen BJ. Recurrence, progression and survival in bladder cancer. A retrospective analysis of 232 patients with greater than or equal to 5-year follow-up. Scand J Urol Nephrol. 1987;21:185–95.
22. Samaratunga H, Makarov DV, Epstein JI. Comparison of WHO/ISUP and WHO classification of noninvasive papillary urothelial neoplasms for risk of progression. Urology. 2002;60:315–9.
23. Busch C, Algaba F. The WHO/ISUP 1998 and WHO 1999 systems for malignancy grading of bladder cancer. Scientific foundation and translation to one another and previous systems. Virchows Arch. 2002;441:105–8.
24. Alsheikh A, Mohamedali Z, Jones E, Masterson J, Gilks CB. Comparison of the WHO/ISUP classification and cytokeratin 20 expression in predicting the behavior of low-grade papillary urothelial tumors. World/Health Organization/Internattional society of urologic pathology. Mod Pathol. 2001;14:267–72.
25. Bertz S, Otto W, Denzinger S, et al. Combination of CK20 and Ki-67 immunostaining analysis predicts recurrence, progression, and cancer-specific survival in pT1 urothelial bladder cancer. Eur Urol. 2014;65(1):218–26.
26. Cina SJ, Lancaster-Weiss KJ, Lecksell K, Epstein JI. Correlation of Ki-67 and p53 with the new world health organization/international society of urological pathology classification system for urothelial neoplasia. Arch Pathol Lab Med. 2001;125:646–51.
27. Kilicli-Camur N, Kilicaslan I, Gulluoglu MG, Esen T, Uysal V. Impact of p53 and Ki-67 in predicting recurrence and progression of superficial (pTa and pT1) urothelial cell carcinomas of urinary bladder. Pathol Int. 2002;52:463–9.
28. Santos L, Amaro T, Costa C, et al. Ki-67 index enhances the prognostic accuracy of the urothelial superficial bladder carcinoma risk group classification. Int J Cancer. 2003;105:267–72.
29. Wolf HK, Stober C, Hohenfellner R, Leissner J. Prognostic value of p53, p21/WAF1, Bcl-2, Bax, Bak and Ki-67 immunoreactivity in pT1 G3 urothelial bladder carcinomas. Tumour Biol. 2001;22:328–36.
30. Kunze E, Schauer A, Schmitt M. Histology and histogenesis of two different types of inverted urothelial papillomas. Cancer. 1983;51:348–58.
31. Fine SW, Epstein JI. Inverted urothelial papillomas with foamy or vacuolated cytoplasm. Human Pathol. 2006;37:1577–82.
32. Fine SW, Chan TY, Epstein JI. Inverted papillomas of the prostatic urethra. A J Surg Pathol. 2006;30:975–9.
33. Broussard JN, Tan PH, Epstein JI. Atypia in inverted urothelial papillomas: pathology and prognostic significance. Human Pathol. 2004;35:1499–504.
34. Sudo T, Irie A, Ishii D, Satoh E, Mitomi H, Baba S. Histopathologic and biologic characteristics of a transitional cell carcinoma with inverted papilloma-like endophytic growth pattern. Urology. 2003;61:837.
35. Amin MB, Gomez JA, Young RH. Urothelial transitional cell carcinoma with endophytic growth patterns: a discussion of patterns of invasion and problems associated with assessment of invasion in 18 cases. A J Surg Pathol. 1997;21:1057–68.

14 Reporting of Bladder Cancer in Transurethral Resection of Bladder Tumor and Cystectomy Specimens

Jesse K. McKenney

Introduction

This chapter focuses on practical issues concerning the reporting of urothelial carcinoma, which should be based on the 7th ed. AJCC Staging Manual and the WHO 2004 classification [1, 2]. The current AJCC cancer staging guidelines are outlined in Table 14.1.

Table 14.1 Current AJCC cancer staging guidelines. (Used with permission from [1])

pT0: No evidence of primary tumor
pTa: Noninvasive papillary carcinoma
pTis: Carcinoma in situ
pT1: Tumor invades subepithelial connective tissue (*lamina propria*)
pT2:Tumor invades muscularis propria
pT2a: Inner half
pT2b: Outer half
pT3: Tumor invades perivesical tissue
pT3a: Microscopically
pT3b: Macroscopically
pT4: Tumor invades any of the following: prostate (does NOT include invasion from the prostatic urethra), uterus, vagina, pelvic wall, abdominal wall

Reporting Stage in Transurethral Resection of Bladder Tumor (TURBT) Specimens

Invasive Carcinomas

In transurethral resection of bladder tumor (TURBT) specimens, the reporting of invasive urothelial carcinomas is critical to subsequent clinical management. It is recommended that bladder biopsy staging evaluation be restricted to pT1 and pT2 disease; pT3 and pT4 disease can only be diagnosed at cystectomy. Adipose tissue is commonly present within the muscularis propria and may even be seen in the lamina propria; therefore, the presence of tumor within adipose tissue does not signify a pT3 tumor. At biopsy evaluation, the most important histologic distinction for invasive urothelial carcinoma is lamina propria invasion versus muscularis propria invasion (i.e., pT1 vs. pT2 disease). Urologists typically favor conservative management with intravesical treatment regimens for high-grade pTa and any pT1 disease. The diagnosis of pT2 carcinoma is generally the threshold for surgical management (e.g., radical cystectomy) and/or radiation therapy. The histologic parameters included in the pathology report should allow the urologist to easily assign a T stage to the patient, and to select the appropriate treatment plan.

Studies suggest that stage is the most important prognostic factor in invasive urothelial carcinoma, independent of grade [3]. This is supported by additional studies documenting the capability of deeply invasive, cytologically bland carcinomas to produce metastases and cause patient

J. K. McKenney (✉)
Department of Pathology, Cleveland Clinic, Robert J. Tomsich Pathology and Laboratory Medicine Institute, Cleveland, OH, USA
e-mail: mckennj@ccf.org

C. Magi-Galluzzi, C. G. Przybycin (eds.), *Genitourinary Pathology,* DOI 10.1007/978-1-4939-2044-0_14,

Table 14.2 Diagnostic template for invasive urothelial carcinoma. (Alternative differentiation (e.g., squamous) or variant subtype should also be included when relevant)

(a) With lamina propria invasion (pT1)
(i) muscularis propria is present, but is not involved or
(ii) muscularis propria is not present for evaluation
(b) With muscularis propria invasion (at least pT2)

mortality [4–6]. In our opinion, invasive urothelial carcinomas are biologically high grade.

Some authors have suggested the utility of substaging lamina propria invasion based on depth measurements or relation to the muscularis mucosae (see Chap. 12). This substaging is difficult in practice because bladder biopsies are frequently sectioned in a tangential plane making orientation difficult to assess. Because of these difficulties and lack of an accepted reproducible method, substaging has not been adopted under the current systems of staging and classification (WHO 2004; 7th edition AJCC).

A simple diagnostic template is shown in Table 14.2 that includes the relevant diagnostic findings needed for patient management. We avoid the use of the term "muscle invasion" because it does not distinguish between carcinomas invading muscularis propria (detrusor muscle) (pT2) from those invading only muscularis mucosae (pT1). It is best to use the more specific anatomic terms "lamina propria" (Fig. 14.1a, b) or "muscularis propria" (Fig. 14.2) to describe depth of invasion. Including the pT stage in the line diagnosis can also help to avoid any misunderstanding with regard to anatomic terms. In a subset of cases, it may be difficult to definitively classify a carcinoma as pT1 or pT2 if fragments of smooth muscle are involved in which the distinction of muscularis propria from muscularis mucosae is problematic. In those cases, we use a diagnostic term such as "invasive urothelial carcinoma, indeterminate depth (see comment regarding stage)" with an appropriate comment section.

Noninvasive Carcinomas

For noninvasive tumors, histologic grade is the most critical factor as discussed in detail in Chap. 13. A diagnostic line such as "non-invasive papillary urothelial carcinoma (pTa), high grade (WHO 2004/ISUP)" is usually sufficient. Even when invasion is not present, we typically report the presence or absence of muscularis propria. Although these papillary tumors are noninvasive, they should not be reported as pTis, which denotes flat urothelial carcinoma.

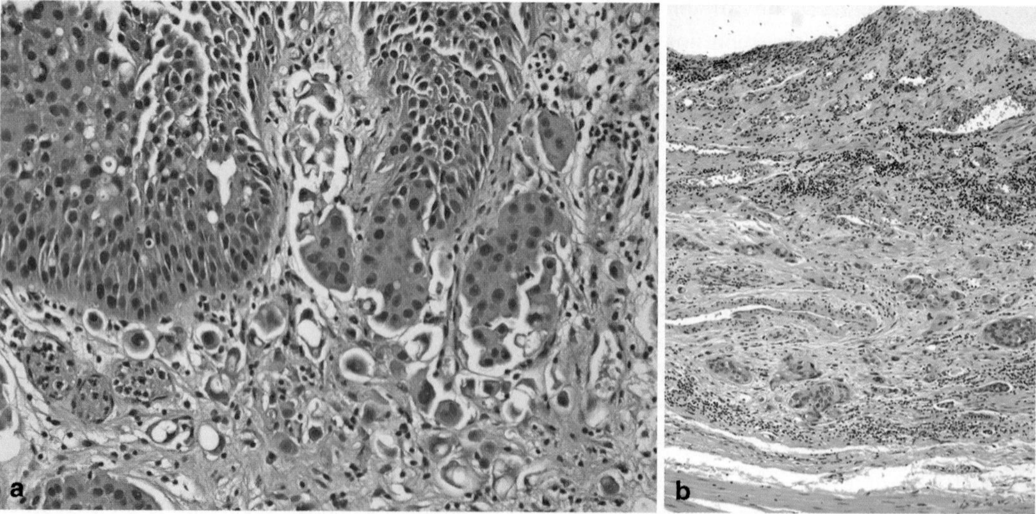

Fig. 14.1 Invasive high-grade urothelial carcinoma with lamina propria invasion (pT1): individual carcinoma cells (**a**) or nests of urothelial carcinoma (**b**) are present within the lamina propria. Notice the presence of stromal retraction surrounding some of the nests of invasive carcinoma (**b**)

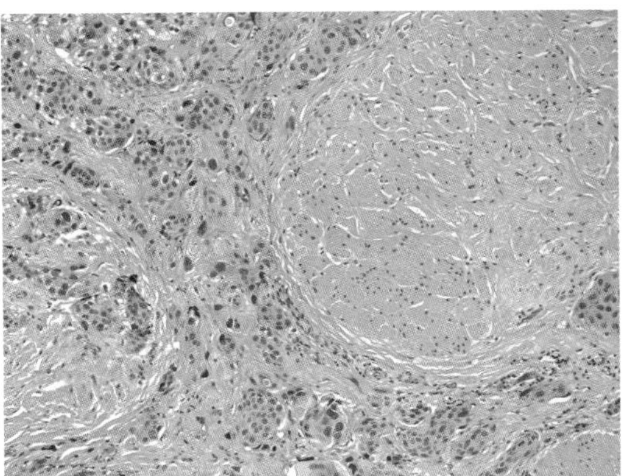

Fig. 14.2 Invasive high-grade urothelial carcinoma with muscularis propria invasion (pT2)

Lymphovascular Invasion

Reporting lymphovascular invasion is problematic because stromal retraction (Fig. 14.1b) is a common feature in invasive urothelial carcinoma that may closely mimic invasion of a blood vessel. There are reports that lymphovascular invasion is an aggressive histologic feature and, although controversial, some urologists will use that finding as rationale for definitive surgical management when a carcinoma is otherwise stage pT1 [7]. It is therefore critical to have a high diagnostic threshold for the diagnosis of vascular invasion to insure distinction from stromal retraction.

Reporting Stage in Cystectomy Specimens

Invasion of Perivesical Tissue

Invasion into perivesical adipose tissue may be assessed in radical cystectomy specimens. This invasion outside the confines of the bladder wall is divided into two types: those that are macroscopically identifiable (pT3b) and those that are seen only after microscopic evaluation (pT3a). Each gross description of a radical cystectomy specimen should include a statement that documents the presence or absence of grossly identifiable invasion into perivesical adipose tissue.

Involvement of Prostate Gland

Reports must be carefully written to address urothelial carcinoma that involves the prostate gland. If urothelial carcinoma invades through the wall of the bladder to involve the prostate gland by direct extension, then it is designated as pT4 disease. Such carcinomas are typically very large with extensive permeative growth. This scenario must be distinguished from urothelial carcinoma that invades into the prostate from a noninvasive urothelial carcinoma of the prostatic urethra (i.e., noninvasive papillary urothelial carcinoma or urothelial carcinoma in situ) or from carcinoma in situ that is colonizing prostatic glands. When the carcinoma invading the prostatic stroma arises from an adjacent urothelial carcinoma of the prostatic urethra (with or without colonization of underlying prostate glands) a separate stage should be assigned (pT2) using the guidelines for a primary urethral carcinoma (i.e., prostatic urethra). Using this approach, two stages may be assigned if there is invasion in both the urinary bladder and the prostatic urethra.

Surgical Margins

The surgical margins for radical cystectomy (or cystoprostatectomy) specimens should be handled and reported separately to include the surrounding soft tissue, the ureters, and the distal urethra.

Reporting Subtypes/Variants of Carcinoma

Since TURBT specimens may provide material that is not completely representative of a given neoplasm, we exercise caution when reporting invasive carcinoma with alternative differentiation (i.e., squamous and glandular histology). If the invasive carcinoma is comprised of only squamous elements without a background of noninvasive urothelial carcinoma in a TURBT specimen, we utilize the diagnostic term "invasive carcinoma with squamous features" and include a comment regarding the difficulty of distinguishing urothelial carcinoma with squamous differentiation from primary vesical squamous cell carcinoma. If adjacent keratinizing metaplasia or dysplasia are present in the biopsy specimen, then that would add support for squamous cell carcinoma. If the carcinoma extends to a location where a human papillomavirus (HPV)-related squamous carcinoma might be considered, we would perform adjunctive HPV in situ hybridization studies for that distinction. The same principles of reporting apply to carcinomas that are purely gland forming on biopsy, where we use the term "invasive carcinoma with glandular features," assuming that secondary involvement by prostatic adenocarcinoma has been excluded when relevant. For cases in which the origin is uncertain, we include a comment to discuss the differential diagnostic possibilities of invasive urothelial carcinoma with glandular differentiation, primary vesical adenocarcinoma, primary carcinomas of the urachus, and direct extension from an adjacent anatomic site such as colorectal. Since colon carcinomas may colonize the luminal surface of the bladder, using the presence of "adenocarcinoma in situ" for this distinction is problematic. Careful radiographic and clinical correlation is needed for these distinctions. If a component of typical urothelial carcinoma is present, then we would render the diagnosis of "invasive urothelial carcinoma with squamous (or glandular) differentiation." In addition, including the percent of neoplasm comprised of the alternative component by visual estimation is helpful.

For other well described subtypes or variant forms of urothelial carcinoma, we generally include the type in the main diagnostic line such as "invasive urothelial carcinoma, micropapillary type" or "invasive urothelial carcinoma with small cell differentiation." Giving the percentage of any subtype patterns, when they are admixed with typical urothelial carcinoma, is useful. As has been discussed in the literature, the changes of micropapillary carcinoma exist over a morphologic continuum due to varying prominence of retraction spaces and tumor nest size such that a subset of cases may be difficult to classify [8]. For borderline cases, we utilize the diagnostic term "invasive urothelial carcinoma with features suspicious for early micropapillary differentiation."

References

1. Edge SB, Byrd DR, Compton CC, Fritz AG, Greene FL, Trotti III A, editors. AJCC cancer staging manual. 7th ed. New York: Springer; 2010.
2. Eble JN, Sauter G, Epstein JI, Sesterhenn IA, editors. World health organization classification of tumours. Pathology and genetics of the urinary system and male genital organs. Lyon: IARC Press; 2004.
3. Jimenez RE, Gheiler E, Oskanian P, Tiguert R, Sakr W, Wood DP Jr., et al. Grading the invasive component of urothelial carcinoma of the bladder and its relationship with progression-free survival. Am J Surg Pathol. 2000;24(7):980–7.
4. Liedberg F, Chebil G, Davidsson T, Gadaleanu V, Grabe M, Mansson W. The nested variant of urothelial carcinoma: a rare but important bladder neoplasm with aggressive behavior. Three case reports and a review of the literature. Urol Oncol. 2003;21(1):7–9.
5. Lin O, Cardillo M, Dalbagni G, Linkov I, Hutchinson B, Reuter VE. Nested variant of urothelial carcinoma: a clinicopathologic and immunohistochemical study of 12 cases. Mod Pathol. 2003;16(12):1289–98.
6. Wasco MJ, Daignault S, Bradley D, Shah RB. Nested variant of urothelial carcinoma: a clinicopathologic and immunohistochemical study of 30 pure and mixed cases. Hum Pathol. 2010;41(2):163–71.
7. Reuter VE. Lymphovascular invasion as an independent predictor of recurrence and survival in node-negative bladder cancer remains to be proven. J Clin Oncol. 2005;23(27):6450–1.
8. Sangoi AR, Beck AH, Amin MB, Cheng L, Epstein JI, Hansel DE, et al. Interobserver reproducibility in the diagnosis of invasive micropapillary carcinoma of the urinary tract among urologic pathologists. Am J Surg Pathol. 2010;34(9):1367–76.

Urothelial Carcinoma Variants: Morphology and Association with Outcomes

15

Gladell P. Paner and Donna E. Hansel

Introduction

Urothelial carcinoma is a challenging diagnostic entity for pathologists. Despite the inherent difficulties in grading and staging of urothelial carcinoma, the additional complexity associated with identifying urothelial carcinoma variants may be daunting. In this chapter, we will describe the 16 morphologic variants of urothelial carcinoma, highlighting unique properties associated with diagnosis and prognosis. In general, urothelial carcinoma variants demonstrate similar demographic and clinical features as conventional urothelial carcinoma, including a male predominance, preponderance in an older patient population, presence of irritative voiding symptoms, and micro/macroscopic hematuria. On gross examination, lesions may appear exophytic or ulcerative, with the rare exception of a more complex appearance in some instances of micropapillary urothelial carcinoma, linitis plastica-like growth in plasmacytoid variant, and possible mucin production if an extensive glandular component is present. It is remarkable though that a higher proportion of some variants is diagnosed at advanced stage. The definitive diagnosis of these urothelial carcinoma variants generally rests on the microscopic analysis of the tumor (Table 15.1). Their unique appearances present a façade of morphologic mimics, both benign and malignant, that further complicates the recognition of these rare tumors. Awareness of variants in this disease process is critical not only in providing accurate patient diagnosis, but also in properly determining patient care and discussions related to prognosis.

Urothelial Carcinoma with Divergent Differentiation

Divergent differentiation in urothelial carcinoma is a common occurrence, with up to 27 % of urothelial carcinomas reported to show this feature, although the reported frequency varies depending on specimen type and study [1–4]. Most commonly, divergent differentiation is represented by squamous change within the neoplasm. The second most common form of divergent differentiation includes glandular change, identified as the presence of glands, small tubules, and occasionally signet ring cells or other glandular-like change. In addition to squamous and glandular differentiation, many other variants of urothelial carcinoma may be present admixed with conventional urothelial carcinoma.

Diagnostic criteria to report "urothelial carcinoma with squamous differentiation" entails identification of clear-cut squamous features within the tumor, including the presence of keratin or desmosomes (Fig. 15.1). These findings are present in a background of otherwise conventional urothelial carcinoma. Documen-

G. P. Paner (✉)
Department of Pathology, University of Chicago Medical Center, Chicago, IL, USA
e-mail: Gladell.paner@uchospitals.edu

D. E. Hansel
Department of Pathology, University of California at San Diego, La Jolla, CA, USA
e-mail: dhansel@ucsd.edu

C. Magi-Galluzzi, C. G. Przybycin (eds.), *Genitourinary Pathology*, DOI 10.1007/978-1-4939-2044-0_15,

Table 15.1 Variant morphologies of urothelial carcinoma of the bladder

Urothelial carcinoma variants	Key morphologic features
Urothelial carcinoma with divergent differentiation	
Urothelial carcinoma with squamous differentiation	Urothelial carcinoma with clear-cut squamous features including keratin production and/or presence of desmosomes
Urothelial carcinoma with glandular differentiation	Gland-forming urothelial carcinoma consisting of columnar, mucinous, signet ring, or intestinal-type cells
Urothelial carcinoma with deceptively benign appearance	Invasive urothelial carcinoma composed of cells with overall bland cytology; it exhibits the following architectures
Nested urothelial carcinoma	Small nests that resemble von Brunn's nests
Large nested urothelial carcinoma	Large nests with pushing border, often connected to surface
Microcystic urothelial carcinoma	Small or large nests with lumina or cysts that resemble cystitis cystica
Urothelial carcinoma with small tubules	Tubular or acinar formation
Micropapillary urothelial carcinoma	Noninvasive surface filiform papillae that lack fibrovascular core and/or invasive small clusters of tightly packed cells in lacunar space with nuclei polarized exteriorly
Urothelial carcinomas with unusual cell morphology	
Plasmacytoid urothelial carcinoma	Discohesive tumor cells with abundant cytoplasm and eccentric nuclei that resemble plasma cells
Urothelial carcinoma with rhabdoid features	Tumor cells with abundant cytoplasm and intracytoplasmic inclusion that indents and peripherally displaces the nucleus
Lipoid urothelial carcinoma	Tumor cells with large or multiple clear cytoplasmic vacuoles that indent the nuclei
Clear cell urothelial carcinoma	Carcinoma cells with clear cytoplasm that resemble clear cell renal cell carcinoma
Urothelial carcinoma with trophoblastic differentiation	Three types: (1) HCG production of morphologically urothelial carcinoma, (2) admixed trophoblasts in urothelial carcinoma, and (3) pure choriocarcinoma of bladder
Lymphoepithelioma-like carcinoma	Syncytium of high-grade undifferentiated cells in dense background of mainly lymphoplasmacytic inflammatory cells
Sarcomatoid urothelial carcinoma	Carcinoma with high-grade spindle cells or malignant heterologous elements (e.g., rhabdomyosarcoma, osteosarcoma, chondrosarcoma)
Urothelial carcinoma with unusual stromal reaction	
Urothelial carcinoma with myxoid stroma and chordoid features	Abundant extracellular mucin and floating carcinoma cells exhibit varied patterns with no glandular differentiation
Undifferentiated urothelial carcinoma, osteoclast rich	Admixture of plump mononuclear cells and large multinucleated osteoclastic giant cells
Undifferentiated urothelial carcinoma	Undifferentiated carcinomas containing multinucleated anaplastic cells

HCG human chorionic gonadotropin

tation of this finding is important, especially in instances where metastatic disease develops that may contain a squamous morphology. In urothelial carcinoma with squamous differentiation, the differential diagnosis includes squamous cell carcinoma of the bladder. The latter is distinguished by the presence of a pure squamous morphology, irrespective of the in situ component present on the surface [5]. In biopsy or transurethral resection specimens, this distinction is difficult since the entire lesion may not be represented in the material submitted [6]. In such instances of incomplete tumor sampling, where an extensive squamous cell carcinoma component is present, a comment should be included with the report that states, "urothelial carcinoma with extensive squamous differentiation cannot be excluded with certainty. Analysis of the entire lesion it is

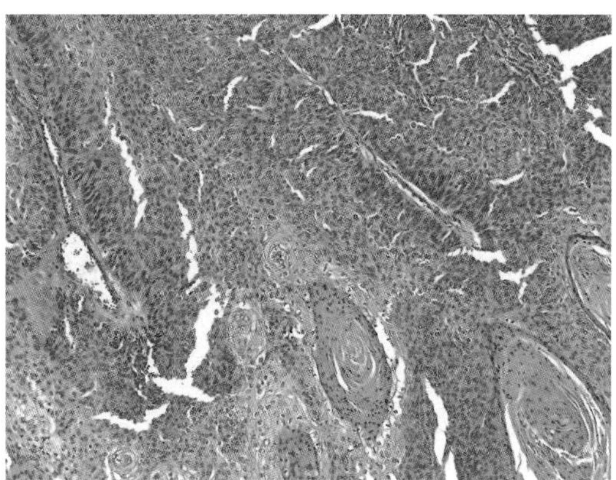

Fig. 15.1 Urothelial carcinoma with squamous differentiation including keratin pearl formation

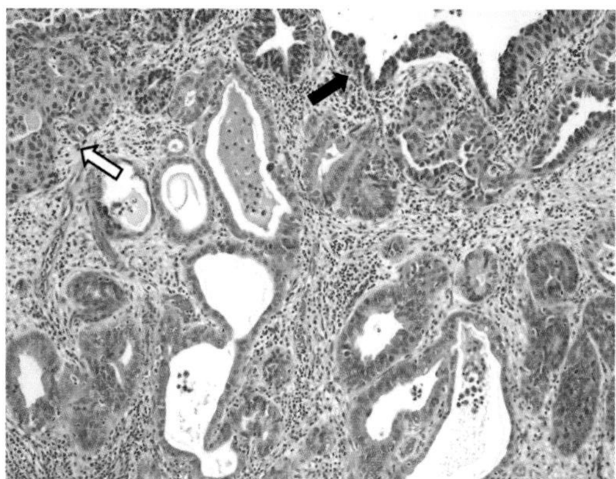

Fig. 15.2 Urothelial carcinoma with glandular differentiation. Note the presence of surface in situ (*dark arrow*) and invasive (*open arrow*) urothelial carcinoma. The malignant glands are lined by columnar cells

required to distinguish urothelial carcinoma with extensive squamous differentiation from pure squamous cell carcinoma of the bladder." Although no diagnostic markers are uniformly useful in distinguishing these two entities, several studies have evaluated markers that can aid in identifying such lesions as being primary to the bladder. Specifically, S100P, GATA3, uroplakin III, cytokeratin 14, and desmoglein-3 have been shown to have utility in many cases in identifying a squamous predominant urothelial lesion as being primary to the bladder [7, 8].

The diagnosis of urothelial carcinoma with glandular differentiation is slightly less problematic. In general, the adenocarcinoma components can show glandular, mucinous, or signet ring cell differentiation in the background of conventional urothelial carcinoma (Fig. 15.2). The primary differential diagnosis in this instance includes either direct spread of a colonic carcinoma or metastatic spread from an adenocarcinoma at a different anatomic location. When approaching this differential, the finding of an in situ component and/or conventional urothelial carcinoma component is helpful in suggesting the lesion is primary to the bladder. In cases in which there is extensive adenocarcinomatous differentiation, a comment should be included stating "we cannot definitely exclude secondary spread from a non-bladder adenocarcinoma, such as colon cancer. Clinical and radiographic assessment of the patient is required."

It remains somewhat unclear in the literature whether divergent differentiation suggests an overall worsened outcome for this patient population. In some studies, it has been suggested that correction for pathologic stage shows similar outcomes for conventional urothelial carcinoma and urothelial carcinoma with divergent differentiation whereas other studies suggest that patients with divergent differentiation have diminished outcomes [9–12]. Further patient-based studies that address this question are needed. A second clinical concern associated with urothelial carcinoma with divergent differentiation is response to therapy. Several studies have shown a reduced response to chemotherapy and radiation therapy; however, the relationship to morphology remains somewhat unclear [13, 14].

Deceptively Benign-Appearing Variants

Nested Urothelial Carcinoma

Archetypical for this group of innocuous-looking carcinomas is the nested variant, which at the surface closely resembles a benign von Brunn's nest proliferation [15–24]. Diagnosis of nested variant can be very difficult in superficial bladder specimens. Nested variant is uncommon,

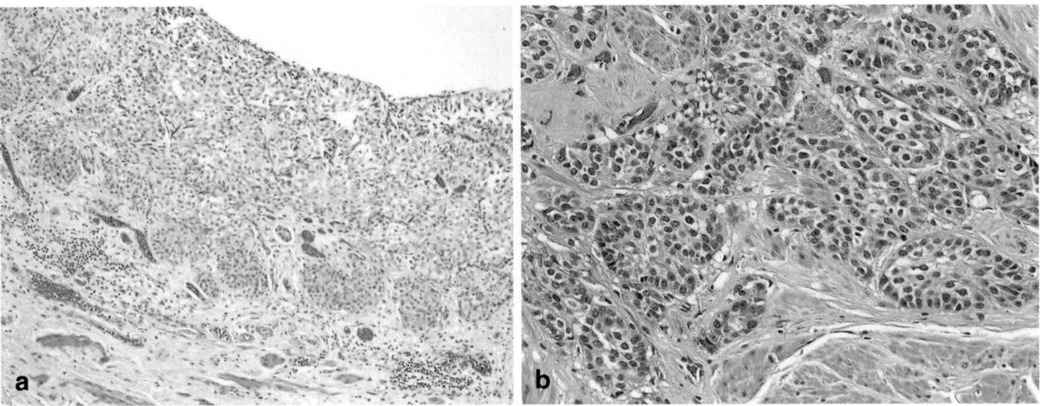

Fig. 15.3 Nested urothelial carcinoma (**a**) at the surface where it resembles von Brunn's nests proliferation and (**b**) invading the muscularis propria

encountered in 0.8–2.4 % of cancer cystectomies [16, 19]. The percentage of nested morphology for diagnosis has not been established, though some requires at least a 50 % component [16, 17]. Some tumors may be encountered as recurrence in patients with prior usual urothelial neoplasm. Most nested variant tumors present with a clinically recognizable bladder mass, of which about two thirds are locally aggressive [16].

Nested urothelial carcinoma is characterized by haphazardly infiltrating nests of bland-appearing urothelial cells that often extends deeply into the muscularis propria (Fig. 15.3a, b). The tumor cells have modest eosinophilic cytoplasm and predominantly show minimal atypia and indistinct nucleoli, although scattered atypical cells are invariably present. Mitoses are typically rare. The nests are usually solid, well delineated, tightly packed, and may show confluence or fusion. The tumor cells may also be arranged into cordlike or trabecular patterns. Occasionally, small lumina may form within the nests producing cysts that may contain eosinophilic secretions and resemble cystitis cystica. Less commonly, focal tubules are also formed intermingled with the infiltrating nests. These microcysts and tubules are similar to those seen in microcytic urothelial carcinoma and urothelial carcinoma with small tubules discussed below. The intervening stroma between the infiltrating tumor nests often shows absent or only minimal tissue reaction. Lymphovascular invasion is often encountered, which can be a helpful hint in the diagnosis. At the deeper aspect of invasion, some neoplastic cells may show greater degree of cytologic atypia exhibiting larger, more irregular and hyperchromatic nuclei. Nested urothelial carcinoma is often encountered admixed with conventional urothelial carcinoma, the latter identified in more than half of tumors with at least 50 % nested morphology [17]. At the surface, no in situ or papillary carcinoma are often identified, where a von Brunn's nest-like proliferation or ulceration is appreciated.

Poorer outcome in nested urothelial carcinoma is attributed to its tendency to high-stage presentation. Compared to conventional urothelial carcinoma, nested variant has a higher rate for locally aggressive disease and nodal involvement at 69–82 % and 19–57 %, respectively [16, 17]. However, when matched stage for stage, behavior of nested variant is not different from conventional urothelial carcinoma. A recent Mayo Clinic study showed a 10-year cancer-specific survival of 41 % for nested urothelial carcinoma versus 46 % for stage-matched conventional urothelial carcinoma [16].

The main differential diagnoses for nested urothelial carcinoma are florid von Brunn's nests and bladder paraganglioma. Morphologic similarities and differences between nested urothelial carcinoma and von Brunn's nests are summarized in Table 15.2. Proliferation markers such as Ki67 and other markers such as p53, p27, and

Table 15.2 Histological features of nested urothelial carcinoma and florid von Brunn's nests

	Nested urothelial carcinoma	Florid von Brunn's nests
Distribution	Haphazard	Orderly
Nests	Some tightly packed, confluent, or fused	Well spaced with regular boundary
Associated microcysts	May be present	May be present (i.e., cystitis cystica)
Associated well-differentiated glands	Absent	May be present (i.e., cystitis glandularis)
Surface in situ or papillary carcinoma	Uncommon	Absent
Cytologic atypia	Random atypia near surface and more conspicuous at deeper aspect	Absent
Muscularis propria invasion	Common	Absent

cytokeratin 20 are not helpful in discriminating these two tumors, except when Ki67 is markedly high (>15 %), which may occur albeit only in a minority of nested urothelial carcinoma and not in von Brunn's nests. Review of cystoscopy findings and close communication with urologists are crucial in the diagnosis of nested urothelial carcinoma, since most tumors present with a clinically appreciable mass concerning for cancer irreconcilable to a von Brunn's nests consideration.

The "zellballen" pattern of bladder paraganglioma mimics the infiltrating nests of nested urothelial carcinoma. Knowledge of clinical information is important, since paraganglioma tends to occur in a wider age range including patients younger than the ones typically affected by urothelial carcinoma, and presents with micturition-associated hypertension, headache, or dizziness. Bladder paragangliomas are often centered deep in the muscularis propria and may not involve the surface (bottom-heavy). Bladder paraganglioma expresses the neuroendocrine markers synaptophysin, chromogranin and CD56, and the intratumoral sustentacular cells can be highlighted by S100.

Large Nested Urothelial Carcinoma

Large nested urothelial carcinoma is characterized by medium-to-large invasive nests with pushing border akin to that of a verrucous carcinoma (Fig. 15.4). A series of 23 cases was reported from John Hopkins Hospital in patients 39–89 years old who were mostly men [25]. Similar to nested urothelial carcinoma, this variant is mainly composed of urothelial cells that lack significant cytologic atypia. Likewise, the tumor nests may also form focal cysts and tubules. Unlike nested urothelial carcinoma, the invasive nests are larger, usually connected to the surface, and separated by intervening stroma; lymphovascular invasion is not common. In addition, a surface papillary urothelial neoplasm component is more often present, seen in 83 % of tumors. The significance of this morphology in terms of tumor biology and behavior is still unclear. Most reported cases were diagnosed with (at least) deep muscle-invasive disease, suggesting similar behavior to nested urothelial carcinoma. The differential diagnosis includes von Brunn's nests and inverted papillary urothelial carcinoma. Unlike von Brunn's nests and inverted papillary urothelial carcinoma, large nested urothelial carcinoma has more variable and irregular nests, have

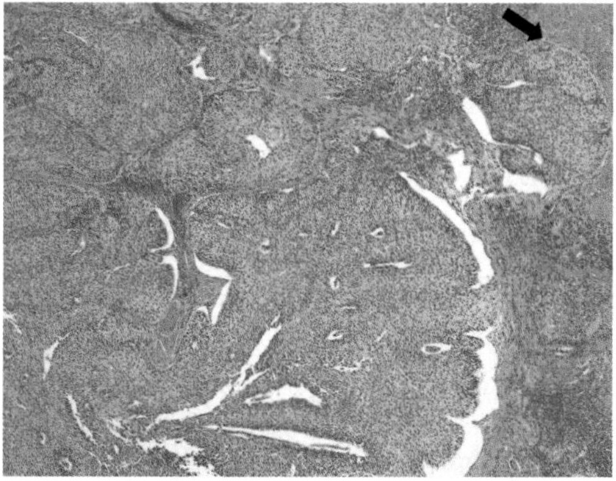

Fig. 15.4 Large nested urothelial carcinoma exhibiting broad front infiltration with involvement of muscularis propria (*arrow*)

intervening stromal reaction, and may extend deep into the muscularis propria. Presence of a surface papillary neoplasm component is helpful to distinguish it from von Brunn's nests.

Microcystic Urothelial Carcinoma

This variant is composed of invasive small and large cysts of bland-appearing cells that closely resemble cystitis cystica (Fig. 15.5) [26–30]. As mentioned above, similar cysts are sometimes seen focally in nested and large nested urothelial carcinomas. There is no established cut-off for the proportion of cysts necessary for the diagnosis. Some authors have proposed at least 25 % cysts formations [31]. The cysts can be small or large (1–2 mm) comprised of transitional cells and occasional flattened cells. Focal mucinous cell change has also been described. Columnar cells are typically not present. The lumens of the microcysts are often filled with eosinophilic secretions or necrotic cellular debris. Behavior of this variant is not known, and probably is similar to nested urothelial carcinoma. Microcystic urothelial carcinoma can be distinguished from cystitis cystica by its more haphazard, variable, and irregular nests, and extension into the muscularis propria.

Urothelial Carcinoma with Small Tubules

Similar to cysts, small tubular or acinar formations may be present focally in nested and large nested urothelial carcinomas (Fig. 15.6). When the invasive tubules predominate, diagnosis of urothelial carcinoma with small tubules is rendered. This variant is very rare with less than a dozen cases reported [26, 32]. The tubules are composed mainly of bland-appearing cuboidal cells with random pleomorphism, similar to nested urothelial carcinoma. Tall columnar cells are generally not appreciated in these tubules. The tubules infiltrate haphazardly and often invade into the muscularis propria. The clinical significance of this variant is unknown, and probably is similar to nested urothelial carcinoma.

The main differential diagnoses of urothelial carcinoma with small tubules include tubules of nephrogenic adenoma, cystitis glandularis, Gleason grade 3 prostatic adenocarcinoma, and primary bladder adenocarcinoma. Careful search for non-tubular urothelial carcinoma component is helpful to distinguish from nephrogenic adenoma and prostate adenocarcinoma. Nephrogenic adenoma is typically superficial and usually has a surface papillary component lined by a single layer of cuboidal, flat, or hobnail cells. The diagnosis of nephrogenic adenoma can be confirmed by Pax2, Pax8, and S100P positivity, and negativity for GATA3 or p63. Prostate

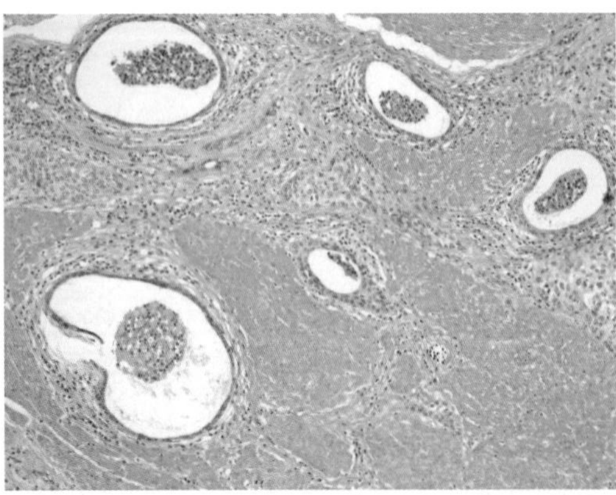

Fig. 15.5 Microcystic urothelial carcinoma invading muscularis propria

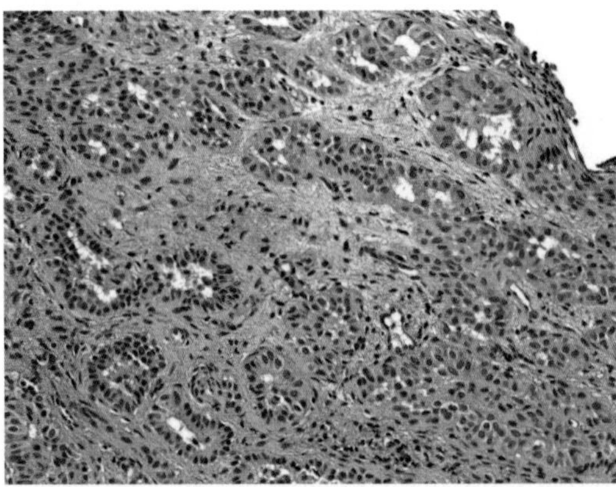

Fig. 15.6 Nested urothelial carcinoma with focal tubular formation

adenocarcinoma can be confirmed by PSA, PAP, NKX3.1, or PSMA positivity. Both cystitis glandularis and primary adenocarcinoma are lined by taller columnar cells and may show Goblet cell or mucinous change. Adenocarcinoma exhibits greater degree of cytologic atypia than urothelial carcinoma with small tubules.

Micropapillary Urothelial Carcinoma

Micropapillary urothelial carcinoma has received significant attention in recent years due to both distinctive pathology features as well as aggressive biologic behavior. Whereas, micropapillary urothelial carcinoma has anecdotally been considered to present at higher pathological stage, a recent study from MD Anderson has confirmed the importance of this clinical diagnosis, reported on the aggressive nature of this variant, and suggested early therapy (radical cystectomy) to be critical to improve patient outcomes [33].

Micropapillary urothelial carcinoma shares morphologic features with micropapillary carcinomas from other sites [34–36]. Specifically, the neoplastic cells form small tight clusters lacking a central fibrovascular core, with the nuclei of the tumor cells polarized to the exterior surface of the clusters (Fig. 15.7a, b). Surrounding the tumor cells is a prominent retraction artifact that gives the appearance of small epithelial nests floating in empty spaces. An in situ variant of micropapillary urothelial carcinoma has been reported, which has been described as thin, filiform exophytic processes on the bladder surface that may be highly branched and glomeruloid on cross section. Despite a relatively clear-cut definition, one recent study has shown that there is significant interobserver variability in the diagnosis of this entity [37]. Although not standard practice at many locations, some studies have shown that the extent of micropapillary urothelial carcinoma present in the background of an otherwise conventional urothelial carcinoma may have prognostic significance; however, this finding varies across studies [38, 39]. Based on these findings, the current convention holds that micropapillary differentiation should be reported regardless of the percentage of this variant present in the tumor [38].

It is important in biopsy and transurethral resection specimens to carefully assess for depth of tumor invasion, as published reports have demonstrated that many of these carcinomas are muscle-invasive (pT2) at the time of diagnosis [34, 38]. Thus, it is critical to report when muscularis propria (detrusor muscle) is absent in the specimen; in such cases, a comment that states "micropapillary urothelial carcinoma may commonly invade the muscularis propria; additional sampling to evaluate muscle invasion is recommended" should be included. In addition, many of these tumors show angiolymphatic invasion that should also be documented in the final pathology report [34].

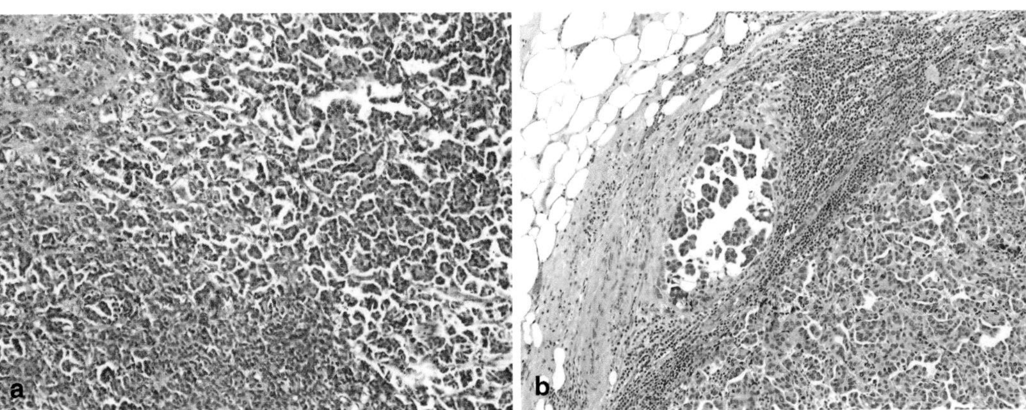

Fig. 15.7 Micropapillary urothelial carcinoma (**a**) shows small tight clusters of urothelial carcinoma cells in retraction spaces. **b** Lymph node metastasis retains the micropapillary architecture

The major differential diagnoses for this variant includes urothelial carcinoma with extensive retraction artifact and metastatic carcinoma with micropapillary morphology, such as papillary serous carcinoma of the ovary. In the latter instance, positive immunohistochemistry for uroplakin and CK20 may aid in the final diagnosis, especially when correlated with patient history and imaging [40]. Additional ancillary tests, including MUC1, HER2, and CA125, have been studied in micropapillary urothelial carcinoma; however, these markers may not reliably distinguish all micropapillary urothelial carcinomas from conventional urothelial carcinoma with extensive retraction artifact [41, 42].

A diagnosis of micropapillary urothelial carcinoma generally denotes that the tumor will behave aggressively. This is supported by the study from MD Anderson that showed that not only does this tumor type respond less well to Bacillus Calmette-Guerin (BCG) and chemotherapy, but that 67% of patients had progression with 22% of patients developing metastatic disease [43]. Based on this study, many sites now advocate for early cystectomy in patients with micropapillary urothelial carcinoma. However, according to a recent study from Memorial Sloan-Kettering Cancer Center a subset of patients with cT1 micropapillary urothelial carcinoma managed conservatively were not found to have significantly worse outcomes compared to patients undergoing early radical cystectomy [44]. It is clear that, based on the inherent challenges in the diagnosis of this entity, further collaborative efforts and research into identifying objective markers for diagnosis are needed.

Plasmacytoid Urothelial Carcinoma

This variant has an unusual composition of infiltrative discohesive cells with eccentrically placed nucleus that resemble plasma cells and poorly differentiated carcinomas [45–55]. The complexity in diagnosis is confounded by their immunopositivity to the usual plasma cell marker CD138. Reported prevalence of this tumor is about 1% among high-grade urothelial carcinomas and

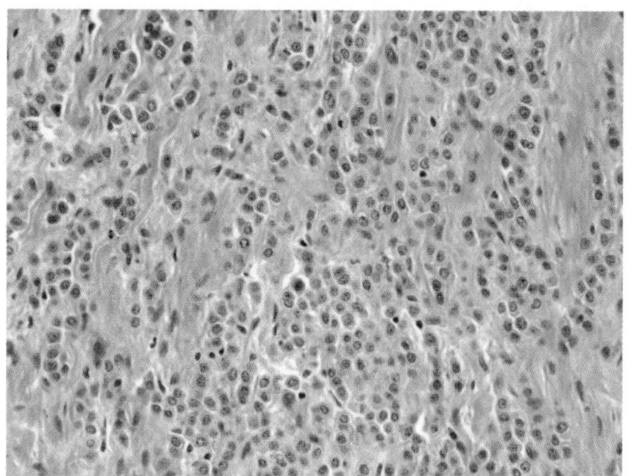

Fig. 15.8 Plasmacytoid urothelial carcinoma

2.7–3.0% of muscle-invasive urothelial carcinomas [53–55]. The tumor may present purely with plasmacytoid morphology, although more often, it is encountered admixed with high-grade conventional urothelial carcinoma. The amount of plasmacytoid morphology varies in published series, with most reports using a 30 or 50% cut-off [45, 47, 50–52].

Although a discrete bladder mass can often be cystoscopically detected, this tumor can also diffusely infiltrate and thicken the bladder wall in a linitis plastica-like manner. The tumor infiltrates the bladder as cords, small nests, or sheet-like growths (Fig. 15.8). Infiltrative cells may also be in a single cell pattern reminiscent of invasive lobular carcinoma of the breast. The tumor cells contain modest to abundant amphophilic to eosinophilic cytoplasm, with low- to intermediate-grade nuclei distinctively displaced to one side. Overall, there is some degree of monotony of the tumor cell infiltrates. Occasionally, intracytoplasmic mucin may be focally present and may loosely resemble signet ring cells [50]. The background stroma often appears edematous or myxoid.

Interestingly, one study showed that FGFR3 and PIK3CA mutations, common in invasive urothelial carcinoma that arises from papillary neoplasm, are not detected in plasmacytoid variant [46]. Unlike conventional urothelial carcinoma, E-cadherin expression is often completely lost in plasmacytoid variant including its concomitant conventional type [46].

Most plasmacytoid urothelial carcinoma presents at a higher stage. A study from MD Anderson reported 85 % of patients with at least muscularis propria invasion and 48 % with metastasis or locally unresectable tumors [47]. The high-stage presentation translates to a poor outcome with a reported median survival of only 17.7 months. Local spread and recurrence is rather unique among urothelial carcinomas where it occurs most commonly in serosal surface including the peritoneum, where it may present as carcinomatosis [47, 48]. Survival of patients with metastatic disease is poor despite of chemotherapy.

The main differential diagnosis for plasmacytoid urothelial carcinoma includes chronic cystitis (or inflammation), plasma cell neoplasm, metastatic poorly differentiated carcinomas, particularly gastric signet ring cell carcinoma and lobular carcinoma of the breast, and primary bladder signet ring cell adenocarcinoma. Diagnosis can be challenging at metastatic sites. Although the plasmacytoid variant is frequently CD138 positive, it does not exhibit kappa or lambda restriction. Keratin AE1/AE3, CK7, or CK20 expression helps distinguish plasmacytoid urothelial carcinoma from hematopoietic cells. It is highly unusual for gastric and breast carcinomas to present as an isolated finding in the urinary tract; when encountered, they are usually part of a widely disseminated disease. The presence of admixed conventional urothelial carcinoma, including the surface in situ component, is helpful in establishing the diagnosis of plasmacytoid urothelial carcinoma. Plasmacytoid variant expresses the urothelial-associated marker GATA3, which may help in the differential diagnosis [49]. Primary signet ring cell adenocarcinoma exhibits predominance of tumor cells with intracytoplasmic mucin, which is only focally present in plasmacytoid urothelial carcinoma.

Urothelial Carcinoma with Rhabdoid Features

This exceedingly rare morphology typically occurs in association with poorly differentiated urothelial carcinomas. Rare examples of "pure" malignant rhabdoid tumors of the bladder have been described in pediatric patients [56–59]. In adults, the only series reported four cases in the bladder of men ages 53–86 years [60]. Rhabdoid morphology comprised at least 60 % of the tumors that also had an in situ or papillary urothelial carcinoma component [60]. The rhabdoid cells are discohesive, infiltrate as single cells, small nests, or diffuse sheets (Fig. 15.9). The tumor cells are plump oval to round with abundant cytoplasm containing intracytoplasmic inclusion that displaces the nucleus. The nuclei are large with vesicular chromatin and prominent nucleoli. High-grade undifferentiated morphology such as small cell and sarcomatoid carcinoma may coexist. Keratin expression (dot-like or diffuse) and negativity for myogenic markers such as desmin, myoD1, or myogenin help establish the epithelial lineage. Ultrastructurally, the cytoplasmic inclusion was shown to be whorls of intermediate filament. In non-vesical carcinomas, the presence of rhabdoid morphology has been associated with poor outcome. The few reported cases of urothelial carcinoma with rhabdoid features suggest an aggressive behavior.

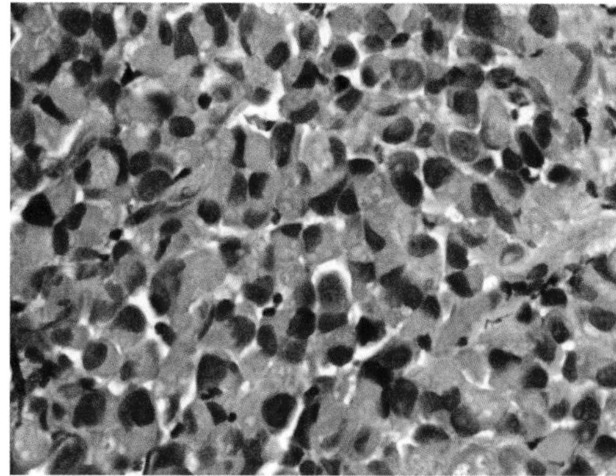

Fig. 15.9 Urothelial carcinoma with rhabdoid features

Lipoid (Lipid-Rich) Urothelial Carcinoma

This variant is characterized by presence of large cells containing large or multiple clear vacuoles that indent the nucleus to resemble lipoblasts or

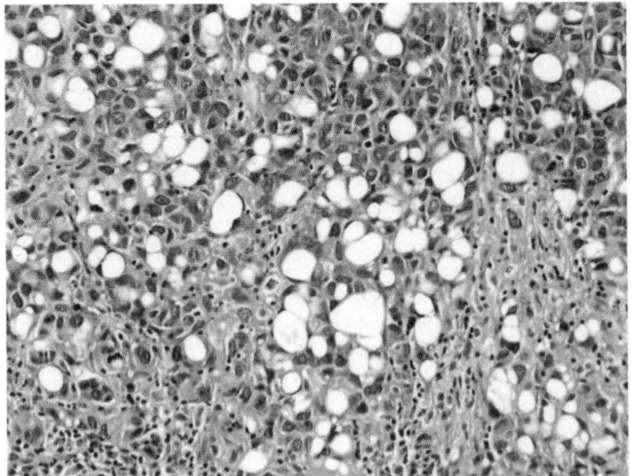

Fig. 15.10 Lipid-rich urothelial carcinoma

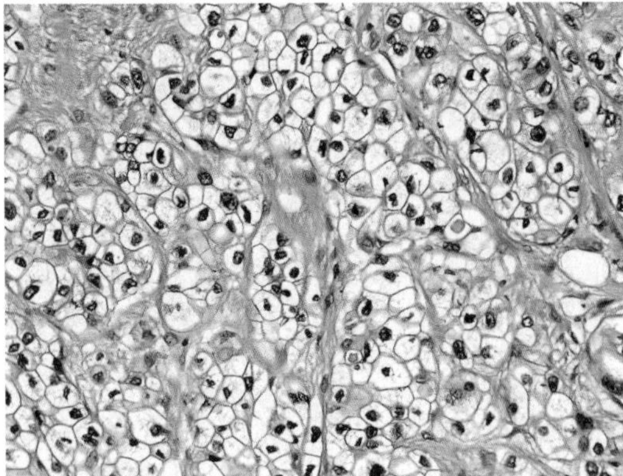

Fig. 15.11 Clear cell urothelial carcinoma

signet ring cells (Fig. 15.10). There are about 35 examples of this variant reported in the literature [61–65]. Almost always, the lipoid carcinoma is admixed with conventional or other variants of urothelial carcinoma. The lipoid cells comprise 10–50 % of the tumor. The overall tumor growth architecture on low-power magnification is similar to conventional urothelial carcinoma. The lipoid cells nuclei show moderate and occasional pleomorphism. The cytoplasmic vacuoles are optically clear and have been shown to have no mucin content. The immunoprofile is similar to that of conventional urothelial carcinoma. Most patients present with higher stage disease, which contributes to a poorer outcome. In a multi-institutional study of 27 cases, 89 % of lipoid urothelial carcinomas were at least deep muscle invasive, 45 % had lymph node metastasis, and 60 % died of disease within 58 months [62].

Clear Cell (Glycogen-Rich) Urothelial Carcinoma

Urothelial carcinoma may contain tumor cells with clear cytoplasm, and very rarely when these cells type predominate, the tumor is considered as clear cell urothelial carcinoma. This carcinoma is exceedingly rare with less than ten cases reported in the bladder [66–70]. The neoplastic cells are large with clear cytoplasm and prominent cell border (Fig. 15.11). The tumor may also exhibit an alveolar growth reminiscent of clear cell renal cell carcinoma. The immunophenotype is similar to conventional urothelial carcinoma and includes expression of the urothelial-associated marker GATA3 [67]. The significance of this variant in terms of behavior is still unclear.

Lymphoepithelioma-Like Carcinoma

Lymphoepithelioma-like carcinoma is a rare variant of urothelial carcinoma, with the largest published series representing 30 cases [71–75]. This variant of urothelial carcinoma demonstrates a distinctive appearance, highlighted by the presence of syncytial nests of carcinoma cells with large vesicular nuclei. The tumor cells are often masked by a dense inflammatory infiltrates consisting of lymphocytes, plasma cells, eosinophils, and occasionally macrophages (Fig. 15.12a, b). Lymphoepithelioma-like carcinoma has been reported in both the bladder as well as the upper urinary tract [76]. Lymphoepithelioma-like carcinoma may be present in pure form or admixed with other elements, including conventional urothelial carcinoma, adenocarcinoma, or squamous cell carcinoma [71, 73].

The primary diagnostic challenge with lymphoepithelioma-like carcinoma is recognizing carcinoma cells in a background of dense inflammation. In this context, immunohistochemical stains for cytokeratins can aid in the diagnosis. In addition, although this variant shares morphologic similarities with Epstein–Barr virus (EBV)

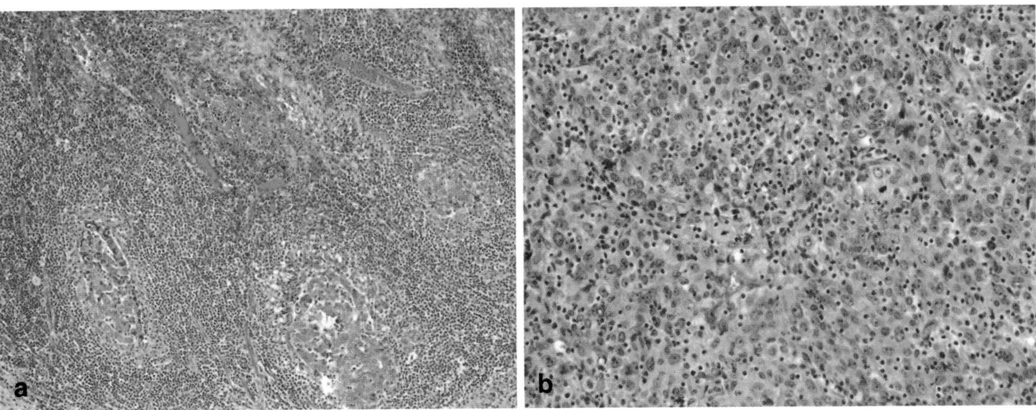

Fig. 15.12 Lymphoepithelioma-like carcinoma (**a**) composed of syncytium of poorly differentiated carcinoma within a dense inflammatory background. **b** Carcinoma cells are high grade with large nuclei and nucleolomegaly

associated carcinoma of the nasopharyngeal tract, the carcinomas arising in the urinary tract are negative for EBV [77, 78].

Although the series reported in the literature are relatively small, it has been suggested that for patients with pure lymphoepithelioma-like carcinoma, the prognosis is more favorable than for patients that have mixed forms of the disease [71, 75]. However, other studies suggest similar outcomes of either pure or mixed lymphoepithelioma-like carcinoma to conventional urothelial carcinoma [73].

Sarcomatoid Urothelial Carcinoma

Sarcomatoid urothelial carcinoma (formerly called carcinosarcoma) is an extremely rare but aggressive variant of urothelial carcinoma. This variant is morphologically defined by the presence of variable amounts of malignant spindled cells that can morphologically mimic a sarcoma (Fig. 15.13) [79]. In many instances, a malignant epithelial component may be identified that can include urothelial carcinoma, squamous cell carcinoma, or other variant morphologies [80, 81]. Occasionally, an in situ component may be present in association with these lesions.

The major category of differential diagnosis of sarcomatoid carcinoma includes malignant mesenchymal neoplasms. This is especially relevant, as sarcomatoid carcinoma can mimic a variety of spindle cell lesions including leiomyosarcoma, angiosarcoma, and malignant fibrous histiocytoma-like lesions among others [81]. Heterologous elements may occasionally be present, such as malignant skeletal muscle (rhabdomyosarcoma), bone (osteosarcoma), cartilage (chondrosarcoma), and others. The diagnosis of sarcomatoid urothelial carcinoma is especially relevant when the tumor lacks clear-cut epithelial differentiation and/or an in situ component. In such cases, immunohistochemistry for pancytokeratin, high molecular weight cytokeratins, and p63 can support the diagnosis of sarcomatoid urothelial carcinoma, although often staining for these markers may be focal [82, 83].

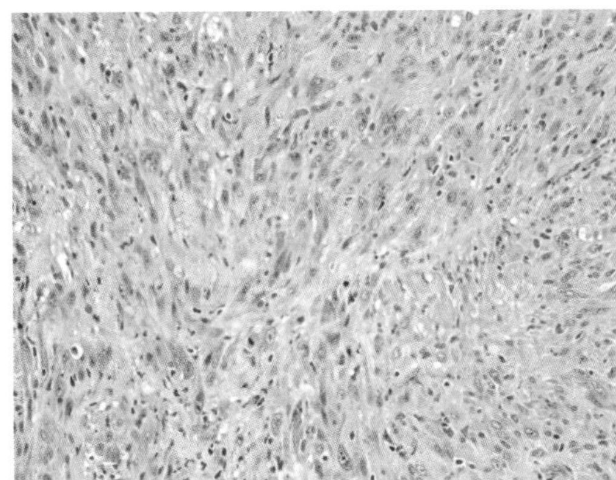

Fig. 15.13 Spindle cell sarcomatoid urothelial carcinoma invading muscularis propria

The outcome for patients with sarcomatoid urothelial carcinoma is poor. Overall survival reported in the literature for this variant was worse than urothelial carcinoma, with some studies reporting a 5-year overall survival of only 17% [84, 85].

Undifferentiated Urothelial Carcinoma with Trophoblastic Differentiation

Trophoblastic differentiation in urothelial carcinoma may occur in three scenarios: (1) by ectopic production of β-human chorionic gonadotropin (β-HCG) of usual urothelial carcinoma [86–93], (2) presence of mixed trophoblastic cells within urothelial carcinoma [86, 94–98], or (3) as rare "pure" choriocarcinoma of the bladder [99–102]. β-HCG production can be detected by immunostaining in urothelial carcinoma or by assays of serum or urine β-HCG level. Positivity to β-HCG was reported in 12–38% of urothelial carcinoma [86–89]. The trophoblastic cells can be syncytiotrophoblasts interspersed among usual urothelial carcinoma cells or as mixed syncytiotrophoblasts and cytotrophoblasts in distinct choriocarcinomatous foci. These neoplastic trophoblasts are thought to arise from metaplastic urothelial cells. This is supported by the fact that these carcinomas develop in the usual older adult age of urothelial carcinoma (rather than younger age of germ cell tumors), syncytiotrophoblasts are intimately admixed with urothelial carcinoma cells, β-HCG positivity is also present in urothelial carcinoma cells, and that bladder choriocarcinoma also occurs with prior urothelial carcinoma. β-HCG is suggested to have an anti-apoptotic effect that may lead to cell proliferation [103]. Interestingly, one report detected isochromosome 12p in pure choriocarcinoma of the bladder, an alteration common in postpubertal germ cell tumors [102].

Most bladder cancers with trophoblastic differentiation present with hematuria; however, some patients may have gynecomastia. Grossly, presence of choriocarcinoma correlates to a hemorrhagic and necrotic tumor. With immunostaining of urothelial carcinomas, β-HCG has propensity to stain the most undifferentiated and pleomorphic areas, although it may also stain usual urothelial carcinoma cells. β-HCG expression also tends to localize at the periphery or forefront of tumor growth. Syncytiotrophoblasts when present are usually randomly distributed among urothelial carcinoma cells. Syncytiotrophoblasts are large multinucleated cells with abundant dense eosinophilic cytoplasm and dark smudgy nuclear chromatin. Other types of giant cells may be present in urothelial carcinoma, but only true syncytiotroblasts are β-HCG positive.

It has been shown that tumors with trophoblastic elements have a poorer outcome, and that β-HCG production correlates with stage and grade [86, 87, 90, 92]. β-HCG positivity is much more common in high-grade urothelial carcinomas, whereas expression is low or absent in low-grade urothelial carcinomas [86, 90]. By stage, β-HCG expression is seen in 63% of muscle-invasive or higher stage tumors and only 24% of noninvasive papillary tumors [87]. β-HCG positivity correlates with greater propensity for metastasis and poorer survival. β-HCG expression was also shown to correlate with poor response to radiotherapy (76% positive), although this was not confirmed by a multivariate analysis [104].

Undifferentiated Urothelial Carcinoma (Including Giant Cell Carcinoma)

This variant of urothelial carcinoma encompasses a broad category that generally includes otherwise unclassifiable types of urothelial carcinoma. The classic definition describes sheets or individual undifferentiated and/or pleomorphic carcinoma cells that do not otherwise fit into conventional categories of bladder cancer or its variants [105, 106]. Included in this category are otherwise undifferentiated tumors that contain multinucleated anaplastic tumor cells with abundant cytoplasm and prominent nucleoli. Tumors may be present in sheets with cells containing prominent cell borders, as well as individual infiltrating cells. Often, an association with conventional urothelial carcinoma or other bladder cancer variants can be identified in the specimen. The most challenging differential diagnosis comes in instances of metastatic disease where only the undifferentiated component is present. In these cases, positive immunohistochemical stains for cytokeratins, thrombomodulin, and uroplakin III, as well as a correlation with a prior bladder cancer histology, can aid in the diagnosis [105, 106].

In general, this variant of urothelial carcinoma is extraordinarily rare, with the largest series consisting of eight cases. All patients reported in the literature demonstrated at least pT3 disease with over 75 % of patients showing lymph node metastasis [105]. It has been reported that up to 75 % of patients diagnosed with this variant will die of disease within approximately 2 years of diagnosis [105, 106].

Urothelial Carcinoma with Myxoid Stroma and Chordoid Features

Urothelial carcinoma may contain abundant extracellular mucin in the absence of glandular differentiation. This morphology is rare with less than 30 cases reported [107–109]. The extracellular mucin is typically associated with tumor cells often arranged in cord-like manner, or as microcysts and small aggregates (Fig. 15.14). The morphology is somewhat reminiscent of extraskeletal myxoid chondrosarcoma, chordoma, or myxomatous yolk sac tumor. The tumor cells in the myxoid areas have "low-grade" cytology and low mitotic count. No intracytoplasmic mucin or glandular differentiation is present. Admixed conventional urothelial carcinoma including surface papillary carcinoma or in situ carcinoma, at least focally, is common. Other morphologies such as micropapillary carcinoma, squamous differentiation, lymphoepithelioma-like carcinoma, and sarcomatoid carcinoma may occur. The immunostaining pattern is similar to conventional urothelial carcinoma including CK7 and p63 positivity. The mucinous material is positive for colloidal iron and Alcian blue and is PAS negative [107].

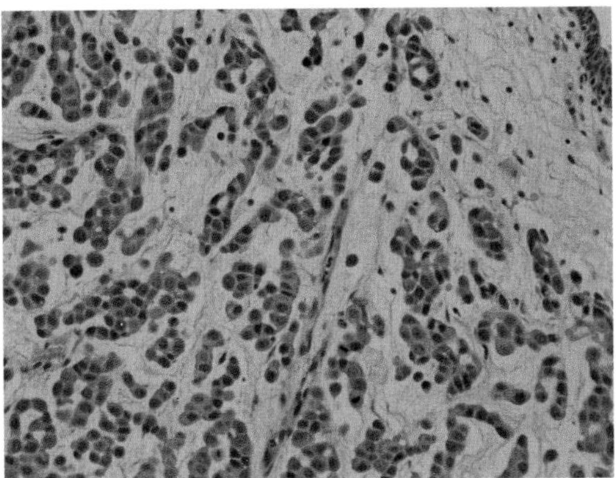

Fig. 15.14 Urothelial carcinoma with myxoid stroma and chordoid features

Most of the cases reported present with high-stage disease: more than 90 % are (at least) muscle invasive and 75 % have already metastasized to lymph nodes [107]. Prognosis is poor and can be attributed to the high-stage presentation. The main differential diagnosis is mucinous adenocarcinoma, which unlike urothelial carcinoma with myxoid stroma shows obvious intracellular mucin and glandular differentiation including positivity for CDX2 and negativity for p63. Myxoid cystitis may have chordoid lymphocytes and mimic urothelial carcinoma with abundant myxoid stroma. Myxoid cystitis, however, contains infiltrates of B-lymphocytes with regular round nuclei admixed with other polymorphous inflammatory cells [110].

Undifferentiated Urothelial Carcinoma, Osteoclast Rich

This unusual morphology in urothelial carcinoma is very rare with less than a hand full of cases reported in elderly male 67–88 years of age [111, 112]. The tumor exhibits a solid infiltrative growth of mononuclear cells with evenly distributed osteoclast giant cells (Fig. 15.15). The mononuclear cells are plump with ovoid to round nuclei, vesicular chromatin, and most with mild atypia. Focal spindling of mononuclear cells may occur. Mitosis is brisk ranging from 5 to 25 per 10 high power fields with occasional atypical mitosis. The proportion of mononuclear cells and osteoclasts varies. The osteoclastic giant cells

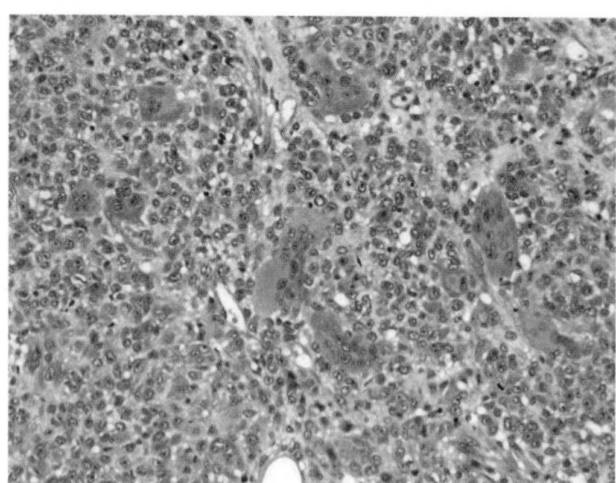

Fig. 15.15 Undifferentiated urothelial carcinoma with osteoclastic giant cells

have abundant dense eosinophilic cytoplasm and nuclei can be plentiful reaching up to 50 per cell. Giant cells have phagocytic features and may contain hemosiderin, erythrocytes, and cellular debris. The tumor is richly vascularized and often with areas of hemorrhage. Aggregates of giant cells can be seen around hemorrhage. The surface urothelium may show in situ and/or papillary urothelial carcinoma, helpful in establishing a diagnosis as primary tumor. The osteoclasts are positive for CD51, CD54, leucocyte common antigen (LCA), and CD68. The biologic significance of this morphology is still unclear.

References

1. Eble JN, Sauter G, Epstein JI, Sesterhenn IA, editors. Pathology and genetics of tumours of the urinary system and male genital organs. Lyon: IARC Press; 2004.
2. Amin MB. Histological variants of urothelial carcinoma: diagnostic, therapeutic and prognostic implications. Mod Pathol. 2009;22(Suppl 2):S96–118.
3. Lopez-Beltran A, Requena MJ, Cheng L, Montironi R. Pathological variants of invasive bladder cancer according to their suggested clinical significance. BJU Int. 2008;101(3):275–81.
4. Bladder Cancer. 2nd international consultation on bladder cancer—Vienna. Vienna: EDITIONS 21; 2012.
5. Lagwinski N, Thomas A, Stephenson AJ, Campbell S, Hoschar AP, El-Gabry E, et al. Squamous cell carcinoma of the bladder: a clinicopathologic analysis of 45 cases. Am J Surg Pathol. 2007;31(12):1777–87.
6. Abd El-Latif A, Watts KE, Elson P, Fergany A, Hansel DE. The sensitivity of initial transurethral resection or biopsy of bladder tumor(s) for detecting bladder cancer variants on radical cystectomy. J Urol. 2013;189(4):1263–7.
7. Gulmann C, Paner GP, Parakh RS, Hansel DE, Shen SS, Ro JY, et al. Immunohistochemical profile to distinguish urothelial from squamous differentiation in carcinomas of urothelial tract. Hum Pathol. 2013;44(2):164–72.
8. Gruver AM, Amin MB, Luthringer DJ, Westfall D, Arora K, Farver CF, et al. Selective immunohistochemical markers to distinguish between metastatic high-grade urothelial carcinoma and primary poorly differentiated invasive squamous cell carcinoma of the lung. Arch Pathol Lab Med. 2012;136(11):1339–46.
9. Antunes AA, Nesrallah LJ, Dall'Oglio MF, Maluf CE, Camara C, Leite KR, et al. The role of squamous differentiation in patients with transitional cell carcinoma of the bladder treated with radical cystectomy. Int Braz J Urol. 2007;33(3):339–45; discussion 46.
10. Rogers CG, Palapattu GS, Shariat SF, Karakiewicz PI, Bastian PJ, Lotan Y, et al. Clinical outcomes following radical cystectomy for primary nontransitional cell carcinoma of the bladder compared to transitional cell carcinoma of the bladder. J Urol. 2006;175(6):2048–53; discussion 53.
11. Martin JE, Jenkins BJ, Zuk RJ, Blandy JP, Baithun SI. Clinical importance of squamous metaplasia in invasive transitional cell carcinoma of the bladder. J Clin Pathol. 1989;42(3):250–3.
12. Black PC, Brown GA, Dinney CP. The impact of variant histology on the outcome of bladder cancer treated with curative intent. Urol Oncol. 2009;27(1):3–7.
13. Scosyrev E, Ely BW, Messing EM, Speights VO, Grossman HB, Wood DP, et al. Do mixed histological features affect survival benefit from neoadjuvant platinum-based combination chemotherapy in patients with locally advanced bladder cancer? A secondary analysis of Southwest oncology group-directed intergroup study (S8710). BJU Int. 2011;108(5):693–9.
14. Logothetis CJ, Dexeus FH, Chong C, Sella A, Ayala AG, Ro JY, et al. Cisplatin, cyclophosphamide and doxorubicin chemotherapy for unresectable urothelial tumors: the M.D. Anderson experience. J Urol. 1989;141(1):33–7.
15. Lin O, Cardillo M, Dalbagni G, Linkov I, Hutchinson B, Reuter VE. Nested variant of urothelial carcinoma: a clinicopathologic and immunohistochemical study of 12 cases. Mod Pathol. 2003;16(12):1289–98.
16. Linder BJ, Frank I, Cheville JC, Thompson RH, Thapa P, Tarrell RF, et al. Outcomes following radical cystectomy for nested variant of urothelial carcinoma: a matched cohort analysis. J Urol. 2013;189(5):1670–5.
17. Wasco MJ, Daignault S, Bradley D, Shah RB. Nested variant of urothelial carcinoma: a clinicopathologic and immunohistochemical study of 30 pure and mixed cases. Hum Pathol. 2010;41(2):163–71.

18. Volmar KE, Chan TY, De Marzo AM, Epstein JI. Florid von Brunn nests mimicking urothelial carcinoma: a morphologic and immunohistochemical comparison to the nested variant of urothelial carcinoma. Am J Surg Pathol. 2003;27(9):1243–52.
19. Holmang S, Johansson SL. The nested variant of transitional cell carcinoma—a rare neoplasm with poor prognosis. Scand J Urol Nephrol. 2001;35(2):102–5.
20. Drew PA, Furman J, Civantos F, Murphy WM. The nested variant of transitional cell carcinoma: an aggressive neoplasm with innocuous histology. Mod Pathol. 1996;9(10):989–94.
21. Dhall D, Al-Ahmadie H, Olgac S. Nested variant of urothelial carcinoma. Arch Pathol Lab Med. 2007;131(11):1725–7.
22. Liedberg F, Chebil G, Davidsson T, Gadaleanu V, Grabe M, Mansson W. The nested variant of urothelial carcinoma: a rare but important bladder neoplasm with aggressive behavior. Three case reports and a review of the literature. Urol Oncol. 2003;21(1):7–9.
23. Xiao GQ, Savage SJ, Gribetz ME, Burstein DE, Miller LK, Unger PD. The nested variant of urothelial carcinoma: clinicopathology of 2 cases. Arch Pathol Lab Med. 2003;127(8):e333–6.
24. Talbert ML, Young RH. Carcinomas of the urinary bladder with deceptively benign-appearing foci. A report of three cases. Am J Surg Pathol. 1989;13(5):374–81.
25. Cox R, Epstein JI. Large nested variant of urothelial carcinoma: 23 cases mimicking von Brunn nests and inverted growth pattern of noninvasive papillary urothelial carcinoma. Am J Surg Pathol. 2011;35(9):1337–42.
26. Young RH, Oliva E. Transitional cell carcinomas of the urinary bladder that may be underdiagnosed. A report of four invasive cases exemplifying the homology between neoplastic and non-neoplastic transitional cell lesions. Am J Surg Pathol. 1996;20(12):1448–54.
27. Sari A, Uyaroglu MA, Ermete M, Oder M, Girgin C, Dincer C. Microcystic urothelial carcinoma of the urinary bladder metastatic to the penis. Pathol Oncol Res. 2007;13(2):170–3.
28. Leroy X, Leteurtre E, De La Taille A, Augusto D, Biserte J, Gosselin B. Microcystic transitional cell carcinoma: a report of 2 cases arising in the renal pelvis. Arch Pathol Lab Med. 2002;126(7):859–61.
29. Paz A, Rath-Wolfson L, Lask D, Koren R, Manes A, Mukamel E, et al. The clinical and histological features of transitional cell carcinoma of the bladder with microcysts: analysis of 12 cases. Br J Urol. 1997;79(5):722–5.
30. Young RH, Zukerberg LR. Microcystic transitional cell carcinomas of the urinary bladder. A report of four cases. Am J Clin Pathol. 1991;96(5):635–9.
31. Zhai QJ, Black J, Ayala AG, Ro JY. Histologic variants of infiltrating urothelial carcinoma. Arch Pathol Lab Med. 2007;131(8):1244–56.
32. Huang Q, Chu PG, Lau SK, Weiss LM. Urothelial carcinoma of the urinary bladder with a component of acinar/tubular type differentiation simulating prostatic adenocarcinoma. Hum Pathol. 2004;35(6):769–73.
33. Kamat AM, Dinney CP, Gee JR, Grossman HB, Siefker-Radtke AO, Tamboli P, et al. Micropapillary bladder cancer: a review of the University of Texas M. D. Anderson Cancer Center experience with 100 consecutive patients. Cancer. 2007;110(1):62–7.
34. Amin MB, Ro JY, el-Sharkawy T, Lee KM, Troncoso P, Silva EG, et al. Micropapillary variant of transitional cell carcinoma of the urinary bladder. Histologic pattern resembling ovarian papillary serous carcinoma. Am J Surg Pathol. 1994;18(12):1224–32.
35. Perepletchikov AM, Parwani AV. Micropapillary urothelial carcinoma: clinico-pathologic review. Pathol Res Pract. 2009;205(12):807–10.
36. Guo CC, Tamboli P, Czerniak B. Micropapillary variant of urothelial carcinoma in the upper urinary tract: a clinicopathologic study of 11 cases. Arch Pathol Lab Med. 2009;133(1):62–6.
37. Sangoi AR, Beck AH, Amin MB, Cheng L, Epstein JI, Hansel DE, et al. Interobserver reproducibility in the diagnosis of invasive micropapillary carcinoma of the urinary tract among urologic pathologists. Am J Surg Pathol. 2010;34(9):1367–76.
38. Comperat E, Roupret M, Yaxley J, Reynolds J, Varinot J, Ouzaid I, et al. Micropapillary urothelial carcinoma of the urinary bladder: a clinicopathological analysis of 72 cases. Pathology. 2010;42(7):650–4.
39. Gaya JM, Palou J, Algaba F, Arce J, Rodriguez-Faba O, Villavicencio H. The case for conservative management in the treatment of patients with non-muscle-invasive micropapillary bladder carcinoma without carcinoma in situ. Can J Urol. 2010;17(5):5370–6.
40. Lotan TL, Ye H, Melamed J, Wu XR, Shih Ie M, Epstein JI. Immunohistochemical panel to identify the primary site of invasive micropapillary carcinoma. Am J Surg Pathol. 2009;33(7):1037–41.
41. Nassar H, Pansare V, Zhang H, Che M, Sakr W, Ali-Fehmi R, et al. Pathogenesis of invasive micropapillary carcinoma: role of MUC1 glycoprotein. Mod Pathol. 2004;17(9):1045–50.
42. Sangoi AR, Higgins JP, Rouse RV, Schneider AG, McKenney JK. Immunohistochemical comparison of MUC1, CA125, and Her2Neu in invasive micropapillary carcinoma of the urinary tract and typical invasive urothelial carcinoma with retraction artifact. Mod Pathol. 2009;22(5):660–7.
43. Kamat AM, Gee JR, Dinney CP, Grossman HB, Swanson DA, Millikan RE, et al. The case for early cystectomy in the treatment of nonmuscle invasive micropapillary bladder carcinoma. J Urol. 2006;175(3 Pt 1):881–5.
44. Spaliviero M, Dalbagni G, Bochner BH, Poon BY, Huang H, Al-Ahmadie HA, et al. Clinical outcome of patients with T1 micropapillary urothelial carcinoma of the bladder. J Urol. 2014;192(3):702–7. doi:10.1016/j.juro.2014.02.2565.
45. Keck B, Wach S, Stoehr R, Kunath F, Bertz S, Lehmann J, et al. Plasmacytoid variant of bladder cancer

defines patients with poor prognosis if treated with cystectomy and adjuvant cisplatin-based chemotherapy. BMC Cancer. 2013;13:71.

46. Keck B, Stoehr R, Wach S, Rogler A, Hofstaedter F, Lehmann J, et al. The plasmacytoid carcinoma of the bladder—rare variant of aggressive urothelial carcinoma. Int J Cancer. 2011;129(2):346–54.
47. Dayyani F, Czerniak BA, Sircar K, Munsell MF, Millikan RE, Dinney CP, et al. Plasmacytoid urothelial carcinoma, a chemosensitive cancer with poor prognosis, and peritoneal carcinomatosis. J Urol. 2013;189(5):1656–61.
48. Ricardo-Gonzalez RR, Nguyen M, Gokden N, Sangoi AR, Presti JC Jr, McKenney JK. Plasmacytoid carcinoma of the bladder: a urothelial carcinoma variant with a predilection for intraperitoneal spread. J Urol. 2012;187(3):852–5.
49. Raspollini MR, Sardi I, Giunti L, Di Lollo S, Baroni G, Stomaci N, et al. Plasmacytoid urothelial carcinoma of the urinary bladder: clinicopathologic, immunohistochemical, ultrastructural, and molecular analysis of a case series. Hum Pathol. 2011;42(8):1149–58.
50. Nigwekar P, Tamboli P, Amin MB, Osunkoya AO, Ben-Dor D, Amin MB. Plasmacytoid urothelial carcinoma: detailed analysis of morphology with clinicopathologic correlation in 17 cases. Am J Surg Pathol. 2009;33(3):417–24.
51. Lopez-Beltran A, Requena MJ, Montironi R, Blanca A, Cheng L. Plasmacytoid urothelial carcinoma of the bladder. Hum Pathol. 2009;40(7):1023–8.
52. Ro JY, Shen SS, Lee HI, Hong EK, Lee YH, Cho NH, et al. Plasmacytoid transitional cell carcinoma of urinary bladder: a clinicopathologic study of 9 cases. Am J Surg Pathol. 2008;32(5):752–7.
53. Fritsche HM, Burger M, Denzinger S, Legal W, Goebell PJ, Hartmann A. Plasmacytoid urothelial carcinoma of the bladder: histological and clinical features of 5 cases. J Urol. 2008;180(5):1923–7.
54. Mai KT, Park PC, Yazdi HM, Saltel E, Erdogan S, Stinson WA, et al. Plasmacytoid urothelial carcinoma of the urinary bladder report of seven new cases. Eur Urol. 2006;50(5):1111–4.
55. Gaafar A, Garmendia M, de Miguel E, Velasco V, Ugalde A, Bilbao FJ, et al. Plasmacytoid urothelial carcinoma of the urinary bladder. A study of 7 cases. Actas Urol Esp. 2008;32(8):806–10. Carcinoma urotelial plasmocitoide de vejiga urinaria. Estudio de 7 casos.
56. Chang JH, Dikranian AH, Johnston WH, Storch SK, Hurwitz RS. Malignant extrarenal rhabdoid tumor of the bladder: 9-year survival after chemotherapy and partial cystectomy. J Urol. 2004; 171(2 Pt 1):820–1.
57. Duvdevani M, Nass D, Neumann Y, Leibovitch I, Ramon J, Mor Y. Pure rhabdoid tumor of the bladder. J Urol. 2001;166(6):2337.
58. Carter RL, McCarthy KP, al-Sam SZ, Monaghan P, Agrawal M, McElwain TJ. Malignant rhabdoid tumour of the bladder with immunohistochemical and ultrastructural evidence suggesting histiocytic origin. Histopathology. 1989;14(2):179–90.
59. Harris M, Eyden BP, Joglekar VM. Rhabdoid tumour of the bladder: a histological, ultrastructural and immunohistochemical study. Histopathology. 1987;11(10):1083–92.
60. Parwani AV, Herawi M, Volmar K, Tsay SH, Epstein JI. Urothelial carcinoma with rhabdoid features: report of 6 cases. Hum Pathol. 2006;37(2):168–72.
61. Kojima Y, Takasawa A, Murata M, Akagashi K, Inoue T, Hara M, et al. A case of urothelial carcinoma, lipid cell variant. Pathol Int. 2013;63(3):183–7.
62. Lopez-Beltran A, Amin MB, Oliveira PS, Montironi R, Algaba F, McKenney JK, et al. Urothelial carcinoma of the bladder, lipid cell variant: clinicopathologic findings and LOH analysis. Am J Surg Pathol. 2010;34(3):371–6.
63. Shimada K, Nakamura M, Konishi N. A case of urothelial carcinoma with triple variants featuring nested, plasmacytoid, and lipoid cell morphology. Diagn Cytopathol. 2009;37(4):272–6.
64. Leroy X, Gonzalez S, Zini L, Aubert S. Lipoid-cell variant of urothelial carcinoma: a clinicopathologic and immunohistochemical study of five cases. Am J Surg Pathol. 2007;31(5):770–3.
65. Soylu A, Aydin NE, Yilmaz U, Kutlu R, Gunes A. Urothelial carcinoma featuring lipid cell and plasmacytoid morphology with poor prognostic outcome. Urology. 2005;65(4):797.
66. Kramer MW, Abbas M, Pertschy S, Becker JU, Kreipe HH, Kuczyk MA, et al. Clear-cell variant urothelial carcinoma of the bladder: a case report and review of the literature. Rare Tumors. 2012;4(4):e48.
67. Rotellini M, Fondi C, Paglierani M, Stomaci N, Raspollini MR. Clear cell carcinoma of the bladder in a patient with a earlier clear cell renal cell carcinoma: a case report with morphologic, immunohistochemical, and cytogenetical analysis. Appl Immunohistochem Mol Morphol. 2010;18(4):396–9.
68. Yamashita R, Yamaguchi R, Yuen K, Niwakawa M, Tobisu K. Urothelial carcinoma (clear cell variant) diagnosed with useful immunohistochemistry stain. Int J Urol. 2006;13(11):1448–50.
69. Kotliar SN, Wood CG, Schaeffer AJ, Oyasu R. Transitional cell carcinoma exhibiting clear cell features. A differential diagnosis for clear cell adenocarcinoma of the urinary tract. Arch Pathol Lab Med. 1995;119(1):79–81.
70. Braslis KG, Jones A, Murphy D. Clear-cell transitional cell carcinoma. Aust New Zeal J Surg. 1997;67(12):906–8.
71. Amin MB, Ro JY, Lee KM, Ordonez NG, Dinney CP, Gulley ML, et al. Lymphoepithelioma-like carcinoma of the urinary bladder. Am J Surg Pathol. 1994;18(5):466–73.
72. Holmang S, Borghede G, Johansson SL. Bladder carcinoma with lymphoepithelioma-like differentiation: a report of 9 cases. J Urol. 1998;159(3):779–82.
73. Tamas EF, Nielsen ME, Schoenberg MP, Epstein JI. Lymphoepithelioma-like carcinoma of the urinary tract: a clinicopathological study of 30 pure and mixed cases. Mod Pathol. 2007;20(8):828–34.

74. Zukerberg LR, Harris NL, Young RH. Carcinomas of the urinary bladder simulating malignant lymphoma. A report of five cases. Am J Surg Pathol. 1991;15(6):569–76.
75. Lopez-Beltran A, Luque RJ, Vicioso L, Anglada F, Requena MJ, Quintero A, et al. Lymphoepithelioma-like carcinoma of the urinary bladder: a clinicopathologic study of 13 cases. Virchows Arch. 2001;438(6):552–7.
76. Allende DS, Desai M, Hansel DE. Primary lymphoepithelioma-like carcinoma of the ureter. Ann Diagn Pathol. 2010;14(3):209–14.
77. Gulley ML, Amin MB, Nicholls JM, Banks PM, Ayala AG, Srigley JR, et al. Epstein-Barr virus is detected in undifferentiated nasopharyngeal carcinoma but not in lymphoepithelioma-like carcinoma of the urinary bladder. Hum Pathol. 1995;26(11):1207–14.
78. Izquierdo-Garcia FM, Garcia-Diez F, Fernandez I, Perez-Rosado A, Saez A, Suarez-Vilela D, et al. Lymphoepithelioma-like carcinoma of the bladder: three cases with clinicopathological and p53 protein expression study. Virchows Arch. 2004;444(5):420–5.
79. Torenbeek R, Blomjous CE, de Bruin PC, Newling DW, Meijer CJ. Sarcomatoid carcinoma of the urinary bladder. Clinicopathologic analysis of 18 cases with immunohistochemical and electron microscopic findings. Am J Surg Pathol. 1994;18(3):241–9.
80. Lopez-Beltran A, Pacelli A, Rothenberg HJ, Wollan PC, Zincke H, Blute ML, et al. Carcinosarcoma and sarcomatoid carcinoma of the bladder: clinicopathological study of 41 cases. J Urol. 1998;159(5):1497–503.
81. Young RH. Carcinosarcoma of the urinary bladder. Cancer. 1987;59(7):1333–9.
82. Hodges KB, Lopez-Beltran A, Emerson RE, Montironi R, Cheng L. Clinical utility of immunohistochemistry in the diagnoses of urinary bladder neoplasia. App Immunohistochem Mol Morphol. 2010;18(5):401–10.
83. Westfall DE, Folpe AL, Paner GP, Oliva E, Goldstein L, Alsabeh R, et al. Utility of a comprehensive immunohistochemical panel in the differential diagnosis of spindle cell lesions of the urinary bladder. Am J Surg Pathol. 2009;33(1):99–105.
84. Wright JL, Black PC, Brown GA, Porter MP, Kamat AM, Dinney CP, et al. Differences in survival among patients with sarcomatoid carcinoma, carcinosarcoma and urothelial carcinoma of the bladder. J Urol. 2007;178(6):2302–6; discussion 7.
85. Wang J, Wang FW, Lagrange CA, Hemstreet Iii GP, Kessinger A. Clinical features of sarcomatoid carcinoma (carcinosarcoma) of the urinary bladder: analysis of 221 cases. Sarcoma. 2010;2010:454792.
86. Shah VM, Newman J, Crocker J, Chapple CR, Collard MJ, O'Brien JM, et al. Ectopic beta-human chorionic gonadotropin production by bladder urothelial neoplasia. Arch Pathol Lab Med. 1986;110(2):107–11.
87. Dirnhofer S, Koessler P, Ensinger C, Feichtinger H, Madersbacher S, Berger P. Production of trophoblastic hormones by transitional cell carcinoma of the bladder: association to tumor stage and grade. Hum Pathol. 1998;29(4):377–82.
88. Rodenburg CJ, Nieuwenhuyzen Kruseman AC, de Maaker HA, Fleuren GJ, van Oosterom AT. Immunohistochemical localization and chromatographic characterization of human chorionic gonadotropin in a bladder carcinoma. Arch Pathol Lab Med. 1985;109(11):1046–8.
89. Martin JE, Jenkins BJ, Zuk RJ, Oliver RT, Baithun SI. Human chorionic gonadotrophin expression and histological findings as predictors of response to radiotherapy in carcinoma of the bladder. Virchows Arch A Pathol Anat Histopathol. 1989;414(3):273–7.
90. Campo E, Algaba F, Palacin A, Germa R, Sole-Balcells FJ, Cardesa A. Placental proteins in high-grade urothelial neoplasms. An immunohistochemical study of human chorionic gonadotropin, human placental lactogen, and pregnancy-specific beta-1-glycoprotein. Cancer. 1989;63(12):2497–504.
91. Iles R. Beta-hCG expression by bladder cancers. Br J Cancer. 1992;65(2):305.
92. Iles RK, Chard T. Human chorionic gonadotropin expression by bladder cancers: biology and clinical potential. J Urol. 1991;145(3):453–8.
93. Iles RK, Purkis PE, Whitehead PC, Oliver RT, Leigh I, Chard T. Expression of beta human chorionic gonadotrophin by non-trophoblastic non-endocrine 'normal' and malignant epithelial cells. Br J Cancer. 1990;61(5):663–6.
94. Regalado JJ. Mixed micropapillary and trophoblastic carcinoma of bladder: report of a first case with new immunohistochemical evidence of urothelial origin. Hum Pathol. 2004;35(3):382–4.
95. Grammatico D, Grignon DJ, Eberwein P, Shepherd RR, Hearn SA, Walton JC. Transitional cell carcinoma of the renal pelvis with choriocarcinomatous differentiation. Immunohistochemical and immunoelectron microscopic assessment of human chorionic gonadotropin production by transitional cell carcinoma of the urinary bladder. Cancer. 1993;71(5):1835–41.
96. Abratt RP, Temple-Camp CR, Pontin AR. Choriocarcinoma and transitional cell carcinoma of the bladder—a case report and review of the clinical evolution of disease in reported cases. Eur J Surg Oncol. 1989;15(2):149–53.
97. Morton KD, Burnett RA. Choriocarcinoma arising in transitional cell carcinoma of bladder: a case report. Histopathology. 1988;12(3):325–8.
98. Wurzel RS, Yamase HT, Nieh PT. Ectopic production of human chorionic gonadotropin by poorly differentiated transitional cell tumors of the urinary tract. J Urol. 1987;137(3):502–4.
99. Minamino K, Adachi Y, Okamura A, Kushida T, Sugi M, Watanabe M, et al. Autopsy case of primary choriocarcinoma of the urinary bladder. Pathol Int. 2005;55(4):216–22.
100. Sievert K, Weber EA, Herwig R, Schmid H, Roos S, Eickenberg HU. Pure primary choriocarcinoma of the urinary bladder with long-term survival. Urology. 2000;56(5):856.

101. Cho JH, Yu E, Kim KH, Lee I. Primary choriocarcinoma of the urinary bladder—a case report. J Korean Med Sci. 1992;7(4):369–72.
102. Hanna NH, Ulbright TM, Einhorn LH. Primary choriocarcinoma of the bladder with the detection of isochromosome 12p. J Urol. 2002;167(4):1781.
103. Butler SA, Ikram MS, Mathieu S, Iles RK. The increase in bladder carcinoma cell population induced by the free beta subunit of human chorionic gonadotrophin is a result of an anti-apoptosis effect and not cell proliferation. Br J Cancer. 2000;82(9):1553–6.
104. Jenkins BJ, Martin JE, Baithun SI, Zuk RJ, Oliver RT, Blandy JP. Prediction of response to radiotherapy in invasive bladder cancer. Br J Urol. 1990;65(4):345–8.
105. Lopez-Beltran A, Blanca A, Montironi R, Cheng L, Regueiro JC. Pleomorphic giant cell carcinoma of the urinary bladder. Hum Pathol. 2009;40(10):1461–6.
106. Lopez-Beltran A, Cheng L, Comperat E, Roupret M, Blanca A, Menendez CL, et al. Large cell undifferentiated carcinoma of the urinary bladder. Pathology. 2010;42(4):364–8.
107. Cox RM, Schneider AG, Sangoi AR, Clingan WJ, Gokden N, McKenney JK. Invasive urothelial carcinoma with chordoid features: a report of 12 distinct cases characterized by prominent myxoid stroma and cordlike epithelial architecture. Am J Surg Pathol. 2009;33(8):1213–9.
108. Gilg MM, Wimmer B, Ott A, Langner C. Urothelial carcinoma with abundant myxoid stroma: evidence for mucus production by cancer cells. Virchows Arch. 2012;461(1):99–101.
109. Tavora F, Epstein JI. Urothelial carcinoma with abundant myxoid stroma. Hum Pathol. 2009;40(10):1391–8.
110. Hameed O. Myxoid cystitis with "chordoid" lymphocytes: another mimic of invasive urothelial carcinoma. Am J Surg Pathol. 2010;34(7):1061–5.
111. Kawano H, Tanaka S, Ishii A, Cui D, Eguchi S, Hashimoto O, et al. Osteoclast-rich undifferentiated carcinoma of the urinary bladder: an immunohistochemical study. Pathol Res Pract. 2011;207(11):722–7.
112. Baydar D, Amin MB, Epstein JI. Osteoclast-rich undifferentiated carcinomas of the urinary tract. Modern Pathol. 2006;19(2):161–71.

16 Independent Predictors of Clinical Outcomes and Prediction Models on Bladder and Upper Urinary Tract Cancer

Maria Carmen Mir, Andrew J. Stephenson and Michael W. Kattan

Introduction

Over the last several decades, breakthroughs in basic and clinical research have led to an evolution in the diagnosis and management of bladder tumors. Our increased understanding of anatomy, tumor biology, and technology has resulted in better staging and treatment of these tumors.

Non-muscle-invasive bladder cancer (NMIBC) is a chronic disease with varying oncologic outcomes requiring frequent follow-up and repeated treatments. Recurrence (in up to 80 %) is the main problem for pTa NMIBC patients, whereas progression (in up to 45 %) is the main threat in pT1 and carcinoma in situ (CIS) NMIBC.

Even though uropathologists have tried to standardize the protocols, still reproducibility of pathologic stage and grade is modest. This is a major concern to clinicians due to the different prognostic implications. Molecular markers are promising for predicting clinical outcome of NMIBC, especially because clinicopathologic variables alone are not always optimal for individual prediction of prognosis. Several obstacles and opportunities have been linked to molecular markers. The role for molecular markers to predict recurrence seems limited because multifocal disease and incomplete treatment probably are more important for recurrence than the molecular features of a removed tumor. Prediction of progression with molecular markers holds considerable promise. Nevertheless, the value of molecular markers over clinicopathologic indexes is still being questioned and their clinical use limited. One of the reasons may be that reproducibility of prognostic (clinical and molecular) markers in NMIBC has been understudied.

As a result of all these difficulties in determining the most appropriate course of action for each patient, the medical community has developed prediction tools to help in the decision-making process.

There are several questions that a patient diagnosed with a bladder tumor and the urologist must answer before deciding upon a management strategy. Firstly, how aggressive is the cancer and which is the associated prognosis. Secondly, is there any further treatment required?

Hitherto, clinical judgment has traditionally formed the basis for risk estimation, patient counseling, and decision making. However, humans have difficulty with outcome prediction due to the biases that exist at all stages of the prediction process. Clinicians do not recall all cases equally, and certain cases can stand

M. C. Mir (✉)
Cleveland Clinic, Glickman Urologic and Kidney Institute, Cleveland, OH, USA
e-mail: mirmare@yahoo.es

A. J. Stephenson
Center for Urologic Oncology, Cleveland Clinic, Glickman Urological and Kidney Institute, Cleveland, OH, USA
e-mail: Stephea2@ccf.org

M. W. Kattan
Department of Quantitative Health Sciences, Cleveland Clinic, Cleveland, OH, USA
e-mail: kattanm@ccf.org

C. Magi-Galluzzi, C. G. Przybycin (eds.), *Genitourinary Pathology,* DOI 10.1007/978-1-4939-2044-0_16,

out and exert a disproportionately large influence when predicting future outcomes. When it comes time to make a prediction, we tend to predict the preferred outcomes rather than the outcome with the highest probability. Finally, when formulating predictions, clinicians can have difficulty weighing the relative importance of each of the many clinical factors that may influence the patient's outcome.

In this chapter, we provide an overview of recent bladder and upper tract predictive tools organized by clinical stage (NMIBC, MIBC) and upper/lower urinary tract. We mention the outcomes of interest, the number of patients, the specific features, and predictive accuracy estimates of each nomogram; as well as if internal/external validation is provided.

Prediction of Disease Recurrence/ Progression in Patients with NMIBC History

Since the early 1990s, many authors have made heroic efforts to improve risk stratification in terms of NMIBC. The British Medical Research Council focused on establishing risk groups to predict recurrence and progression of Ta and T1 tumors [1]. These authors demonstrated the importance of disease status at the 3 months cystoscopy and tumor multifocality as most important predictors for recurrence.

In early 2000, a Spanish group [2] assessed predictors of recurrence, progression, and cancer-specific mortality among 1529 patients with NMIBC. Three risk groups were described, with tumor grade being the strongest predictor of progression and thus cancer-specific mortality. Unfortunately, this cohort never underwent external validation of the results (Table 16.1).

Recently, the European Association of Urology (EAU) utilized a larger cohort of patients (2596) with NMIBC randomized who received all kinds of postoperative intravesical chemotherapy. Three risk groups were identified (low risk: single lesion, Ta, grade 1 and ≤3 cm), intermediate risk (Ta–T1, grade 1–2, multifocal, >3 cm) and high risk (any T1, grade 3, multifocal or highly recurrent, CIS). Unfortunately, the outcomes generated from this risk stratification tool are difficult to interpret in the present situation. Only 200 patients received bacillus Calmette–Guerin (BCG) as an immediate postoperative treatment (gold standard in the treatment of NMIBC), no standard second TURBT was performed, and less than 20% of patients actually received an additional intravesical treatment. Several authors have tried to externally validate this cohort showing an overestimation of the recurrence and progression rates [3]. The software for this model is available on line at http://www.eortc.be/tools/bladdercalculator.

In 2008, the Spanish Urological Club for Oncological Treatment published a similar stratification model. A total of 1062 patients treated with intravesical BCG were included in the study. Recurrence and progression scores were created. The BCG maintenance protocol was standardized among the different institutions; however, treatments lasted only up to 6 months. Furthermore, the series was graded according to 1987 TNM classification and the WHO 1973 grading system. Neither second transurethral resection (TUR) nor immediate instillation was performed. Approximately 20% of the patients had high-grade (HG) T1 disease and less than 10% had CIS at biopsy, the population where this kind of predictive model is mostly needed [3].

The first nomogram in bladder cancer was published in 2005 [4]. It was a multi-institutional collaboration were the authors estimated the risk of recurrence and progression in 2861 patients with NMIBC using a urine marker NMP22 (nuclear matrix protein 22) and urine cytology. The performance of the nomogram was increased by adding the urine marker for the three endpoints evaluated: any transitional cell carcinoma (TCC) recurrence, recurrence of HG Ta/T1, and recurrence higher than T2. The main clinical application in this setting for NMP22 is that it could provide a means to individualize the cystoscopy follow-up in patients with Ta or T1 TCC or CIS by determining the best timing for repeated cystoscopy (delay in cystoscopy follow-up if negative test). The limitations of the study are that it does not consider relevant factors such as previous history of TCC

Table 16.1 Summary of available predictive models in bladder cancer

Patient population	Reference	Prediction form	Outcome	No. of patients	Variables	Accuracy	Validation
NMIBC	Parmar	Risk grouping	RFS	919	# Tumors, cystoscopy at 3 months	Not reported	Not performed
NMIBC	MillanRodriguez	Risk grouping	RFS, PFS, ACS	1529	# Tumors, tumor size, T category, CIS grade, intravesical BCG	Not reported	Not performed
NMIBC	Shariat	Probability nomogram	RFS, PFS	2681	Age, gender, urine cytology, NMP22 Y/N	84% recurrence any BC, 87% recurrence HGBC, 86% progression	Internal
NMIBC	Sylvester	Look-up table	RFS, PFS	2596	# Tumors, tumor size, prior recurrence rate, T category, CIS, grade	Not reported	External
NMIBC	CUETO	Look-up table	RFS, PFS	1062	Age, gender, recurrence (Y/N), # tumors, T category, CIS, grade	Not reported	Internal
NMIBC	Ali-El-Dein	Probability nomogram	RFS, PFS	1019	Therapy, arm, stage, multiplicity, recurrence (Y/N)		Internal
NMIBC	Quershi	Artificial neural network	TaT1 (Recurrence at 6 months) TaT1 (PFS) T2T4 (CSS at 1 year)	56 105 40	EGFR, c-erbB2, p53, stage, grade, tumor size, number of tumors, gender, smoking status, histology of mucosal biopsies, CIS, metaplasia, architecture, location	75% 80% 82%	Internal Internal Internal
NMIBC	Catto	Neuro-fuzzy modeling	Ta–T4 (RFS)	109	p53, mismatch repair proteins, stage, grade, age, smoking status, previous cancer	88–95%	Internal
MIBC	Karakiewi cz	Probability nomogram	Radical cystectomy (Cystectomy T and N)	731	Age, TUR stage, TUR grade, CIS	76% for T, 63% for N	Internal
MIBC	Karakiewi cz	Probability nomogram	Radical cystectomy (RFS at 2, 5, 8 years)	731	Age, T stage, N stage, grade, LVI, CIS, adjuvant radiotherapy, adjuvant chemotherapy, neoadjuvant chemotherapy	78%	Internal

Table 16.1 (continued)

Patient population	Reference	Prediction form	Outcome	No. of patients	Variables	Accuracy	Validation
MIBC	Shariat	Probability nomogram	Radical cystectomy (CSS at 2, 5, 8 years)	731	Age, T stage, N stage, grade, LVI, CIS, adjuvant radiotherapy, adjuvant chemotherapy, neoadjuvant chemotherapy	79% for all-cause survival, 73% for CSS	Internal
MIBC	Bochner	Probability nomogram	Radical cystectomy (RFS at 5 years)	9064	Age, gender, T stage, N stage, grade, histology, time from diagnosis to surgery	75%	Internal
MIBC	Bassi	Artificial neural network	Radical cystectomy (ACS at 5 years)	369	Age, gender, T stage, N stage, LVI, grade, concomitant prostate cancer, history of UTTCC	76%	Internal
MIBC	Cohen	Probability nomogram	TURBT + Radiotherapy (T2–T4)	325	CR to induction therapy: hydronephrosis, age, complete TURBT, gender CSS: T stage, grade, hydronephrosis	68% 60%	Internal Internal
MIBC	Xylinas	Risk grouping	Radical cystectomy (T1–T3)	2145	Bladder intact disease free survival: T stage, age, hydronephrosis, complete TURBT Recurrence: pT stage, LVI, SM, CSM: T stage, LVI, SM	60% 67% recurrence, 64 mortality	Internal External

MIBC muscle-invasive bladder cancer, *NMIBC* non-muscle-invasive bladder cancer, *RFS* relapse-free survival, *PFS* progression-free survival, *ACS* all-cause survival, *CSS* cancer-specific survival, *CIS* carcinoma in situ, *BCG* bacillus Calmette–Guerin, *TUR* transurethral resection, *LVI* lymphovascular invasion, *UTTCC* upper tract transitional cell carcinoma, *TURBT* transurethral resection of bladder tumor, *EGFR* epidermal growth factor receptor, *SM* surgical margin, *CSM* cancer-specific mortality, *CR* complete remission/complete response (recurrences and grades) and previous history of intravesical therapy. Moreover, the performance of the nomogram varied significantly among the participant institutions, emphasizing the need for external validation of all tools.

Recently, an Egyptian group published nomograms for NMIBC patients from a single institution [5]. Approximately 74 % of patients received intravesical BCG (induction and maintenance). It included patients over a 25-year period. The second TUR protocol was established in 2003, and the grading system includes WHO1973/TNM 1987. In the analysis no sub-grouping between patients prior to 2003 is shown. The accuracy of the model for predicting recurrence is less than 70 %; thus, the clinical applicability of these nomograms is moderate, making us wonder if the year of TURBT could be actually a predictive factor of recurrence.

Preoperative Predictions of Pathologic Features at Radical Cystectomy

Inaccuracy of clinical staging (TURBT and CT scan) is well documented but still remains the main determinant in decision making in these patients [6]. Thus, developing accurate risk models in the pre-cystectomy setting would allow accurately determining patients with advanced stage and enabling better selection for neoadjuvant chemotherapy administration. For this purpose, Karakiewicz et al. [7] analyzed 958 patients undergoing radical cystectomy and pelvic lymph node dissection with curative intent in order to determine factors that could predict advanced stage or lymph node positivity. When patient age, TUR stage, grade, and presence of CIS were included in the nomogram, 75 % accuracy was recorded in predicting advanced stage (>T3) versus 71 % if TUR alone was used. In terms of predicting lymph node positivity 63 versus 61 % accuracy was shown.

The pre-cystectomy nomograms provide only a modest increase in accuracy. However, there are several variables implied in this prediction that may have contributed to the suboptimal results of the prediction models, such as differences in the TUR technique, restaging, and pathological evaluation.

Postoperative Predictions After Radical Cystectomy

Several post-cystectomy nomograms have been developed to predict the natural history of surgically treated patients and assist in the decision-making process regarding the use of adjuvant therapy after cystectomy [8–10].

The Bladder Cancer Research Consortium (BCRC) in 2006 developed a nomogram for prediction of recurrence after radical cystectomy. A total of 731 evaluable patients undergoing radical cystectomy and pelvic lymph node dissection were included from multiple institutions. No central pathology review was performed. The 2002 TNM classification and WHO 1973 grading system were used. The accuracy of the AJCC (American Joint Committee on Cancer) was exceeded by 3 % when grouping the different variables. The recurrence nomogram relied on age, pT, pN, lymphovascular invasion (LVI), postoperative CIS, neoadjuvant chemotherapy, adjuvant chemotherapy, and adjuvant radiotherapy. The recurrence probabilities are dictated at 2, 5, and 8 years.

In the same period, the International Bladder Cancer Nomogram Consortium (IBCNC) published a nomogram with the predicted risk of recurrence after radical cystectomy and lymph node dissection at 5 years. It was a multicentric study with more than 9000 patients included. Age, gender, grade, pathologic stage, histologic subtype, lymph node status, and time from diagnosis to surgery were significant contributing factors to the nomogram. The predictive accuracy was in this case 75 % (vs 68 % for AJCC). The clear advantage of this IBCNC nomogram is that it includes all histologic variants in the decision making. The BCRC is best suited only for Western populations with urothelial carcinoma.

There are several limitations to the above-mentioned nomograms. Multi-institutional analysis and nonuniform data collection can make final conclusions inaccurate. In addition, all of these data have been obtained from excellent referral centers where radical cystectomy is a cancer operation performed on a daily basis; caution should be used when applying these results to the real world.

Recently, Xylinas et al. published a nomogram to counsel patients after radical cystectomy about adjuvant chemotherapy [10]. Two endpoints were analyzed, recurrence and cancer-specific mortality. A total of 2145 patients with pT1–3 N0 urothelial bladder cancer who were chemotherapy naïve were included. Median follow-up was less than 5 years. The recurrence probability was determined at 2, 5, and 7 years. The nomogram's accuracy for recurrence was 64–67 %, while for cancer-specific survival (CSS) was 65–69 %. Once more, the clinical applicability of the nomogram is questionable. Moreover, the majority of patients included in this study currently would be candidates for neoadjuvant chemotherapy, which has shown a 5 % overall survival improvement, instead of adjuvant chemotherapy.

Only one nomogram has been published regarding bladder-sparing treatment in MIBC [11], a single center analysis including 325 patients with cT2–4a disease treated with radiotherapy. The endpoint of the nomogram was prediction of complete response rate, disease-specific survival, and the likelihood of remaining free of recurrence within the bladder or having had a cystectomy. For all three endpoints the accuracy was below 70 %. Once again, the clinical applicability of these nomograms is modest in decision making in order to preserve or remove the bladder as a treatment for curative intent.

As an alternative to nomogram-based modeling, Bassi et al. [12] developed an artificial neural network (ANN) to overcome the shortcomings of conventional statistical methods. ANNs are based on software that is easy to use, logical and fast, and that imitates low-level brain function to "learn" from data used as an example (training dataset) and make intelligent predictions given new, limited data. In oncology, ANNs have been mainly investigated to resolve the diagnostic, staging, and prognostic problems of prostate cancer. In this model, the authors developed an ANN using gender, age at surgery, LVI, pT, pN, grade, presence of concomitant prostatic adenocarcinoma, and history of upper tract urothelial tumors as input variables for prediction of 5-year all-cause survival after cystectomy. In a single institution cohort with 369 patients, the prognostic accuracy of the ANN was slightly superior to the logistic regression model. Unfortunately, the comparison of the accuracy of both models was performed on the same population that served for model development.

Nomograms in Upper Tract Transitional Cell Carcinoma

Scattered nomograms have been published for upper tract TCC (UTTCC). Unfortunately, because the incidence of this disease is very low, determining survival outcomes is only possible by joining data from various institutions. CSS rates for UTTCC patients vary among series; however, when tumor is outside the kidney boundaries CSS rates decline to less than 25 %. Nomogram predictions endeavor to better stratify patients with this disease and thus improve multimodal therapy.

The first UTTCC nomogram was published in 2010 by Margulis et al. [13] as a multi-institutional study with a total of 1453 patients who underwent radical nephroureterectomy with bladder cuff resection during a 20-year period. The purpose of the nomogram is determining presurgery features that could help identify which patients are going to show a non-organ-confined UTTCC and thus would be candidates for neoadjuvant chemotherapy or deserve retroperitoneal lymphadenectomy. On average, 40 % of the patients in this report had non-organ-confined UTTCC at radical nephroureterectomy, 28 % had systemic and/or local recurrence, and 24 % died of the UTTCC. No external validation of this cohort has been published.

In the same period, another group showed the results of a multicenter population-based assessment of the perioperative mortality (90 days) related to radical nephroureterectomy [14]. A total of 3039 patients obtained from the SEER database

Table 16.2 Summary of available predictive models in upper tract TCC

Reference	Prediction form	Outcome	No. of patients	Variables	Accuracy	Validation
Roupret	Probability nomogram	Radical nephroureterectomy (CSS)	3387	Age, T stage, N stage, architecture, LVI Recurrence: T stage, LN, LVI, architecture, CIS;	80%	External
Cha	Probability nomogram	Radical nephroureterectomy (RFS, CSS)	2244	CSS: T stage, LN, LVI, architecture	76% recurrence, 81% mortality	External
Jeldres	Probability nomogram	Radical nephroureterectomy (CSS)	5918	Age, T stage, N stage, tumor grade	75%	External
Jeldres	Probability nomogram	Radical nephroureterectomy (90 dM)	6078	90 dM after NUx	73%	External
Margulis	Probability nomogram	Radical nephroureterectomy (Nonconfined disease)	1453	Tumor location, tumor grade, tumor architecture	76%	Internal

CSS cancer-specific survival, *RFS* relapse-free survival, *dM* day mortality, *LVI* lymphovascular invasion, *LN lymph node*, *CIS* carcinoma in situ, *NUx* nephroureterectomy, *TCC* transitional cell carcinoma

were studied. Age and clinical stage at surgery were the most important predictors of perioperative mortality in this population. These factors should be taken into consideration in the decision-making process of aging patients with this disease.

In terms of prediction of survival outcomes, two nomograms have reported some light into this decision web. Similar SEER database as previously reported was used to identify predictors of CSS [15]; once more age and pathological stage after radical nephroureterectomy as well as tumor architecture and lymphovascular invasion were the most important determinants of cancer-specific death. These data bring to the clinical decision process a tool to make decisions on further treatment requirements after radical surgery. Finally, an updated report of the latest multi-institutional datasets that includes a total of 3387 patients with radical nephroureterectomy only (patients with neoadjuvant or adjuvant chemotherapy were excluded). This data set reports similar results as the previous set with age, tumor stage, architecture, and LVI as the most relevant predictors [16]. See Table 16.2.

Conclusions

Nomograms in TCC, as in any other subgroup of diseases, represent a very powerful tool to be taken into consideration when in the decision-making process of a multidisciplinary approach. Nomograms currently represent the most accurate and discriminating tool for predicting outcomes in patients with bladder and UTTCC. In this chapter, we reviewed the most relevant nomograms published in the literature regarding TCC especially focusing on the clinical relevance of its components. Patients with bladder cancer need to be involved in the decision-making process; they should be aware of the available options and the consequences of their choices. Nomograms are not perfect, but they give us a better understanding of the aggressiveness of the tumor that we are facing and the odds for cure.

References

1. Parmar MK, et al. Prognostic factors for recurrence and followup policies in the treatment of superficial bladder cancer: report from the British medical research council subgroup on superficial bladder cancer (Urological Cancer Working Party). J Urol. 1989;142(2 Pt 1):284–8.
2. Millan-Rodriguez F, et al. Primary superficial bladder cancer risk groups according to progression, mortality and recurrence. J Urol. 2000;164(3 Pt 1):680–4.
3. Fernandez-Gomez J, et al. Predicting nonmuscle invasive bladder cancer recurrence and progression in patients treated with bacillus Calmette-Guerin: the CUETO scoring model. J Urol. 2009;182(5):2195–203.
4. Shariat SF, et al. Nomograms including nuclear matrix protein 22 for prediction of disease recurrence and progression in patients with Ta, T1 or CIS transitional cell carcinoma of the bladder. J Urol. 2005;173(5):1518–25.

5. Ali-El-Dein B, et al. Construction of predictive models for recurrence and progression in >1000 patients with non-muscle-invasive bladder cancer (NMIBC) from a single centre. BJU Int. 2013;111(8):E331–41.
6. Shariat SF, et al. Discrepancy between clinical and pathologic stage: impact on prognosis after radical cystectomy. Eur Urol. 2007;51(1):137–49; discussion 149–51.
7. Karakiewicz PI, et al. Precystectomy nomogram for prediction of advanced bladder cancer stage. Eur Urol. 2006;50(6):1254–60; discussion 1261–2.
8. Karakiewicz PI, et al. Nomogram for predicting disease recurrence after radical cystectomy for transitional cell carcinoma of the bladder. J Urol. 2006;176(4 Pt 1):1354–61; discussion 1361–2.
9. Bochner BH, et al. Postoperative nomogram predicting risk of recurrence after radical cystectomy for bladder cancer. J Clin Oncol. 2006;24(24):3967–72.
10. Xylinas E, et al. Risk stratification of pT1–3N0 patients after radical cystectomy for adjuvant chemotherapy counselling. Br J Cancer. 2012;107(11):1826–32.
11. Coen JJ, et al. Nomograms predicting response to therapy and outcomes after bladder-preserving trimodality therapy for muscle-invasive bladder cancer. Int J Radiat Oncol Biol Phys. 2013;86(2):311–6.
12. Bassi P, et al. Prognostic accuracy of an artificial neural network in patients undergoing radical cystectomy for bladder cancer: a comparison with logistic regression analysis. BJU Int. 2007;99(5):1007–12.
13. Margulis V, et al. Preoperative multivariable prognostic model for prediction of nonorgan confined urothelial carcinoma of the upper urinary tract. J Urol. 2010;184(2):453–8.
14. Jeldres C, et al. A population-based assessment of perioperative mortality after nephroureterectomy for upper-tract urothelial carcinoma. Urology. 2010;75(2):315–20.
15. Jeldres C, et al. Highly predictive survival nomogram after upper urinary tract urothelial carcinoma. Cancer. 2010;116(16):3774–84.
16. Roupret M, et al. Prediction of cancer specific survival after radical nephroureterectomy for upper tract urothelial carcinoma: development of an optimized postoperative nomogram using decision curve analysis. J Urol. 2013;189(5):1662–9.

17 Familial Urothelial Carcinomas

Christopher G. Przybycin and Jesse K. McKenney

Introduction

The majority of urothelial carcinomas (UCs) are considered to be sporadic, often occurring in association with environmental risk factors (e.g., smoking, exposure to aromatic amines). The past few decades, however, have seen recognition of an inherited basis for a small but increasing proportion of these tumors. Candidate gene studies have found that polymorphisms in two genes involved in metabolism of toxic compounds, N-acetyltransferase 2 (*NAT2*) and glutathione S-transferase μ1 (*GSTM1*), play a role in bladder carcinogenesis [1]. The slow-acetylator phenotype of *NAT2* and the *GSTM1* null phenotype are associated with a 1.4-fold and 1.5-fold increase in bladder cancer risk, respectively [2]. Subsequent genome-wide association studies have identified numerous susceptibility loci for bladder cancer [1]. In other cases, inherited UCs have been associated with one of several specific syndromes, namely, the Hereditary Non-Polyposis Colorectal Carcinoma (HNPCC)/Lynch syndrome (LS), hereditary retinoblastoma, and Costello syndrome.

It has been suggested that the proportion of UCs with a hereditary basis is underestimated. Applying a specific set of clinical criteria to define suspected hereditary UC (age at diagnosis less than 60 years with no previous history of bladder cancer, previous history of HNPCC-related cancer regardless of age, one first-degree relative with HNPCC-related cancer diagnosed before 50 years of age, or two first-degree relatives diagnosed regardless of age), one group estimates that 21 % of patients presenting with upper urinary tract UCs may have a hereditary cause (specifically HNPCC) [3].

Recognition of a familial basis for UC in a given patient has important implications not only for the patient's family members, but also for the patient himself: he may be at risk for other malignancies for which he should be evaluated (as in HNPCC), and there is some evidence to suggest a possible difference in treatment response. Specifically, when the above-mentioned clinical criteria for suspected hereditary UC are applied to upper urinary tract UCs, one study has shown that patients with these "hereditary-like" cancers have improved overall survival and cancer specific survival after radical nephroureterectomy and adjuvant cisplatin-based chemotherapy as compared with patients with sporadic upper urinary tract UCs [4].

Familial Risk of Urothelial Carcinoma

Several case-control studies and cohort studies have examined the relative risk of UC in patients with a family history of UC. A recent review

C. G. Przybycin (✉) · J. K. McKenney
Department of Pathology, Cleveland Clinic, Robert J. Tomsich Pathology and Laboratory Medicine Institute, Cleveland, OH, USA
e-mail: przybyc@ccf.org

J. K. McKenney
e-mail: mckennj@ccf.org

C. Magi-Galluzzi, C. G. Przybycin (eds.), *Genitourinary Pathology*, DOI 10.1007/978-1-4939-2044-0_17,

article on the subject [5] showed that most of these studies reported a relative risk between 1.4 and 1.9, with the largest case-control study reporting a relative risk of 1.5 [6] (95% CI=1.2–1.8). This increased risk among patients with a positive family history remains even after controlling for smoking; a large Dutch cohort reported a smoking-adjusted risk of 1.8 (95% CI=1.3–2.7) [7]. Thus, the increase in UC risk among patients with a family history of UC is not likely due to shared environmental exposures alone.

HNPCC (Lynch Syndrome)

LS is the most common syndrome with familial UC as a feature. Inherited in an autosomal dominant fashion, LS is caused by a germline mutation in one allele of a gene encoding one of a group of DNA mismatch repair proteins, including *MSH2*, *MLH1*, *MSH6*, and *PMS2*. When the functional allele is inactivated by mutation or epigenetic silencing, replication errors are propagated, resulting in eventual tumorigenesis [8, 9]. Lack of mismatch repair proteins can be detected by loss of immunohistochemical expression, or by observing novel alterations in microsatellite regions of DNA (microsatellite instability), an artifact of the resultant genetic instability.

Although LS is most commonly associated with colorectal carcinomas and endometrial carcinomas, UCs of the upper urinary tract are the third most common tumor subtype found in this population [10, 11]. One of the earliest studies of extra-colonic cancers in patients with LS found a relative risk of ureteral cancer of 22 times over that of the general population [12]. Upper urinary tract UC has been reported as the presenting malignancy in up to 21% of LS patients [11]. The increased risk of upper urinary tract UC in LS patients has been shown in several studies to be more strongly associated with *MSH2* mutations than *MLH1* mutations [8, 11, 13].

Upper tract UCs associated with HNPCC have a slightly different epidemiologic profile than sporadically occurring tumors, with a median age at presentation of 56 years (10–15 years earlier than usual) [14]. The male-to-female ratio is closer to 1:1 as compared with 2:1 for upper tract UC in the general population, and ureteral tumors seem to predominate over renal pelvis tumors (1.3:1), in contrast to the threefold to fourfold preponderance of renal pelvis tumors over ureteral tumors in the general population [11].

The pathologic characteristics of upper urinary tract UCs in HNPCC patients overlap substantially but not completely with those occurring sporadically. In one study of 39 HNPCC patients with upper tract UCs, the majority (88%) were high grade, a finding compatible with that seen in sporadic tumors, and 23% were found to be high stage (pT3 or higher) [11].

While no distinctive morphologic feature has been definitively associated with HNPCC-associated upper urinary tract UCs, the presence of an inverted growth pattern has been reported in this setting. Although it remains to be proven whether inverted growth is definitively associated with HNPCC per se, inverted growth has been shown to be predictive of microsatellite instability in upper tract UCs in general. In one study [15] of 132 upper tract UCs that were tested for microsatellite instability by PCR, 35 (26.5%) were found to be microsatellite unstable. The majority (65.7%) of the microsatellite unstable tumors had an inverted growth pattern accounting for at least 20% of the tumor volume, a finding that was seen in only 17.5% of the microsatellite stable tumors. Although microsatellite instability is not always predictive of HNPCC, given this strong association between inverted growth and microsatellite instability, it seems reasonable to consider screening patients with inverted upper urinary tract UCs for loss of mismatch repair proteins by immunohistochemistry or PCR in an effort to diagnose HNPCC, as is currently done in colonic and endometrial carcinomas with key histologic features.

Initial data suggested that the predisposition to UC in patients with LS was limited to upper tract disease, with an incidence of bladder cancer in LS patients similar to that seen in the general population [12] and low rates of microsatellite instability in UCs of the bladder [16, 17]. More recently, however, an increased risk for bladder cancer has also been found in LS patients, specifically those who carry mutations in *MSH2*. In a Dutch cohort of families with a germline mutation in *MLH1, MSH2,* or *MSH6* and their first-degree relatives, van der Post et al. [18] found a relative risk of bladder cancer in *MSH2* carriers and their first-degree relatives of 7.0 for men ($p<0.001$) and 5.8 for women ($p<0.15$). Nine of the 11 bladder tumors (82 %) in that study lacked immunohistochemical expression of *MSH2*, and six of the seven (86 %) whose microsatellite instability (MSI) status was successfully tested were MSI high (MSI-H). A more recent study on a Canadian population [8] reported similar findings. This group found an increased rate of bladder cancer in patients with MSH2 mutations compared with lifetime risks for the general population (6.21 %, as compared with the expected 3.6 % for men and 1.2 % for women). They likewise demonstrated loss of *MSH2* expression by immunohistochemistry in 9 of the 11 tumors (82 %), and found MSI-H status in 6 of the 8 (75 %) bladder tumors successfully studied for MSI. Most of these bladder UCs were high grade and either noninvasive (pTa) or invaded the lamina propria (pT1). Patients with *MLH1* mutations had a bladder cancer incidence similar to the lifetime risk of the general population.

Hereditary Retinoblastoma

A study by Fletcher et al. [19] identified five subsequent UCs of the bladder from among 144 hereditary retinoblastoma survivors. This increased incidence of bladder cancer appears to be associated with the presence of the germline RB mutation, as these patients did not receive high-dose radiation or chemotherapy for treatment of their retinoblastomas. A subsequent study [20] found four bladder UCs arising in hereditary retinoblastoma survivors, for a standardized incidence ratio of 124 (95 % CI = 34.0–319). An increased risk of bladder cancer in hereditary retinoblastoma patients is consistent with the finding that RB gene mutations play a significant role in urothelial carcinogenesis [21].

Costello Syndrome

Costello syndrome is a rare genetic disorder associated with postnatal growth deficiency, mental retardation, coarse facial features (macrocephaly, sparse and curly hair, low set ears, depressed nasal bridge, bulbous nose with anteverted nostrils, and thick lips), loose skin, cardiac abnormalities, and papillomas. Three patients with Costello syndrome have been reported to have UCs of the bladder, presenting at age 10, 11, and 16. Hematuria was the presenting symptom in two cases [22, 23]; the third case presented as a bladder mass detected by transabdominal ultrasound in a patient with a history of recurrent urothelial papillomas [24]. In all three patients, the tumors were low-grade papillary UCs (reported as grade 1). Recurrences occurred in two of these patients; one a low-grade recurrence and one recurrence whose grade was not reported.

As the findings of genome-wide association studies are further analyzed and tested by clinical studies, it is hoped that additional genetic factors predisposing to UCs (which are the basis for at least some of the familial aggregation of these tumors) will be identified, and that means of reducing that risk will be found.

References

1. Grotenhuis AJ, Vermeulen SH, Kiemeney LA. Germline genetic markers for urinary bladder cancer risk, prognosis and treatment response. Future Oncol. 2010;6:1433–60.
2. Garcia-Closas M, Malats N, Silverman D, et al. NAT2 slow acetylation, GSTM1 null genotype, and risk of bladder cancer: results from the Spanish Bladder Cancer Study and meta-analyses. Lancet. 2005;366:649–59.
3. Audenet F, Colin P, Yates DR, et al. A proportion of hereditary upper urinary tract urothelial carcinomas are misclassified as sporadic according to a multi-institutional database analysis: proposal of patient-specific risk identification tool. BJU Int. 2012;110:E583–9.
4. Hollande C, Colin P, de La Motte Rouge T, et al. Hereditary-like urothelial carcinomas of the upper urinary tract benefit more from adjuvant cisplatin-based chemotherapy after radical nephroureterectomy than do sporadic tumours. BJU Int. 2014;113(4):574–80.

5. Mueller CM, Caporaso N, Greene MH. Familial and genetic risk of transitional cell carcinoma of the urinary tract. Urol Oncol. 2008;26:451–4.
6. Kantor AF, Hartge P, Hoover RN, et al. Familial and environmental interactions in bladder cancer risk. Int J Cancer. 1985;35:703–6.
7. Aben KK, Witjes JA, Schoenberg MP, et al. Familial aggregation of urothelial cell carcinoma. Int J Cancer. 2002;98:274–8.
8. Skeldon SC, Semotiuk K, Aronson M, et al. Patients with Lynch syndrome mismatch repair gene mutations are at higher risk for not only upper tract urothelial cancer but also bladder cancer. Eur Urol. 2013;63:379–85.
9. Hartmann A, Cheville JC, Dietmaier W, et al. Hereditary nonpolyposis colorectal cancer syndrome in a patient with urothelial carcinoma of the upper urothelial tract. Arch Pathol Lab Med. 2003;127:E60–63.
10. Maul JS, Warner NR, Kuwada SK, et al. Extracolonic cancers associated with hereditary nonpolyposis colorectal cancer in the Utah Population Database. Am J Gastroenterol. 2006;101:1591–96.
11. Crockett DG, Wagner DG, Holmang S, et al. Upper urinary tract carcinoma in Lynch syndrome cases. J Urolo. 2011;185:1627–30.
12. Watson P, Lynch HT. Extracolonic cancer in hereditary nonpolyposis colorectal cancer. Cancer. 1993;71:677–85.
13. Watson P, Vasen HF, Mecklin JP, et al. The risk of extra-colonic, extra-endometrial cancer in the Lynch syndrome. Int J Cancer. 2008;123:444–9.
14. Watson P, Lynch HT. The tumor spectrum in HNPCC. Anticancer Res. 1994;14:1635–9.
15. Hartmann A, Dietmaier W, Hofstadter F, et al. Urothelial carcinoma of the upper urinary tract: inverted growth pattern is predictive of microsatellite instability. Hum Pathol. 2003;34:222–7.
16. Mongiat-Artus P, Miquel C, Flejou JF, et al. Spectrum of molecular alterations in colorectal, upper urinary tract, endocervical, and renal carcinomas arising in a patient with hereditary non-polyposis colorectal cancer. Virchows Arch. 2006;449:238–43.
17. Bonnal C, Ravery V, Toublanc M, et al. Absence of microsatellite instability in transitional cell carcinoma of the bladder. Urology. 2000;55:287–91.
18. van der Post RS, Kiemeney LA, Ligtenberg MJ, et al. Risk of urothelial bladder cancer in Lynch syndrome is increased, in particular among MSH2 mutation carriers. J Med Genet. 2010;47:464–70.
19. Fletcher O, Easton D, Anderson K, et al. Lifetime risks of common cancers among retinoblastoma survivors. J Natl Cancer Inst. 2004;96:357–63.
20. Marees T, Moll AC, Imhof SM, et al. Risk of second malignancies in survivors of retinoblastoma: more than 40 years of follow-up. J Natl Cancer Inst. 2008;100:1771–9.
21. Mitra AP, Birkhahn M, Cote RJ. p53 and retinoblastoma pathways in bladder cancer. World J Urol. 2007;25:563–71.
22. Franceschini P, Licata D, Di Cara G, et al. Bladder carcinoma in Costello syndrome: report on a patient born to consanguineous parents and review. Am J Med Genet. 1999;86:174–79.
23. Gripp KW, Scott CI Jr., Nicholson L, et al. Second case of bladder carcinoma in a patient with Costello syndrome. Am J Medal Genet. 2000;90(3):256–9.
24. Urakami S, Igawa M, Shiina H, et al. Recurrent transitional cell carcinoma in a child with the Costello syndrome. J Urol. 2002;168:1133–4.

18 New Molecular Markers with Diagnostic and Prognostic Values in Bladder Cancer

Hikmat A. Al-Ahmadie and Gopa Iyer

Immunohistochemical Markers With Diagnostic Value in Bladder Cancer

Immunohistochemistry

In the majority of cases, an accurate diagnosis of urothelial carcinoma as well as the presence and extent of invasion is achieved by regular histological examination without the need for ancillary studies such as immunohistochemistry (IHC). As discussed below, however, there are situations where IHC might be helpful. The following are some of the common scenarios. Details about new or relevant markers for urothelial differentiation will be reported following the section.

Distinction of Reactive Atypia from Urothelial Carcinoma In Situ

In flat urothelial lesions, IHC with CK20, CD44, p53, and Ki-67 may be utilized to aid in the distinction of reactive flat urothelial lesions from urothelial carcinoma in situ (CIS) [1–3]. In the normal state, CK20 (Fig. 18.1a) expression is limited to the umbrella cell layer and CD44 (Fig. 18.1b) stains predominantly the basal cell layer. Urothelial CIS is expected to express CK20 (Fig. 18.2a) in the majority of tumor cells (full thickness) with total loss of CD44 expression (Fig. 18.2b). CIS is also expected to exhibit diffuse labeling with p53 and the proliferation marker Ki-67. On the other hand, reactive urothelial lesions are expected to express CD44 with the other markers exhibiting limited expression. This pattern has been recently shown to aid in the differential diagnosis of radiation-induced atypia versus urothelial CIS [4].

It is important to note that none of these markers should be used individually to establish a malignant or benign diagnosis. Aberrant expression of these markers is well established and their interpretation must be made in the correct context. Moreover, IHC should not be used in all cases as a screening test, but rather as an adjunctive tool to aid in the histological classification of atypical flat urothelial lesions or in the de novo diagnosis of CIS where the morphologic features are questionable.

Differentiating Urothelial Carcinoma (with or Without Divergent Differentiation) from Other Carcinomas that Secondarily Involve the Urinary Bladder

Distinguishing invasive urothelial carcinoma from carcinomas secondarily involving the urinary bladder is of paramount significance and can at times be difficult due to significant morphologic overlap. Prostatic adenocarcinoma, colorectal adenocarcinoma, squamous cell carcinoma of

H. A. Al-Ahmadie (✉)
Department of Pathology, Memorial Sloan Kettering Cancer Center, New York, NY, USA
e-mail: alahmadh@mskcc.org

G. Iyer
Department of Medicine, Memorial Sloan Kettering Cancer Center, New York, NY, USA
e-mail: iyerg@mskcc.org

C. Magi-Galluzzi, C. G. Przybycin (eds.), *Genitourinary Pathology*, DOI 10.1007/978-1-4939-2044-0_18,

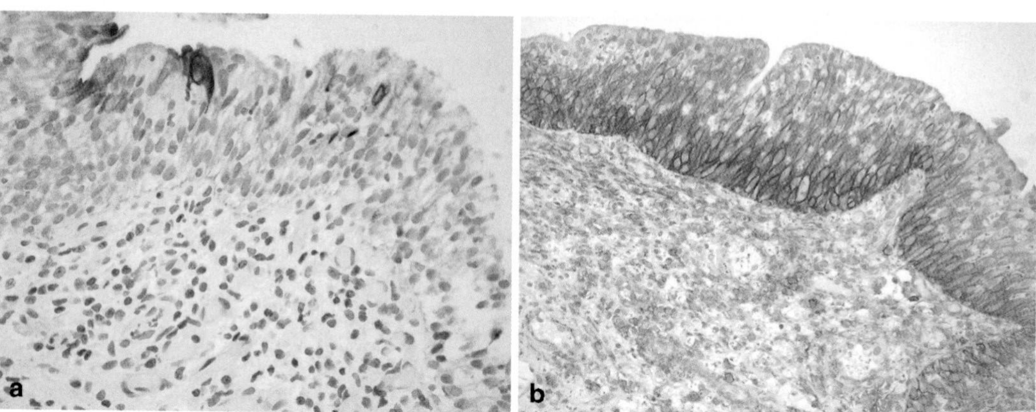

Fig. 18.1 In normal urothelium and in reactive atypia CK20 expression is limited to the umbrella cell layer (**a**); CD44 stains predominantly the basal cell layer, although patchy positivity can be seen in all layers (**b**)

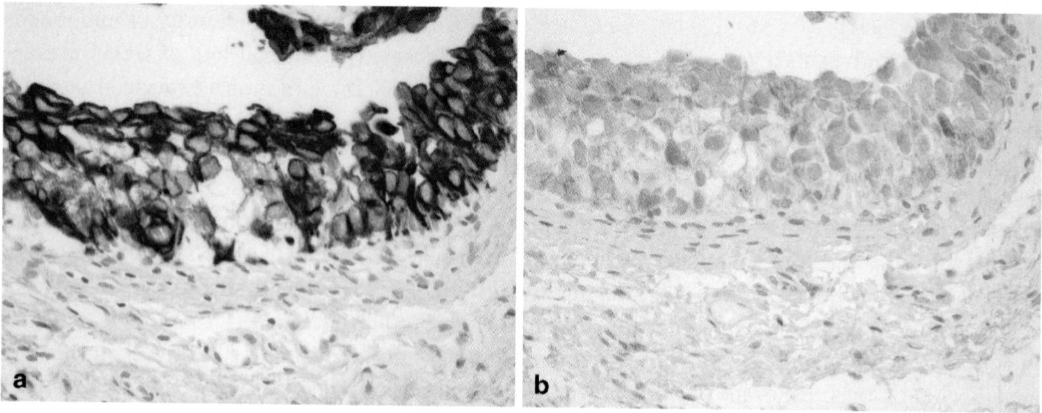

Fig. 18.2 Urothelial carcinoma in situ is expresses CK20 in the majority of tumor cells (full thickness) (**a**), with loss of CD44 expression (**b**)

the uterine cervix, and to a lesser extent, carcinomas of the uterus or ovary, and rarely those from breast, lung, stomach, and skin [5, 6], can involve the bladder during their course and may present a diagnostic challenge primarily in the absence of a relevant clinical history regarding the potential primary site of origin.

It is important to keep in mind that both squamous and glandular differentiations are common findings in primary urothelial carcinoma of the bladder but the diagnostic dilemmas can arise in cases of pure adenocarcinoma or squamous cell carcinoma involving the bladder. The best way to solve any potential misdiagnosis is to think of the possibility that these tumors can present in the bladder and to explore the clinical situation of the patient. Having a similar tumor in a site where it is more common to have tumors with the given morphology is perhaps the strongest clue favoring a metastatic origin of the bladder tumor.

Poorly Differentiated Prostatic Adenocarcinoma Versus Urothelial Carcinoma

These two entities might have morphologic overlap and the clinical management implications are significant. The history of prostatic adenocarcinoma might not be provided or might be overlooked. Additionally, some of these patients might have received treatments that affected the morphological appearance of the prostate cancer, further complicating its recognition.

Generally, a panel of markers is useful in separating the two entities in the majority of the cases. Markers that are supportive of prostatic differentiation (Fig. 18.3a) include prostate-specific antigen (PSA) (Fig. 18.3b), prostate-specific acid phosphatase (PSAP), prostate-specific membrane antigen (PSMA), P501s (Fig. 18.3c), NKX3.1 (Fig. 18.3d), and erythroblast transformation-specific-related gene (ERG); whereas, markers favoring urothelial differentiation (Fig. 18.4a) and origin include high molecular weight cytokeratin (34βe12), CK7 (Fig. 18.4b), p63 (Fig. 18.4c), thrombomodulin, uroplakin III, and recently GATA3 (Fig. 18.4d) [7–12].

Obviously not all of these markers are needed in any individual case. It is recommended to start with a few markers with high sensitivity and specificity and then use additional markers as needed. PSA, CK34βe12, and p63 are very useful as a start in the majority of cases.

A unique scenario is the presence of prostatic adenocarcinoma with extensive squamous differentiation involving the bladder. This is a rare situation that occurs primarily postradiation or hormone therapy for prostate cancer. The clues to the prostatic origin of such a tumor is the clinical suspicious based on the clinical history which should prompt careful and extensive examination of the tumor to find even the slightest glandular differentiation, which would then be confirmed by any of the prostatic markers mentioned above. It is only logical to keep in mind that these prostatic markers will not be expressed in the component with pure squamous differentiation.

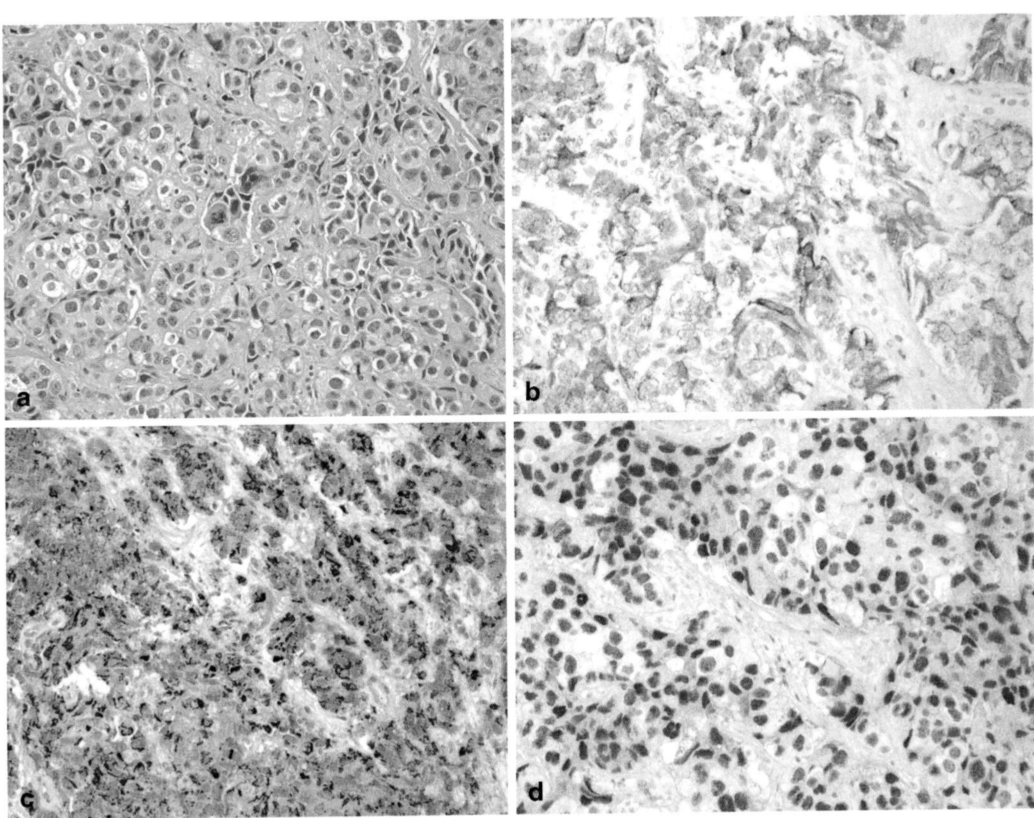

Fig. 18.3 Bladder neck tumor from a 70-year-old man with urine cytology positive for urothelial carcinoma (**a**). Tumor cells are positive for PSA (**b**), P501s (**c**), and NKX3.1 (**d**), supporting the diagnosis of prostatic adenocarcinoma

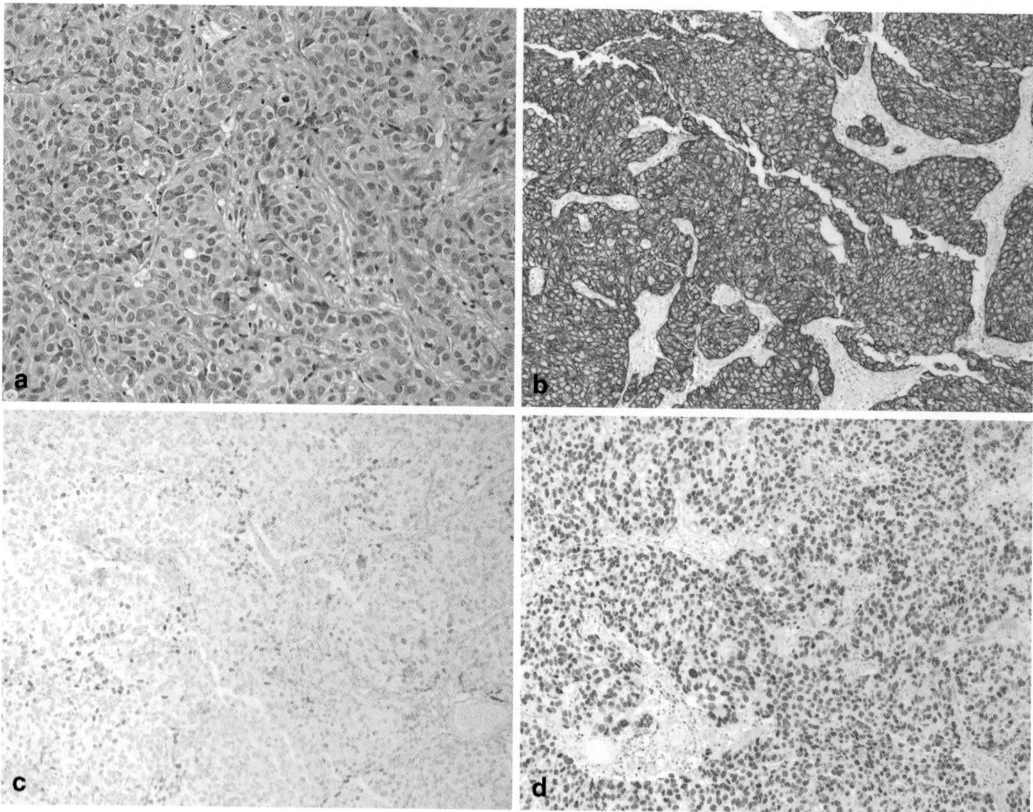

Fig. 18.4 Bladder mass from a 67-year-old man with urine cytology positive for urothelial carcinoma (**a**). Tumor is diffusely positive for CK7 (**b**), focally positive for p63 (**c**), and diffusely positive for GATA3 (**d**), supporting the diagnosis of urothelial carcinoma

Colorectal Adenocarcinoma Involving the Bladder by Direct Extension or Metastasis Versus Primary Bladder Adenocarcinoma (Enteric Morphology)

For this differential diagnosis, the clinical history is also extremely important which should include knowledge of the presence of a prior or current tumor of the colorectal region, its grade, and stage. These tumors may even colonize the bladder mucosa giving the impression of a "precursor" or "in situ" lesion. Unfortunately, IHC currently is of limited value in this differential diagnosis as tumors with enteric phenotype will generally stain similarly regardless of the site of origin. There have been suggestions that β-catenin might be of value in this scenario as it will not label the nuclei of primary bladder adenocarcinoma compared to those originating from the colorectal region [13–16]. While this pattern seems to be of value, nuclear localization of β-catenin was still reported in cases of primary bladder adenocarcinoma in some of these studies. Moreover, nuclear localization of β-catenin is not universal to all cases of primary colorectal adenocarcinoma, and a negative stain (i.e., only membranous and or cytoplasmic expression) will not exclude a colorectal primary. It is therefore, very important to always inquire about the clinical history of the patient for the possibility of a primary in the colorectal region when facing the diagnosis of enteric adenocarcinoma in the urinary bladder.

Squamous Cell Carcinoma of Uterine Cervix Involving the Bladder by Direct Extension or Metastasis Versus Primary Squamous Cell Carcinoma of the Bladder (or Urothelial Carcinoma with Squamous Differentiation)

Bladder involvement by squamous cell carcinoma of uterine cervical origin is admittedly rare but can still be diagnostically challenging when encountered, especially considering that squamous differentiation is rather common in urothelial carcinoma.

A number of markers have shown strong correlation with squamous neoplasms but unfortunately, these markers will not be able to point to a specific site of origin for these squamous carcinomas. Examples of such markers include desmogelin-3, MAC387, and TRIM29, which although sensitive markers for squamous phenotype, can be positive in squamous cell carcinoma of the cervix as well as that of the bladder. These markers can also be expressed in the squamous component of urothelial carcinoma with squamous differentiation and less commonly within the classical urothelial component [17, 18]. This is why these markers are not reliable as the sole means of establishing a site of origin for a tumor with squamous differentiation.

The role of the human papillomavirus (HPV) is well established in the vast majority of cervical squamous cell carcinoma for which p16 serves as a surrogate marker for the detection of HPV in these tumors [19, 20]. The expression of p16 in squamous cell carcinoma of the bladder has been shown to be less specific with little if any association with HPV infection in such setting [21]. There were, however, rare cases of true HPV-associated squamous cell carcinoma of the bladder and at least in some of them the tumors exhibited basaloid morphology and were associated with a history of neurogenic bladder or other situations that required repeated catheterization of the bladder [22, 23].

A number of *other carcinomas* may rarely involve the bladder during their course such as mammary carcinoma, endometrial or ovarian carcinoma, gastric carcinoma, etc. It is prudent to review the primary tumor alongside the metastasis. Immunostains might be ordered according to the suspected primary tumor, particularly if the status of such markers is known in the primary site.

Markers for the Differential Diagnosis of Spindle Cell Lesions of the Bladder

Many entities exist in the bladder in which spindle cell morphology predominates and range from reactive myofibroblastic lesions to frankly malignant (sarcomatous) entities. The main categories include inflammatory myofibroblastic tumor/pseudosarcomatous myofibroblastic proliferations (IMT/PMP), sarcomatoid urothelial carcinoma, and sarcomas with spindle cell morphology (leiomyosarcoma, rhabdomyosarcoma). There is marked overlap in morphology and immunoprofile among these entities and a judicious use of IHC in the context of morphology plays an important supportive role in this differential diagnosis.

Establishing the diagnosis of IMT can be aided by the expression of ALK by IHC or the presence of *ALK* rearrangement by fluorescence in situ hybridization (FISH) or other molecular technique. Since this expression or rearrangement is not present in all cases, a negative test does not rule out the diagnosis of IMT [24]. The overall morphologic features and the expression of other markers such as smooth muscle actin and cytokeratins may help. The challenge remains to differentiate this entity from a reactive myofibroblastic proliferation, which can be exuberant in the bladder.

For sarcomatoid urothelial carcinoma, finding an unequivocal epithelial component would be the ideal scenario but when this is not feasible, the presence of epithelial differentiation by IHC might be helpful in pointing toward the diagnosis of sarcomatoid UC. This can be achieved by a number of epithelial markers such as wide spectrum cytokeratins (AE1/AE3, CAM5.2...), epithelial membrane antigen (EMA), high molecular weight keratins, and p63. GATA3 might be helpful as well but we still do not know its full functions in spindle cell lesions in general and more studies are needed to assess its value in this setting.

For true sarcomas with specific lineage or differentiation such as leiomyosarcoma and rhabdomyosarcoma, the diagnosis can be confirmed by the markers related to these entities such as actin, desmin, myogenin, etc.

The Confirmation of Urothelial Differentiation at a Metastatic Site

Generally, urothelial carcinoma presents at metastatic sites with the morphology of a poorly differentiated carcinoma without specific morphologic features. It could be particularly difficult to distinguish metastatic urothelial carcinoma from metastatic squamous cell carcinoma (or from primary squamous cell carcinoma in the example of a lung tumor). What might be helpful in pointing to an origin of a urothelial primary include (1) prior history of bladder cancer, which should warrant review of the primary tumor if available and (2) the presence of divergent differentiation (squamous, glandular, etc.).

In these settings, IHC can play a role in establishing the urothelial origin of such tumors.

Antibodies that can be used to confirm urothelial differentiation/origin include GATA3, cytokeratins 7 and 20, high molecular weight cytokeratin, p63, uroplakin III, thrombomodulin, cytokeratin CK5/6, and S100P [25–28].

It is important to keep in mind that, despite their relative specific pattern of expressions, none of these markers is by itself diagnostic of a primary urothelial carcinoma as certain degree of overlap still exists and it may take more than one marker to help in this differential.

The Role of IHC in Confirming the Presence of Lymphovascular Invasion (LVI)

LVI in urothelial carcinoma has been reported to be an independent prognostic factor for metastasis, recurrence, and survival [29–31]. Identifying LVI, however, can be complicated by the presence of peri-tumoral stromal retraction, which is a relatively common finding in invasive urothelial carcinoma that mimics LVI. This is particularly problematic within the lamina propria. As a result, assessing LVI suffers from a considerable lack of diagnostic reproducibility, which limits its utility as a prognostic finding [32, 33]. If LVI is to retain its clinical significance, it should be reported with caution and after applying rigid criteria for its identification. In this regard, a number of endothelial/vascular IHC markers can be used to confirm the presence of LVI such as CD31, CD34, D2-40, and ERG [34, 35]. It is not recommended, however, to use these markers as a screening tool in all cases of invasive urothelial carcinoma and they should be used only in histologically equivocal cases for confirmation.

The Role of IHC in Staging of Bladder Cancer

For the majority of cases, documenting invasion in bladder cancer is not problematic by following well-established and recognized criteria [36]. In cases of ambiguity, however, such as thermal artifact, marked inflammation, or disrupted anatomy due to a prior biopsy, applying IHC may be helpful. The most commonly used markers are cytokeratins (AE1/AE3, CK7, CK8/18). An important caveat is the potential staining of stromal myofibroblasts with such epithelial markers.

Documenting tumor invasion of the muscularis propria (MP) is an important parameter in staging urothelial carcinoma, upon which major management decisions depend, such as proceeding to radical cystectomy or the administration of neoadjuvant chemotherapy. The distinction between MP and muscularis mucosae (MM), although readily achieved by light microscopy in most cases, may be challenging in some situations, such as extensive tumor infiltration of tissue fragments, post-biopsy changes that mask the normal anatomy, marked thermal artifact of tumor-bearing tissue, or hyperplastic MM. Several muscle markers have been tried in the past but were found to be of limited utility such as smooth muscle actin, desmin, and caldesmon. Recent reports have identified a new marker, smoothelin, expressed by terminally differentiated smooth muscle cells, to be differentially expressed in smooth muscle of the MP compared to that of the MM [37–41]. It should be noted, however, that other studies reported overlap of staining intensity of smoothelin between MM and MP [42]. Hence, it is still early to determine the exact role of smoothelin as a diagnostic marker to determine tumor invasion into MP and should be used with caution.

Immunohistochemical Markers with Prognostic Value in Bladder Cancer

In papillary urothelial tumors, a number of markers have shown promising results, particularly in distinguishing between low-grade and high-grade papillary urothelial carcinoma and decreasing the interobserver variability in this category. Ki-67 and survivin were two markers that have been frequently studied and whose increased expression correlates with recurrence and progression of papillary tumors [43, 44]. Similar results were reported when the mRNA levels of survivin were measured both in urine cytology and tumor tissue [43, 45–48].

Despite the great advancement in the molecular biology of urothelial carcinoma, there has not been to date a molecular marker that outperforms a combination of established morphologic and clinical markers such as grade, histologic type, and stage, in predicting clinical outcome. This has been the case with the tumor suppressor genes p53 and Rb, which are known to be involved in urothelial neoplasia. Although they have been shown by several investigators to be accurate predictors of progression, metastasis, survival, and possibly response to systemic chemotherapy [49–53], others have challenged these results which have not been validated prospectively.

On the other hand, IHC can serve as a surrogate marker for underlying molecular aberrations that can be used in targeted therapy. In particular, alterations in receptor tyrosine kinases present promising opportunities for targeted therapy in urothelial carcinomas, such as those targeting *ERBB2* (Her2) amplifications or mutations and *FGFR3* mutations; as well as aberrations in the mTOR/Akt/PI3K pathway that are known to affect subsets of urothelial carcinoma [54–57].

GATA3 is a transcription factor of the GATA family whose functions include regulating genes involved in the luminal differentiation of breast epithelium, genes related to T-cell development, gene regulation in the development or maintenance of skin, trophoblasts, and some endothelial cells [12, 58]. GATA3 has been identified as an IHC marker for mammary and urothelial carcinomas in both primary and metastatic setting. It has been suggested useful in the distinction between urothelial versus prostatic adenocarcinoma and metastatic urothelial versus squamous cell carcinoma in the lung. Despite the early promising specificity and sensitivity, however, more recent studies have shown that not all non-urothelial squamous cell carcinomas or prostate cancers to be negative [12, 18, 25–27]. GATA3 can still be of use in the workup of a neoplasm with possible urothelial origin if used with the right context and right combination with other antibodies.

Uroplakins are widely regarded as urothelium-specific proteins of terminal urothelial cell differentiation and have been reported positive in both primary and metastatic urothelial carcinoma [59–62]. Despite being specific to urothelial differentiation, they are not very sensitive as some urothelial carcinomas are not positive for these markers, which limits their practical use and requires the addition of other markers in the workup for a potential urothelial tumor.

Thrombomodulin is a surface glycoprotein involved in the regulation of intravascular coagulation that has been reported to be expressed in a variety of tumors including mesothelioma, endothelial vascular tumors, squamous carcinomas, urothelial carcinoma, and various adenocarcinomas in primary and metastatic setting [63]. The lack of specificity of this marker to urothelial differentiation limits its use in this setting. But as it has been shown in a number of studies mentioned in this section, this marker can be useful when used in combination with other markers in the workup of a potential urothelial tumor.

S100P is a member of the S100 family of proteins that was first discovered in placenta and was thus designated S100P (it is different from the S100 that is widely used in the melanocytic and nerve sheath tumors). Although it was initially identified in the placenta, expression of S100P by IHC has also been described in benign and malignant urothelial cells, pancreatic carcinoma, esophageal squamous mucosa, and breast carcinoma [11].

Urine-Based Markers for Diagnosis of Bladder Cancer

Fluorescence In Situ Hybridization (UroVysion®, Abbott Molecular, Abbott Park, IL, USA)

UroVysion® is a FISH probe set with Food and Drug Administration (FDA) approval for use in monitoring tumor recurrence and primary detection of UC in voided urine specimens from patients with gross or microscopic hematuria, but no previous history of UC. The UroVysion® test probe set contains a mixture of four fluorescent labeled DNA probes; a locus-specific probe to the 9p21 band on chromosome 9 and to the centromere of chromosomes 3, 7, and 17. The individual sensitivity of the centromeric probes for chromosome 3, 7, 17 is reported to be 73.7, 76.2, and 61.9%, respectively, while the sensitivity of homozygous 9p21 deletion for UC has been reported as 28.6% [64]. The UroVysion® test is based on combination of these probes and the sensitivity and specificity has been reported to be 72 and 83%, respectively [65]. This test, however, is not free of false positive and false negative results [66]. Inflammation may interfere with proper interpretation of the test.

The Bladder Tumor Antigen (BTA) Tests

This test is based on the detection of the human complement factor H-related protein, which is reported to be expressed only in bladder tumor cells [67, 68]. There are two types of BTA tests, one can be used in the physician's office or even in the patient's home (BTA stat), while the other has to be sent to a reference laboratory for analysis (BTA trak). The sensitivity of the BTA stat is reported to be 50% for low-grade urothelial carcinomas, which is higher than cytology. Conversely, the specificity of BTA stat is reportedly lower than cytology [69, 70]. The BTA stat test is FDA-approved for use by patients undergoing monitoring for recurrent bladder cancer.

Nuclear Matrix Protein 22 (NMP22)

This test is based on the detection of NMP22, which is a member of a family of proteins that is part of the structural framework of the nucleus and provide support for the nuclear shape. It is also involved in DNA replication, RNA transcription, and regulation of gene expression [71]. This protein is reported to have a concentration as high as 25 times in UC as compared to normal urothelial cells [71, 72]. This assay is FDA-approved for both the detection of new cancers and the follow-up of patients with a prior history of urothelial carcinoma. The reported sensitivity ranges are 34.6–100%, and 49.5–65.0%, but false positive results have been reported [73, 74].

Bladder Cancer Immunofluorescence Assay (Former Immunocyt®)

This is an immunofluorescence assay designed to improve the sensitivity of urine cytology. It employs a cocktail of three monoclonal antibodies; M344, LDQ10, and 19A211 [75]. The first two detect a mucin-like antigen, while the third one recognizes a high molecular weight glycosylated form of carcinoembryonic antigen in exfoliated tumor cells. This assay is FDA approved only for use as a surveillance test if used in conjunction with cytology. The overall sensitivity of the combined Bladder Cancer Immunofluorescence Assay and cytology is approximately 84%, which is better than either test alone. It performs better at the detection of low-grade UC [76, 77].

Telomerase

Telomeres are repetition sequences at the end of chromosomes that protect genetic stability during DNA replication. As a result of telomeric loss during each cell division, chromosomal instability and cell senescence develops. Bladder cancer cells express telomerase, which is an enzyme that regenerates telomeres at the end of each DNA replication. The detection of the ribonucleoprotein telomerase (the telomerase subunits human telomerase RNA [hTR] and human telomerase reverse transcriptase [hTERT]) in urine samples may offer diagnostic applications as the activity of this enzyme is generally limited to malignant cells and tissues. Detection of telomerase activity is available by the TRAP-assay (telomeric repeat amplification protocol), which is a polymerase chain reaction (PCR)-based method [78, 79]. Most studies on telomerase activity in bladder cancer report good sensitivity of the tests but low specificity. Moreover, test results can be influenced by the patient's age and inflammatory conditions of the urinary system, making this assay a suboptimal test for the detection of bladder cancer [78, 80].

In a recent comprehensive review of the role of urine biomarkers in the detection and surveillance of bladder cancer, there were several markers that showed higher sensitivity compared with cytology but were less specific. Hence, they remain insufficient to replace cystoscopy approach to establish the diagnosis of urothelial carcinoma [81].

There is a need for well-designed protocols and prospective, controlled trials to provide the basis to integrate biomarkers into clinical decision making for bladder cancer detection and screening in the future.

Acknowledgement Microphotographs provided by Dr. Magi-Galluzzi

References

1. McKenney JK, Desai S, Cohen C, Amin MB. Discriminatory immunohistochemical staining of urothelial carcinoma in situ and non-neoplastic urothelium: an analysis of cytokeratin 20, p53, and CD44 antigens. Am J Surg Pathol. 2001;25(8):1074–8.
2. Kunju LP, Lee CT, Montie J, Shah RB. Utility of cytokeratin 20 and Ki-67 as markers of urothelial dysplasia. Pathol Int. 2005;55(5):248–54.
3. Mallofre C, Castillo M, Morente V, Sole M. Immunohistochemical expression of CK20, p53, and Ki-67 as objective markers of urothelial dysplasia. Mod Pathol. 2003;16(3):187–91.
4. Oliva E, Pinheiro NF, Heney NM, Kaufman DS, Shipley WU, Gurski C, et al. Immunohistochemistry as an adjunct in the differential diagnosis of radiation-induced atypia versus urothelial carcinoma in situ of the bladder: a study of 45 cases. Hum Pathol. 2013;44(5):860–6.
5. Coleman JF, Hansel DE. Utility of diagnostic and prognostic markers in urothelial carcinoma of the bladder. Adv Anat Pathol. 2009;16(2):67–78.
6. Bates AW, Baithun SI. Secondary neoplasms of the bladder are histological mimics of nontransitional cell primary tumours: clinicopathological and histological features of 282 cases. Histopathology. 2000;36(1):32–40.
7. Genega EM, Hutchinson B, Reuter VE, Gaudin PB. Immunophenotype of high-grade prostatic adenocarcinoma and urothelial carcinoma. Mod Pathol. 2000;13(11):1186–91.
8. Chuang AY, DeMarzo AM, Veltri RW, Sharma RB, Bieberich CJ, Epstein JI. Immunohistochemical differentiation of high-grade prostate carcinoma from urothelial carcinoma. Am J Surg Pathol. 2007;31(8):1246–55.
9. Hameed O, Humphrey PA. Immunohistochemistry in diagnostic surgical pathology of the prostate. Semin Diagn Pathol. 2005;22(1):88–104.
10. Liu H, Shi J, Wilkerson ML, Lin F. Immunohistochemical evaluation of GATA3 expression in tumors and normal tissues: a useful immunomarker for breast and urothelial carcinomas. Am J Clin Pathol. 2012;138(1):57–64.
11. Higgins JP, Kaygusuz G, Wang L, Montgomery K, Mason V, Zhu SX, et al. Placental S100 (S100P) and GATA3: markers for transitional epithelium and urothelial carcinoma discovered by complementary DNA microarray. Am J Surg Pathol. 2007;31(5):673–80.
12. Miettinen M, McCue PA, Sarlomo-Rikala M, Rys J, Czapiewski P, Wazny K, et al. GATA3: a multispecific but potentially useful marker in surgical pathology: a systematic analysis of 2500 epithelial and nonepithelial tumors. Am J Surg Pathol. 2014;38(1):13–22.
13. Wang HL, Lu DW, Yerian LM, Alsikafi N, Steinberg G, Hart J, et al. Immunohistochemical distinction between primary adenocarcinoma of the bladder and secondary colorectal adenocarcinoma. Am J Surg Pathol. 2001;25(11):1380–7.
14. Paner GP, McKenney JK, Barkan GA, Yao JL, Frankel WL, Sebo TJ, et al. Immunohistochemical analysis in a morphologic spectrum of urachal epithelial neoplasms: diagnostic implications and pitfalls. Am J Surg Pathol. 2011;35(6):787–98.
15. Roy S, Smith MA, Cieply KM, Acquafondata MB, Parwani AV. Primary bladder adenocarcinoma versus metastatic colorectal adenocarcinoma: a persisting diagnostic challenge. Diagn Pathol. 2012;7:151.
16. Rao Q, Williamson SR, Lopez-Beltran A, Montironi R, Huang W, Eble JN, et al. Distinguishing primary adenocarcinoma of the urinary bladder from secondary involvement by colorectal adenocarcinoma: extended immunohistochemical profiles emphasizing novel markers. Mod Pathol. 2013;26(5):725–32.
17. Huang W, Williamson SR, Rao Q, Lopez-Beltran A, Montironi R, Eble JN, et al. Novel markers of squamous differentiation in the urinary bladder. Hum Pathol. 2013;44(10):1989–97.

18. Gulmann C, Paner GP, Parakh RS, Hansel DE, Shen SS, Ro JY, et al. Immunohistochemical profile to distinguish urothelial from squamous differentiation in carcinomas of urothelial tract. Hum Pathol. 2013;44(2):164–72.
19. Dehn D, Torkko KC, Shroyer KR. Human papillomavirus testing and molecular markers of cervical dysplasia and carcinoma. Cancer. 2007;111(1):1–14.
20. Agoff SN, Lin P, Morihara J, Mao C, Kiviat NB, Koutsky LA. p16(INK4a) expression correlates with degree of cervical neoplasia: a comparison with Ki-67 expression and detection of high-risk HPV types. Mod Pathol. 2003;16(7):665–73.
21. Alexander RE, Hu Y, Kum JB, Montironi R, Lopez-Beltran A, Maclennan GT, et al. p16 expression is not associated with human papillomavirus in urinary bladder squamous cell carcinoma. Mod Pathol. 2012;25(11):1526–33.
22. Blochin EB, Park KJ, Tickoo SK, Reuter VE, Al-Ahmadie H. Urothelial carcinoma with prominent squamous differentiation in the setting of neurogenic bladder: role of human papillomavirus infection. Mod Pathol. 2012;25(11):1534–42.
23. Chapman-Fredricks JR, Cioffi-Lavina M, Accola MA, Rehrauer WM, Garcia-Buitrago MT, Gomez-Fernandez C, et al. High-risk human papillomavirus DNA detected in primary squamous cell carcinoma of urinary bladder. Arch Pathol Lab Med. 2013;137(8):1088–93.
24. Shanks JH, Iczkowski KA. Spindle cell lesions of the bladder and urinary tract. Histopathology. 2009;55(5):491–504.
25. Zhao L, Antic T, Witten D, Paner GP, Taxy JB, Husain A, et al. Is GATA3 expression maintained in regional metastases?: a study of paired primary and metastatic urothelial carcinomas. Am J Surg Pathol. 2013;37(12):1876–81.
26. Gruver AM, Amin MB, Luthringer DJ, Westfall D, Arora K, Farver CF, et al. Selective immunohistochemical markers to distinguish between metastatic high-grade urothelial carcinoma and primary poorly differentiated invasive squamous cell carcinoma of the lung. Arch Pathol Lab Med. 2012;136(11):1339–46.
27. Chang A, Amin A, Gabrielson E, Illei P, Roden RB, Sharma R, et al. Utility of GATA3 immunohistochemistry in differentiating urothelial carcinoma from prostate adenocarcinoma and squamous cell carcinomas of the uterine cervix, anus, and lung. Am J Surg Pathol. 2012;36(10):1472–6.
28. Parker DC, Folpe AL, Bell J, Oliva E, Young RH, Cohen C, et al. Potential utility of uroplakin III, thrombomodulin, high molecular weight cytokeratin, and cytokeratin 20 in noninvasive, invasive, and metastatic urothelial (transitional cell) carcinomas. Am J Surg Pathol. 2003;27(1):1–10.
29. Gondo T, Nakashima J, Ozu C, Ohno Y, Horiguchi Y, Namiki K, et al. Risk stratification of survival by lymphovascular invasion, pathological stage, and surgical margin in patients with bladder cancer treated with radical cystectomy. Int J Clin Oncol. 2012;17(5):456–61.
30. Lotan Y, Gupta A, Shariat SF, Palapattu GS, Vazina A, Karakiewicz PI, et al. Lymphovascular invasion is independently associated with overall survival, cause-specific survival, and local and distant recurrence in patients with negative lymph nodes at radical cystectomy. J Clin Oncol. 2005;23(27):6533–9.
31. Bolenz C, Herrmann E, Bastian PJ, Michel MS, Wulfing C, Tiemann A, et al. Lymphovascular invasion is an independent predictor of oncological outcomes in patients with lymph node-negative urothelial bladder cancer treated by radical cystectomy: a multicentre validation trial. BJU Int. 2010;106(4):493–9.
32. Algaba F. Lymphovascular invasion as a prognostic tool for advanced bladder cancer. Curr Opin Urol. 2006;16(5):367–71.
33. Reuter VE. Lymphovascular invasion as an independent predictor of recurrence and survival in node-negative bladder cancer remains to be proven. J Clin Oncol. 2005;23(27):6450–1.
34. Park K, Tomlins SA, Mudaliar KM, Chiu YL, Esgueva R, Mehra R, et al. Antibody-based detection of ERG rearrangement-positive prostate cancer. Neoplasia. 2010;12(7):590–8. P
35. Kahn HJ, Marks A. A new monoclonal antibody, D2–40, for detection of lymphatic invasion in primary tumors. Lab Invest. 2002;82(9):1255–7.
36. Epstein JI, Amin MB, Reuter VR, Mostofi FK. The world health organization/international society of urological pathology consensus classification of urothelial (transitional cell) neoplasms of the urinary bladder. Bladder consensus conference committee. Am J Surg Pathol. 1998;22(12):1435–48.
37. Paner GP, Shen SS, Lapetino S, Venkataraman G, Barkan GA, Quek ML, et al. Diagnostic utility of antibody to smoothelin in the distinction of muscularis propria from muscularis mucosae of the urinary bladder: a potential ancillary tool in the pathologic staging of invasive urothelial carcinoma. Am J Surg Pathol. 2009;33(1):91–8.
38. Council L, Hameed O. Differential expression of immunohistochemical markers in bladder smooth muscle and myofibroblasts, and the potential utility of desmin, smoothelin, and vimentin in staging of bladder carcinoma. Mod Pathol. 2009;22(5):639–50.
39. Paner GP, Brown JG, Lapetino S, Nese N, Gupta R, Shen SS, et al. Diagnostic use of antibody to smoothelin in the recognition of muscularis propria in transurethral resection of urinary bladder tumor (TURBT) specimens. Am J Surg Pathol. 2010;34(6):792–9.
40. Hansel DE, Paner GP, Nese N, Amin MB. Limited smoothelin expression within the muscularis mucosae: validation in bladder diverticula. Hum Pathol. 2011;42(11):1770–6.
41. Khayyata S, Dudas M, Rohan SM, Gopalan A, Fine SW, Reuter VE, et al. Distribution of smoothelin expression in the musculature of the genitourinary tract. Lab Invest. 2009;89:175a–a.

42. Miyamoto H, Sharma RB, Illei PB, Epstein JI. Pitfalls in the use of smoothelin to identify muscularis propria invasion by urothelial carcinoma. Am J Surg Pathol. 2010;34(3):418–22.
43. Chen YB, Tu JJ, Kao J, Zhou XK, Chen YT. Survivin as a useful adjunct marker for the grading of papillary urothelial carcinoma. Arch Pathol Lab Med. 2008;132(2):224–31.
44. Yin W, Chen N, Zhang Y, Zeng H, Chen X, He Y, et al. Survivin nuclear labeling index: a superior biomarker in superficial urothelial carcinoma of human urinary bladder. Mod Pathol. 2006;19(11):1487–97.
45. Karam JA, Lotan Y, Ashfaq R, Sagalowsky AI, Shariat SF. Survivin expression in patients with non-muscle-invasive urothelial cell carcinoma of the bladder. Urology. 2007;70(3):482–6.
46. Schultz IJ, Kiemeney LA, Karthaus HF, Witjes JA, Willems JL, Swinkels DW, et al. Survivin mRNA copy number in bladder washings predicts tumor recurrence in patients with superficial urothelial cell carcinomas. Clin Chem. 2004;50(8):1425–8.
47. Moussa O, Abol-Enein H, Bissada NK, Keane T, Ghoneim MA, Watson DK. Evaluation of survivin reverse transcriptase-polymerase chain reaction for noninvasive detection of bladder cancer. J Urol. 2006;175(6):2312–6.
48. Eissa S, Badr S, Barakat M, Zaghloul AS, Mohanad M. The diagnostic efficacy of urinary survivin and hyaluronidase mRNA as urine markers in patients with bladder cancer. Clin Lab. 2013;59(7–8):893–900.
49. Dalbagni G, Presti JC Jr., Reuter VE, Zhang ZF, Sarkis AS, Fair WR, et al. Molecular genetic alterations of chromosome 17 and p53 nuclear overexpression in human bladder cancer. Diagn Mol Pathol. 1993;2(1):4–13.
50. Fujimoto K, Yamada Y, Okajima E, Kakizoe T, Sasaki H, Sugimura T, et al. Frequent association of p53 gene mutation in invasive bladder cancer. Cancer Res. 1992;52(6):1393–8.
51. Sidransky D, Von Eschenbach A, Tsai YC, Jones P, Summerhayes I, Marshall F, et al. Identification of p53 gene mutations in bladder cancers and urine samples. Science. 1991;252(5006):706–9.
52. Cordon-Cardo C, Wartinger D, Petrylak D, Dalbagni G, Fair WR, Fuks Z, et al. Altered expression of the retinoblastoma gene product: prognostic indicator in bladder cancer. J Natl Cancer Inst. 1992;84(16):1251–6.
53. Cairns P, Proctor AJ, Knowles MA. Loss of heterozygosity at the RB locus is frequent and correlates with muscle invasion in bladder carcinoma. Oncogene. 1991;6(12):2305–9.
54. Iyer G, Al-Ahmadie H, Schultz N, Hanrahan AJ, Ostrovnaya I, Balar AV, et al. Prevalence and co-occurrence of actionable genomic alterations in high-grade bladder cancer. J Clin Oncol. 2013;31(25):3133–40.
55. Milowsky MI, Iyer G, Regazzi AM, Al-Ahmadie H, Gerst SR, Ostrovnaya I, et al. Phase II study of everolimus in metastatic urothelial cancer. BJU Int. 2013;112(4):462–70.
56. Iyer G, Hanrahan AJ, Milowsky MI, Al-Ahmadie H, Scott SN, Janakiraman M, et al. Genome sequencing identifies a basis for everolimus sensitivity. Science. 2012;338(6104):221.
57. Al-Ahmadie HA, Iyer G, Janakiraman M, Lin O, Heguy A, Tickoo SK, et al. Somatic mutation of fibroblast growth factor receptor-3 (FGFR3) defines a distinct morphological subtype of high-grade urothelial carcinoma. J Pathol. 2011;224(2):270–9.
58. Chou J, Provot S, Werb Z. GATA3 in development and cancer differentiation: cells GATA have it! J Cell Physiol. 2010;222(1):42–9.
59. Olsburgh J, Harnden P, Weeks R, Smith B, Joyce A, Hall G, et al. Uroplakin gene expression in normal human tissues and locally advanced bladder cancer. J Pathol. 2003;199(1):41–9.
60. Kageyama S, Yoshiki T, Isono T, Tanaka T, Kim CJ, Yuasa T, et al. High expression of human uroplakin Ia in urinary bladder transitional cell carcinoma. Jpn J Cancer Res. 2002;93(5):523–31.
61. Mhawech P, Uchida T, Pelte MF. Immunohistochemical profile of high-grade urothelial bladder carcinoma and prostate adenocarcinoma. Hum Pathol. 2002;33(11):1136–40.
62. Xu X, Sun TT, Gupta PK, Zhang P, Nasuti JF. Uroplakin as a marker for typing metastatic transitional cell carcinoma on fine-needle aspiration specimens. Cancer. 2001;93(3):216–21.
63. Ordonez NG. Thrombomodulin expression in transitional cell carcinoma. Am J Clin Pathol. 1998;110(3):385–90.
64. Sokolova IA, Halling KC, Jenkins RB, Burkhardt HM, Meyer RG, Seelig SA, et al. The development of a multitarget, multicolor fluorescence in situ hybridization assay for the detection of urothelial carcinoma in urine. J Mol Diagn. 2000;2(3):116–23.
65. Hajdinjak T. UroVysion FISH test for detecting urothelial cancers: meta-analysis of diagnostic accuracy and comparison with urinary cytology testing. Urol Oncol. 2008;26(6):646–51.
66. Ferra S, Denley R, Herr H, Dalbagni G, Jhanwar S, Lin O. Reflex UroVysion testing in suspicious urine cytology cases. Cancer. 2009;117(1):7–14.
67. Burchardt M, Burchardt T, Shabsigh A, De La Taille A, Benson MC, Sawczuk I. Current concepts in biomarker technology for bladder cancers. Clin Chem. 2000;46(5):595–605.
68. Heicappell R, Wettig IC, Schostak M, Muller M, Steiner U, Sauter T, et al. Quantitative detection of human complement factor H-related protein in transitional cell carcinoma of the urinary bladder. Eur Urol. 1999;35(1):81–7.
69. Murphy WM, Rivera-Ramirez I, Medina CA, Wright NJ, Wajsman Z. The bladder tumor antigen (BTA) test compared to voided urine cytology in the detection of bladder neoplasms. J Urol. 1997;158(6):2102–6.
70. Sanchez-Carbayo M, Herrero E, Megias J, Mira A, Espasa A, Chinchilla V, et al. Initial evaluation

of the diagnostic performance of the new urinary bladder cancer antigen test as a tumor marker for transitional cell carcinoma of the bladder. J Urol. 1999;161(4):1110–5.
71. Berezney R, Coffey DS. Identification of a nuclear protein matrix. Biochem Biophys Res Commun. 1974;60(4):1410–7.
72. Fey EG, Krochmalnic G, Penman S. The nonchromatin substructures of the nucleus: the ribonucleoprotein (RNP)-containing and RNP-depleted matrices analyzed by sequential fractionation and resinless section electron microscopy. J Cell Biol. 1986;102(5):1654–65.
73. Budman LI, Kassouf W, Steinberg JR. Biomarkers for detection and surveillance of bladder cancer. Can Urol Assoc J. 2008;2(3):212–21.
74. Chang YH, Wu CH, Lee YL, Huang PH, Kao YL, Shiau MY. Evaluation of nuclear matrix protein-22 as a clinical diagnostic marker for bladder cancer. Urology. 2004;64(4):687–92.
75. Fradet Y, Lockhard C. Performance characteristics of a new monoclonal antibody test for bladder cancer: immunoCyt trade mark. Can J Urol. 1997;4(3):400–5.
76. Tetu B, Tiguert R, Harel F, Fradet Y. ImmunoCyt/uCyt+ improves the sensitivity of urine cytology in patients followed for urothelial carcinoma. Mod Pathol. 2005;18(1):83–9.
77. Sullivan PS, Nooraie F, Sanchez H, Hirschowitz S, Levin M, Rao PN, et al. Comparison of immunoCyt, UroVysion, and urine cytology in detection of recurrent urothelial carcinoma: a "split-sample" study. Cancer. 2009;117(3):167–73.
78. Muller M. Telomerase: its clinical relevance in the diagnosis of bladder cancer. Oncogene. 2002;21(4):650–5.
79. Kim NW, Piatyszek MA, Prowse KR, Harley CB, West MD, Ho PL, et al. Specific association of human telomerase activity with immortal cells and cancer. Science. 1994;266(5193):2011–5.
80. Weikert S, Krause H, Wolff I, Christoph F, Schrader M, Emrich T, et al. Quantitative evaluation of telomerase subunits in urine as biomarkers for noninvasive detection of bladder cancer. Int J Cancer. 2005;117(2):274–80.
81. Xylinas E, Kluth LA, Rieken M, Karakiewicz PI, Lotan Y, Shariat SF. Urine markers for detection and surveillance of bladder cancer. Urol Oncol. 2014;32(3):222–9.

Intraoperative Consultation for Bladder Tumors: Challenges and Implications for Treatment

19

Hiroshi Miyamoto and Steven S. Shen

Introduction

Urothelial neoplasm is by far the most common urinary bladder tumor (comprising more than 90%). Other less common histologic types of tumor include squamous cell carcinoma, adenocarcinoma, and neuroendocrine carcinomas. Patients with bladder tumor often present with hematuria, with or without other urinary symptoms such as dysuria and urgency, and the diagnosis is usually made after cystoscopic examination followed by transurethral resection (TUR) of the lesion. Almost all neoplastic lesions of the bladder are biopsied or resected before intravesical therapy or definitive surgery, but intraoperative diagnosis remains important in selected situations. It is also important to know that the utilization of intraoperative frozen section assessment (FSA) during bladder surgery also varies in different institutions and depends on urologists.

To provide an appropriate frozen section diagnosis, the pathologist should be familiar with clinical history, imaging and prior biopsy findings, history of prior treatment, and surgeon's operative plan. The following examples illustrate the value of clinicopathologic correlation:

S. S. Shen (✉)
Department of Pathology and Genomic Medicine, Houston Methodist Hospital, Houston, TX, USA
e-mail: stevenshen@houstonmethodist.org

H. Miyamoto
Departments of Pathology and Urology, The Johns Hopkins Medical Institutions, Baltimore, MD, USA
e-mail: hmiyamo1@jhmi.edu

- Clinical aspects of the case may help to increase the chance of identifying invasive carcinoma or carcinoma in-situ (CIS) at the surgical margins (e.g., imaging studies suggest a neoplasm in one of the ureters, there is extensive biopsy-proven CIS).
- The prior TUR observations may help to interpret unusual findings in a biopsy of an extravesical nodule (e.g., a spindle cell lesion is not dismissed as reactive fibroblastic tissue if the patient is known to have a sarcomatoid urothelial carcinoma).
- It is important to know the operative plan (e.g., an FSA of extravesical positive lymph node or visceral lesion may dissuade the surgeon from completing radical cystectomy).

Common Indications for Intraoperative Consultation

- The status of surgical margins at the ureter, urethra, and soft tissue during radical cystectomy
- The status of surgical margins during partial cystectomy
- Histopathologic diagnosis of extravesical masses or lesions incidentally detected during cystectomy
- Initial diagnosis of primary bladder lesion
- Lymph node metastatic status during cystectomy

C. Magi-Galluzzi, C. G. Przybycin (eds.), *Genitourinary Pathology,* DOI 10.1007/978-1-4939-2044-0_19,

Assessment of Surgical Margins During Radical Cystectomy or Cystoprostatectomy

Radial cystectomy, combined with pelvic lymph node dissection, is the standard treatment for muscle-invasive bladder carcinomas, as well as high-grade non-muscle-invasive urothelial carcinomas that are resistant to conventional intravesical therapy or show adverse prognostic features (e.g., extensive lymphovascular invasion, aggressive histologic variants including micropapillary urothelial carcinoma). Intraoperative assessment of ureteral, urethral, and radial/perivesical soft tissue margins during radical cystectomy are important because negative margins reduce the risk of tumor recurrence and may influence decision making regarding the choice of urinary diversion [1, 2]. The incidence of marked atypia or CIS found at the ureteral margins has been reported to range from 4.8 to 9% [1, 2], whereas the apical urethral margin is rarely positive [3]. As a result, the ureteral margins are often routinely submitted for FSA, and the distal urethral margin much less frequently. However, FSA of the urethral margin is commonly performed in cases without pre-cystectomy prostatic urethra biopsies. Additionally, if there are changes of concern for malignancy in the perivesical soft tissue, a biopsy is submitted for FSA as this may influence whether total cystectomy is undergone.

When a short segment (i.e., <0.5 cm) of the ureter is submitted, the lumen should be identified and entire specimen should be embedded for FSA. For longer segments of ureter, the true margin is usually designated by the surgeon with a suture or ink, and this end should be amputated from the specimen and embedded for FSA. Changes at the ureteral margin should be reported as nondysplastic (normal or reactive), atypia not further classified, high-grade dysplasia/CIS, or invasive carcinoma. Reactive atypia is relatively common in patients with bladder cancer, possibly induced by prior therapy, and is often associated with inflammation, edema, or fibrosis of lamina propria (Fig. 19.1). The diagnosis of "low-grade dysplasia" should be avoided if possible because of the poor reproducibility between pathologists particularly on FSA and the uncertainty about how this lesion should be treated. The diagnosis of CIS is based on both architectural and cytologic features (Fig. 19.2), but full thickness atypia is not required to make the diagnosis; for instance, partial involvement or pagetoid spread is

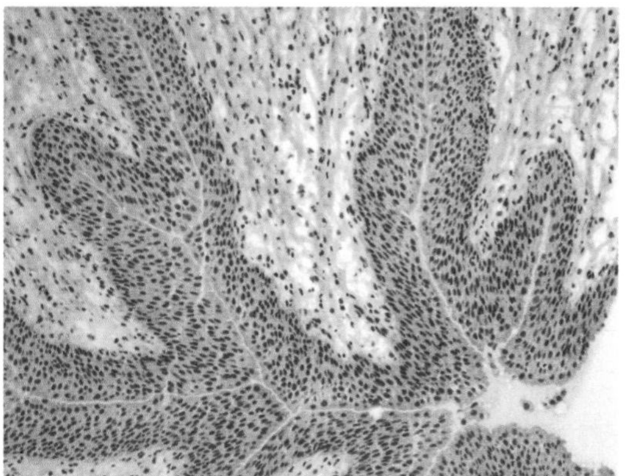

Fig. 19.1 Frozen section of a ureteral margin showing urothelium with reactive atypia associated with subepithelial edema and mild chronic inflammation. Slight, but uniform, nuclear enlargement is seen, but the nuclear polarity is maintained. Original magnification × 100

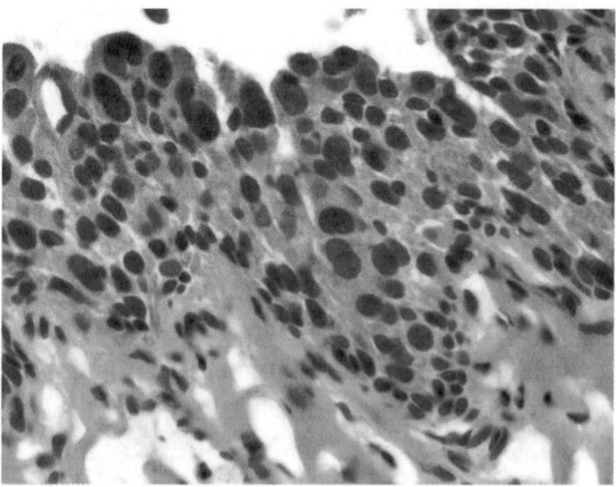

Fig. 19.2 Frozen section of a ureteral margin positive for urothelial carcinoma in-situ (*CIS*). On frozen section, the most reliable criteria for diagnosis of urothelial *CIS* is marked cytologic atypia with nuclear enlargement, increased nuclear to cytoplasmic ratio, hyperchromasia, and frequent mitoses. Original magnification × 400

Fig. 19.3 Frozen section of the ureter showing largely denuded and attenuated urothelium with scattered in-situ carcinoma cells. Original magnification × 200

sufficient for the diagnosis of CIS. Dilatation of the ureter, vascular proliferation, and chronic inflammation of the subepithelial connective tissue are often associated with CIS, and the presence of these findings should alert the pathologist to have more critical assessment of the urothelium. In addition, urothelial CIS frequently undergoes complete or partial sloughing of neoplastic cells (Fig. 19.3). When this is encountered, deeper levels should be prepared so that diagnostic changes of CIS can be seen.

Because of retraction of the urethral mucosa, multiple levels of the specimen for intraoperative FSA may be necessary to identify the mucosa. The urothelium is often denuded due to intravesical therapy or intubation, special attention should be paid to the periurethral glands or ducts; pagetoid spread with a few high-grade malignant cells is sufficient for the diagnosis of urothelial CIS (Fig. 19.4).

A biopsy of perivesical fat may be submitted for FSA to determine if there is extravesical extension or invasion of the tumor. Fat necrosis with associated fibrosis is not uncommonly seen, which is usually not too difficult to distinguish from carcinoma (Fig. 19.5). Reactive endothelial cells can sometimes be problematic, especially when they show cautery artifact. Thus, familiarity of preoperative diagnosis, intraoperative findings, and careful assessment of cytologic details are necessary for an accurate diagnosis.

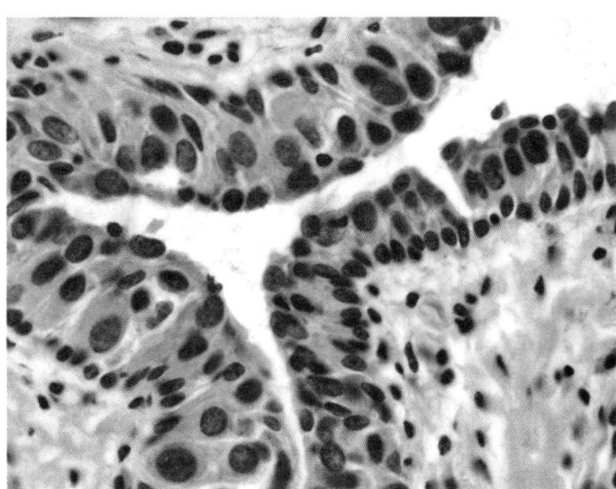

Fig. 19.4 Frozen section of the urethra showing a prominent pagetoid spread of urothelial *CIS* characterized by individual large atypical tumor cells peculating in the urothelium. Notice the marked nuclear enlargement of tumor cells compared with the adjacent normal basal cells. Original magnification × 400

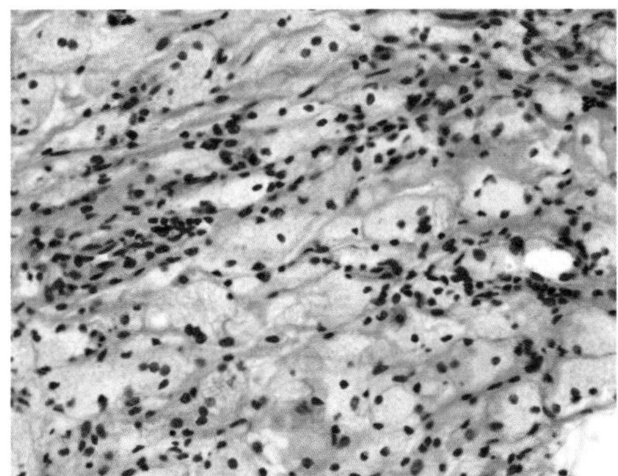

Fig. 19.5 Frozen section of a nodule on the peritoneal surface of the bladder showing fat necrosis and plump endothelial cells which may mimic infiltrating carcinoma. Original magnification × 200

Assessment of Surgical Margins During Partial Cystectomy

Partial cystectomy, without a separate urinary diversion, is reserved for localized tumors, including solitary, primary urothelial carcinoma that does not involve specific regions of the bladder (e.g., trigone, bladder neck) and that can be resected with adequate (i.e., 1–2 cm) surgical margins. The classically described indication for partial cystectomy included carcinoma arising in a bladder diverticulum and urachal adenocarcinoma [4]. Partial cystectomy is also adequate for some high-risk patients and palliative situations. If it is done in properly selected patients, it has some advantages over radical cystectomy, such as the preservation of a functionally continent native urinary bladder and sexual potency in men.

The diagnosis of the bladder tumor is almost always established prior to cystectomy, and the purpose of intraoperative consultation is generally to evaluate surgical margins. This is an example that surgeon's help in orientation of specimen is particularly critical. The margins should be inked, often with different colors when entire partial cystectomy specimen is submitted for FSA. How the sections are taken (i.e., parallel or perpendicular to the margins) is dependent on the gross findings. If a visible lesion is seen within 0.5 cm of the margin, it is advisable to take multiple serial sections perpendicular to that margin. Otherwise, sections may be taken parallel to the margin. Before taking sections parallel to the margin, tissue layers should be lined up so that all the layers could be visible in frozen section slides.

It is much easier to interpret the frozen section findings when the pathologist is familiar with the histologic characteristics of the tumor. For example, mucin pools at the surgical margin in a patient with mucinous carcinoma would be interpreted as a positive margin even if epithelial cells are absent. Likewise, a spindle cell process would be viewed with suspicion in a patient who has a biopsy diagnosis of sarcomatoid carcinoma.

Assessment of Incidental Serosal and Extravesical Lesions

During radical cystectomy, the surgeon may encounter nodules or areas of thickening or discoloration on the peritoneal surface of the bladder or in the perivesical fat, which often prompts a request for FSA. The diagnosis may not alter the surgical procedure if it is in close proximity to the bladder, but extensive extravesical spread of invasive carcinoma may lead to abandonment of radical cystectomy.

Commonly encountered lesions include mesothelial hyperplasia, fibrous nodules, chronic inflammation, calcification, endometriosis, endocervicosis, endosalpingiosis, and rarely metastatic tumor of a nonbladder origin.

Initial Diagnosis of Primary Lesions

Rarely, FSA is requested on a bladder lesion that has an unusual appearance on cystoscopic examination or for which prior biopsies have been unsuccessful. The surgeon's goal is to confirm that the specimen contains diagnostic tissue and, when appropriate, to ensure that muscularis propria (detrusor muscle) is present in the specimen.

If the biopsy consists of one or a few small fragment(s), the entire specimen should be embedded for FSA. If the TUR specimen consists of multiple pieces of tissue, the firmer areas should be selected as they are more likely to contain muscularis propria. A specific diagnosis should be made if it is possible, but a diagnosis such as "high-grade carcinoma with invasion into muscularis propria" is sufficient for immediate management of the patient. However, it is occasionally difficult or even impossible to determine whether the muscle fibers invaded by the tumor in TUR specimens represent true muscularis propria. Under no circumstances should definitive radical surgery be performed on the basis of an equivocal intraoperative consultation diagnosis. Malignant neoplasms, such as lymphoma and metastasis, which do not warrant radical surgery, should be excluded, although this is best done on permanent sections with ancillary tests. Intraoperative communication between the surgeon and pathologist should be clearly documented, and any uncertainty of the diagnosis in terms of histology and staging should be informed and resolved on permanent sections.

Assessment of Pelvic Lymph Nodes During Cystectomy

Pelvic lymph node dissection is performed routinely during radical cystectomy because it not only provides prognostic information but also appears to offer therapeutic benefits. Furthermore, data suggest that higher lymph node numbers

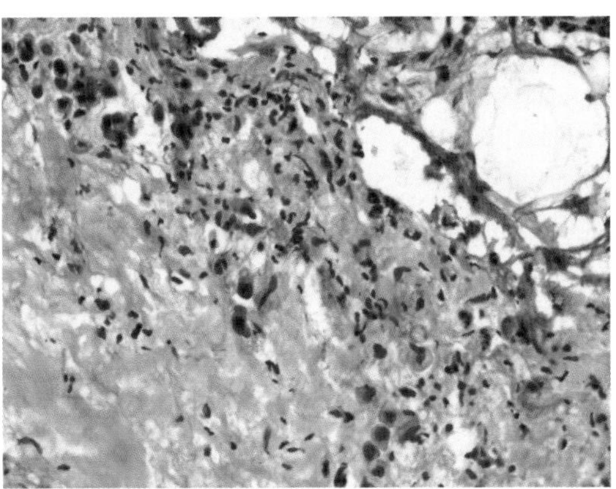

Fig. 19.6 Frozen section of a pelvic lymph node showing rare clusters of atypical tumor cells following neoadjuvant therapy. Original magnification × 200

correlate with improved survival, although node count can depend on multiple factors including surgical techniques and the extent of node dissection as well as surgical pathology processing [5]. Some urologists routinely perform an extended pelvic lymph node dissection and submit the specimens in formalin for evaluation on permanent sections, whereas others perform a limited dissection using intraoperative FSA to guide the extent of the lymph node dissection.

The pathologist should know what is at stake when asked to examine pelvic lymph nodes in a patient with bladder carcinoma, and every effort should be made to determine if there are nodal metastases. If one or more of the lymph nodes are grossly abnormal, a cytoscrape preparation can be made, which may be all that is necessary. If, however, the cytologic findings are negative, the lymph nodes should be embedded in their entirety for FSA, and multiple levels may need to be prepared in an attempt to identify small foci of metastases. It is usually not difficult to identify metastatic urothelial carcinoma on cytologic preparations or FSA, although neoadjuvant therapy may complicate the changes (Fig. 19.6). Pathologists should also be aware of unusual variants when evaluating a lymph node, such as lymphoma-like or plasmacytoid urothelial carcinoma, in which false negative results can occur.

References

1. Raj GV, Tal R, Vickers A, Bochner BH, Serio A, Donat SM, Herr H, Olgac S, Dalbagni G. Significance of intraoperative ureteral evaluation at radical cystectomy for urothelial cancer. Cancer. 2006;107(9):2167–72.
2. Schumacher MC, Scholz M, Weise ES, Fleischmann A, Thalmann GN, Studer UE. Is there an indication for frozen section examination of the ureteral margins during cystectomy for transitional cell carcinoma of the bladder? J Urol. 2006;176(6):2409–13.
3. Stein JP, Clark P, Miranda G, Cai J, Groshen S, Skinner DG. Urethral tumor recurrence following cystectomy and urinary diversion: clinical and pathological characteristics in 768 male patients. J Urol. 2005;173(4):1163–8.
4. Ashley RA, Inman BA, Sebo TJ, Leibovich BC, Blute ML, Kwon ED, Zincke H. Urachal carcinoma: clinicopathologic features and long-term outcomes of an aggressive malignancy. Cancer. 2006;107(4):712–20.
5. Gordetsky J, Scosyrev E, Rashid H, Wu G, Silvers C, Golijanin D, Messing EM, Yao JL. Identifying additional lymph nodes in radical cystectomy lymphadenectomy specimens. Mod Pathol. 2012;25(1):140–4.

20 Genetic and Epigenetic Alterations in Urothelial Carcinoma

Hikmat A. Al-Ahmadie and Gopa Iyer

Introduction

It is estimated that more than 70,000 new cancer cases are caused by urinary bladder cancer in 2013, resulting in nearly 18,000 cancer-related deaths [1]. Until recently, management approaches to these tumors have not incorporated molecular biomarkers in the diagnosis, risk stratification, and treatment, in contrast to what has become an integral component of the clinical management in other tumors such as lung, colon, and breast cancer. Recent major advances in cancer genetics and genomics are changing the landscape and rapidly affecting the clinical management of solid tumors, which undoubtedly includes cancers of the urinary bladder.

Genetic Alterations in Urothelial Carcinoma

Many genetic alterations have been described in bladder cancer including deletions and amplifications of chromosomal regions (wide or focal) as well as many mutations in significant cancer-related genes and pathways. In fact, in a recent comprehensive analysis by The Cancer Genome Atlas (TCGA) Project across several cancer types, bladder cancer (at least invasive into muscularis propria per TCGA inclusion criteria) was one of the cancers with the highest rate of somatic mutations [2]. On average, there were 302 exonic mutations, 204 segmental alterations in genomic copy number, and 22 genomic rearrangements per sample [3].

There is evidence to support viewing bladder cancer as developing through two distinct molecular pathways that correspond to two main groups of tumors with generally distinct treatment considerations: superficial bladder cancer, including noninvasive papillary and flat urothelial carcinoma (UC) and UC invasive into lamina propria and/or muscularis propria (detrusor muscle) [4–8].

Most studies of low-grade papillary UC show few molecular alterations in addition to deletions involving chromosome 9 and mutations of *FGFR3* and *HRAS* [9–20]. These tumors are often near-diploid with loss of chromosome 9 being by far the most common cytogenetic finding [21–23]. In a recent study utilizing whole-exome sequencing, it was reported that *KDM6A* (*UTX)*, one of the genes involved in chromatin remodeling, was significantly more frequently mutated in low-grade and low-stage UC [24]. Another genetic aberration recently reported at a higher frequency in noninvasive papillary UC compared to invasive UC is an inactivating mutation in *STAG2,* a gene which regulates sister

H. A. Al-Ahmadie (✉)
Department of Pathology, Memorial Sloan Kettering Cancer Center, New York, NY, USA
e-mail: alahmadh@mskcc.org

G. Iyer
Department of Medicine, Memorial Sloan Kettering Cancer Center, New York, NY, USA
e-mail: iyerg@mskcc.org

C. Magi-Galluzzi, C. G. Przybycin (eds.), *Genitourinary Pathology,* DOI 10.1007/978-1-4939-2044-0_20,

chromatid cohesion and segregation and has a role in controlling chromosome number and cell division [25–27]. The majority of the mutations reported in *STAG2* were truncating (~85 %) or missense (~15 %), and predicted to result in inactivation of the gene. It was suggested that *STAG2* mutations represent an early event in the development of bladder cancer. It is worth noting that another recent publication reported stronger association between inactivating mutations in *STAG2* and increased tumor aneuploidy and worse outcome compared to tumors without such aberrations [28]. This view, however, was not shared by other investigators [25–27].

Urothelial carcinoma in situ (CIS) is characterized by a high frequency of *TP53* mutations but a relatively low frequency of chromosome 9 loss, unless it is associated with a papillary lesion, in which case loss of chromosome 9 is more frequent [29].

Many genetic alterations have been reported in invasive UC in addition to frequent chromosome 9 deletions, involving dysregulation of several oncogenes and tumor suppressor genes [4–6]. Multiple regions of somatic copy number alteration (CNA) have been reported including amplification of *PPARG*, *E2F3*, *EGFR*, *CCND1,* and *MDM2*, as well as loss of *CDKN2A* and *RB1* [30–32]. Sequencing of candidate pathways has identified recurrent mutations in *TP53*, *FGFR3*, *PIK3CA*, *TSC1*, *RB1,* and *HRAS* [30, 32]. It has been recently shown that tumors with aberrations in *TP53, MDM2, RB1, and E2F3* are associated with more genomic instability compared to tumors without such aberrations [33].

The most comprehensive molecular analysis of invasive UC to date has been conducted by the TCGA which performed an integrated in-depth profiling of DNA copy number, somatic mutation, mRNA and miRNA (miR) expression, protein and phosphorylated protein expression, DNA methylation, and viral integration [3]. This study included samples from 19 tissue source sites and consisted of 131 chemotherapy naive, at least muscle-invasive (pT2), high-grade UC without significant amount of any divergent histology.

By assessing somatic CNAs (SCNAs), multiple aberration were identified including 22 significant arm-level copy number changes, 27 amplified, and 30 deleted recurrent focal SCNAs. The most common recurrent focal deletion contained *CDKN2A* (9p21.3, in 47 % of samples). Other focal deletions involved regions containing *PDE4D*, *RB1*, *FHIT*, *CREBBP*, *IKZF2*, *FOXQ1*, *FAM190A*, *LRP1B,* and *WWOX*. Focal amplifications involved genes previously reported to be altered in bladder cancer such as *E2F3/SOX4*, *CCND1*, *CCNE1*, *EGFR*, *ERBB2*, *PPARG,* and *MDM2* [30–32], but also some that have not been previously reported such as *PVRL4*, *BCL2L1,* and *ZNF703*.

Whole-exome sequencing of tumors along with matched germline samples identified 32 genes with statistically significant levels of recurrent somatic mutation. The most frequently mutated gene was *TP53* (49 %), which was found to be altered in a mutually exclusive relationship with *MDM2* amplification (9 %) or overexpression (29 %). Most *RB1* mutations were inactivating and were mutually exclusive with *CDKN2A* deletions. *PIK3CA* mutations were also relatively common (20 %).

A number of genes involved in epigenetic regulation were significantly mutated such as *MLL2*, *ARID1A*, *KDM6A,* and *EP300*, with truncating mutations being the most common and indicating both a functional significance for these genes and a potential role in tumorigenesis. Other chromatin-regulating genes with less frequent mutations in UC include *MLL3*, *MLL*, *CREBBP*, *CHD7,* and *SRCAP*. Some of these mutations have previously been reported in bladder cancer [24, 28].

When compared with other epithelial cancers in the TCGA Project, bladder cancer was found to be significantly more enriched for mutations in chromatin-regulatory genes. By using low-pass paired-end, whole-genome sequencing, and RNA sequencing, numerous structural aberrations including some that involve gene–gene fusions of different types were detected (e.g., interchromosomal, intrachromosomal, fusions resulting from inversions or deletions). One of the recurrent translocations of probable pathogenic significance was an intrachromosomal translocation on chromosome 4 involving *FGFR3* and *TACC3* in three tumors, which confirms a previously reported finding [28, 34, 35].

Integrated analysis of the mutation and copy number data revealed frequent dysregulation in major cancer pathways including cell cycle regulation (93 %), kinase and phosphatidylinositol-3-kinase (PI3K) signaling (72 %), and chromatin remodeling (histone-modifying genes, 89 % and the SWItch/Sucrose NonFermentable (SWI/SNF) nucleosome remodeling complex, 64 %). By applying network analysis, increased activity in other important signaling hubs was identified including *MYC/MAX*, *FOXA2*, *SP1*, and *HSP90AA1*.

Looking at the recently generated and reported data, it is notable that multiple druggable targets have been identified in UC [31, 32, 34–39]. These targets include activating *FGFR3* mutations, amplification and activating mutations in *ERBB2* and *ERBB3*, and alterations in the PI3K/mTOR/AKT/TSC1 pathway. Possible targets also include alterations in epigenetic regulatory pathways due to the high frequency of such aberrations in UC and merit further investigation. In summary, the molecular profile of bladder cancer identified through TCGA and other efforts has opened a number of exciting therapeutic avenues in the treatment of this disease. Clinical trials based upon the genetics of bladder cancer are already underway in an attempt to exploit these aberrations.

Epigenetics of Bladder Cancer

Epigenetic changes are defined as heritable, reversible alterations in gene expression that are not due to DNA sequence alterations [40–42]. This level of regulation of gene expression occurs in both normal and tumor cells and involves DNA methylation, typically at the cytosine 5 position within CpG repeat sequences, posttranslational modification of histones, and microRNA regulation [43–46]. Early studies examined the methylation status of specific genes while the more recent advent of global methylation profiling technologies has helped to define the methylome in tumors of specific grades and stages of development [47, 48]. These investigations have identified both global hypomethylation and gene-specific promoter hyper- and hypomethylation as characteristic changes across numerous tumor types that impact tumor progression, invasion, and prognosis [49, 50].

Methylation

DNA hypermethylation of CpG repeats in the promoter region of specific genes with subsequent repression of expression has been reported in UC. In one study, methylation-specific polymerase chain reaction (PCR) of ten genes implicated in tumorigenesis was performed in 98 bladder tumors from both transurethral resection (TUR) and cystectomy specimens, revealing high methylation frequencies of >20 % for *CDH1*, *CDH13*, *RASSF1A*, and *APC* [51]. *CDH1* and *FHIT* methylation was associated with inferior survival, with *CDH1* methylation status remaining an independent prognostic factor in a multivariate analysis; additionally, a methylation index was calculated for each tumor, representing the methylation fraction for all ten genes, and those tumors with a high methylation index displayed worse survival. Another study screened for methylation of seven genes commonly implicated in tumorigenesis in 98 bladder tumor specimens consisting of both primary and recurrent tumors removed by TUR [52]. Using methylation-specific PCR, *RARβ*, *DAPK*, *CDH1*, and *p16Ink4a* were found to be methylated from 26.5 to 87.8 %, and at least one of these four genes was methylated in all 98 samples. *RARβ* was methylated in three of seven normal urothelial samples obtained from patients without UC; none of the other genes was found to be methylated. Four CIS samples were analyzed in which *DAPK*, *CDH1*, and *RARβ* were found to be methylated at high frequency. No clinical or pathologic correlation was found based upon the methylation status of any of the genes screened. In this same study, the methylation status of *DAPK1*, *CDH1*, *RARβ*, and *p16Ink4a* was defined in 22 voided urine specimens. While the methylation frequency of these four genes was generally lower than in the corresponding tumor specimens, methylation of at least one of these four genes was detected in 90.9% of samples. In contrast, cancer cells were detected by urine cytology in 45.5% of these 22 samples, suggesting that detection of methylated genes in urine is more sensitive than traditional cytologic approaches as a screening tool for UC. Additional evidence for the utility of methylated gene detection within urine as a screening biomarker for the presence of urothelial tumors stems from another study of 51 bladder tumors and 47 matched urine samples [53]. The methylation status of four genes (*CDH1*, *p16*, *p14*, and *RASSF1A*) was defined using methylation-specific PCR. The sensitivity of urine methylation marker detection was 83% when using *RASSF1A*, *p14*, and *CDH1* methylation status, while that for urine cytology was 28%. Moreover, 90% of superficial low-grade tumors that were not detected by urine cytology contained hypermethylation. Methylation-mediated inactivation of p16, which is part of the *CDKN2A* locus on chromosome 9p21, may contribute to loss of heterozygosity at this locus, since *CDKN2A* loss by both mutations and deletions is an early and common genetic alteration in UC. Loss of p16 function results in cell cycle dysregulation and uncontrolled proliferation. Furthermore, E-cadherin, the protein encoded by *CDH1*, is implicated in suppression of the Wnt/β-catenin pathway which is involved in promoting cell growth [54]; therefore, loss of E-cadherin expression by promoter methylation leads to constitutive activation of this pathway and excessive cell proliferation. Methylation patterns have been reported to vary based upon the location of urothelial tumors (upper tract vs. bladder) as well as stage and mortality [55]. Hypermethylation at CpG islands in the promoter regions of 11 genes was performed using methylation-specific PCR in 116 bladder tumors and 164 tumors of the upper tract. Promoter methylation was more common in upper tract tumors (94 vs. 76%, $p<0.0001$) as well as muscle-invasive tumors compared to pTa specimens. Notably, tumors harboring methylation at any of the 11 genes exhibited higher rates of progression, including pTa tumors with a high methylation index. Global hypomethylation has been correlated with noninvasive tumors while widespread hypermethylation seems to occur in invasive tumors [56]. Using the Illumina GoldenGate methylation platform, Wolff et al. interrogated 784 genes for methylation status in 49 noninvasive and 38 invasive tumors. Thirty-eight percent of loci were hypermethylated in invasive tumors versus 10% in noninvasive tumors as compared to normal urothelial tissue from patients without UC. In contrast, hypomethylated loci were predominantly found in the noninvasive tumors (16 vs. 3% invasive), and these regions of hypomethylation were frequently observed in non-CpG island regions of the genome. Notably, normal-appearing urothelium sampled at varying distances from invasive tumors also showed an abnormal pattern of hypermethylation in 12% of loci with a significant overlap with the hypermethylated loci identified within invasive tumors, suggesting that epigenetic alterations may precede the development of histologic changes within the bladder. Such alterations may contribute to the well-described field effect in UC, an increased propensity for tumor development within the urinary tract of patients with disease.

Histone Modification

Covalent modification of histones, the packaging units of chromosomes, is another mechanism of epigenetic alteration commonly observed in cancer, including methylation and acetylation of specific amino acid residues. Such modifications regulate transcription of downstream genes. Mutations within histone modifiers have recently been detected at high frequency in UC [36]. Specifically, nine muscle-invasive urothelial tumors were subjected to whole-exome sequencing followed by targeted sequencing of 328 somatically mutated genes from a validation set of 88 tumors. Notably, mutations within the histone demethylase UTX as well as ARID1A, a member of the SWI/SNF nucleosome remodeling complex, were present in 21 and 13% of all samples, respectively, and alterations within a panel of additional chromatin remodeling genes were found in

59 % of specimens, suggesting a significant role for epigenetic alterations in bladder cancer.

MicroRNA Regulation

miRs are short, noncoding strands of RNA that control gene expression at the posttranscriptional level through binding to specific 3′ UTR sequences within mRNA and subsequent transcript degradation. miR expression is frequently altered in neoplastic tissue when compared to its normal counterpart due to epigenetic silencing, and mounting evidence suggests that altered miR expression plays a role in malignant transformation [57]. In one study, the expression levels of 322 miRs were profiled in a cohort of 72 UC samples comprised of high- and low-grade, invasive and noninvasive specimens and compared to normal urothelium from patients with and without UC [58]. Low-grade tumors displayed a reduction in expression of certain miR species involved in downregulation of FGFR3 and HRAS mRNA levels. In contrast, high-grade tumors harbored elevated levels of miR species that downregulate p53, suggesting that the differential expression profile of miRs is linked to the disparate molecular pathways which characterize high- and low-grade disease. Epigenetic regulation of miR expression frequently occurs through hypermethylation of upstream CpG islands and this mechanism has been shown to occur in UC. The role of miRs as tumor markers of UC in urine has also been investigated; specifically, miR-96 and miR-183 were evaluated for diagnostic utility in urine. In a cohort of 78 patients with UC, 43.6 % were found to have positive urine cytology as compared to 69.2 % with detectable miR-96 levels. The sensitivity to detect UC improved from 43.6 % using cytology alone to 78.2 % with a combination of mIR-96 plus cytology. Additionally, miR-96 was detected in 50 % of patients with low-grade and noninvasive disease as compared to 11 % with positive urine cytology. Both miR-96 and miR-183 expression levels increased with higher grade and stage of tumor and in 17 patients who underwent surgical resection of disease by cystectomy or nephroureterectomy, urine miR levels were substantially reduced postoperatively as compared to presurgical levels.

Summary

In summary, multiple mechanisms for epigenetic regulation of gene expression exist in normal cells, which undergo dysregulation during oncogenesis. These include aberrant methylation of CpG repeats, mutations within histone modifiers and chromatin remodelers, as well as abnormal variations in miR expression. Examples of anomalies within all three of these mechanisms of gene regulation have been observed in all stages and grades of bladder cancer and preliminary data suggest that such alterations may serve as biomarkers of tumor recurrence that can be detected noninvasively in urine. Additionally, further insight into the biologic consequences of such aberrations should lead to novel therapeutic advances in the treatment of UC.

References

1. Siegel R, Naishadham D, Jemal A. Cancer statistics, 2013. CA Cancer J Clin. 2013;63(1):11–30.
2. Lawrence MS, et al. Mutational heterogeneity in cancer and the search for new cancer-associated genes. Nature. 2013;499(7457):214–8.
3. The Cancer Genome Atlas Research Network. Comprehensive molecular characterization of urothelial bladder carcinoma. Nature. 2014;507(7492):315–22.
4. Castillo-Martin M, et al. Molecular pathways of urothelial development and bladder tumorigenesis. Urol Oncol. 2010;28(4):401–8.
5. Knowles MA. Molecular subtypes of bladder cancer: Jekyll and Hyde or chalk and cheese? Carcinogenesis. 2006;27(3):361–73.
6. Mitra AP, Datar RH, Cote RJ. Molecular pathways in invasive bladder cancer: new insights into mechanisms, progression, and target identification. J Clin Oncol. 2006;24(35):5552–64.
7. Pollard C, Smith SC, Theodorescu D. Molecular genesis of non-muscle-invasive urothelial carcinoma (NMIUC). Expert Rev Mol Med. 2010;12:e10.
8. Wu XR. Urothelial tumorigenesis: a tale of divergent pathways. Nat Rev Cancer. 2005;5(9):713–25.
9. Tsai YC, et al. Allelic losses of chromosomes 9, 11, and 17 in human bladder cancer. Cancer Res. 1990;50(1):44–7.

10. Cairns, P., Shaw ME, Knowles MA. Initiation of bladder cancer may involve deletion of a tumour-suppressor gene on chromosome 9. Oncogene. 1993;8(4):1083–5.
11. Habuchi T, et al. Detailed deletion mapping of chromosome 9q in bladder cancer: evidence for two tumour suppressor loci. Oncogene. 1995;11(8):1671–4.
12. Linnenbach AJ, et al. Characterization of chromosome 9 deletions in transitional cell carcinoma by microsatellite assay. Hum Mol Genet. 1993;2(9):1407–11.
13. Cappellen D, et al. Frequent activating mutations of FGFR3 in human bladder and cervix carcinomas. Nat Genet. 1999;23(1):18–20.
14. Billerey C, et al. Frequent FGFR3 mutations in papillary non-invasive bladder (pTa) tumors. Am J Pathol. 2001;158(6):1955–9.
15. van Rhijn BW, et al. The fibroblast growth factor receptor 3 (FGFR3) mutation is a strong indicator of superficial bladder cancer with low recurrence rate. Cancer Res. 2001;61(4):1265–8.
16. Al-Ahmadie HA, et al. Somatic mutation of fibroblast growth factor receptor-3 (FGFR3) defines a distinct morphological subtype of high-grade urothelial carcinoma. J Pathol. 2011;224(2):270–9.
17. Theodorescu D, et al. Overexpression of normal and mutated forms of HRAS induces orthotopic bladder invasion in a human transitional cell carcinoma. Proc Natl Acad Sci U S A. 1990;87(22):9047–51.
18. Czerniak B, et al. Concurrent mutations of coding and regulatory sequences of the Ha-ras gene in urinary bladder carcinomas. Hum Pathol. 1992;23(11):1199–204.
19. Knowles MA, Williamson M. Mutation of H-ras is infrequent in bladder cancer: confirmation by single-strand conformation polymorphism analysis, designed restriction fragment length polymorphisms, and direct sequencing. Cancer Res. 1993;53(1):133–9.
20. Zhang ZT, et al. Role of Ha-ras activation in superficial papillary pathway of urothelial tumor formation. Oncogene. 2001;20(16):1973–80.
21. Fadl-Elmula I, et al. Karyotypic characterization of urinary bladder transitional cell carcinomas. Genes Chromosomes Cancer. 2000;29(3):256–65.
22. Aboulkassim TO, et al. Alteration of the PATCHED locus in superficial bladder cancer. Oncogene. 2003;22(19):2967–71.
23. Simoneau M, et al. Four tumor suppressor loci on chromosome 9q in bladder cancer: evidence for two novel candidate regions at 9q22.3 and 9q31. Oncogene. 1999;18(1):157–63.
24. Gui Y, et al. Frequent mutations of chromatin remodeling genes in transitional cell carcinoma of the bladder. Nat Genet. 2011;43(9):875–8.
25. Solomon DA, et al. Frequent truncating mutations of STAG2 in bladder cancer. Nat Genet. 2013;45(12):1428–30.
26. Taylor CF, et al. Frequent inactivating mutations of STAG2 in bladder cancer are associated with low tumour grade and stage and inversely related to chromosomal copy number changes. Hum Mol Genet. 2014;23(8):1964–74.
27. Balbas-Martinez C, et al. Recurrent inactivation of STAG2 in bladder cancer is not associated with aneuploidy. Nat Genet. 2013;45(12):1464–9.
28. Guo G, et al. Whole-genome and whole-exome sequencing of bladder cancer identifies frequent alterations in genes involved in sister chromatid cohesion and segregation. Nat Genet. 2013;45(12):1459–63.
29. Hopman AH, et al. Identification of chromosome 9 alterations and p53 accumulation in isolated carcinoma in situ of the urinary bladder versus carcinoma in situ associated with carcinoma. Am J Pathol. 2002;161(4):1119–25.
30. Iyer G, et al. Prevalence and co-occurrence of actionable genomic alterations in high-grade bladder cancer. J Clin Oncol. 2013;31(25):3133–40.
31. Forbes SA, et al. COSMIC: mining complete cancer genomes in the catalogue of somatic mutations in cancer. Nucleic Acids Res. 2011;39(Database issue):D945–50.
32. Goebell PJ, Knowles MA. Bladder cancer or bladder cancers? Genetically distinct malignant conditions of the urothelium. Urol Oncol. 2010;28(4):409–28.
33. Lindgren D, et al. Combined gene expression and genomic profiling define two intrinsic molecular subtypes of urothelial carcinoma and gene signatures for molecular grading and outcome. Cancer Res. 2010;70(9):3463–72.
34. Williams SV, Hurst CD, Knowles MA. Oncogenic FGFR3 gene fusions in bladder cancer. Hum Mol Genet. 2013;22(4):795–803.
35. Wu YM, et al. Identification of targetable FGFR gene fusions in diverse cancers. Cancer Discov. 2013;3(6):636–47.
36. Gui Y, et al. Frequent mutations of chromatin remodeling genes in transitional cell carcinoma of the bladder. Nat Genet. 2011;43(9):875–8.
37. Hurst CD, et al. Novel tumor subgroups of urothelial carcinoma of the bladder defined by integrated genomic analysis. Clin Cancer Res. 2012;18(21):5865–77.
38. Lindgren D, et al. Integrated genomic and gene expression profiling identifies two major genomic circuits in urothelial carcinoma. PLoS One. 2012;7(6):e38863.
39. Iyer G, et al. Genome sequencing identifies a basis for everolimus sensitivity. Science. 2012;338(6104):221.
40. Jones PA, Baylin SB. The epigenomics of cancer. Cell. 2007;128(4):683–92.
41. Tsai HC, Baylin SB. Cancer epigenetics: linking basic biology to clinical medicine. Cell Res. 2011;21(3):502–17.
42. Portela A, Esteller M. Epigenetic modifications and human disease. Nat Biotechnol. 2010;28(10):1057–68.

43. Laird PW. Principles and challenges of genome-wide DNA methylation analysis. Nat Rev Genet. 2010;11(3):191–203.
44. Rodriguez-Paredes M, Esteller M. Cancer epigenetics reaches mainstream oncology. Nat Med. 2011;17(3):330–9.
45. Gronbaek K, Hother C, Jones PA. Epigenetic changes in cancer. APMIS. 2007;115(10):1039–59.
46. Baylin SB, Jones PA. A decade of exploring the cancer epigenome—biological and translational implications. Nat Rev Cancer. 2011;11(10):726–34.
47. Nagarajan RP, et al. Methods for cancer epigenome analysis. Adv Exp Med Biol. 2013;754:313–38.
48. Hansen KD, et al. Increased methylation variation in epigenetic domains across cancer types. Nat Genet. 2011;43(8):768–75.
49. Suzuki MM, Bird A. DNA methylation landscapes: provocative insights from epigenomics. Nat Rev Genet. 2008;9(6):465–76.
50. Fernandez AF, et al. A DNA methylation fingerprint of 1628 human samples. Genome Res. 2012;22(2):407–19.
51. Maruyama R, et al. Aberrant promoter methylation profile of bladder cancer and its relationship to clinicopathological features. Cancer Res. 2001;61(24):8659–63.
52. Chan MW, et al. Hypermethylation of multiple genes in tumor tissues and voided urine in urinary bladder cancer patients. Clin Cancer Res. 2002;8(2):464–70.
53. Lin HH, et al. Increase sensitivity in detecting superficial, low grade bladder cancer by combination analysis of hypermethylation of E-cadherin, p16, p14, RASSF1A genes in urine. Urol Oncol. 2010;28(6):597–602.
54. Gottardi CJ, Wong E, Gumbiner BM. E-cadherin suppresses cellular transformation by inhibiting beta-catenin signaling in an adhesion-independent manner. J Cell Biol. 2001;153(5):1049–60.
55. Catto JW, et al. Promoter hypermethylation is associated with tumor location, stage, and subsequent progression in transitional cell carcinoma. J Clin Oncol. 2005;23(13):2903–10.
56. Wolff EM, et al. Unique DNA methylation patterns distinguish noninvasive and invasive urothelial cancers and establish an epigenetic field defect in premalignant tissue. Cancer Res. 2010 70(20):8169–78.
57. Croce CM. Causes and consequences of microRNA dysregulation in cancer. Nat Rev Genet. 2009;10(10):704–14.
58. Catto JW, et al. Distinct microRNA alterations characterize high- and low-grade bladder cancer. Cancer Res. 2009;69(21):8472–81.

Urine Cytology

21

Jordan P. Reynolds

Introduction

This chapter describes the spectrum of abnormalities seen in urine cytology specimens. The focus is on the detection of bladder cancer with special consideration for evaluation of upper tract specimens. Ancillary testing to increase the sensitivity of urine cytology is also discussed in detail.

Urine cytology is useful for the diagnosis of urothelial carcinoma in situ and high-grade carcinoma, but not as useful in detecting low-grade papillary lesions. The main purpose of urine cytology is to detect high-grade urothelial carcinoma. Urine cytology may be performed in patients who initially present with hematuria, either grossly or on microscopic urine examination. Alternatively, cytology may be performed for surveillance on patients who are already diagnosed with bladder cancer and may have received treatment with transurethral resection of the bladder, bacillus Calmette–Guérin (BCG) therapy, or cystectomy.

Bladder cancer continues to be the fourth most common malignancy and ninth common cause of cancer death. The National Cancer Institute predicted that, in 2012 in the USA, 55,000 men and 18,000 women would be diagnosed with bladder cancer [1]. Treatment with BCG or transurethral resection of bladder tumor (TURBT) is the preferred treatment of non-muscle-invasive bladder cancer [2]. Once the tumor invades the muscularis propria, surgical resection (radical cystectomy) with or without neoadjuvant chemotherapy is necessary [3]. The purpose of urine cytology screening is to detect bladder cancer prior to invasion of the muscularis propria to decrease patient morbidity and mortality [4].

Microscopic hematuria is the typical initial presentation. Patients visiting their physician for another reason may provide a urine sample showing microscopic hematuria on routine urinalysis [5]. Screening urine cytology for patients with asymptomatic microscopic hematuria may detect bladder cancer in 16% of patients [6]. Patients with macroscopic hematuria showed evidence of bladder cancer in 20% of cases [7]. Patients with hematuria warrant urine cytology with cystoscopy, and imaging of the upper urothelial tract is recommended [8].

Evaluation of the urinary tract involves examination of both the upper and lower tract. Upper tract urothelial cancer (UTUC) evaluation involves a computed tomography (CT) urogram while lower tract evaluation involves cystoscopy. Cystoscopy evaluation is successful in detecting papillary UC, but may miss flat urothelial carcinoma in situ [9]. The role of urine cytology is to detect the poorly visualized high-grade carcinoma including urothelial carcinoma in situ.

J. P. Reynolds (✉)
Department of Pathology, Cleveland Clinic, Robert J. Tomsich Pathology and Laboratory Medicine Institute, Cleveland, OH, USA
e-mail: Reynolj4@ccf.edu

C. Magi-Galluzzi, C. G. Przybycin (eds.), *Genitourinary Pathology,* DOI 10.1007/978-1-4939-2044-0_21,

Specimen Type

Voided urine is the most common sample provided, as it is a noninvasive way to collect urine for cytology. The first morning urine should be discarded as it may contain more inflammation from urinary stasis from the previous night. A second voided collection is more appropriate. Obtaining voided urine cytology specimens is not without challenges, however; the specimen must be provided by a competent patient and may contain abundant contamination with squamous mucosal cells from the penile urethra and vagina.

Instrumented or catheterized urine samples can provide a more cellular specimen; however, this manner of collection is more invasive than collecting voided urine. Bladder washings use forced saline water to wash urothelial mucosal cells from the epithelial surface. The pressure of the washing action releases the cells from the urothelial mucosa and causes clustering of cells [10]. Clusters of urothelial cells may lead to increased diagnosis of atypical or more false positive diagnoses in urine cytologic specimens (Fig. 21.1) [11].

Postcystectomy patients present special consideration for urine cytology, as ileal conduit, bladder augmentation, and urethral washings are used for surveillance. In cases where there is a neobladder or ileal conduit, there may be abundant acute inflammation as well as organisms native to the gastrointestinal (GI) tract such as *Candida* species. Searching for neoplastic urothelial cells may be more difficult due to obscuring inflammation and bacterial colonies [12]. The utility of urine cytology in ileal conduit specimens has come into question, as atypical cells present in these specimens have poor positive predictive value in detecting recurrent urothelial carcinoma [13].

Adequacy in urine cytology is somewhat controversial. Although some samples are paucicellular, the cellularity of a voided urine sample is beyond the control of the provider. Normal urine has few urothelial cells and a clean background with few leukocytes. Squamous cells may be present in men and women from squamous metaplasia of the trigone or contamination from the urethra. A paucicellular sample in a symptomatic patient should be reported as limited cellularity. An overabundance of bacteria or blood may inhibit interpretation [14].

Clusters of urothelial cells in urine cytology can be attributed to the presence of bladder calculi, low-grade papillary urothelial carcinoma, or instrumentation effect, such as catheterization (Fig. 21.2). Correlation of the cytologic findings

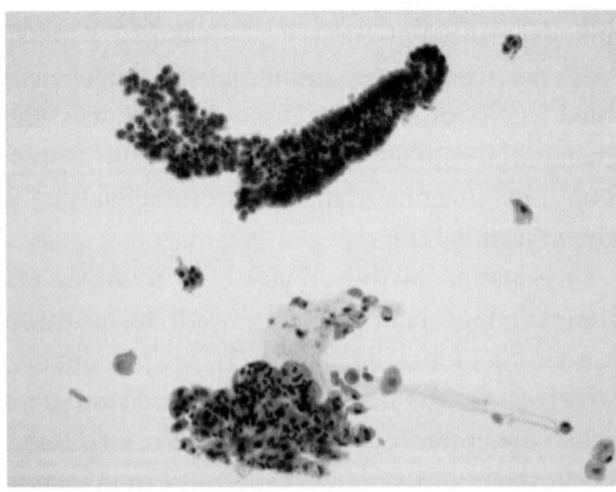

Fig. 21.1 Pap stain 20×. Bladder washing specimen obtained from a patient with a history of urothelial CIS. The instrumentation effect from the washing may slough off epithelial fragments and give them a papillary appearance. These clusters should not be overcalled as low-grade papillary urothelial carcinoma. One should search for high-grade features

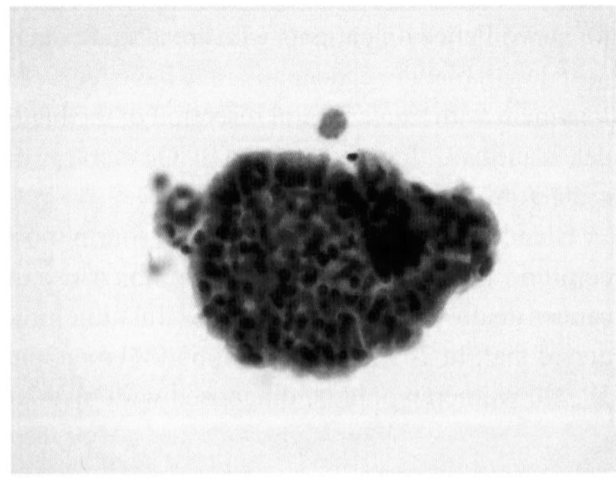

Fig. 21.2 Pap stain 40×—Urine sample from a patient who was paralyzed in a motor vehicle accident who subsequently had long-term indwelling catheterization. The cells show columnar morphology with stratification and mucin formation. The histology showed cystitis cystica et glandularis

with the cystoscopy report with special attention to the presence of tumor, tumor size, and multifocal lesions increases the sensitivity for finding low-grade papillary urothelial carcinoma [15].

Normal Urine

Urothelial mucosal cells exhibit a wide morphologic spectrum. Superficial umbrella cells have one or more nuclei and may measure between 20 and 30 μm in diameter. Multinucleated cells are common, and these cells may raise alarm in urine cytology interpretation. A low nuclear to cytoplasmic ratio and an absence of nuclear hyperchromasia indicates the presence of benign umbrella cells. The cytoplasm can be hard, dense, and solid similar to the cytoplasm of squamous cells, but may also exhibit vacuolization and granularity.

Cells from beneath the umbrella cell layer are comprised of smaller single cells in the urine. They usually contain a single round nucleus measuring between 8 and 10 microns with a smooth nuclear contour. The cytoplasm is thick and exhibits a low nuclear to cytoplasmic ratio. These cells resemble parabasal squamous cells from the cervix in that they are round to almost ovoid with a basophilic cytoplasm. Under more reactive conditions such as inflammation, the chromatin will become more open and contain 1–2 micronucleoli.

The presence of squamous cells in urine can pose a diagnostic challenge. Most squamous cells in the urine are usually present as contamination from squamous-lined mucosa from the gynecologic tract in females, or penile urethra in males. Less commonly, these cells may arise from the squamous metaplasia of the bladder trigone, especially if the patient is in a state of urinary stasis, or has a history of an indwelling urinary catheter (Fig. 21.3). In patients with urothelial carcinoma, the presence of atypical squamous cells may be associated with urothelial carcinoma with squamous features, or invasive squamous cell carcinoma (Fig. 21.4) [16].

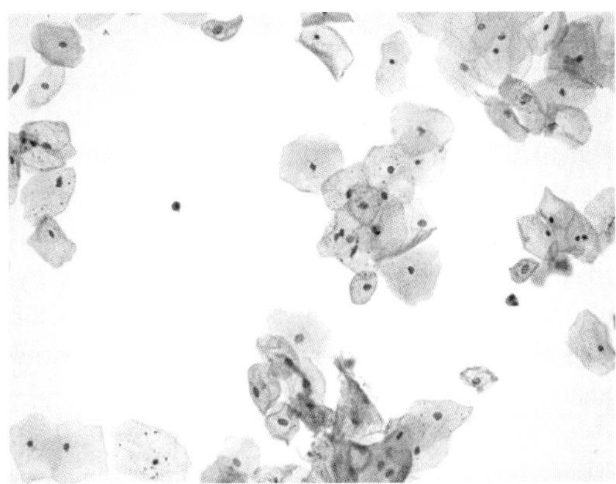

Fig. 21.3 Pap stain 20×. This is a normal urine sample with abundant benign squamous cells in a 72-year-old male. These squamous cells could arise from urethral contamination or squamous metaplasia of the bladder trigone

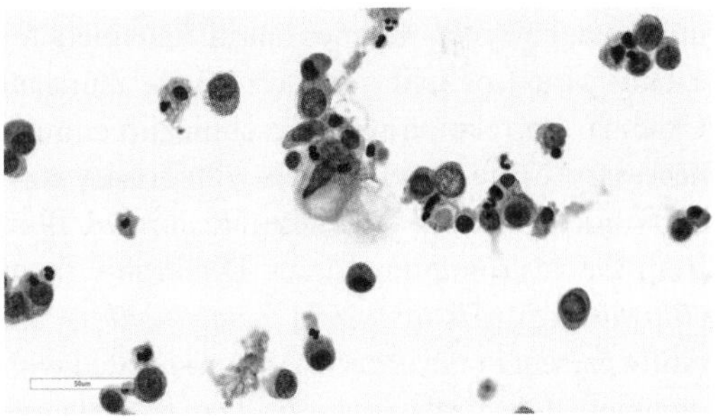

Fig. 21.4 Pap stain 40×—Squamous differentiation in high-grade papillary urothelial carcinoma. The orangeophilic cell with the elongated, hyperchromatic nucleus may occur in squamous cell carcinoma, urothelial carcinoma with squamous differentiation, or high-grade urothelial carcinoma. Correlation with biopsy findings is needed

The background of the normal urine can contain squamous cells, bacteria, blood, and inflammatory cells. These features in the background are not essential to the diagnosis, nor are they necessarily in concordance with the patient's clinical picture. Acute inflammation may not correspond to an acute cystitis. However, reporting of these features may help the clinician explain some of the clinical findings. Patients with urinary stasis may have abundant acute inflammation. An immunocompromised patient with anucleated squames may have malakoplakia.

Bacteria

Bacterial colonies present in urine typically consist of gram negative rods, usually from bacteria native to the colon. When present, they are usually associated with mixed acute and chronic inflammatory cells and macrophages. Urine cytology is neither a sensitive nor specific means of detecting bacterial infection. Urine dipstick analysis and culture are more suitable.

Fungi

Fungal organisms affecting the bladder can be seen in the urine and usually consist of *Candida* species. Overgrowth of many Candida organisms may be present in patients with a urinary fungal infection; however, samples left in containers for a long period of time may also grow abundant Candida. Correlation with the clinical picture is necessary. Cystectomy patients with urinary conduits have *Candida* but these are normal flora from the gastrointestinal tract. Dimorphic fungi (*Blastomyces*, *Histoplasma*, *Coccidioides*) are rarely present in the urine and are associated with granulomatous inflammation. The specific organism is dependent on the geographic residence or travel history of the patient. The main fungal diagnostic value in urine specimens lies in analysis for polysaccharide detection of Histoplasma antigen [17].

Viruses

Viral organisms can cause significant cytologic changes in the form of viral cytopathic effect. HPV viral changes can be present in the form of contamination from squamous mucosa, HPV changes present in squamous metaplasia of the bladder trigone, or in urothelial carcinoma with squamous differentiation [18, 19]. Herpes simplex can cause nuclear molding, multinucleation, and margination of the chromatin to give the classic "ground glass" appearance [20]. The bizarre cytopathic changes should be recognized to prevent misdiagnosis of malignancy. Cytomegalovirus inclusions can be seen in immunocompromised (e.g., HIV, transplant) patients and contain large cells with large blue intranuclear inclusions. Polyoma virus is the most common virus seen in urine cytology. Cells infected with this virus have characteristic viral inclusions showing nuclear enlargement, margination of the nuclear material around the nuclear membrane, and a disorganized cobweb-like stranding of the nuclear material [21]. Ancillary techniques are available including the SV40 immunocytochemistry stain as well as fluorescence in situ hybridization (FISH) for the BK virus [22–24]. The viral load of the blood can be detected and correlated with the BK viral inclusions in the bladder [25]. While these are often found in transplant patients, they can be present in any type of immunocompromised patients, and rarely, in immunocompetent patients [26].

Malignant Changes in the Urine

Urine cytology has low sensitivity (35 % on meta-analysis) and high specificity (99 %) for detecting high-grade urothelial carcinoma (in situ or invasive) [27]. Urothelial carcinoma cells in the urine are enlarged, have a decreased nuclear to cytoplasmic ratio, are hyperchromatic, and show nuclear irregularity (Figs. 21.5 and 21.6) [28]. Absence of any of these features would lead to a diagnosis of suspicious for urothelial carcinoma. Clinical information provided by the cystoscopy report, for example, the presence of a bladder mass or erythematous areas further strengthens the diagnosis. Unfortunately, this information is sometimes unavailable and may leave a diagnostic void [28].

Atypical diagnoses are frustrating for clinicians. Many etiologies could cause cytologic atypia, including presence of bladder calculi, inflammation, chemotherapy for another neoplasm, or radiation of the prostate or rectum for carcinoma (Fig. 21.7). A diagnosis of atypical is more worrisome in upper tract specimens as compared to lower tract samples and should be more thoroughly investigated [29].

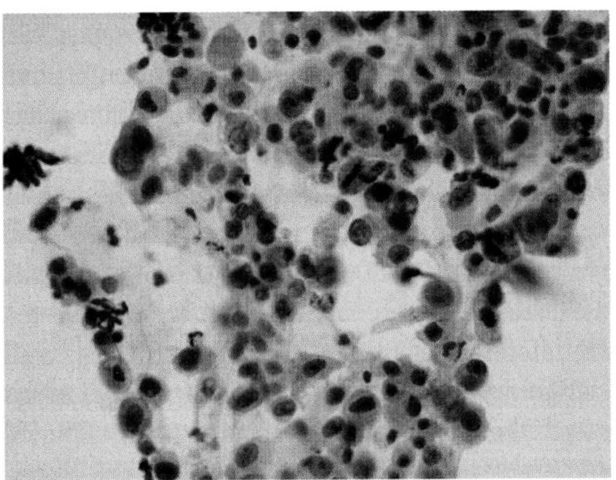

Fig. 21.5 Pap stain 40×—High-grade urothelial carcinoma with nuclear enlargement, hyperchromasia, anisonucleosis, and increased nuclear to cytoplasmic ratio. Whether this patient has urothelial carcinoma in situ or invasive, high-grade urothelial carcinoma must be determined with bladder biopsies

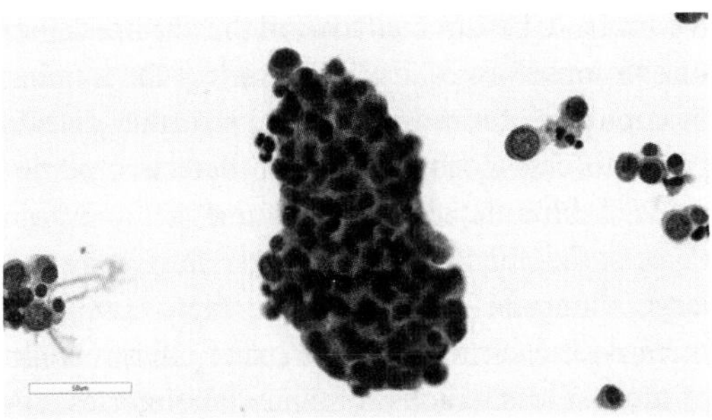

Fig. 21.6 Pap stain 40×—Papillary high-grade urothelial carcinoma. Similar nuclear features to Fig. 21.5. Cystoscopy revealed papillary lesions and biopsy confirmed invasive high-grade papillary urothelial carcinoma

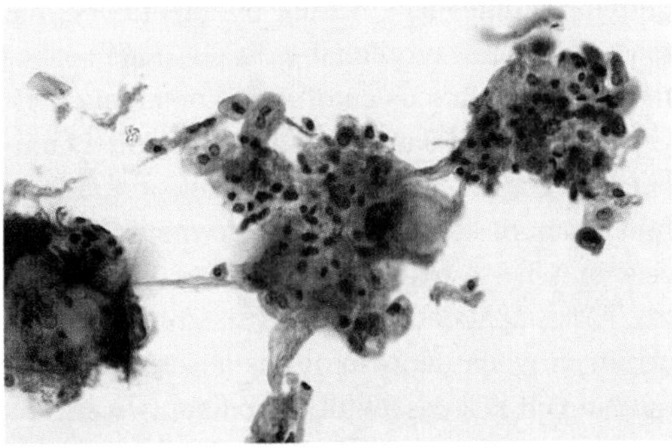

Fig. 21.7 Pap stain 40×. Radiation cystitis in a patient with a history of adenocarcinoma of the prostate treated with radiation. Note the multinucleation and marked cytomegaly while maintaining a normal nuclear to cytoplasmic ratio

Upper Urothelial Tract Carcinoma

Samples of the upper urothelial tract are usually obtained by bladder washing. Upper tract specimens carry their own set of diagnostic and clinical management dilemmas as they are harder to visualize. Endoureteroscopy is necessary to fully visualize the ureters. Retrograde pyelography and CT urograms in conjunction with upper tract samples are useful in detecting urothelial carcinoma [30]. Biopsies of the ureter are difficult since they are usually performed through a very thin instrument. As a result, ureteral cytology may often be the key to the diagnosis.

Ureteral cytology specimens can, however, prove diagnostically challenging. They can be subject to overinterpretation, particularly when obtained from patients with a previous stent for obstruction. Reactive urothelial atypia and clusters are more prevalent in these specimens due to contact with the stent which leads to reactive epithelial changes. In addition, cancers of the bladder may detach and wash into the ureter, rendering a false positive result [15, 31]. It is important to be cognizant of the presence of a prior bladder cancer when interpreting ureter specimens. When evaluating a ureter specimen it is extremely helpful to the cytologist if bladder urine and bilateral ureter samples are provided. Bilateral examination may allow for comparison between the normal and atypical samples. Malignant-appearing cells in one ureter and negative findings in the contralateral ureter with correlating clinical and radiographic information would substantiate a diagnosis of positive for malignancy. However, if atypical/malignant-appearing cells are present in both ureter specimens and a bladder urine sample, contamination by bladder UC may cause a false positive diagnosis.

Detection of low-grade cytology is difficult in urine cytologic specimens. As mentioned previously, clusters of bland-appearing urothelial cells are seen in instrumentation effect or stones (Fig. 21.8). Even in patients with cystoscopic evidence of a low-grade papillary neoplasm, the urine cytology may not correspond to the tumor load [15]. Papillary clusters with true vascular cores may indicate the presence of a low-grade papillary carcinoma if it is in concordance with the cystoscopy report [15, 32].

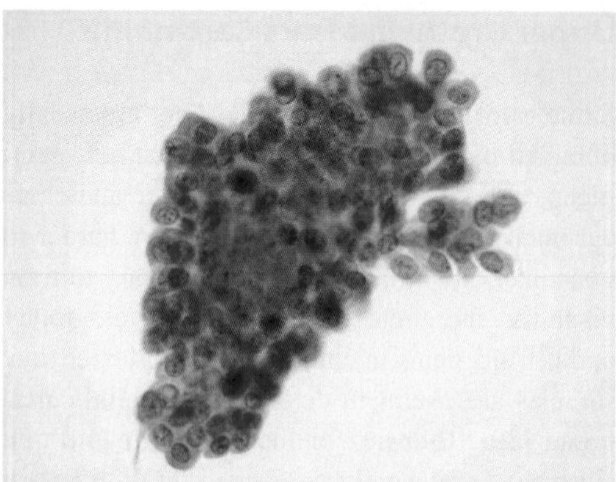

Fig. 21.8 Pap stain 40×—Low-grade papillary urothelial carcinoma in a patient who had small papillary lesions. He underwent transurethral resection of the tumor and had urine cytology collected prior to the procedure. No definitive vascular core is present and the cells do not have high-grade morphology. These cells are nearly identical to those found in an instrumented urine specimen

Non-urothelial Carcinomas in the Urine

Renal cell carcinoma can rarely shed cells into the urine if it invades the renal pelvis. This is a rare occurrence and should be confirmed with immunohistochemistry staining [33, 34].

Adenocarcinoma of the prostate presenting in the urine is also rare [34]. One study reported four cases in 10,000; these positive cases were characterized by acinar cell clusters with large pale nuclei and prominent nucleoli. These groups can be overlooked as clusters of urothelial cells or misinterpreted as low-grade papillary urothelial carcinoma [35].

Ancillary Testing in Urine Cytology

Fluorescence In Situ Hybridization UroVysion™

Since the sensitivity and negative predictive value of screening urine cytology are so low, testing that would increase detection would make urine cytology more effective. Urothelial carcinoma is an aneuploid cancer, showing multiple copies of chromosomes [36]. FISH utilizes probes to detect the DNA content of urothelial cells. Centromere enumeration probes (CEP) for chromosome 3, 7, and 17 label the centromere of the chromosome. The presence of more than one signal indicates an abnormal DNA content.

The DAPI stain (4′6-diamidino-2-phenylindole) is used to stain the nucleus blue under fluorescence microscopy. Normal urothelial cells will show a homogeneous stain, reflecting even chromatin distribution in a cell with normal DNA content. Malignant cells show a heterogeneous staining pattern with large nuclei and a clumped chromatin pattern. This reflects an aneuploid cell with coarse chromatin distribution, characteristic of epithelial neoplasms on cytology. These can be detected manually by a molecular technologist or cytotechnologist or with the use of automated screening systems [37].

Once an abnormal cell is detected on the DAPI stain, various filters can be used to detect the probe. CEP directed toward the chromocenter of chromosomes 3, 7, and 17 reflect the number of copies of chromosomes. The red filter detects probe to chromosome 3, green detects chromosome 7, blue detects chromosome 17, and gold detects the locus-specific 9p21. Screening for large abnormal cells on DAPI, then examining them with each filter would make interpretation of the test less tedious. In many laboratories, cytotechnologists, who are already trained to screen for abnormal cells on light microscopy, can be trained to examine the cells through the various filters.

The minimum number of urothelial cells required for adequacy varies by laboratory, but most accept 25 urothelial cells. Different laboratories have various cutoffs for abnormal cases. Generally, when one cell with an abnormal number of probes is found, the tech looks for at least four or more abnormal cells, at which time the case may be signed out as “Positive for aneusomy.” These patients are at increased risk for cancer, even when the cytology is negative. An abnormal cell is a case with more than two signals in two or more probes. For instance, three signals in chromosome 3, and 5 in chromosome 7 would be considered an abnormal cell. Special cases to consider are when all probes contain four signals, or show tetrasomy. These cells may represent malignant change; however, they may represent a dividing urothelial cell, which may be 2N. Tetrasomic cells are found more frequently in the upper urothelial tract and should be interpreted with caution [38]. Some laboratories may count 100 consecutive urothelial cells and provide a percentage of abnormal cells. Previous literature suggests that higher percentage of abnormal cells would indicate a higher tumor load.

The locus-specific 9q21 is completely lost in low-grade papillary urothelial carcinoma. In most cases, this probe is the first to fade away and true "loss" is difficult to assess. If the probe is absent in every cell, the signal may have faded. True 9p21 loss occurs in clusters of urothelial cells, which may represent low-grade papillary lesions of the bladder.

FISH in the upper urothelial tract should be interpreted with caution, if at all. Tetrasomic cells in the upper tract are more frequently found due to more mitotically active cells present in the upper tract and pelvis [38, 39]. Tetrasomic cases should be interpreted as suspicious for malignancy, but not as outright positive. In addition, concomitant urothelial carcinoma of the bladder may cause a false positive result.

ImmunoCyt/uCyt+ testing is an immunofluorescence-based technique to detect bladder cancer in the urine. Cell membrane fluorescence for high molecular weight glycosylated carcinogenic embryonic antigen and bladder cancer mucin are evaluated [40]. The presence of five or more positive cells confirms a positive diagnosis. Five hundred epithelial cells lacking fluorescence is considered negative. ImmunoCyt has about twofold sensitivity for detecting bladder cancer compared to urine cytology, but lower specificity [27].

NMP22 is a marker of urothelial cell death expressed in the urine of patients with urothelial carcinoma. It also has twofold sensitivity for detection of urothelial carcinoma compared to urine cytology [41, 42].

Conclusion

Overall, urine cytology and FISH carry decent sensitivity in the detection of urothelial carcinoma. The specificity is high and further evaluation of the urinary tract with biopsy confirmation is warranted in positive cases. In equivocal cases, ancillary testing to increase the sensitivity of the test or clarify these atypical cases may help the clinician make further management decisions.

References

1. Siegel R, Naishadham D, Jemal A. Cancer statistics, 2012. CA Cancer J Clin. 2012;62(1):10–29.
2. Smith ZL, Christodouleas JP, Keefe SM, Malkowicz SB, Guzzo TJ. Bladder preservation in the treatment of muscle-invasive bladder cancer (MIBC): a review of the literature and a practical approach to therapy. BJU Int. 2013;112(1):13–25. Epub 2013/01/30.
3. Grossman HB, Natale RB, Tangen CM, et al. Neoadjuvant chemotherapy plus cystectomy compared with cystectomy alone for locally advanced bladder cancer. N Engl J Med. 2003;349(9):859–66.
4. Bastacky S, Ibrahim S, Wilczynski SP, Murphy WM. The accuracy of urinary cytology in daily practice. Cancer Cytopathol. 1999;87(3):118–28.
5. Cohen RA, Brown RS. Microscopic hematuria. N Engl J Med. 2003;348(23):2330–8.
6. Khadra MH, Pickard RS, Charlton M, Powell PH, Neal DE. A prospective analysis of 1,930 patients with hematuria to evaluate current diagnostic practice. J Urol. 2000;163(2):524–7.
7. Blick CGT, Nazir SA, Mallett S, et al. Evaluation of diagnostic strategies for bladder cancer using computed tomography (CT) urography, flexible cystoscopy and voided urine cytology: results for 778 patients from a hospital haematuria clinic. BJU Int. 2012;110(1):84–94.
8. Grossfeld GD, Litwin MS, Wolf JS, et al. Evaluation of asymptomatic microscopic hematuria in adults: the American urological association best practice policy—part II: patient evaluation, cytology, voided markers, imaging, cystoscopy, nephrology evaluation, and follow-up. Urology. 2001;57(4):604–10.
9. Brien JC, Shariat SF, Herman MP, et al. Preoperative hydronephrosis, ureteroscopic biopsy grade and urinary cytology can improve prediction of advanced upper tract urothelial carcinoma. J Urol. 2010;184(1):69–73.
10. Raab SS, Grzybicki DM, Vrbin CM, Geisinger KR. Urine cytology discrepancies—frequency, causes, and outcomes. Am J Clin Pathol. 2007;127(6):946–53.
11. Kapur U, Venkataraman G, Wojcik EM. Diagnostic significance of 'atypia' in instrumented versus voided urine specimens. Cancer Cytopathol. 2008;114(4):270–4.
12. Huguet-Perez J, Palou J, Millan-Rodriguez F, Salvador-Bayarri J, Villavicencio-Mavrich H, Vicente-Rodriguez J. Upper tract transitional cell carcinoma following cystectomy for bladder cancer. Eur Urol. 2001;40(3):318–23.

13. Yoshimine S, Kikuchi E, Matsumoto K, et al. The clinical significance of urine cytology after a radical cystectomy for urothelial cancer. Int J Urol. 2010;17(6):527–32.
14. Mody DR. Defining adequacy in nongynecologic specimens. CAP Today. 2003;17:68–70.
15. Jackson J, Barkan GA, Kapur U, Wojcik EM. Cytologic and cystoscopic predictors of recurrence and progression in patients with low-grade urothelial carcinoma. Cancer Cytopathol. 2013;121(7):398–402.
16. Rosa M. Clinical significance of dysplastic squamous cells in exfoliative urine cytology. Diagn Cytopathol. 2010;38(6):468–9.
17. Wheat LJ, Kohler RB, Tewari RP. Diagnosis of disseminated histoplasmosis by detection of histoplasma-capsulatum antigen in serum and urine specimens. N Engl J Med. 1986;314(2):83–8.
18. Aggarwal S, Arora VK, Gupta S, Singh N, Bhatia A. Koilocytosis: correlations with high-risk HPV and its comparison on tissue sections and cytology, urothelial carcinoma. Diagn Cytopathol. 2009;37(3):174–7.
19. Jong EE, Mulder JW, van Gorp ECM, et al. The prevalence of human papillomavirus (HPV) infection in paired urine and cervical smear samples of HIV-infected women. J Clin Virol. 2008;41(2):111–5.
20. LeBlanc RE, Maleki Z. Herpes simplex viral cytopathic effect in urine cytology. Diagn Cytopathol. 2013;41(1):61–2.
21. Singh HK, Bubendorf L, Mihatsch MJ, Drachenberg CB, Nickeleit V. Urine cytology findings of polyomavirus infections. In: Ahsan N, editor. Polyomaviruses and human diseases. New York: Springer; 2006. pp. 201–12.
22. Drachenberg CB, Beskow CO, Cangro CB, et al. Human polyoma virus in renal allograft biopsies: morphological findings and correlation with urine cytology. Hum Pathol. 1999;30(8):970–7.
23. Wang Z, Portier BP, Hu B, et al. Diagnosis of BK viral nephropathy in the renal allograft biopsy role of fluorescence in situ hybridization. J Mol Diagn. 2012;14(5):494–500.
24. Li RM, Mannon RB, Kleiner D, et al. BK virus and SV40 co-infection in polyomavirus nephropathy. Transplantation. 2002;74(11):1497–504.
25. Randhawa P, Vats A, Shapiro R. Monitoring for polyomavirus BK and JC in urine: comparison of quantitative polymerase chain reaction with urine cytology. Transplantation. 2005;79(8):984–6.
26. Egli A, Infanti L, Dumoulin A, et al. Prevalence of Polyomavirus BK and JC infection and replication in 400 healthy blood donors. J Infect Dis. 2009;199(6):837–46.
27. Lotan Y, Roehrborn CG. Sensitivity and specificity of commonly available bladder tumor markers versus cytology: results of a comprehensive literature review and meta-analyses. Urology. 2003;61(1):109–18.
28. Koss LG, Deitch D, Ramanathan R, Sherman AB. Diagnostic-value of cytology of voided urine. Acta Cytol. 1985;29(5):810–6.
29. Ubago JM, Mehta V, Wojcik EM, Barkan GA. Evaluation of atypical urine cytology progression to malignancy. Cancer Cytopathol. 2013;121(7):387–91.
30. Williams SK, Denton KJ, Minervini A, et al. Correlation of upper-tract cytology, retrograde pyelography, ureteroscopic appearance, and ureteroscopic biopsy with histologic examination of upper-tract transitional cell carcinoma. J Endourol. 2008;22(1):71–6.
31. Raj GV, Bochner BH, Serio AM, et al. Natural history of positive urinary cytology after radical cystectomy. J Urol. 2006;176(5):2000–5.
32. Whisnant RE, Bastacky SI, Ohori NP. Cytologic diagnosis of low-grade papillary urothelial neoplasms (low malignant potential and low-grade carcinoma) in the context of the 1998 WHO/ISUP classification. Diagn Cytopathol. 2003;28(4):186–90.
33. Dubal SB, Pathuthara S, Ajit D, Menon S, Kane SV. Case report of renal cell carcinoma diagnosed in voided urine confirmed by CD10 immunocytochemistry. Acta Cytol. 2011;55(4):372–6.
34. Sathiyamoorthy S, Ali SZ. Urinary cytology of prostatic duct adenocarcinoma—a clinicopathologic analysis. Acta Cytol. 2013;57(2):184–8.
35. Tyler KL, Selvaggi SM. Morphologic features of prostatic adenocarcinoma on ThinPrep(R) urinary cytology. Diagn Cytopathol. 2011;39(2):101–4.
36. Dalquen P, Kleiber B, Grilli B, Herzog M, Bubendorf L, Oberholzer M. DNA image cytometry and fluorescence in situ hybridization for noninvasive detection of urothelial tumors in voided urine. Cancer Cytopathol. 2002;96(6):374–9.
37. Daniely M, Rona R, Kaplan T, et al. Combined analysis of morphology and fluorescence in situ hybridization significantly increases accuracy of bladder cancer detection in voided urine samples. Urology. 2005;66(6):1354–9.
38. Keay S, Warren JW, Zhang CO, Tu LM, Gordon DA, Whitmore KE. Antiproliferative activity is present in bladder but not renal pelvic urine from interstitial cystitis patients. J Urol. 1999;162(4):1487–9.
39. Wu CF, Pang ST, Shee JJ, et al. Identification of genetic alterations in upper urinary tract urothelial carcinoma in end-stage renal disease patients. Genes Chromosomes Cancer. 2010;49(10):928–34.
40. Mian C, Pycha A, Wiener H, Haitel A, Lodde M, Marberger M. Immunocyt: a new tool for detecting transitional cell cancer of the urinary tract. J Urol. 1999;161(5):1486–9.
41. Schlake A, Crispen PL, Cap AP, Atkinson T, Davenport D, Preston DM. NMP-22, urinary cytology, and cystoscopy: a 1 year comparison study. Can J Urol. 2012;19(4):6345–50.
42. Mansoor I, Calam RR, Al-Khafaji B. Role of urinary NMP-22 combined with urine cytology in follow-up surveillance of recurring superficial bladder urothelial carcinoma. Anal Quant Cytol Histol. 2008;30(1):25–32.

Part III

Update on Renal Tumor Pathology

22 Anatomy of the Kidney Revisited: Implications for Diagnosis and Staging of Renal Cell Carcinoma

Stephen M. Bonsib

Abbreviation

RCC Renal cell carcinoma

Introduction

Pathologic stage is the single most important prognostic parameter for renal cell carcinoma (RCC). The tumor, nodes, and metastases (TNM) staging system has two renal-limited categories: a category for local spread outside of the kidney and a category for metastatic disease. The primary mission of the pathologist in evaluation of a tumor nephrectomy is to determine if the tumor is renal limited, or if it has extended locally into veins or into one of the two perinephric fat compartments. Metastatic disease is largely the domain of the clinician (adrenal metastasis excluded). To fulfill this charge, the pathologist must understand the gross and microscopic nuances of the kidney and its environs in order to optimize the dissection strategies, and to permit recognition of invasive behaviors so critical to tissue sampling. Although the basic gross and microscopic anatomy of the kidney is familiar to most pathologists, there are anatomical points that merit specific emphasis with respect to renal neoplasia. This chapter reviews the basic anatomy of the kidney, its neighboring structures within the retroperitoneum, and the numerous potential avenues for distant spread.

Retroperitoneum

The kidneys reside in the retroperitoneum. The retroperitoneum is a large compartment enclosed anteriorly by the peritoneum, posteriorly by the transversalis fascia, and vertebrae superiorly by the 12th rib, and inferiorly by the iliac crest and base of the sacrum [1, 2]. The retroperitoneum is spacious compared to the size of the kidneys, often permitting neoplasms to grow to a large size prior to clinical detection. Thus, symptomatic renal tumors typically are of high stage and have a very poor outcome.

The retroperitoneum is divided into three fascia-invested compartments or spaces: the anterior pararenal space, the perirenal space, and the posterior pararenal space. The anterior pararenal space contains several organs and major vessels, including the pancreas, duodenal loop, ascending and descending colon, and the hepatic, splenic, and proximal superior mesenteric arteries. In large widely invasive tumors, this compartment is occasionally breached leading to composite multiorgan resections. The posterior pararenal space contains fat but no organs.

The perirenal space is home to the kidneys. In addition to the kidneys, it contains the adrenal glands, hilar structures such as the vascular pedicle and its venous tributaries, renal pelvis and ureter, a variable number of hilar lymph nodes and two fat-containing compartments important in renal staging, the peripheral and the central

S. M. Bonsib (✉)
Nephropath, Little Rock, AR, USA
e-mail: Stephen.bonsib@nephropath.com

C. Magi-Galluzzi, C. G. Przybycin (eds.), *Genitourinary Pathology,* DOI 10.1007/978-1-4939-2044-0_22,

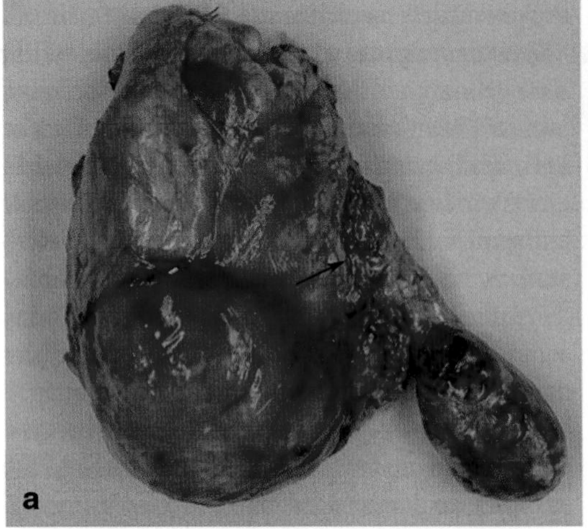

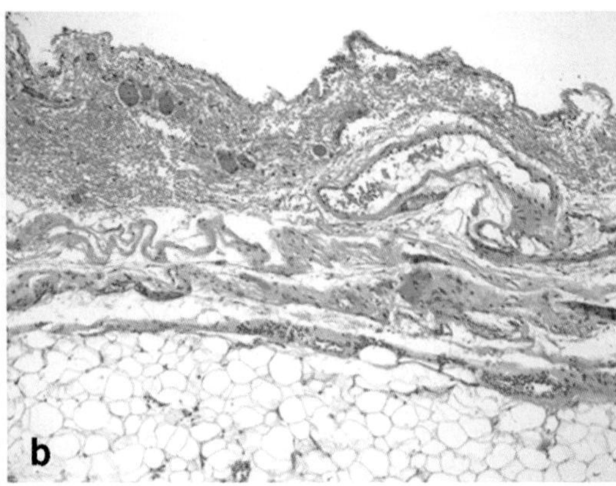

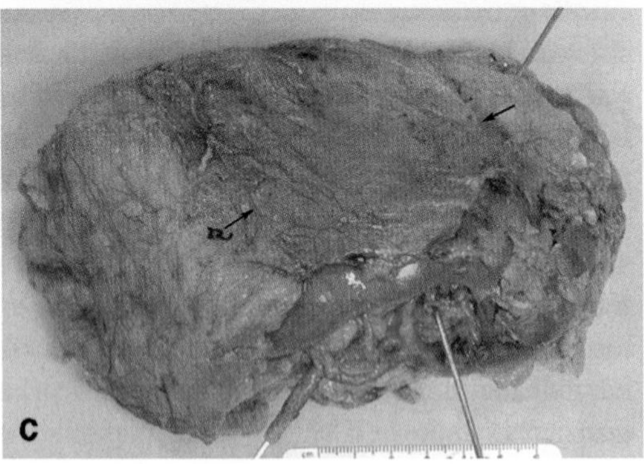

Fig. 22.1 **a** This is a perifascial radical nephrectomy with massive main renal vein involvement by clear cell renal cell carcinoma. Gerota's fascia is intact and visible as a thin delicate connective tissue envelope for the kidney and adrenal. It has been incised medially (*arrow*) exposing more clearly the hilar-perinephric fat. **b** This section shows Gerota's fascia. It is a thin vascularized connective tissue layer that invests the peripheral perinephric fat located below. **c** The anterior pararenal space is thin, overlying the kidneys. Anterior to it is the peritoneum. In this radical nephrectomy, there is a portion of the peritoneum (between *arrows*) covering Gerota's fascia

sinus fat compartments. The anterior and posterior fascial investments of the perirenal spaces are known as Gerota's fascia—a thin connective tissue envelope that provides surgical dissection planes employed during radical perifascial nephrectomy (Fig. 22.1a, b). The posterior layer is a well-defined layer. The anterior layer, however, is more delicate and often adheres to the peritoneum which may be included in radical nephrectomy specimens (Fig. 22.1c). The perirenal space is bounded medially by dense fat and the adventitial connective tissues of the aorta and vena cava that impede communication across the midline of perinephric processes such as urine leaks, hemorrhage, infection, and even neoplastic infiltration.

Peripheral Perinephric Fat Compartment

The peripheral perinephric fat contains the adrenal gland, and the hilar structures already mentioned. It surrounds the outer aspect of the kidney and is separated from the kidney by the fibrous renal capsule. The quantity of peripheral perinephric fat varies substantially in nephrectomy specimens, especially since adrenal-sparing procedures are often employed. Although it is common practice to weigh nephrectomy specimens, these data provide little useful information. For RCC to qualify as extending into this perinephric compartment, it should be in contact with adipocytes, or in loose connective tissue containing adipocytes.

Renal Parenchyma

The kidney consists of two basic components—the renal cortex and the renal medulla, also known as the renal pyramids because of their distinctive shape [3] (Fig. 22.2). The cortical tissue includes the columns of Bertin, portions of the cortex that dip deeply between the renal pyramids toward the renal sinus fat as mentioned above. The kidney is partially invested by the renal capsule, a dense fibrous tissue layer that covers the peripheral aspects of the kidney and extends a short distance into the renal hilum where it terminates (Figs. 22.2 and 22.3a). The cortical columns of Bertin that extend between the renal pyramids are in direct contact with the renal sinus without an intervening fibrous capsule (Fig. 22.3b). Assuming that the renal capsule provides some resistance to tumor extension outside the kidney into the peripheral perirenal fat, the absence of a capsule between the columns of Bertin and the sinus fat may represent a preferential site for extrarenal extension into the central perinephric sinus fat. This may be especially pertinent for tumors arising in the column of Bertin.

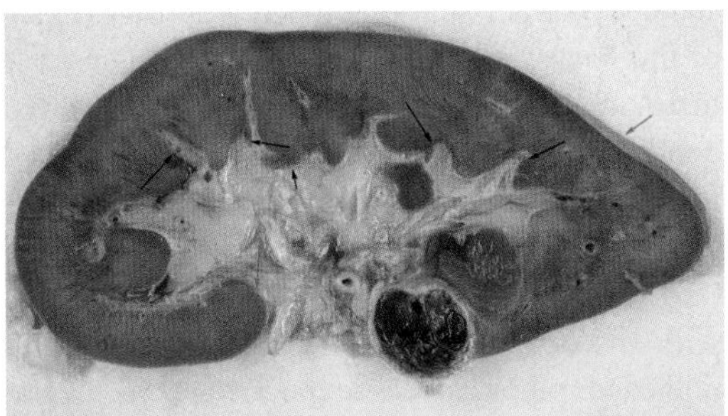

Fig. 22.2 This nephrectomy was bivalved through the lateral mid plane. Most of the perinephric fat was removed. A small portion of the renal capsule is visible to the *upper right* (*red arrow*). The renal capsule curves into the renal sinus a short distance then terminates (*red arrow*). The renal parenchyma consists of the renal cortex and medulla. The cortical columns of Bertin extend between the pyramids and are in direct contact with the renal sinus (*short arrow*). The renal sinus is the central fatty compartment. Wedges of sinus fat extend toward the cortex between the papilla and the columns of Bertin (*long arrows*)

The renal cortex consists of two histological compartments—the cortical labyrinth and the medullary rays. The cortical labyrinth contains glomeruli, proximal and distal convoluted tubules, and the initial portion of the collecting ducts, as well as the renal arteries, veins, and lymphatics. The medullary rays contain parallel tubular segments that course down into the medulla and travel back up to the cortex. It is important to be familiar with the normal histology

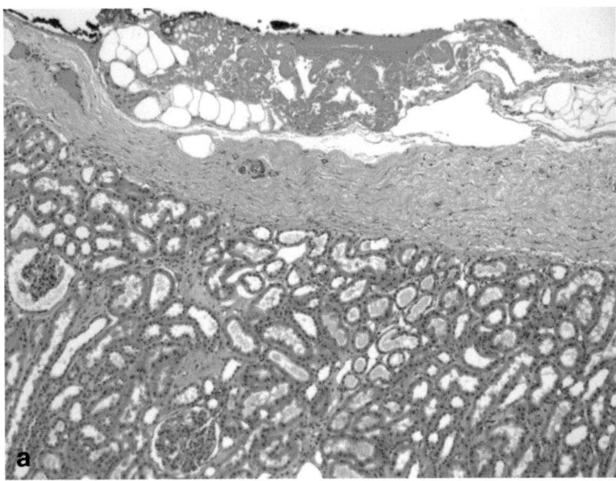

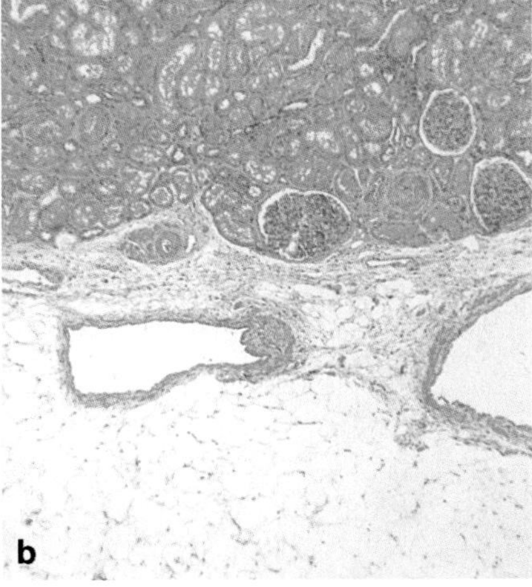

Fig. 22.3 **a** This section shows the dense fibrous renal capsule. It represents a fibrous barrier between the peripheral perinephric fat and the peripheral renal cortex. **b** This image shows the interface between a column of Bertin and the renal sinus fat. Notice the absence of a fibrous capsule. The renal sinus fat with two veins is visible *below*. It is not uncommon for a delicate connective tissue layer to be present between the cortical tissue and the sinus fat as shown here. Involvement of this connective tissue layer is regarded as extension beyond the kidney (pT3a)

of the kidney because the nonneoplastic cortex provides a window into the presence of systemic diseases. Especially important are the common systemic diseases hypertension and diabetes—conditions, that when detected, may have greater prognostic implications than the neoplasm itself. The reader is referred to the recent reviews on this topic that have led to reporting recommendations regarding findings in the nonneoplastic cortex [4, 5].

Central Perinephric Sinus Fat Compartment

The renal sinus is the fatty compartment located within the central confines of the kidney (Fig. 22.2). Involvement of the renal sinus veins was recognized as the primary route of tumor dissemination in nephroblastoma in the early 1980s [6]. A similar role in tumor dissemination for RCC, however, was not shown until 2000 [7]. Inclusion of renal sinus involvement in RCC staging was first codified in the 2002 TNM formulation [8]. Extension into this perinephric compartment is now known to be the most common site of extrarenal extension by RCC. Therefore, understanding the anatomy and histology of this compartment is critical to the accurate staging of RCC [9, 10].

The renal sinus begins at the renal hilum and fills the space between the pelvicalyceal system and the renal parenchyma. The renal sinus has a complex three-dimensional structure [1, 2, 11]. There are pyramidal extensions of the sinus containing fat and interlobar vessels between the renal pyramids that separate the minor calyces from the columns of Bertin (Fig. 22.2). These slender cords of sinus approach within 1–1.5 cm of the renal capsule. Therefore, it is no surprise that sinus tissue is commonly present in partial nephrectomy specimens. This should be looked for grossly at the partial nephrectomy resection margin and when the specimen is sectioned (Fig. 22.4a, b) because sinus fat and sinus veins will occasionally be involved. Most renal pyramids and minor calyces angle toward the central portion of the renal sinus from the anterior and posterior planes of the kidney. Therefore, in a bivalved specimen and in kidney sections, the sinus tissue can be encountered completely surrounded by renal parenchyma (Fig. 22.5a, b).

The renal cortex of the columns of Bertin is in direct contact with the renal sinus without an intervening capsule in contrast to the peripheral renal cortex as previously mentioned (Figs. 22.2 and 22.3b). The renal tubules of the cortical column of Bertin tissue may contact adipocytes directly, or may be separated by loose connective tissue fibers. Involvement of either constitutes the renal sinus involvement. The renal pyramids,

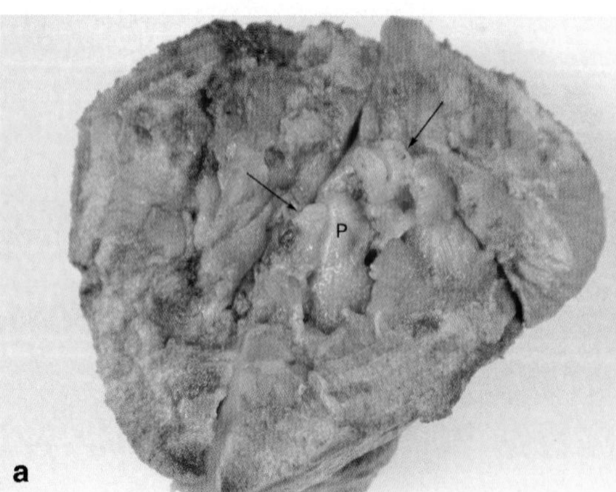

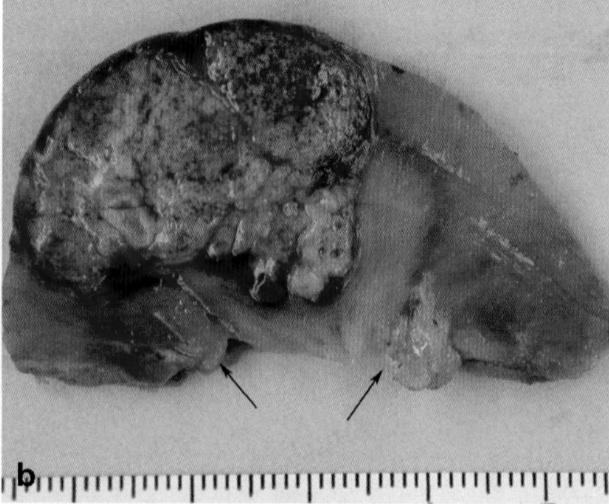

Fig. 22.4 **a** This image shows the surgical resection margin of a partial nephrectomy. Several renal papillae (*P*) can be seen. In addition, two wedges of renal sinus fat are also visible (*arrows*). **b** This cut surface of the above specimen shows a papillary RCC. Notice the two wedges (*arrows*) of sinus fat flanking the renal pyramid

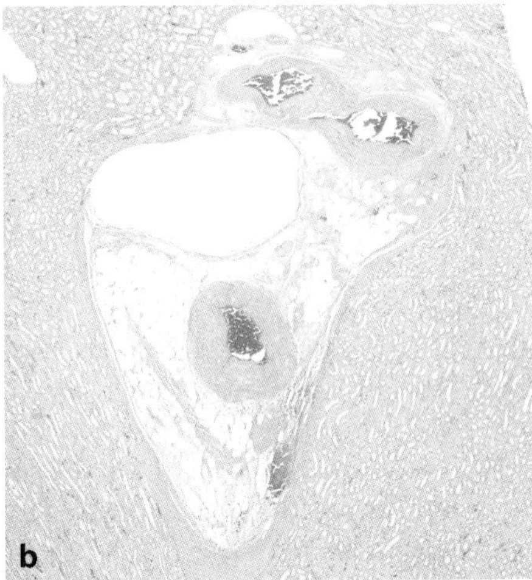

Fig. 22.5 **a** This bivalved kidney shows a compound renal pyramid in the center with two islands of renal sinus (*arrows*) seen in cross section that are completely surrounded by renal parenchyma. **b** In this section of the kidney, there is an island of renal sinus surrounded by the cortex to the top and renal pyramids on both sides. There is a thin-walled interlobar vein adjacent to the cortex that would be easily accessible to a RCC if developing in this area

by contrast, are nested within minor calyces and are not in direct contact with the renal sinus. When RCC involves the collecting system, it usually indicates sinus involvement because it would be uncommon, but not impossible, for a slender cord of tumor to breach only the papillary tip without also invading the renal sinus. The renal sinus' defining attribute is its lush vascularity discussed in detail below.

Renal Parenchymal Vasculature

The renal parenchymal vasculature has two components [1–3, 11–14]. There is a minor system of small vessels, the stellate arteries and veins, which supply and drain, respectively, the superficial cortex through the renal capsule (Fig. 22.6a). These arteries and veins are themselves supplied by, and drain into, the major hilar vessels. An in-

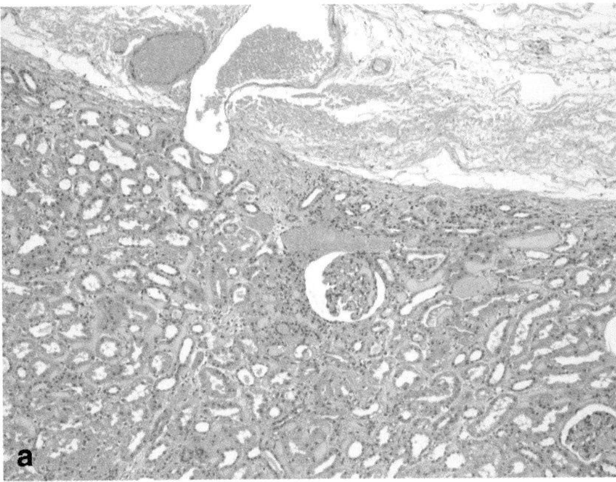

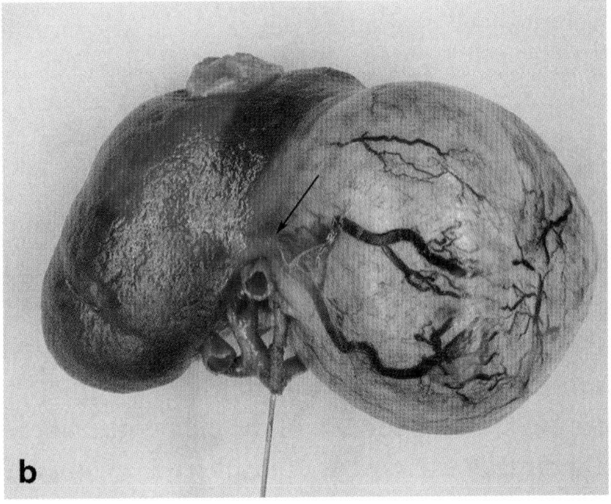

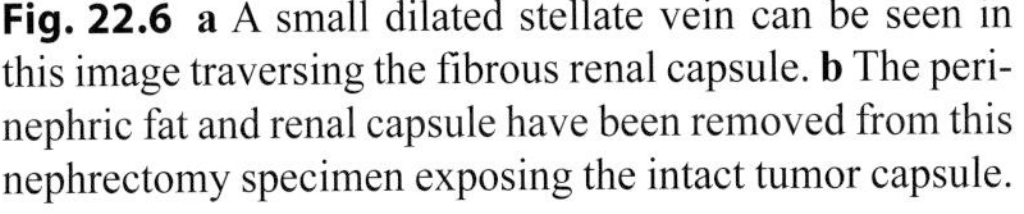

Fig. 22.6 **a** A small dilated stellate vein can be seen in this image traversing the fibrous renal capsule. **b** The perinephric fat and renal capsule have been removed from this nephrectomy specimen exposing the intact tumor capsule. Notice the engorged veins that drape across the tumor capsule. They disappear (*arrow*) as they approach the hilum to drain into hilar veins

travenous tumor in the peripheral perinephric fat represents a tumor that has gained access to the stellate system or may be there by retrograde extension from the hilar connection of the stellate veins (see below). It may be that the venous engorgement occasionally observed in tumor capsules represents this system of veins (Fig. 22.6b).

The major renal parenchymal vasculature resides in the central cortical labyrinth. The arteries and veins travel in parallel as they ascend from, and descend to, the renal sinus, respectively. The renal parenchymal veins are distinctive compared to veins in most other organs because they lack a smooth muscle media (Fig. 22.7a, b). They are essentially very large capillaries. The absence of a smooth muscle media assumes importance with respect to the recognition of retrograde cortical venous invasion and the possibility of multifocal tumors, issues addressed in Chap. 24.

The interlobular veins of the cortex progressively enlarge as they approach the corticomedullary junction to form the arcuate veins. The arcuate veins drain into the interlobar veins that travel between the pyramid and enter the renal sinus. There are elaborate anastomoses between these large veins that encircle the renal pyramids and minor calyces. The interlobar veins converge within the renal sinus forming segmental veins that course anterior to the renal pelvis. Once veins enter the sinus, they acquire a smooth muscle media as discussed below. There are no arteries or veins in the renal medulla, only arterioles, venules, and capillaries.

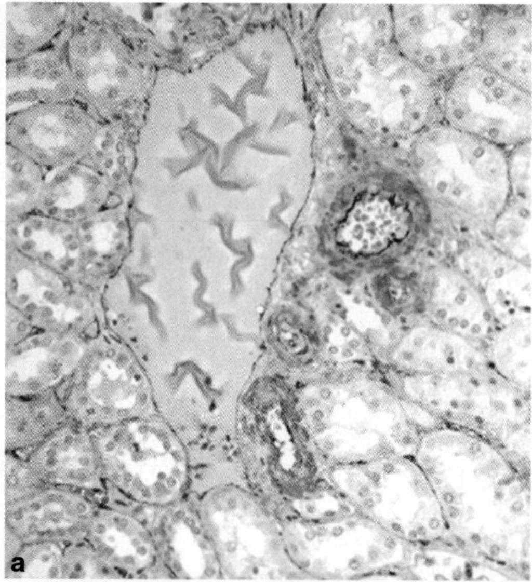

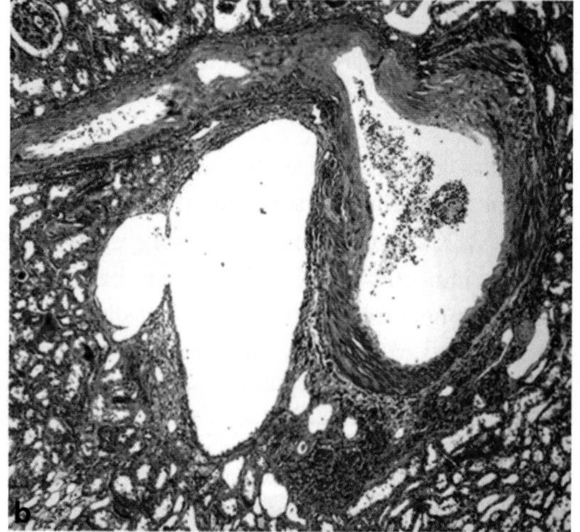

Fig. 22.7 **a** This image shows a cortical interlobular vein to the *left* with small interlobular arteries and arterioles to the *right*. The arteries and veins are always adjacent. Notice that the vein lacks a smooth muscle media and resembles the peritubular capillaries in the surrounding cortex. *Red:* actin smooth muscle; *brown:* CD 31 immunoperoxidase stains. **b** This is the corticomedullary junction. The cortex is to the *top*. Abundant smooth muscle can be seen in the media of the artery to the *right*. However, the arcuate vein to the *left* is devoid of medial smooth muscle. Masson's trichrome stain

Arterial Supply to the Kidney

The kidney's blood supply is disproportionately high compared to that of other organs. Although the kidneys represent only 1 % of the body mass, they receive 25 % of the cardiac output, five times the blood flow through the coronary arteries [15]. Since only 1 % of the glomerular filtrate is normally excreted as urine, there is a comparably impressive venous return that exits the renal sinus through the renal veins. Thus, tumors arising within the kidney are heavily perfused with a voluminous venous return that potentiates venous metastases.

One of the first observations in a nephrectomy for RCC is examination of the vascular hilum, and in particular, assessment of the hilar vessels. Although there are countless variations in the organization of the renal arteries (and veins as discussed below), there are a few generaliza-

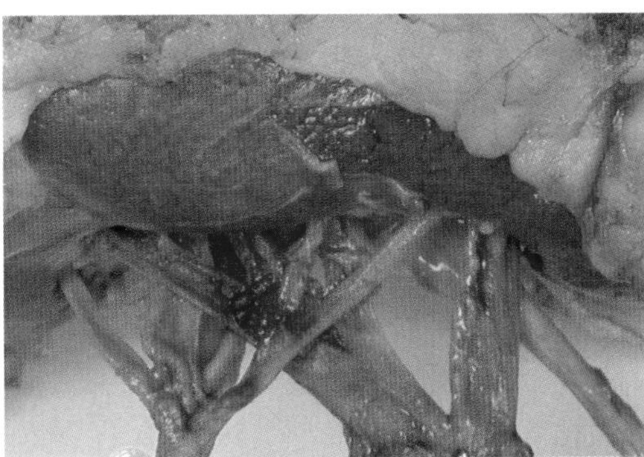

Fig. 22.8 This image shows the vascular hilum of a left kidney. Notice that the arteries and vein are located anterior to the renal pelvis. The artery on the *left* has five segmental branches. The main renal vein on the *right* is formed by the confluence of four tributaries. Notice that the segmental renal arteries and veins interdigitate

tions that apply to most nephrectomy specimens [3, 11–14]. The most common arterial arrangement is for the main renal artery to give rise to an anterior and posterior division. Four segmental arteries arise from the anterior division to supply the upper and lower poles and the anterior kidney. The posterior division continues as the posterior segmental artery. The segmental arteries sequentially branch into the interlobar arteries that enter the renal parenchyma giving rise to six to eight arcuate arteries, from which the interlobular arteries are derived that ascend to the renal capsule. These arteries are all end arteries. There is a vascular junction between the anterior and posterior blood supply 1–2 cm posterior to the lateral convex border of the kidney. This is known as "Brödel's bloodless line of incision," a useful landmark for surgical entry to the kidney [11].

Although the arteries play no role in tumor dissemination or staging, documentation of significant atherosclerotic disease is important because of its role in nephrosclerosis. The major grossing issue related to renal arteries is their frequent tendency to intertwine with the major tributaries of the main renal vein at the renal hilum (Fig. 22.8). This complicates the dissection of the renal veins and may explain the all too frequent occurrence of stapling of arteries and veins together, especially with laparoscopic resections.

Renal Sinus Veins

Once the interlobar veins enter the renal sinus fat, they lose their association with the renal arteries and acquire a smooth muscle media [10]. The smooth muscle of the sinus veins is remarkably variable in quantity and organization. The sinus veins may have a thick layer of smooth muscle that abruptly transitions into a thin layer or no muscle, or the muscle may have only a loose association with the actual vascular lumen (Fig. 22.9a, b). This is noteworthy because the TNM staging definition of sinus vein involvement employs the term "muscular containing vein" [8].

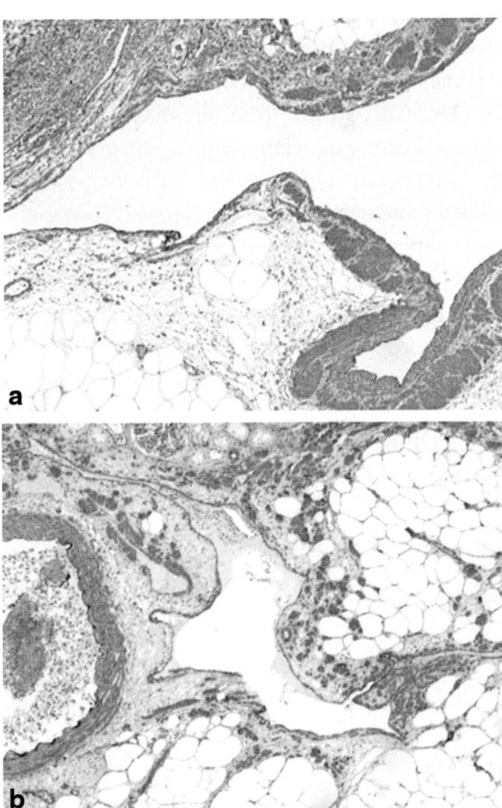

Fig. 22.9 **a** This large sinus vein has just exited the renal parenchyma. Notice the abrupt transition from scant to nonexistent smooth muscle on the *left,* to a very thick smooth muscle media on the *right*. Does only the portion to the *right* qualify as a "muscle containing vein"? What if the tumor was present only in the portion to the *left*? **b** This large sinus vein has a large quantity of smooth muscle in the vicinity on the *right* and to the *bottom,* but no muscle to the *left*. Is this a "muscle-containing vein"? Fully expanded it would be at least 1 cm in size, possibly even larger

Since large caliber sinus veins may have little or no muscle, or the muscle may become attenuated or destroyed when involved by a tumor, this qualification is counterproductive. Furthermore, it has been clearly demonstrated that at least in clear cell RCC, venous involvement begins with entry into large veins that drain the tumor [10]. Therefore, the author contends that any sinus vein involved regardless of size, or quantity of smooth muscle, should be regarded as significant and assigned a pT3a stage designation.

The multiple proximal tributaries of the main renal vein within the renal sinus are large veins that may normally range up to 1–2 cm in diameter. They can become much larger when involved by a tumor. Gross appreciation of the impressive sinus venous system, however, requires sectioning the kidney though its "venous plane." The venous plane is offset from the mid plane of the kidney. There are no large sinus veins posterior to the renal pelvis. The veins that drain the posterior kidney cross over the minor calyces anterior to the renal pelvis, to join the anterior veins before exiting through the renal hilum to form the main renal vein. The venous plane will be missed with sectioning through the lateral mid plane or sectioning through the collecting system. Compare the kidney in Fig. 22.2 sectioned along the lateral mid plane in which the sinus veins are inconspicuous and cut in cross section, with the kidney in Fig. 22.10, which was sectioned through the venous system along probes placed within the major renal veins.

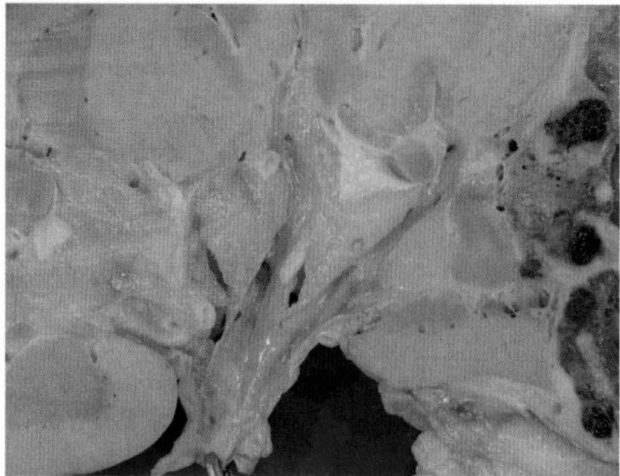

Fig. 22.10 This nephrectomy specimen was venous perfusion fixed allowing visualization of the sinus venous system. The specimen was opened through the venous plane by placing probes within the primary tributaries of the main renal vein and cutting along that plane. The pelvis would be deep to this plane

Main Renal Veins and Their Systemic Venous Connections

The right renal vein is shorter than the left renal vein by 2–4 cm because the vena cava lies to the right of the aorta (Fig. 22.11a). Although there are important differences between the left and

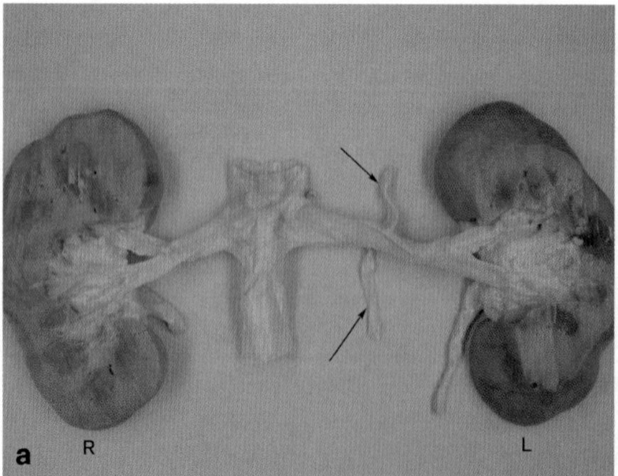

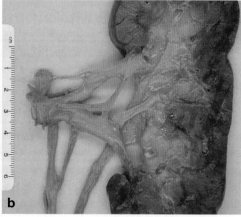

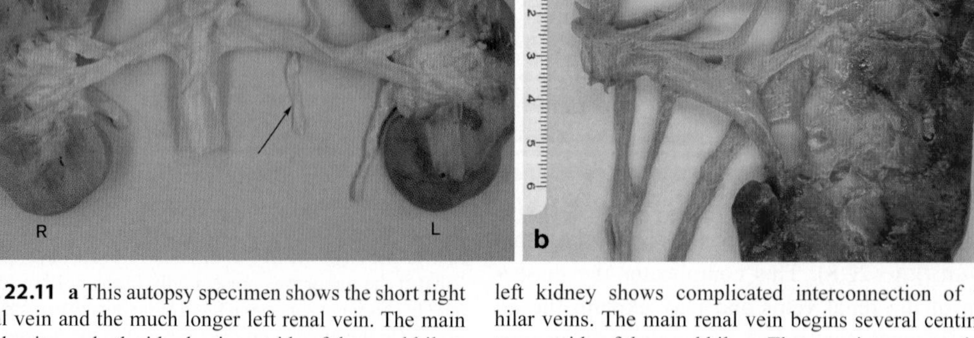

Fig. 22.11 **a** This autopsy specimen shows the short right renal vein and the much longer left renal vein. The main renal veins on both sides begin outside of the renal hilum as two large primary tributaries merge. The left renal vein (*right side*) is fed by the left adrenal vein to the *top* and the left gonadal vein to the *bottom* (*arrows*). **b** This autopsy left kidney shows complicated interconnection of the hilar veins. The main renal vein begins several centimeters outside of the renal hilum. There are interconnections between the primary tributaries of the main renal vein and a thin connection to the large left adrenal vein pointing upwards. The gonadal veins are to the *bottom*

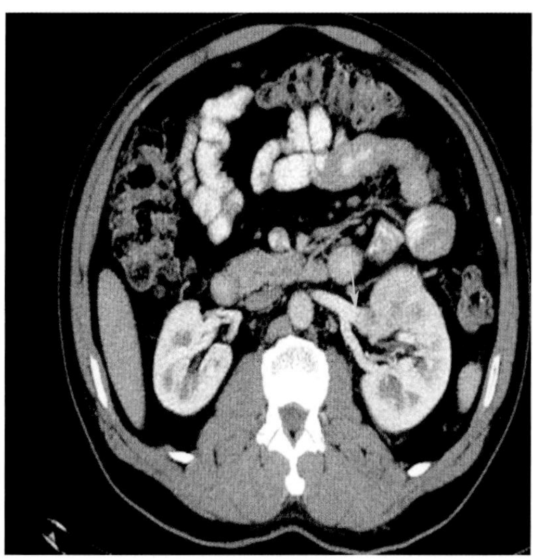

Fig. 22.12 This computed tomography (CT) scan shows a RCC in the left kidney. The tumor extends into a large primary tributary of the left main renal vein (*arrow*). The author reported this as a positive left main renal vein, unaware that it was only a tributary and another branch vein was present draining the opposite pole

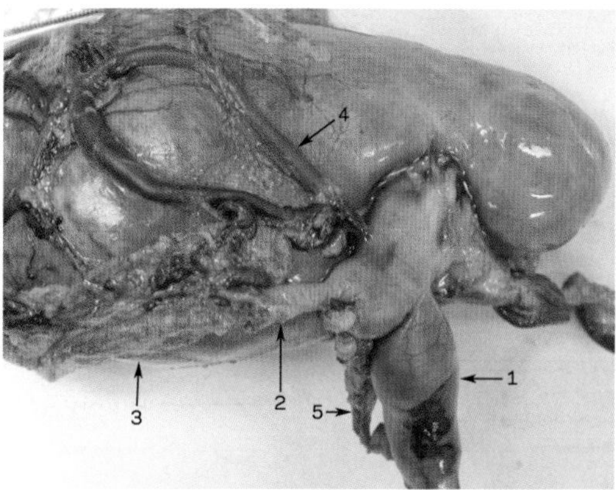

Fig. 22.13 This is a left radical nephrectomy showing venous engorgement due to the main renal vein involvement (*1*). Notice the adrenal vein (*2*) and adrenal gland (*3*), capsular veins (*4*) posterior lumbar vein (*5*), ureteral veins to the *right*. It is easy to envision once the tumor occludes the main renal vein for the tumor to preferentially extend into the other veins and metastasize to the adrenal gland, vertebral venous plexus via the lumbar vein or down the ureter to the pelvis. In addition, when a tumor is found in the capsular vein in the perinephric fat, it is conceivable that it arrived via retrograde flow from the main renal vein

right main renal veins, a feature that they have in common is the frequent occurrence of anomalies. This seems to make every nephrectomy specimen a unique developmental experiment and a dissection challenge for the pathologist.

It is common for more than one major vein to be present at the vascular resection margin of a nephrectomy specimen because the convergence of the primary tributaries of the right and left segmental veins to form the main renal vein often occurs outside of the renal hilum (Figs. 22.8 and22.11a, b). This is more common on the left side where there may be two to three large renal vein tributaries to examine for venous involvement [13–15]. Unfortunately, when there are large main renal vein tributaries located outside of the renal hilum, this can result in disagreement between the pathologist and the radiologist about the status of the main renal vein (Fig. 22.12). The radiologist will report the main renal vein involvement when the tumor is within the final point of convergence of all venous tributaries forming a single vein which may be several centimeters beyond the renal hilum. However, the pathologist will often report a main renal vein involvement when a large caliber renal vein at the renal hilum is occluded by a tumor, often unaware that on imaging studies this vein was only a large tributary of the main renal vein. A similar conundrum is created when multiple "main" renal veins attach directly to the vena cava. This is also common. Approximately 24–30 % of right renal veins will have two to three separate vena cava attachments, while 10 % of left renal veins will have two separate vena cava attachments [13–15].

The renal veins frequently receive one or more extrarenal venous tributaries, such as the adrenal, ureteric, gonadal, lumbar, and segmental veins (Fig. 22.13). The left adrenal vein drains into the main renal vein or one of its large tributaries while the right adrenal vein drains directly into the vena cava (Figs. 22.11a, b and 22.14). The gonadal vein and lumbar vein frequently join the main renal veins after they exit the renal sinus (Fig. 22.14). This occurs in 58 % of cases on the left side, but only 3 % of cases on the right side. When these veins do not drain into the main renal vein, they drain directly into the vena cava and are close to the origin of the main renal vein and represent potential avenues for intravenous

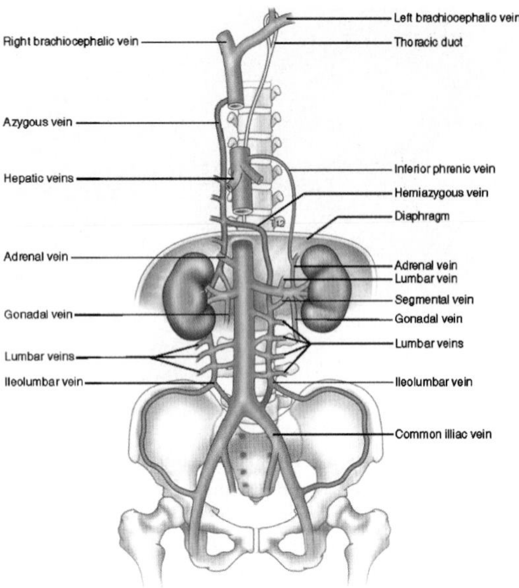

Fig. 22.14 This diagram shows the diverse venous interconnections between the renal veins and the hemiazygous and azygous systems which communicate with the iliac veins and the lumbar veins at each intervertebral space providing avenues for metastatic spread to pelvic and vertebral venous systems

dissemination of a tumor to pelvic or more widespread locations when the main renal vein is involved.

The multiple venous connections of the main renal veins are significant because they communicate with the hemiazygous veins on the left side and azygous veins on the right side which are in turn connected with the common iliac veins (Fig. 22.14). The lumbar veins at every intervertebral disc connect to the vertebral venous system. The vertebral venous system consists of a venous labyrinth within each disc and several longitudinal sinuses that extend along the entire spinal column. Inferiorly, this system communicates with the sacral, pelvic and prostatic veins. Superiorly, it communicates with the intracranial venous system which is composed of the cortical veins, the dural sinuses, the cavernous sinuses, and the ophthalmic veins. The subsequent venous drainage of the intracranial systems ultimately flows into the jugular veins to the superior vena cava.

In 1940, Batson employing intravenous injection with X-rays studies demonstrated that the vertebral venous system was a low pressure, valveless system that permits bidirectional blood flow [16, 17]. With changes in intracranial pressure, blood flows into the vertebral venous system. With the valsalva maneuver, or straining, coughing, sneezing, etc., blood flows from intrathoracic, abdominal, and retroperitoneal veins into the vertebral venous plexus and the intracranial venous system. Thus, cancers of the kidney can spread to the pelvic bones and organs, the vertebral skeleton, and demonstrate the seemingly paradoxical behavior of bypassing the heart and lungs to metastasize to the skull, brain, and head and neck sites [16, 18–20]. Batson commented about the vertebral venous system: "We have a vast intercommunicating system of veins…constantly and physiologically the site of frequent reversals of flow. During these reversals a pathway up and down the spine exists which does not involve the heart or lungs. It provides a ready vehicle for the explanation of 'aberrant' metastatic patterns and removes the stumbling block of the absence of lung involvement." Some of these complex venous interconnections are demonstrated in a left nephrectomy (Fig. 22.13) and in a venous diagram provided (Fig. 22.14).

Renal Lymphatics

Hematogenous dissemination is the principle invasive pathway for RCCs. However, it is important to be familiar with the lymphatic drainage of the kidney and the diverse nodal stations that lymphatic metastases may involve because lymph node dissections have demonstrated that from 7 to 17% of patients have hilar or locoregional lymph node metastases [19, 20]. This occurs more commonly with certain RCC types, particularly papillary and chromophobe RCCs [19].

There are two lymphatic systems in the kidney [21, 22]. Similar to the stellate arteries and veins, there is a minor capsular lymphatic system

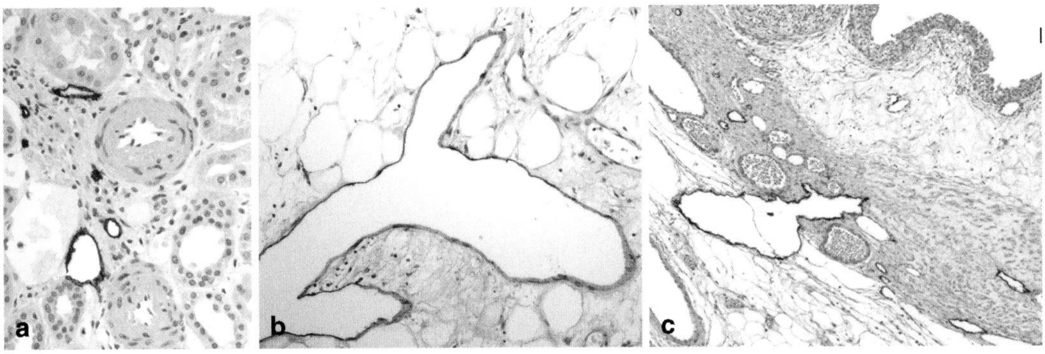

Fig. 22.15 **a** This image is from the superficial cortical labyrinth. It shows multiple small cortical lymphatic endothelia stained with podoplanin. The lymphatics are associated with the arterial-venous system. The vein on the *left* is larger than the several stained lymphatics. **b** This is a lymphatic within the sinus fat. It consists of an endothelial cell lining without a smooth muscle media. **c** The pelvis mucosa is invested with numerous lymphatics. These allow the intralymphatic tumor to spread along a pelviureteral pathway

that drains the superficial cortex and courses toward the renal hilum to join the major lymphatic system that exists through the renal sinus. The major lymphatic system travels with the arterial-venous structures. In the mid to upper cortex, one or more small lymphatics of the caliber of peritubular capillaries are located within the connective tissue investment of interlobular arteries (Fig. 22.15a). Lymphatics lack smooth muscle so they are indistinguishable from capillaries and veins unless stained with a marker specific for lymphatic endothelium.

The small lymphatics enlarge and become more numerous as they descend along the interlobular vessels to the corticomedullary junction. As the corticomedullary junction is approached, the lymphatics stray from the arterial adventitia although they remain associated with the arterial-venous structures. The cortical lymphatics are invariably smaller than the adjacent veins. The lymphatics continue to travel with the arcuate and interlobar vessels until they enter the renal sinus. There are no lymphatics among the glomeruli and renal cortical tubules, or in the renal medulla, unless inflammation-associated neo-lymphangiogenesis occurs [23]. It is not known if such new lymphatics are actually functional and connected to the native lymphatics.

The largest caliber lymphatics occur within the renal sinus where they appear to lose a vascular association and are scattered throughout the sinus fat (Fig. 22.15b). Sinus lymphatics may have an interrupted smooth muscle media, but most often the lymphatics consist solely of a thin endothelial cell layer as the lymphatics within the renal parenchyma. There are numerous lymphatics within the renal pelvic muscularis allowing pelviureteral lymphatic spread of RCC (Fig. 22.15c).

Most Lymph exit through the renal hilum and flows to the hilar lymph nodes and/or the locoregional lymph nodes. That said, most radical nephrectomy specimens will not contain any hilar lymph nodes. In a recent study in which all of the hilar fat was examined histologically, only 20% of cases had lymph node tissue identified [24]. The primary locoregional drainage for the right kidney are the precaval, postcaval, and interaortocaval lymph nodes, while the primary locoregional drainage for the left kidney are the para-aortic, postcaval, and postaortic lymph nodes [22, 25].

Lymphatic involvement in RCC is very unpredictable. Only a third of patients with positive locoregional nodes will have positive hilar lymph nodes because the renal lymph may follow a number of alternate routes and not only bypass hilar lymph nodes, but may even bypass locoregional lymph nodes and flow to more distal nodal stations, such as the pelvic and thoracic lymph nodes [25, 26]. As shown in the drawing from the classic lymphatic injection studies of Parker in

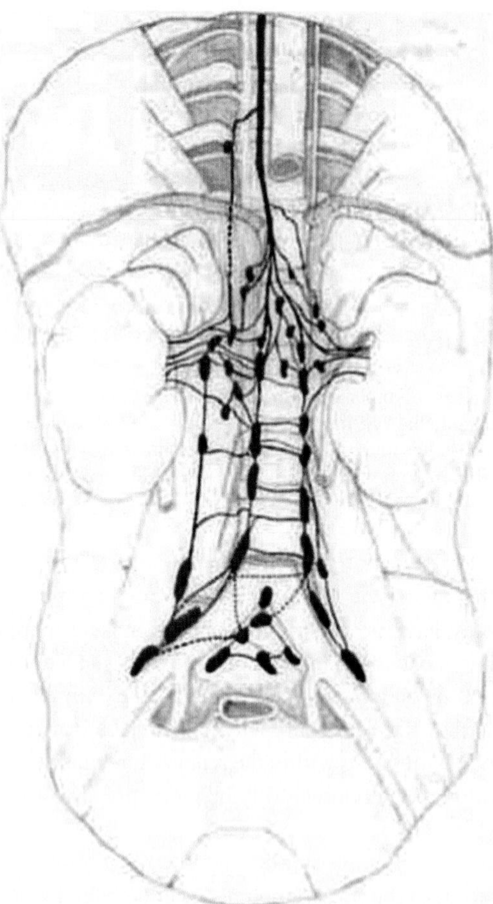

Fig. 22.16 This diagram by Parker shows the elaborate lymphatic intercommunications between the locoregional nodal stations and the pelvic and thoracic nodal stations. Notice the most superior lymphatic pathway to the thoracic duct that allows the lymph to flow from the kidneys directly into the brachiocephalic vein potentially bypassing all nodal stations. (Used with permission from Parker [22])

1935, there are three parallel tracks that an intralymphatic tumor can follow up and down the aorta and the vena cava [22] (Fig. 22.16). Renal lymphatics may connect directly to the thoracic duct without passing through any intervening lymph node stations (Fig. 22.16). This occurs more often on the right side than the left side (38 versus 15 %). This allows intralymphatic RCC to flow into the left brachiocephalic vein and metastasize to the lungs without nodal involvement. The unpredictability of lymphatic spread may explain the lack of survival advantage afforded by lymph node dissections resulting in a decreasing incidence of routine regional lymph node dissection in RCC treatment [26]. It has also hampered implementation of sentinel lymph node biopsy in operative staging of RCC which is technically feasible [27].

Conclusion

The kidneys and their environs are complex and important to understand not only for specimen handling and pathologic staging purposes, but also for understanding the phenomenal potential of RCC to spread to seemingly anomalous sites. The kidneys have four coverings—the renal capsule, the perinephric fat, Gerota's fascia, and the anterior and posterior pararenal spaces. They are cushioned internally and externally by perirenal fat compartments. These many layers would seem to impart numerous barriers to distant spread. However, the kidney's uniquely voluminous arterial blood supply, with its equally impressive venous return, allows RCC to circumvent these barriers because the majority of RCCs gain access to the venous outflow prior to any another type of extrarenal extension. This becomes an even greater liability since the renal veins not only drain directly into the largest caliber vein of the body, the vena cava, but also freely interconnect with the azygous and hemiazygous systems and the large volume, low pressure, and the valveless bidirectional cerebrospinal venous system. Collectively, these interconnected venous highways allow metastases to travel to the liver and lungs, descend into the pelvis, or bypass the abdominal and thoracic organs with seemingly paradoxical metastases to the brain, head, and neck.

The renal lymphatics, although representing a minor metastatic pathway, not only flow into the hilar and locoregional nodes but may directly connect to the pelvic and thoracic nodal stations allowing the lymphatic tumor spread to bypass the more proximal nodal stations. This compromises the ability of the urologist to surgically control locoregional lymphatic spread. Direct lymphatic connections to the thoracic duct bypassing nodal stations allows the intralymphatic tumor to spread via hematogenous routes to the lung, even in the absence of intravenous invasion by the primary tumor.

The countless number of venous and lymphatic pathways available to RCC explains why no bone, organ, or body site is immune to RCC metastases. Furthermore, these anatomic complexities underscore the fact that when we generate a pathologic stage, it represents the least stage of the process, but not necessarily the true stage of the process. The tumor may have already escaped the confines of the specimen and its environs by the time of our examination.

References

1. Kaye KW, Goldberg ME. Applied anatomy of the kidney and ureter. Urol Clin North Am. 1982;9(1): 3–13.
2. Sampaio FJB. Renal anatomy endourologic considerations. Urol Clin North Am. 2000;27(4):585–607.
3. Bonsib SM. Renal anatomy and histology. In: Jennette JC, Olson JL, Schwartz MM, Silva FG, editors. Heptinstall'spathology of the kidney. 6th ed. Philadelphia: Lippincott Williams & Wilkins; 2007.
4. Bonsib SM, Pei Y. The non-neoplastic kidney in tumor nephrectomy specimens: what can it show and what is important? Adv Anat Pathol. 2010;17(4): 235–50.
5. Henriksen KJ, Meehan SH, Chang A. Non-neoplastic renal diseases are often unrecognized in adult tumor nephrectomy specimens: a review of 246 cases. Am J kid Dis. 2007;31:575–84.
6. Beckwith JB. National Wilmstumor study: an update for pathologists. Pediatr Dev Pathol. 1998;1:79–84.
7. Bonsib SM, Gibson D, Greene GF, Mhoon M. Renal sinus involvement in renal cell carcinomas. Am J Surg Pathol. 2000;24:451–8.
8. Edge SB, Byrd DR, Compton CC, Fritz AG, Greene FL, Trotti A III, editors. Kidney. AJCC cancer staging handbook. 7th ed. New York: Springer; 2010.
9. Bonsib SM. The renal sinus is the principal invasive pathway: a prospective study of 100 renal cell carcinomas. Am J Surg Pathol. 2004;28:1594–600.
10. Bonsib SM. Renal veins and venous extension in clear cell renal cell carcinoma. Mod Pathol. 2007;20: 44–53.
11. Hodson CJ. The renal parenchyma and its blood supply. Curr Prob Diagn Radiol. 1978;7:1–32.
12. Molema G, Aird WC. Vascular heterogeneity in the kidney. Semin Nephrol. 2012;32(2):145–55.
13. Brödel M. The intrinsic blood-vessels of the kidney and their significance in nephrotomy. Johns Hopkins Hosp Bull. 1901;12:10–3.
14. Satyapal KS. Classification of the drainage patterns of the renal veins. J Anat. 1995;186:329–33.
15. Raman SS, Pojchamarnwipugh S, Muangsomboon K, Schulam PG, Gritsch HA, Lu DSK. Surgically relevant normal and variant renal parenchymal and vascular anatomy in preoperative 16-MDCT evaluation of potential laparoscopic renal donors. Am J Radiol. 2007;188(1):105–14.
16. Batson OV. The function of the vertebral veins and their role in the spread of metastases. Ann Surg. 1940;112:138–49.
17. Nathoo N, Caris EC, Wiener JA, Mendel E. History of the vertebral venous plexus and the significant contributions of Breschet and Batson. Neurosurgery. 2011;69(5):1007–114.
18. Oeppen RS, Tung K. Retrograde venous invasion causing vertebral metastases in renal cell carcinoma. Brit J Radiol. 2001;74:759–61.
19. Hoffmann NE, Gillett MD, Cheville JC, Loshe CM, Leibovich BC, Blute ML. Differences in organ system of distant metastases by renal cell carcinoma subtype. J Urol. 2009;179(2):474–7.
20. Weiss L, Harlos JP, Torhorst J, Gunthard B, Hartveit F, Svendsen E, et al. Metastatic patterns of renal carcinoma: an analysis of 687 autopsies. J Cancer Res Clin Oncol. 1988;114:605–12.
21. Bonsib SM. Renal lymphatics, and lymphatic involvement in sinus invasive (pT3b) clear cell renal cell carcinoma. Mod Pathol. 2006;19:746–53.
22. Parker AE. Studies on the main posterior lymph channels of the abdomen and their connections with the lymphatics of the genito-urinary system. Am J Anat. 1935;56:409–43.
23. Seeger H, Bonani M, Segerer S. The role of lymphatics in renal inflammation. Nephrol Dial Transpl. 2012;27:2634–41.
24. Phan DC, McKenney JK, Cox RM, Madi R, Greene GF, Gokden N. Should hilar lymph nodes be expected in radical nephrectomy specimens? Pathol Res Pract. 2010;206(5):310–3.
25. Phillips CK, Taneja SS. The role of lymphadenectomy in the surgical management of renal cell carcinoma. Urol Oncol. 2004;22:214–24.
26. Kates M, Lavery HJ, Brajtbord J, Samadi D, Palese MA. Decreasing rates of lymph node dissection during radical nephrectomy for renal cell carcinoma. Ann Surg Oncol. 2012;19:2693–9.
27. Bex A, Vermeeron L, Meinhardt W, Prevoo W, Horenblas S, Olmos RAV. Intraoperative sentinel node identification and sampling in clinically node-negative renal cell carcinoma: initial experience in 20 patients. World J Urol. 2011;29:793–9.

Classification of Adult Renal Tumors and Grading of Renal Cell Carcinoma

23

William R. Sukov and John C. Cheville

Introduction

The first major unifying classification system for renal cell carcinoma (RCC) and other adult renal tumors was developed at an international consensus conference in Heidelberg, Germany, in 1996 [1]. In the Heidelberg classification, RCC was divided into conventional RCC, chromophil (papillary) RCC, chromophobe RCC, collecting duct RCC (including medullary carcinoma) and RCC, unclassified types. Benign tumors included oncocytoma, papillary adenoma, and metanephric adenoma. This classification system was endorsed in a subsequent consensus conference held in Rochester, MN in 1997 [2]. Since that time, refinements have been made in the classification system with the additional description of unique and rarer subtypes that was endorsed at an International Society of Urologic Pathology (ISUP) consensus conference in 2012 in Vancouver, Canada, (Table 23.1), and this tumor classification is discussed in this chapter [3].

Grading of Renal Cell Carcinoma

The first major study on RCC grading was published in 1932 by Drs. Hand and Broder from the Mayo Clinic. Their grading system was based on nuclear features and correlated with patient outcome. Since that time, three notable studies addressing RCC grading have been published, and with the exception of the 2012 ISUP consensus conference grading system, all were reported prior to the Heidelberg and Rochester classifications. The work by Skinner et al. is of particular note as these authors analyzed their experience with a large cohort of surgically treated patients and found that a four-tier nuclear grading system based on the worst grade of a tumor stratified patients into four prognostic groups [4]. The 309 patients in their series treated by nephrectomy and with at least 5 years follow-up had 5-year survival for grades 1, 2, 3, and 4 of 75, 65, 56, and 26 %, respectively. Skinner et al. also reported for the first time that grade remained prognostic within the various RCC stages (Robson) including advanced stages. The authors also realized at that time that little was known of the various types of RCC, and divided tumors into clear cell, clear cell or granular, and spindle cell types. Subsequently, the most cited paper on RCC grading was published by Fuhrman et al. in 1982 [5]. Their study consisted of 103 patients, 84 treated by nephrectomy and with at least 5 years of follow-up. The grading system had four tiers and was based on nuclear features (size, shape, nucleoli) and the highest grade within a tumor was designated as the overall grade identical to

W. R. Sukov (✉) · J. C. Cheville
Department of Pathology, Mayo Clinic,
Rochester, MN, USA
e-mail: Sukov.william@mayo.edu

J. C. Cheville
e-mail: Cheville.john@mayo.edu

C. Magi-Galluzzi, C. G. Przybycin (eds.), *Genitourinary Pathology,* DOI 10.1007/978-1-4939-2044-0_23,

Table 23.1 Classification of adult renal tumors

Renal cell carcinoma (RCC)	Benign
Clear cell RCC	Oncocytoma
Multilocular cystic RCC	Papillary adenoma
Papillary RCC	Metanephric adenoma
Chromophobe RCC	Angiomyolipoma
Collecting duct RCC	Epithelioid AML
Medullary carcinoma	Cystic nephroma
RCC, unclassified type	Mixed epithelial andstromal tumor
Clear cell papillary RCC[a]	
Xp11 translocation associated RCC[a]	
Mucinous tubular and spindle cell carcinoma[a]	
Tubulocystic carcinoma[a]	
Thyroid-like follicular carcinoma[a]	

AML angiomyolipoma
[a]Denotes new RCC variant not recognized in 1996 Heidelberg and 1997 Rochester classifications

Skinner et al. Fuhrman et al. made the additional observation of nucleolar size evident at various microscopic magnifications as an additional objective measure of nuclear grade. In their survival analysis, only three groups that differed in outcome were identified. Fuhrman grade 1 tumors had a survival of 65% compared to grades 2 and 3 at 30% and grade 4 at less than 10%. Prior to 2012, the Fuhrman grading system was recommended for clinical use.

Shortcomings in the Fuhrman grading system have been well documented, and in 2012, a consensus conference of the ISUP developed grading system recommendations that were specific to the classification of RCC. Studies examining the prognostic impact of grade on outcome have been limited to clear cell, papillary, and chromophobe RCC as the other RCC types are too infrequent to analyze or have a relatively defined clinical behavior. In clear cell and papillary RCC, the ISUP recommended that the grade is determined exclusively by nucleolar prominence in grades 1–3, that grade 4 includes pleomorphic cells or sarcomatoid and rhabdoid differentiation (Table 23.2 and Fig. 23.1), and that chromophobe RCC should not be graded [6]. In clear cell RCC, the ISUP system shows a strong association with cancer-specific outcome among surgically treated patients at the Mayo Clinic (Fig. 23.2) [7]. A study subsequent to the ISUP consensus conference found that the addition of coagulative tumor necrosis in the clear cell RCC grading system improved the prognostic ability of the ISUP grading system particularly for grade 3 tumors where grade 3 clear cell RCC without necrosis has a 5-year cancer specific survival of 62% compared to 30% for tumors that have necrosis [7].

Table 23.2 2012 ISUP grading system for clear cell and papillary RCC

ISUP grade	Feature
Grade 1	Absent or inconspicuous nucleoli
Grade 2	Nucleoli evident at 400x but inconspicuous or invisible at 100x
Grade 3	Nucleoli visible at 100x
Grade 4	Nuclear pleomorphism or rhabdoid or sarcomatoid differentiation

ISUP International Society of Urologic Pathology

Classification of Adult Renal Tumors

Clear Cell Renal Cell Carcinoma

Clear cell RCC accounts for approximately 70% of all RCC [8]. The highest incidence occurs in the sixth and seventh decades but there is a wide age distribution, and males are affected twice as frequently as women. Presenting signs and symptoms include hematuria, abdominal pain or discomfort, scrotal varicocele, or generalized symptoms such as weight loss, fever, anorexia, or fatigue. Tumors are frequently identified incidentally by imaging for unrelated issues. Clear cell RCC is cortically based and are generally solitary, and multiple lesions should raise the consideration of von Hippel–Lindau disease caused by a germ-line mutation of the Von Hippel–Lindau (VHL) tumor suppressor gene at chromosome 3p25.

Clear cell RCC generally exhibits a round to lobulated growth pattern with pushing borders and formation of a fibrous pseudocapsule. High-grade clear cell RCC may have infiltrative margins. Low-grade tumors have a distinctive golden yellow appearance due to high lipid content that may be lost in higher grade tumors. Areas of hemorrhage, fibrosis and cystic degeneration are frequent. Clear cell RCC exhibits a sheet-like

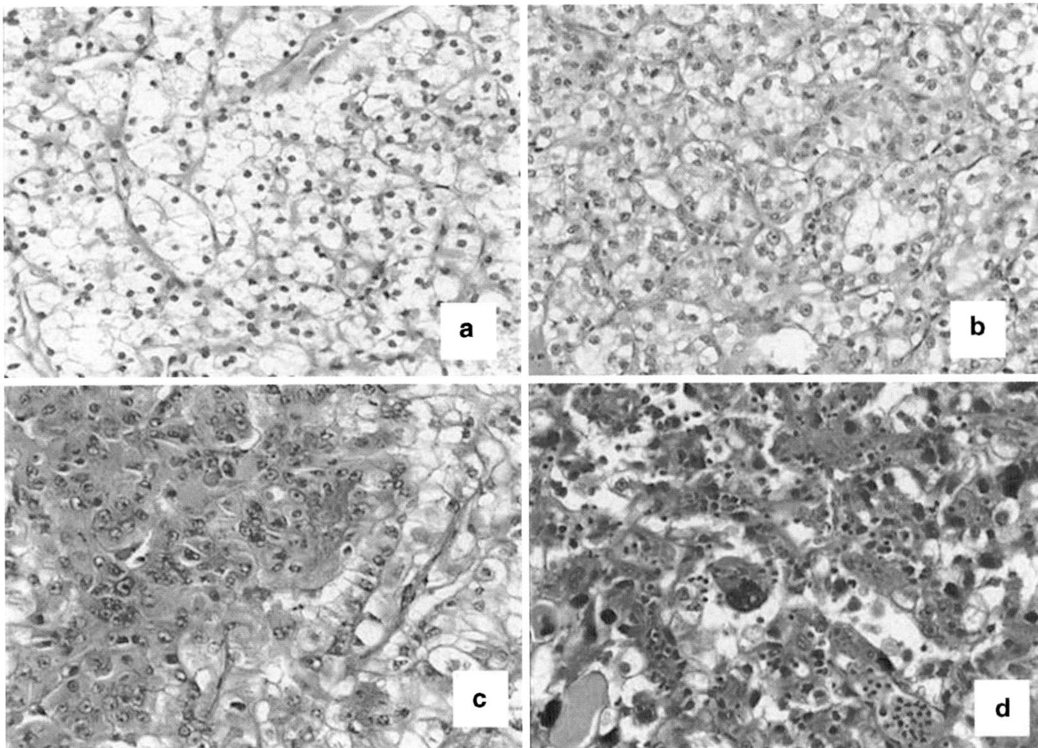

Fig. 23.1 ISUP grading for clear cell RCC. Grade 1 (**a**), 2 (**b**), and 3 (**c**) are defined by nucleolar prominence while grade 4 (**d**) contains pleomorphic cells

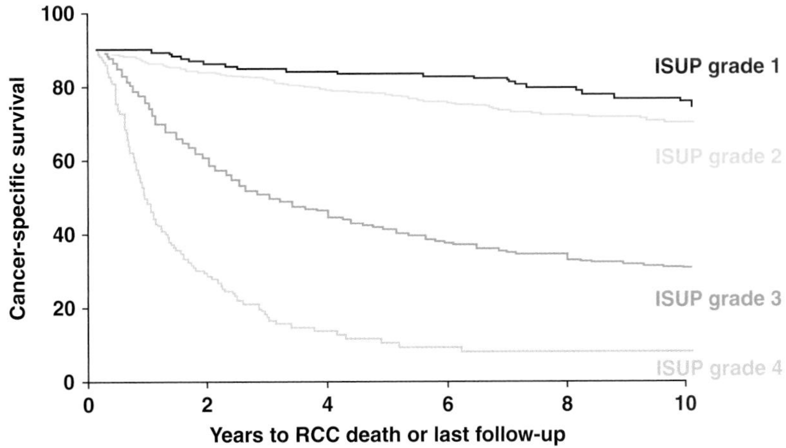

Fig. 23.2 Kaplan-Meier curve of patients treated by nephrectomy at the Mayo Clinic between 1970 and 2008 for clear cell renal cell carcinoma (*RCC*). International Society of Urologic Pathology (*ISUP*) grade is significantly associated with the outcome

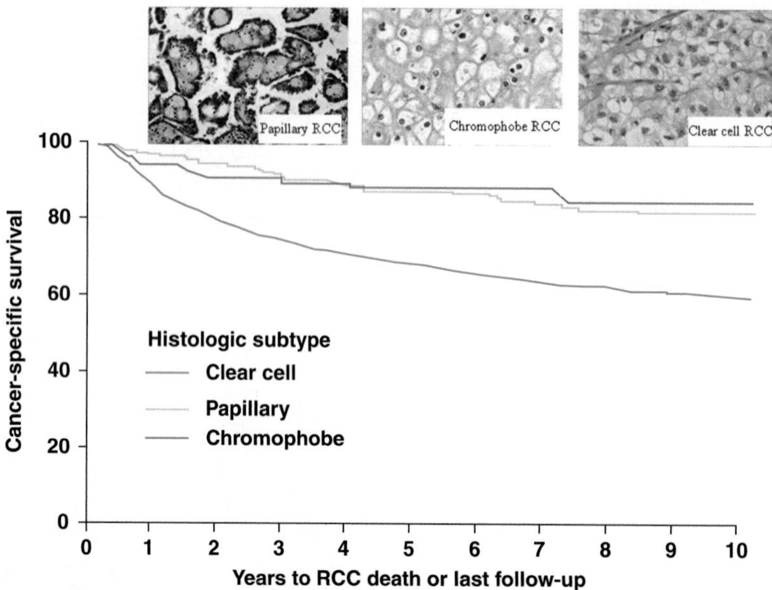

Fig. 23.3 Patients with clear cell renal cell carcinoma (*RCC*) have a significantly worse outcome than patients with papillary and chromophobe *RCC*. The Kaplan-Meier curve shows the outcome difference between all patients with these tumor types treated surgically at the Mayo Clinic. This outcome difference is also seen within the various tumor nodes metastasis (TNM) stages

or nested growth pattern interspersed by a rich network of delicate thin-walled vessels. The cells within clear cell RCC typically have an abundant clear cytoplasm and prominent cell membranes. Higher grade tumors may lose this lipid production and show populations of cells having a more eosinophilic or granular appearance. Most clear cell RCCs show reactivity using antibodies against low-molecular-weight keratins, vimentin, RCC antigen, epithelial membrane antigen (EMA) carbonic anhydrase IX (CA IX), and CD10. Clear cell RCC is usually not positive for cytokeratin 7 (CK7) or alpha-methylacyl CoA racemase (AMACR), features that can be helpful separating clear cell from papillary RCC. CD117 and e-cadherin are negative in clear cell RCC in contrast to chromophobe RCC. Immunohistochemical stains may be useful in separating clear cell RCC from other subtypes on needle core biopsy specimens using a panel that includes CA IX, CD117, AMACR, CK7 and CD10 [9]. Genetic testing of clear cell RCC is characterized by structural alterations of the short arm of chromosome 3 (3p) resulting in the loss of genomic material at 3p21 and 3p12–14 or 3p25.

The outcome of patients with clear cell RCC is dependent on grade, stage, tumor size, coagulative tumor necrosis, and the presence of sarcomatoid and rhabdoid differentiation [10]. A number of clinical nomograms are available based on these features to predict outcome [11]. In regard to the three most common RCC subtypes, stage for stage and grade for grade, clear cell RCC has a worse outcome than papillary and chromophobe RCC (Fig. 23.3) [12].

Multilocular Cystic Renal Cell Carcinoma

Multilocular cystic RCC is an uncommon variant of clear cell RCC accounting for less than 2% of RCC. This tumor is multicystic, and cysts are lined by cells with low grade nuclear features and clear cytoplasm in addition to small nests of clear cells in the cyst walls. Expansile nests of clear cells, however, disqualify a tumor from this diagnosis. The distinction of multilocular cystic RCC from a benign renal cortical cyst is made by the presence of multiple cell layers lining the cysts or more frequently and more dependably, by the presence of nests of clear cells in the cyst wall. Patients have an excellent outcome following tumor excision, and in our experience, none of these tumors has exhibited aggressive behavior.

Papillary Renal Cell Carcinoma

Papillary type RCC is the second most common type of RCC, and accounts for 10% of adult RCC [8]. The age distribution, male to female ratio, and presenting signs and symptoms are similar to patients with clear cell RCC. Papillary RCC (PRCC) is typically solitary, but multifocal or bilateral lesions are not uncommon, and rarely indicative of an inherited RCC syndrome. Grossly, PRCC is lobulated and circumscribed and frequently show degenerative changes with hemorrhage and friability. PRCC demonstrates a wide variety of morphologic features but are characterized by a papillary or tubulo-papillary growth pattern. Papillary structures are composed of fibrovascular cores that contain lipid-laden histiocytes. Some tumors have a more solid and tubular growth pattern mimicking metanephric adenoma. Psammomatous calcifications, areas of hemosiderin deposition (that can be present within the cytoplasm of tumor cells) and necrosis are also frequent findings.

The cells comprising PRCC can be quite variable showing a range of minimal to abundant eosinophilic, basophilic, or clear cytoplasm. This variability in cytoplasmic appearance has resulted in the categorization of PRCC into two types based in part on these cytoplasmic differences (Fig. 23.4) [13]. Tumors classified as type 1 are comprised of cells with a minimal amount of pale to basophilic cytoplasm and small oval nuclei with inconspicuous nucleoli. Cells of type 1 tumors tend to be distributed in a single layer along the papillary structures and commonly show lipid-laden macrophages and psammomatous calcifications. Type 2 tumors are comprised of cells with more abundant eosinophilic cytoplasm and larger, round nuclei with visible nucleoli, showing a pseudostratified organization along the papillary structures. Classifying a particular PRCC as type 1 or 2 can be problematic at times as there can be areas demonstrating features of both types within a single tumor. Cells with clear cytoplasm can be seen in PRCC, though generally they do not show the clarity of clear cell RCC but have a suggestion of granularity within the cytoplasm. The presence in a tumor with a papillary growth pattern of a significant proportion of cells with clear cytoplasm should raise the possibility of a translocation-associated RCC. Immunohistochemically, tumors are positive for low molecular weight keratin, RCC, CD10 and P504S,

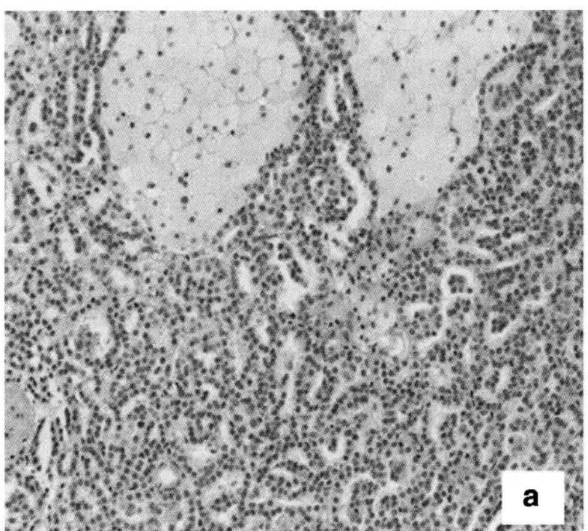

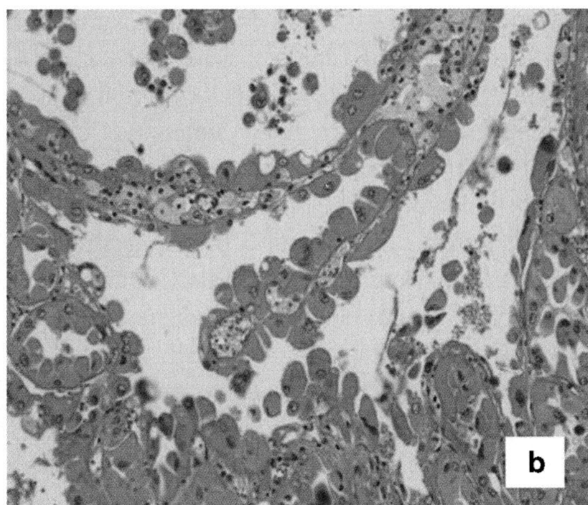

Fig. 23.4 Two examples of papillary RCC showing the wide spectrum in histologic appearance. The tumor (**a**) is type 1, grade 1, while the tumor (**b**) is type 2, grade 3

and CK7 is present in a significant proportion of PRCC with type 1 morphology. In cases of low-grade papillary RCC with basophilic features that resembles metanephric adenoma, WT-1 and CK7 are particularly helpful, as PRCC is WT1 negative and CK7 positive in contrast to metanephric adenoma. Immunohistochemistry (transcription factor E3/transcription factor EB, TFE3/TFEB) and molecular genetic analysis can be used to differentiate from translocation-associated tumors. The most reproducible genetic abnormality in PRCC is trisomy of chromosomes 7 and 17. Patients with PRCC have a better outcome grade for grade and stage for stage when compared to patients with clear cell RCC. Features predictive of outcome include tumor grade and stage. Although it is recommended to report the type of PRCC, the grade is a stronger prognostic feature than the type [14].

Clear Cell Papillary Renal Cell Carcinoma

Clear cell PRCC (also known as clear cell tubulopapillary RCC) is a relatively recently described subtype of RCC that displays features of both clear cell and PRCC. This entity, along with other recently described entities addressed in this chapter, is covered in greater detail in Chap. 26 of this book. These tumors are typically circumscribed, encapsulated, and solitary although multiple tumors have been described in patients. They show areas of papillary, acinar, or tubular growth with a cystic component common. The cells have a small to moderate amount of clear cytoplasm and small, compact nuclei. A helpful diagnostic feature is the orientation of the nuclei towards the apical aspect of cells lining tubules or papillary structures. Unlike PRCC, clear cell papillary RCC does not contain clusters of lipid-laden histiocytes or exhibit necrosis.

Clear cell papillary RCC demonstrates a distinct immunophenotype. Tumor cells are strongly positive for CK7 and CA IX, and are typically negative for CD10 and AMACR [15]. Molecular studies have shown that clear cell papillary RCC represents an entity distinct from either papillary or clear cell RCC as it does not exhibit trisomy 7 or 17 or alteration of chromosome 3p. Based on reports thus far, clear cell papillary RCC is an indolent tumor. Nearly all tumors are low grade (ISUP grade 1 and 2) and low stage, and no reports of death have been reported although in our experience, rare tumors have acted aggressively.

Chromophobe Renal Cell Carcinoma

Chromophobe RCC constitutes approximately 5–10 % of RCC [8, 10]. Signs and symptoms, age distribution and male to female ratio are similar to other RCC subtypes. Chromophobe RCC can be quite large and most are circumscribed, homogenous, and lack necrosis (Fig. 23.5). Higher stage tumors and tumors with necrosis should raise concern for sarcomatoid differentiation. Chromophobe RCC has a characteristic histologic appearance with solid growth and cells that have distinct cell membranes, abundant clear to eosinophilic cytoplasm with perinuclear clearing and irregular nuclei imparting a "plant cell" appearance to the tumor. Some tumors are composed of cells with eosinophilic cytoplasm, the so-called eosinophilic variant of chromophobe RCC. The nuclei in chromophobe RCC have a characteristic appearance and are particularly helpful in separating from other tumors, particularly oncocytoma. The nuclei have irregular

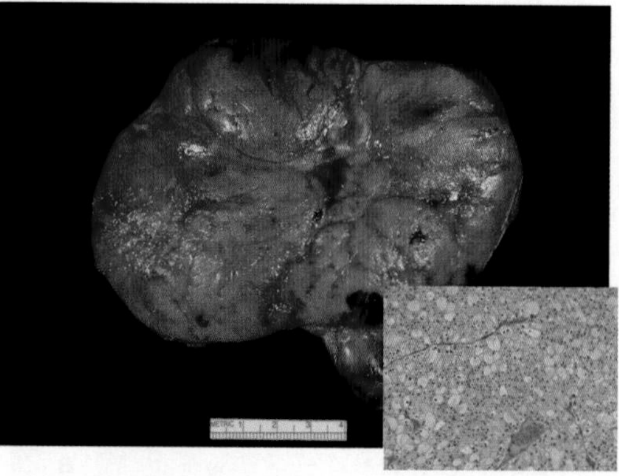

Fig. 23.5 Chromophobe RCC can be quite large, and the histologic appearance shows a classic "plant cell" appearance

wrinkled contours, often described as "raisinoid" or "koilocytotic" with condensed chromatin and inconspicuous nucleoli. Chromophobe RCC usually demonstrate reactivity with antibodies against pan keratins, CK7, CD117 and e-cadherin and are usually negative for CD10 and vimentin. The most common recurrent genetic abnormalities described in chromophobe RCC are losses of whole chromosomes 1, 2, 6, 10, 13, 17, and 21. Outcome for chromophobe RCC is similar to patients with papillary RCC. Features associated with outcome include stage, tumor necrosis, and presence of sarcomatoid component [10]. The ISUP recommends that tumors that share features of chromophobe and oncocytoma be designated as "hybrid" oncocytic chromophobe tumor and be classified as chromophobe RCC [3].

Collecting Duct Carcinoma

Collecting duct RCC (or carcinoma of the collecting ducts of Bellini) accounts for less than 1 % of RCCs [8]. There is a slight male predominance. The mean age at presentation is around 55 years with a wide age distribution ranging from the first to the ninth decades. Signs and symptoms leading to discovery are similar to those of other renal epithelial malignancies. Collecting duct carcinoma has been associated with renal allografts.

Collecting duct RCC is medullary in origin, although this feature may be difficult to appreciate in large tumors. Collecting duct RCC tends to be poorly circumscribed with ill-defined borders and infiltration into the adjacent tissue. Therefore, the gross appearance can at times give the impression that it is arising from the cortex or the renal pelvis. The cut surface is firm and white to tan in color with areas of necrosis often present. Collecting duct RCC is high grade and characterized by a combination of tubules, angulated glands, tubulopapillary structures, and solid growth. There is often a marked desmoplastic and inflammatory (neutrophilic) response associated with infiltrative growth. Immunohistochemical analysis shows collecting-duct RCC to be variably reactive with antibodies against high molecular weight keratins, CK7, and CD117, and to typically lack reactivity with antibodies against CD10, RCC antigen, and p504S. Some collecting duct RCCs may show loss of SWI/SNF-Related, Matrix-Associated, Actin-Dependent Regulator of Chromatin, Subfamily B, Member 1 (SMARCB1) staining suggesting a role of the *SMARCB1/INI-1* gene in the development of some of these tumors [16]. Separation from urothelial carcinoma can be difficult. Collecting duct carcinoma is an aggressive malignancy that often is quite advanced at the time of presentation. Regional lymph node metastases are seen in around half of patients and distant metastases in approximately a third of patients at diagnosis. Cancer-specific survival is poor.

Renal Medullary Carcinoma

Renal medullary carcinoma is a rare renal epithelial malignancy that occurs almost exclusively in patients with sickle cell trait or sickle cell disease [17]). The Heidelberg and Rochester Classification systems classified this tumor a variant of collecting duct carcinoma. Due to the association with sickle cell disease, renal medullary carcinoma is overwhelmingly seen in patients with some degree of African or Middle Eastern ancestry. Rare cases have been reported in Caucasian patients. Patients also tend to be younger with the mean age at the time of presentation around 25 years, although there is a wide age distribution (5–70 years). There is a marked male predominance with a male to female ratio of approximately 2:1 in patients younger than ten and approximately 5:1 in older patients. Patients present with symptoms that overlap with symptoms associated with sickle cell disease such as hematuria, pain or abdominal discomfort, and dysuria.

Most renal medullary carcinomas are solitary lesions that arise in the medullary region of the kidney. Tumors are infiltrative and frequently exhibit necrosis and hemorrhage. Microscopically, renal medullary carcinoma shows areas of solid growth, anastomosing angulated tubules and cords, and microcysts producing a reticular or cribriform growth pattern associated with a marked desmoplastic stromal response and inflammatory reaction. Tumor cells have eosinophilic cytoplasm and show high grade nuclear features. Erythrocytes within the tumor and adjacent kidney often show sickling. Tumors tend to be diffusely immunoreactive with antibodies against pan keratin and vimentin with moderate reactivity with antibodies against CK7 and some weak reactivity to high molecular weight keratin. Recent studies have identified frequent loss of nuclear staining for INI1 as well as deletion of the *INI1* tumor suppressor gene in a subset of tumors. Examples of renal medullary carcinoma harboring chromosomal rearrangement involving the anaplastic lymphoma kinase (ALK) locus at 2p23 have been reported. Renal medullary carcinoma is associated with a poor prognosis with 95 % of patients demonstrating metastatic disease at the time of presentation. Mean survival from the time of presentation is approximately 19 weeks.

Renal Cell Carcinoma, Unclassified Type

RCC, unclassified type, is not a unique variant of RCC but encompasses a heterogeneous group of tumors that do not fit into one of the currently described RCC types. This group also includes sarcomatoid RCC where an underlying subtype cannot be identified. These tumors are usually high grade with poorer outcome, but similar to other RCC types, this is dependent on grade and stage [18]. RCC, unclassified type, accounts for less than 5 % of RCC.

Mucinous Tubular and Spindle Cell Carcinoma

Mucinous tubular and spindle cell carcinoma (MTSC) was first described in 1997 as low-grade collecting duct carcinoma. Subsequently, it was also reported under various other names until it was identified as a unique entity in the 2004 World Health Organization classification and renamed mucinous tubular and spindle cell carcinoma [8, 19, 20]. This tumor is uncommon with a distinct female predominance and wide age range. Occasionally, MTSC presents with hematuria or pain, but often is identified incidentally.

Grossly, MTSC is usually well circumscribed, cortically, or centrally based. The cut surface is smooth and white or tan in color; necrosis and hemorrhage are rare. These tumors are generally small ranging from 2 to 4 cm. Histologically, the MTSC has a distinct appearance consisting of long straight or curved branching tubules lined by a single layer of cuboidal epithelial cells with minimal cytoplasm and small uniform nuclei with inconspicuous nucleoli. The tubules are often separated by intervening stroma that contains areas of spindle cell growth and basophilic extracellular mucin. The overall composition with regard to proportion of tubular and spindle cell growth and quantity of extracellular mucin can vary and cause some heterogeneity in histologic appearance. Mucinous tubular and spindle cell carcinoma has low-grade nuclear features although cases showing high-grade features including sarcomatoid change and necrosis have been reported. Immunohistochemical studies have shown a large proportion of MTSC to express CK7 and AMACR and to lack expression of CD10 and RCC. Genetic studies have demonstrated the losses of chromosomes 1, 4, 6, 8, 9, 13, 14, 15, and 22 to be recurrent abnormalities in MTSC. Despite the morphologic similarities between these tumors and papillary RCC, trisomy of chromosomes 7 and 17, abnormalities typically observed in papillary RCC, are not a recurrent finding in MTSC. These tumors generally behave in an indolent manner. However, metastatic cases have been reported.

Tubulocystic Carcinoma

Tubulocystic carcinoma was initially considered a low-grade collecting duct carcinoma, but in 2009, these were reported as a distinct RCC type. Tubulocystic carcinoma has been reported in patients with a wide age distribution (34–94 years of age) and shows a male predominance with a male to female ratio of 7:1 [21].

Tubulocystic carcinomas are typically solitary unencapsulated but well-circumscribed tumors with a median size of 4.0 cm, ranging from 0.5 to 17 cm. The cut surface is tan with a multicystic or spongy appearance. Tubulocystic carcinoma shows a distinct morphology consisting of tubules and cystic structures with intervening fibrous septae. The stroma within the septae has a low degree of cellularity. Spaces are lined by a single layer of cuboidal cells with eosinophilic cytoplasm. Nuclei are typically large which can give the epithelium a hobnail appearance. Nucleoli are usually prominent. By immunohistochemistry, tubulocystic carcinoma typically shows reactivity with antibodies against low molecular weight keratins, CD10, CK7, and AMACR.

Genetic studies have identified trisomy of chromosomes 7 and 17 to be a recurrent abnormality. Interestingly, some examples of tubulocystic carcinoma are found in association with classic papillary RCC. Considering this finding in the context of the genetic, immunophenotypic and morphologic features, tubulocystic carcinoma likely represents a group of PRCC with a particular growth pattern. This tumor has an indolent behavior and nearly all patients are cured by excision; however, metastases have been reported.

MiTF Family Translocation RCC

Translocation-associated RCCs are the recently identified subtypes of RCC that are defined by recurrent chromosomal rearrangements and encompass Xp11 and t(6:11) RCC. These tumors represent the majority of RCC identified in children and young adults, and account for 1–4% of tumors in adults with patients reported in their 70s [22, 23]. There is a distinct female predominance with male to female ratio of 3:1. Translocations that define this tumor result in rearrangement of *TFEB* and *TFE3*, members of the micropthalmia transcription factor (MiTF) subfamily of genes, resulting in fusion with another gene partner. Chromosomal rearrangements involving the *TFE3* gene at chromosome Xp11.2 comprise greater than 90% of translocation-associated RCC. *TFE3* is typically fused with *ASPSCR1* at 17q25 or *PRCC* at 1q21; however, numerous other pairing partners have been identified. The remaining tumors exhibit rearrangements involving the *TFEB* locus at chromosome 6p21 and various partner genes. The gross appearance of translocation-associated RCC is often similar to that of clear cell RCC, a well-circumscribed, soft yellow-brown mass with degenerative changes. The microscopic appearance of the tumors can be quite variable and dependent on whether the lesion is associated with a *TFE3* or *TFEB* rearrangement. The typical example of *TFE3* translocation-associated RCC shows a papillary architecture populated by cells with abundant clear to eosinophilic cytoplasm and large round nuclei with prominent nucleoli. However, some tumors may have a predominantly solid or nested growth pattern, and may be comprised solely of cells with granular eosinophilic cytoplasm or clear cytoplasm. Psammoma bodies, hemorrhage, hemosiderin deposition and hyaline deposits are common. Nuclei are generally large and round with prominent nucleoli.

The original reports of *TFEB* translocation-associated RCC described a biphasic pattern consisting of large epithelioid cells with eosinophilic cytoplasm associated with smaller epithelial cells centered round hyaline material. However, as more cases accumulated, it was evident that the morphology is variable with tumors showing a spectrum of papillary and solid growth and cells with clear to eosinophilic cytoplasm. The defining feature is the presence of chromosomal rearrangements involving either the *TFE3* or *TFEB* gene. Rearrangements can be detected by conventional cytogenetic, fluorescence in situ hybridization, or polymerase chain reaction (PCR)-based assays. Identification can also be made by immunohistochemistry to detect nuclear expression of either TFE3 or TFEB protein. *TFE3* rearrangement-associated RCCs generally show reactivity using antibodies against CD10, P504S, variable reactivity with CK7 and negativity for EMA, whereas *TFEB* rearrangement-associated RCCs show reactivity with antibodies against HMB45 and Melan-A which is less commonly seen in tumors with rearranged *TFE3*. Original reports of *TFE3* rearrangement-associated RCC in children suggested an indolent clinical course. However, recent studies of adult patients suggest that these tumors can be aggressive. The number of cases of *TFEB* rearrangement-associated RCC is thus far too small to clarify clinical behavior.

Thyroid-Like Follicular Renal Cell Carcinoma

Thyroid-like follicular renal carcinoma is a rare and recently described entity characterized by a distinct morphologic appearance closely resembling follicular carcinoma of the thyroid. This is a provisional ISUP subtype of RCC. To date, 13 cases have been reported in the literature. A slightly greater number of cases have been described in women than in men with a wide age distribution (29–83 years) [24].

Thyroid-like follicular RCC is typically small (2–4 cm) but larger tumors up to 12 cm have been described. The tumors are comprised of tightly packed, variably sized follicles, most of which are filled with colloid-like material. Areas of papillary growth are not present. The cells lining the follicles are generally cuboidal with a moderate or scant amount of cytoplasm. Nucleoli are inconspicuous and mitotic activity rare. By immunohistochemical studies, these tumors have shown a great amount of variability; however, they are consistently negative for thyroid transcription factor 1 (TTF-1) and thyroglobulin excluding metastatic follicular carcinoma from the thyroid. Most reports indicate the tumor has an indolent behavior; however, regional lymph node and distant metastases are reported.

Oncocytoma (Fig. 23.6)

Oncocytoma is a benign tumor that represents approximately 5 % of all renal tumors [8]. Most are asymptomatic and discovered incidentally by imaging, although sometimes oncocytoma presents with flank pain or hematuria. Tumors vary widely in size (up to 15 cm), and are usually solitary but can be multiple, including cases of oncocytosis. Tumors are characteristically mahogany brown and nearly half have a central stellate scar. Some cases contain abundant blood that mimics hemangioma, microscopically correlating with extravasated red blood cells in dilated tubules. Oncocytomas are composed of cells arranged in oval nests as well as solid areas and variably sized tubules. Nests can be closely packed or separated by an intervening stroma that is often paucicellular, hyalinized, or edematous. The cells show an abundant eosinophilic cytoplasm and nuclei are round and regular with visible nucleoli. Discrete foci of cells with enlarged hyperchromatic smudged nuclei are common and believed to be degenerative. Tumors can extend into perinephric fat in up to 15 % of cases but are not associated with a stromal response. Features that are distinctly unusual in oncocytoma and should raise the possibility of RCC include mitotic activity, coagulative tumor necrosis, and vascular invasion. By immunohistochemistry, oncocytomas are CD117 and e-cadherin positive, and negative for CD10, vimentin, and P504S. They are also negative to focally positive for CK7. Some tumors may show nonspecific diffuse granular staining for antibodies not typically positive in oncocytoma. Oncocytoma demonstrates several recurrent genetic abnormalities including loss of the *p*-arm or entire chromosome 1, loss of the Y chromosome in men and rearrangements of the *CCND1* locus at 11q13.

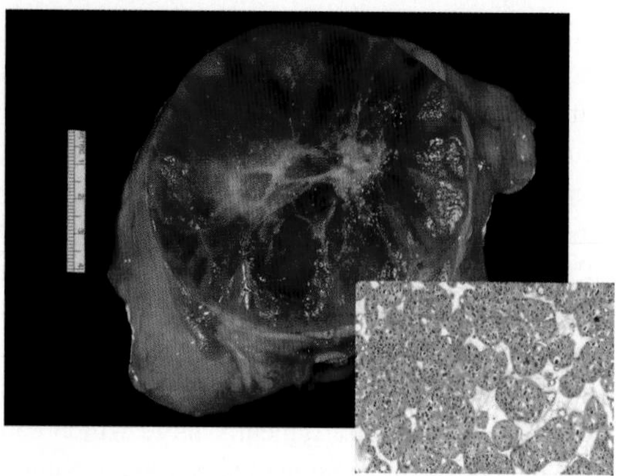

Fig. 23.6 The classic appearance of oncocytoma includes mahogany brown color and central scar. The gross appearance can be very helpful in separating from other tumors. The oval nest pattern is also characteristic

Papillary Adenoma

Papillary adenoma is an incidental finding, identified in resection specimens for RCC where they are frequently associated with papillary RCC. They are also common in kidneys removed for other reasons such as end-stage renal disease. Papillary adenomas are papillary neoplasms that are low grade (ISUP grade 1 and 2), and 0.5 cm or less in greatest dimension. They share cytogenetic and immunohistochemical features with type 1 papillary RCC but exhibit fewer cytogenetic abnormalities.

Metanephric Adenoma

Metanephric adenoma (MA) is a benign neoplasm accounting for approximately 0.5% of all renal tumors (Fig. 23.7) [8, 25]. Most are incidental findings, but rarely they can produce abdominal pain, hypertension, erythrocytosis, or hematuria. There is a female predominance with a wide age distribution (from children to the elderly) with a mean age in the fifth decade. In the largest series of cases, median tumor size was 5.5 cm, and the largest was 15 cm. Metanephric adenoma is variably encapsulated, has a tan-yellow appearance, and may be calcified. Cystic areas and hemorrhage may be present. Microscopically, the tumor is composed of small tight tubules, glomeruloid structures, and small papillary and polypoid structures with a variably edematous acellular stroma. Microcystic patterns have been described. The cells have very scant cytoplasm, and overlapping small lymphocyte-sized nuclei with smooth chromatin. Related tumors include metanephric adenofibroma and metanephric stromal tumor. The differential diagnosis for MA includes type 1 PRCC (with glomeruloid growth pattern) and epithelial Wilms tumor. PRCC tends to have large nonoverlapping nuclei with more abundant cytoplasm and larger nucleoli. Foamy macrophages are also more common, and PRCC lacks the edematous polypoid papillae of MA. In regard to epithelial Wilms tumor, the MA has smaller nucleoli and lacks the mitotic activity of Wilms tumor. Immunohistochemical stains can be helpful as MA is positive for WT1 and negative for CK7, EMA, and AMACR in contrast to papillary RCC. Metanephric adenoma has a disomy of chromosome 7 and 17. Recently, V-RAF Murine Sarcoma Viral Oncogene Homolog B1 (BRAF) mutations have been identified in the majority of MA. Although there are reports with MA with regional lymph node involvement, we agree with others that this is likely the result of displacement of benign tumor cells into the regional nodes, and not indicative of metastases.

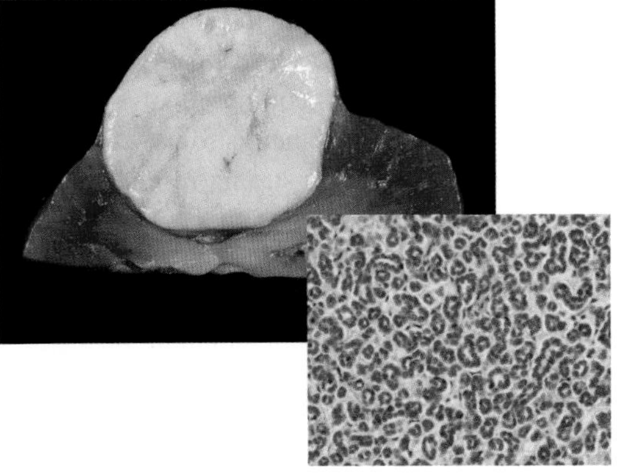

Fig. 23.7 Metanephric adenoma with solid tan yellow appearance and discrete tubules with small cells

Angiomyolipoma

Angiomyolipoma (AML) is a benign mesenchymal neoplasm of the kidney that constitutes up to 2% of renal neoplasms and can be sporadic or a manifestation of the tuberous sclerosis complex. While 80% of patients with germ line alterations of the tuberous sclerosis-related genes *TSC1* at chromosome 9q34 and *TSC2* at chromosome 16p13.3 will develop AML, the majority of patients with AML will not have a germ line abnormality in either gene. These tumors are believed to arise from the perivascular epithelioid cells (PEC) and are considered to be related to other PEC-associated tumors such as PEComas, lymphangioleiomyomatosis, clear cell sugar tumor of the lung, and cardiac rhabdomyoma. Most AMLs are discovered incidentally or as part of a workup for tuberous sclerosis. There is a female predominance, and the age at presentation differs depending on whether the lesion is sporadic or related to tuberous sclerosis, with tuberous sclerosis patients presenting a younger age. Most AMLs arise in the renal parenchyma but can arise in association with the renal capsule. Size can vary greatly. Most sporadic lesions are solitary, while lesions associated with tuberous sclerosis are multiple.

Grossly, AML can be variable in appearance depending on composition, with tumors of high adipose tissue content being yellow, while those with more smooth muscle content being white to tan in color. Hemorrhage is not uncommon. Microscopically, AML is composed of variable quantities of smooth muscle, blood vessels, and adipose tissue. The adipose tissue is mature in appearance and may show fat necrosis. The blood vessels are generally thick walled and have a population of vesicular smooth muscle cells that appear to originate from and radiate away from the vessel. Away from vessels, the smooth muscle forms large fascicles coursing between islands of adipose tissue and vessels. Smooth muscle cells may show some degree of nuclear atypia and mitotic activity. Some tumors may contain epithelial-lined cysts. The tumor is positive for actin and desmin in the smooth muscle component, and the melanocytic markers, melan-A and HMB45, are positive. Cytokeratin is negative. It may be present in draining lymph nodes, a finding that should not be considered metastatic tumor.

Epithelioid Angiomyolipoma

Epithelioid AML (EAML) is a rare morphologically and clinically distinct subset of AML [26]. Like AMLs, EAML are associated with tuberous sclerosis but can be sporadic. In patients with tuberous sclerosis, EAML represents a larger proportion of all AMLs relative to those found in patients without tuberous sclerosis, with EAML representing 25 versus 8% of AMLs in tuberous sclerosis and nontuberous sclerosis patients, respectively. As such, these tend to be more common in younger patients with a mean age at presentation of 38 years and are more likely to be associated with additional AMLs.

EAMLs are typically solid to partially cystic and well circumscribed with a hemorrhagic cut surface. Necrosis can be present. Microscopically, EAMLs are comprised predominantly of sheets or nests of tumor cells with abundant eosinophilic to slightly clear and granular cytoplasm. Nuclei are often large and pleomorphic with prominent nucleoli. Multinucleated cells are often present. The level of mitotic activity may be quite high. The tumors may show necrosis and infiltration into the perinephric tissues. Areas showing features of traditional AML may be present; however a definition of maximal amount of classic AML features allowable to classify a lesion as EAML has been a point of controversy. Although early studies suggested aggressive behavior in up to half of patients with EAML, a recent study on nonconsultative cases showed that malignant behavior was uncommon with metastases occurring in less than 10% of patients [27].

Renal Epithelial Stromal Tumors

The group of renal tumors classified as mixed epithelial stromal tumor (MEST) and cystic nephroma (CN) are cystic tumors with significant histologic and clinical similarity that have recently been the source of some controversy regarding classification [28]. Cystic nephroma was defined in 1998, while MEST was first reported in 1973 as an adult congenital mesoblastic nephroma. Both tumors occur primarily in middle-aged women, and are composed of cysts with MEST showing a prominent stromal component in contrast to CN. This stroma resembles ovarian stroma and is positive for estrogen receptor, particularly the pericystic stromal component. It now seems likely that these two entities represent two extreme ends along a continuum of features for a single entity categorized under the unifying term renal epithelial and stromal tumor (REST). Most cases of REST are clinically and histologically benign. However, several examples of malignant REST have been reported, and malignant transformation has been reported arising from both the mesenchymal and epithelial components.

References

1. Kovacs G, Akhtar M, Beckwith JB, et al. The Heidelberg classification of renal cell carcinoma. J Pathol. 1997;183:131–3.
2. Storkel S, Eble JN, Adlakha K, et al. Classification of renal cell carcinoma workgroup No. 1 Union Internationale Contre Cancer (UICC) and American Joint Committee on Cancer (AJCC). Cancer. 1997;80:987–9.
3. Srigley JR, Delahunt B, Eble JN, et al. The International Society of Urological Pathology (ISUP) vancouver classification of renal neoplasia. Am J Surg Pathol. 2013;37:1469–89.
4. Skinner DG, Colvin RB, Vermillion CD, et al. Diagnosis and management of renal cell carcinoma: a clinical and pathologic study of 309 cases. Cancer. 1981;28:1165–77.
5. Fuhrman AS, Lasky LC, Limas C, et al. Prognostic significance in morphologic parameters in renal cell carcinoma. Am J Surg Pathol. 1982;6:656–63.
6. Delahunt B, Chevill JC, Martignoni G, et al. The International Society of Urological Pathology (ISUP) grading system for renal cell carcinoma and other prognostic parameters. Am J Surg Pathol. 2013;37:1490–1504.
7. Delahunt B, McKenney JK, Lohse CM, et al. A novel grading system for clear cell renal cell carcinoma incorporating tumor necrosis. Am J Surg Pathol. 2013;37:311–22.
8. Tumors of the kidney. In: Eble JN, Sauter G, Epstein JI, Sesterhenn IA, editors. Pathology and genetics. Tumors of the urinary system and male genital organs. Lyon: IARC Press; 2004. pp. 9–87.
9. Al-Ahmadie HA, Alden D, Fine SW, et al. Role of immunohistochemistry in adult renal tumors: an ex vivo study. Am J Surg Pathol. 2011;35:949–61.
10. Cheville JC, Lohse CM, Zincke H, et al. Comparison of outcomes and prognostic features among the histological subtypes of renal cell carcinoma. Am J Surg Pathol. 2003;27:612–24.
11. Lohse CM, Cheville JC. A review of prognostic pathologic features and algorithms for patients treated surgically for renal cell carcinoma. Clin Lab Med. 2005;25:433–64.
12. Leibovich BC, Lohse CM, Crispen PL, et al. Histological subtype is an independent predictor of outcome for patients with renal cell carcinoma. J Urol. 2010;183:1309–15.
13. Delahunt B, Eble JN. Papillary renal cell carcinoma: a clinicopathologic and immunohistochemical study of 105 cases. Mod Pathol. 1997;10:537–44.
14. Sukov WR, Lohse CM, Leibovich BC, et al. Clinical and pathological features associated with prognosis in patients with papillary renal cell carcinoma. J Urol. 2011;187:54–9.
15. Williamson SR, Eble JN, Cheng L, Grignon DJ. Clear cell papillary renal cell carcinoma: differential diagnosis and extended immunohistochemical profile. Mod Pathol. 2013;26:697–708.
16. Elwood H, Chaux A, Schultz L, et al. Immunohistochemical analysis of SMARCB1/INI-1 expression in collecting duct carcinoma. Urology. 2011;78(474):e1–5.
17. Davis CJ, Mostofi FK, Sesterhenn IA. Renal medullary carcinoma: the seventh sickle syndrome. Am J Surg Pathol. 1995;19:1–11.
18. Crispen PL, Tabidian MR, Almer C, et al. Unclassified renal cell carcinoma: impact on survival following nephrectomy. Urology. 2010;76:580–6.
19. Fine SW, Argani P, DeMarzo A, et al. Expanding the histologic spectrum of mucinous tubular and spindle cell carcinoma of the kidney. Am J Surg Pathol. 2006;30:1154–60.
20. Rakozy C, Schmahl GE, Bogner S, Storkel S. Low-grade tubular-mucinous renal neoplasms: morphologic, immunohistochemical and genetic features. Mod Pathol. 2002;15:1162–71.
21. Amin BM, MacLennan GT, Gupta R, et al. Tubulocystic carcinoma of the kidney. Clinicopathologic analysis of 31 cases of a distinctive rare subtype of renal cell carcinoma. Am J Surg Pathol. 2009;33:384–92.
22. Ellis CL, Elbe JN, Subhawong AP, et al. Clinical heterogeneity of Xp11 translocation renal cell carcinoma: impact of fusion subtype, age and stage. Mod Pathol. 2014;27(6):875–86.
23. Argani P, Olgac S, Tickoo SK, et al. Xp11 translocation renal cell carcinoma in adults: expanded clinical, pathologic and genetic spectrum. Am J Surg Pathol. 2007;31:1149–60.
24. Amin MB, Gupta R, Ondrej H, et al. Primary thyroid-like follicular carcinoma of the kidney: report of 6 cases of a histologically distinctive adult renal epithelial neoplasm. Am J Surg Pathol. 2009;33:393–400.
25. Davis CJ Jr., Barton JH, Sesterhenn IA, et al. Metanephric adenoma. Clinico-pathologic study of fifty patients. Am J Surg Pathol. 1995;19:1101–14.
26. Eble JN, Amin MB, Young RH. Epithelioid angiomyolipoma of the kidney: a report of five cases with a prominent and diagnostically confusing epithelioid smooth muscle component. Am J Surg Pathol. 1997;21:1123–30.
27. He W, Cheville JC, Sadow PM, et al. Epithelioid angiomyolipoma of the kidney: pathologic features and clinical outcome in a series of consecutively resected tumors. Mod Pathol. 2013;26:1355–64.
28. Turbiner J, Amin MB, Humphrey PA, et al. Cystic nephroma and mixed epithelial and stromal tumor of the kidney: a detailed clinico-pathologic analysis of 34 cases and proposal for renal epithelial and stromal tumor (REST) as a unifying term. Am J Surg Pathol. 2007;31:489–500.

Tumor Staging for Renal Pathology

24

Stephen M. Bonsib

Abbreviations

RCC	Renal cell carcinoma
TNM	Tumor nodes metastasis
ISUP	International Society of Urological Pathologists
SEER	Surveillance epidemiology and end results
NCDB	National cancer data base
RVI	Retrograde venous invasion
LND	Lymph node dissection

Introduction

It has been almost 100 years since Albert Broders, MD, and Cuthbert Dukes, MD, introduced the concepts of tumor grading and anatomic extent of disease (stage) in the prognostication of cancer [1]. These seminal concepts have withstood the test of time for tumors of diverse organ systems. With respect to renal cell carcinoma (RCC) an additional powerful prognosticator is tumor type exemplified by the extremely favorable outcome for chromophobe cell RCC that contrasts with extremely aggressive forms of RCC such as collecting duct carcinoma and sarcomatoid forms of RCC. A number of additional prognostic anatomic and clinical features are emerging such as tumor necrosis, clinical presentation, and performance status whose prognostic merit is further enhanced when coupled with grade and stage in the form of nomograms [2]. However, for the pathologist, our first and foremost responsibility in handling a tumor nephrectomy is to establish an accurate pathologic stage.

Historical Review of Staging Systems

Establishing the anatomic extent of disease is critically important in cancer treatment. As commented by Greene and Sobin "Staging provides a format for the uniform exchange of information among clinicians regarding the extent of disease, and a basis for their selection of initial therapeutic approaches and consideration of the possible need for adjuvant treatment" [3]. There have been multiple staging systems proposed for RCC over the past 55 years. Each system has had four pathologic stages that recapitulate a common three-tiered theme that encompasses renal-limited, local extension, and distant spread categories. In the hands of most investigators each has demonstrated prognostic utility.

The first staging system for RCC was formulated by Flocks and Kadesky in 1958 (Table 24.1) [4]. Their classification system consisted of one category for renal-limited disease, two categories for local spread (perinephric fat and/or veins, or lymph nodes), and one category for distant metastases. Although their publication was more about treatment than stage, the concept that a

S. M. Bonsib (✉)
Nephropath, 10810 Executive Center Drive, Suite 100, Little Rock, AR 72211, USA
e-mail: stephen.bonsib@nephropath.com

C. Magi-Galluzzi, C. G. Przybycin (eds.), *Genitourinary Pathology,* DOI 10.1007/978-1-4939-2044-0_24,

Table 24.1 The first staging systems for renal cell carcinoma

Stage	Flocks and Kadesky—1958		Petkovic—1959		Robson—1969	
		5-year survival (%)		5-year survival (%)		5-year survival (%)
1	Limited to renal capsule	55	Renal limited and encapsulated	75	Renal limited	66
2	Renal pedicle ± fat invasion	40.5	Renal limited with capsular invasion	55	Perirenal fat but within Gerota's fascia	64
3	Regional lymph nodes	9.5	Extrarenal into fat, veins, lymphatics	4	3a. Gross renal vein or inferior Vena Cava (VC)	
					3b. Lymphatics	
					3c. Veins and lymphatics	42
4	Distant metastasis	3.5	Distant metastasis	6	4a adjacent organs	11
					4b distant metastasis	

stage allows outcome stratification in RCC was launched.

The second staging system was formulated by Petkovic a year later (Table 24.1) [5]. Curiously, he did not cite the Flocks and Kadesky paper even though they were both published in The Journal of Urology. In contrast to Flocks and Kadesky's staging system, Petkovic's staging system had two renal-limited categories, one category for local spread and one for distant metastases. Petkovic provided drawings to illustrate his tumor stages. Use of such visual aids is helpful to pathologist and surgeon alike, a practice currently followed by TNM staging. Petkovic commented that tumor growth characteristics are more important than tumor size, and noted that even patients with apparently renal-limited tumors may have metastases, a vexing problem with all staging systems.

The third staging system was formulated by Robson in 1969 (Table 24.1) [6]. The Robson's system was similar to Flocks and Kadesky having a single renal-limited stage and two stage designations for local extension. Robson emphasized the additional prognostic factor of tumor grade in addition to stage. This system was popular well into the 1980s despite the existence of the TNM staging system for more than a decade, possibly because the Robson system was featured in the first Armed Forces Institute of Pathology (AFIP) fascicle.

The Tumor-Node-Metastasis (TNM) Classification

The fourth and internationally utilized staging system is the Tumor-Node-Metastasis (TNM) Classification of Malignant Tumors. The TNM system was developed between 1943 and 1952 by Pierre Denoix, a French surgeon [3]. The International Union Against Cancer (UICC) published ten manuals between 1956 and 1967 that incorporated his TNM staging recommendations for tumors of two dozen body sites. In 1968, these were collated into the first edition of the TNM Classification. Kidney was one organ, however, that was not included in this initial formulation. It did appear in the second edition published in 1974. The initial inclusion of kidney almost seems like an afterthought based upon the definitions of the pT1 and pT2 categories in both the 1974 TNM and the 1978 TNM editions which were listed as "small" and "large" [7]. In 1959, the American Joint Commission on Cancer (AJCC) was founded. Since the 1980s, the UICC and AJCC have worked together and simultaneously published the TNM Classification of Malignant Tumors by the UICC, and the Cancer Staging Manual by the AJCC. The revision cycle is 6–8 years. From 1968 to 2009, seven iterations of the TNM Classification have appeared; an eighth iteration can be expected soon [3, 7–9].

The TNM system classifies extent of disease based on anatomic information about the primary tumor (pT stage), regional lymph nodes (pN stage) and metastases (pM stage) [3, 9]. These are combined into four stage groups. These can be purely clinical groupings, pathological groupings, or a combination of data may be employed. The latter is common in RCC since regional lymph node dissections are infrequently performed. The complete 2009 TNM pT, pN, and pM stage definitions and the stage groupings are provided at the end of this chapter.

Tables 24.2 and 24.3 list the staging parameters for most of the TNM formulations so that the evolution of TNM for RCC can be appreciated. The recurrent themes of tumor size stratification, the definitions of local extension, and the optimum handling of vena cava (VC) invasion represent the ongoing attempts to optimize stage prognostication, struggles inherent to the evolutionary process that characterizes TNM staging. The evolution of stage definition is important to keep in mind when comparing stage-related outcome data over time because a change in stage

Table 24.2 Evolving definition of the TNM renal cell carcinoma staging system

UICC/ AJCC	pT1		pT2	
1968 TNM excluded the kidney				
1978	Small, without enlargement of kidney, limited distortion pelvis, calyces or vessels		Large, with enlargement of kidney, or pelvi-calyceal involvement	
1987	<2.5 cm renal limited		>2.5 cm renal limited	
1997	<7.0 cm renal limited		>7.0 cm renal limited	
	pT1a	pT1b	pT2	
2002	4 cm or less renal limited	>4–7.0 cm renal limited	>7.0 cm renal limited	
			pT2a	pT2b
2009	4 cm or less renal limited	>4.7.0 cm renal limited	>7–10 cm renal limited	>10 cm renal limited

UICC International Union Against Cancer, *AJCC* American Joint Commission on Cancer, *TNM* tumor nodes metastasis

Table 24.3 Evolving definition of the TNM renal cell carcinoma staging system

UICC/ AJCC	pT3			pT4	
1968 excluded kidney					
1978	Involvement of perinephric fat or hilar vessels			Involvement of neighboring organs or abdominal wall	
	pT3a	pT3b	pT3c	pT4a	pT4b
1987	Perinephric fat or adrenal	RV involvement	VC below diaphragm	Beyond Gerota's fascia	VC above diaphragm
				pT4	
1997	Perinephric fat or adrenal	RV or IVC below diaphragm	VC above diaphragm	Beyond Gerota's fascia	
2002	Perinephric fat includes sinus fat or adrenal	RV includes muscular sinus veins or VC below diaphragm	VC above diaphragm	Beyond Gerota's fascia	
2009	Gross involvement of RV or segmental muscle containing branches, perinephric and/or sinus fat	Gross extension into VC below diaphragm	Gross extension into VC above diaphragm or invades VC wall	Beyond Gerota's fascia, or contiguous extension into adrenal gland	

UICC International Union Against Cancer, *AJCC* American Joint Commission on Cancer, *RV* renal vein, *VC* vena cava, *IVC* inferior vena cava

definition affects the tumor composition of the stage groupings. A notable example was the major change in tumor size criteria for pT1 versus pT2 between the 1987 TNM and 1997 TNM when the pT1/2 break point was shifted from 2.5 to 7 cm. This drastically increased the proportion of stage I tumors and reduced the proportion of stage II tumors.

Several notable modifications appeared in the 2002 and 2009 TNM formulations relating to the size and local extension Tables 24.2 and 24.3. Substages for the pT1 and pT2 categories were introduced in the 2002 and 2009 TNMs, respectively. However, possibly the most significant modification occurred in the 2002 TNM with incorporation of renal sinus invasion into the pT3 category [9]. This mandated a paradigm shift in specimen handling.

Additional important modifications in 2009 TNM recognized the importance of direct adrenal extension, and added VC wall invasion.

In 2012, the International Society of Urological Pathology (ISUP) convened a Consensus Conference at the US and Canadian Academy of Pathology annual meeting. Over 130 urologic pathologists from around the world participated. This was preceded by a comprehensive survey that included queries relating to specimen handling and TNM staging, and many other topics. The survey documented diagnostic criteria and practice behaviors while the Consensus Conference led to practice recommendations based upon achieving a 65% consensus threshold among participants [10]. Issues failing to achieve consensus provided topics for future investigation and possible subsequent incorporation into the next TNM formulation.

pT1 and pT2 Substages

The prognostic relationship between size and outcome has been known for almost a century. In 1937, ET Bell, MD, published a seminal study of 71 RCCs in which he found that only one of 38 tumors less than 3 cm developed metastases [11]. This subsequently led to the long-lived, but now defunct 3 cm rule, used to distinguish so-called adenomas from carcinomas. Recently, the Mayo Clinic Group examined a much larger number of patients and found an even lower incidence of metastases; only one of 781 patients with M1 disease had an RCC 3 cm or less [12].

Dr. Bell also found that with increasing tumor size the metastatic rate increased, findings repeatedly confirmed. Multiple large series of RCC have demonstrated that tumor size is an independent predictor of cancer-specific survival, risk of metastases at presentation, recurrence rates, and patient outcomes [7, 13–15]. However, for size to retain its prognostic importance size determination must not only be accurate but measurements must be made in a standard fashion.

The ISUP Consensus Conference recommends that size be determined following multiple parallel sections through the tumor [10]. The primary tumor measurement should include perinephric fat extension, both peripheral perinephric fat and central sinus fat. Satellite nodules, renal vein, and VC involvement, however, should not be included.

The introduction of the first size subgroup of renal-limited RCC involved pT1 tumors and appeared in 2002 TNM [8]. It divided pT1 into pT1a, defined as RCC 4 cm or less, and pT1b, defined as RCC >4–7 cm. This 4 cm cutoff was originally introduced to identify a group of tumors suitable for nephron sparing surgery, a procedure initially heavily weighted toward tumors 4 cm or less. However, this clinical relevance is diminishing since much larger tumors are now similarly treated. Although multiple large studies of RCC have noted a difference in patient outcomes with breakpoints in the 4–5.5 cm size range validating a pT1 subgrouping, Delahunt et al. suggest that size may actually represent a continuous variable [14]. They have shown a 3.51x risk of cancer-related death for each doubling in tumor size.

The second size subgroup introduced affected pT2 tumors and appeared in the 2009 TNM [9]. Its implementation was based primarily upon a study from the Mayo Clinic of 544 patients treated for RCC (77.7% clear cell type) [15]. They found a survival difference for tumors "renal limited" in the 7–10 cm versus "renal-limited" tumors > 10 cm. Stage pT2 tumors are now stratified in 2009 TNM into pT2a, defined as renal-limited tumors >7–10 cm, and pT2b, defined as renal-limited tumors >10 cm. More recently, however, Waalkes et al. in a validation study of 2009 TNM restaged 5122 patients with pT2 tumors and found no difference in cancer-specific survival for pT2a versus pT2b [16]. Novara et al. in a recent European multi-institutional validation study of 2009 TNM that included 5339 patients, found excellent stratification in 5- and 10-year cancer-specific survival for most stages [17]. However, both pT1a and pT1b, and pT2b and pT3a had similar Cancer specific survival (CSS) (Fig. 24.1). These data raise concern that substage definitions may be somewhat arbitrary and that large tumor size may be a surrogate marker for undetected extrarenal spread, espe-

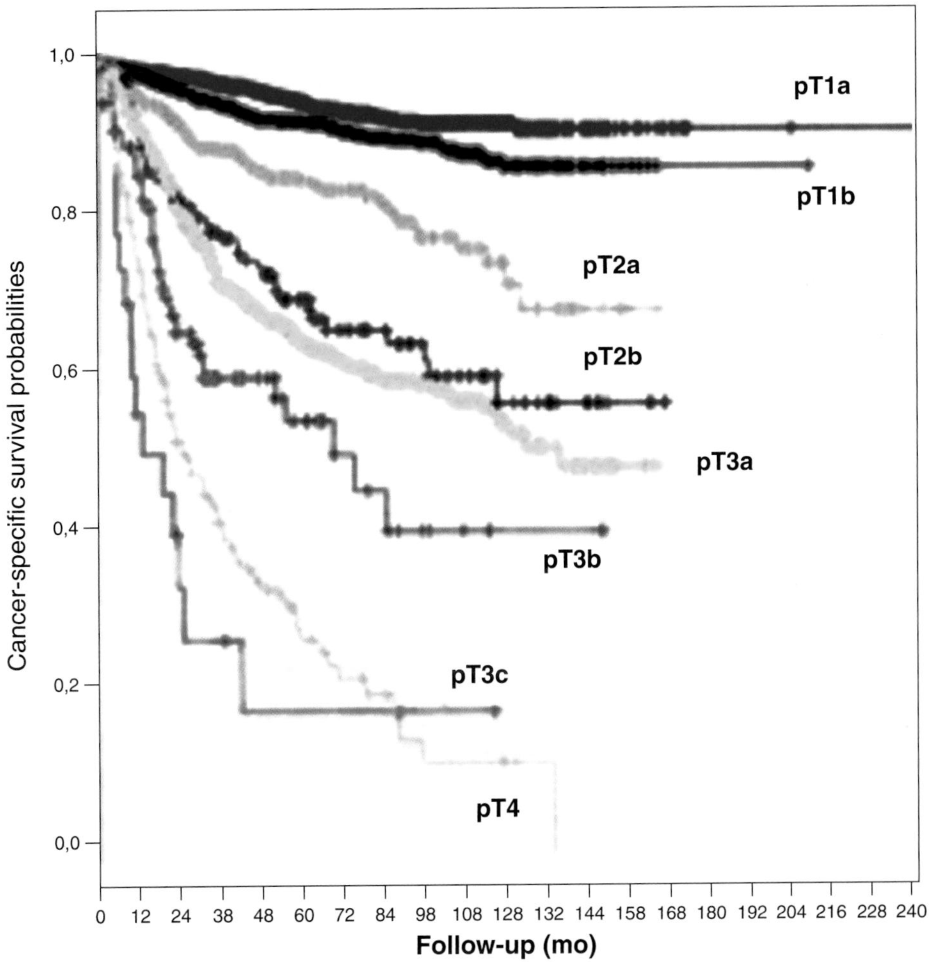

Fig. 24.1 Cancer-specific survival (CSS) probability according to the 2009 TNM staging system (log-rank pooled over strata $p<0.0001$). Five-year CSS was 94.9% in pT1a (*blue curve*), 92.6 in pT1b (*green curve*), 85.4% in pT2a (*gray curve*), 70% in pT2b (*violet curve*), 64.7% in pT3a (*yellow curve*), 54.7% in pT3b (*red curve*), and 27.1% in pT4 (*lightgray curve*). All the pairwise survival differences among the different pT stages were statistically significant with the exception of those observed between pT2b and pT3a cancers (log-rank pairwise $p=34$) and between pT3c and pT4 cancers (log-rank pairwise $p=26$). (Used with permission from [17])

cially invasion of the renal sinus. The 7 cm cut-off for pT2 tumors may have another unintended consequence, the selection of a more indolent subset of RCCs enriched for certain RCC types. Using the Surveillance Epidemiology and End Results (SEER) data, Rothman et al. found that 70% of pT2 tumors over 7 cm were not only low grade, they were overrepresented for the more indolent RCC types of papillary RCC and chromophobe cell RCC [18].

pT3a Regional Extension

Robson stated in 1969 "…the hope for a cure lies in the hands of the surgeon" [6]. However, the hope for accurate tumor prognostication lies in the hands of the pathologist. A lofty goal for a RCC staging system, and possibly the "holy grail" for a specimen examination protocol, is to stratify those cases in which a surgical cure can be expected from those cases with risk of residual disease. Renal-limited tumors, pT1 and pT2, represent the only stage categories in which a surgical cure is feasible. Regrettably, every staging system, from Flocks and Kadesky to the 2009 TNM, fall short of predicting surgical cures. The National Cancer Data Base (NCDB) indicates that for 37,166 tumors resected for years 2001 and 2002, there was an 81 and 74% observed survival (cancer deaths plus death due to other causes) for stage I and stage II RCC, respectively (Fig. 24.2) [9]. Many stage I and II patients whose deaths are attributable to metastatic disease had RCCs that were not renal limited at the time of nephrectomy.

In 1969, the National Wilms Tumor Study (NWTS) was initiated in the hope of identifying the optimal therapy for Wilms tumor. From the onset of the NWTS, there was standardized specimen handling and central review of the nephrectomy findings by Bruce Beckwith, MD. One of Dr. Beckwith's many contributions to the understanding of Wilms tumor and other pediatric renal neoplasms was the recognition that the renal sinus was the principal metastatic pathway

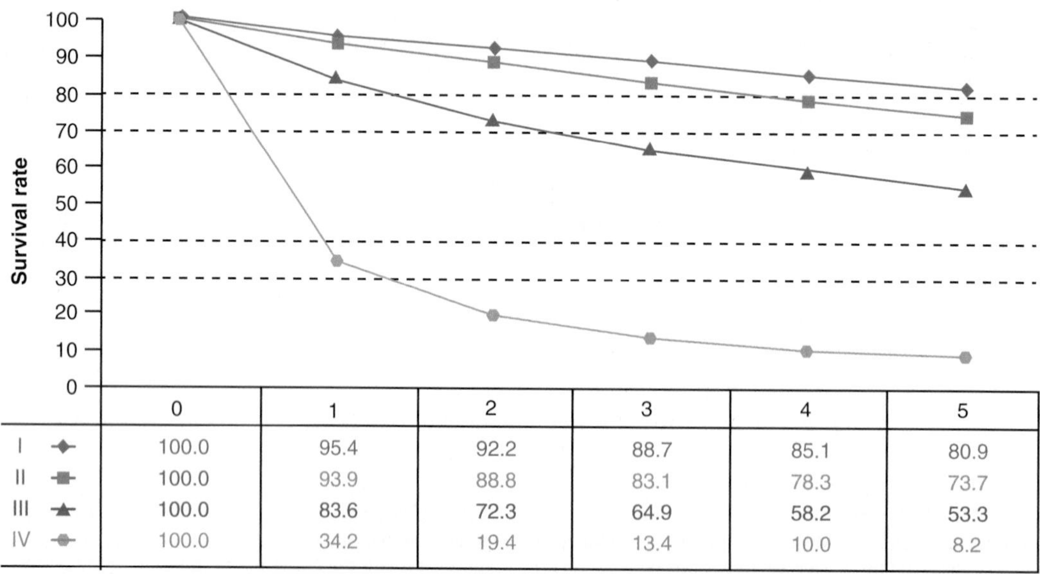

	0	1	2	3	4	5
I	100.0	95.4	92.2	88.7	85.1	80.9
II	100.0	93.9	88.8	83.1	78.3	73.7
III	100.0	83.6	72.3	64.9	58.2	53.3
IV	100.0	34.2	19.4	13.4	10.0	8.2

Fig. 24.2 Observed survival rates for 37,166 patients with kidney cancer classified by the 2009 AJCC staging classification. Data taken from the National Cancer Data Base (Commission on Cancer of the American College of Surgeons and the American Cancer Society) for the years 2001–2002. Stage I includes 18,912 patients; stage II 4443; stage III 5952; and stage IV 7859. (Used with permission from [9])

[19]. This seems now intuitive since the majority of the renal parenchymal venous and lymphatic outflow pass through the renal sinus as detailed in Chap. 22. Initially, the NWTS threshold for upstaging from renal-limited stage I to extrarenal stage II was extension of tumor beyond the "hilar plane." This was a difficult judgment to make for the primary prosector, and even more challenging to validate on central review. In the NWTS-5, the fifth clinical trial launched in 1995, involvement of sinus vessels or extensive sinus fat involvement qualified for stage 2 designation. At that time, a similar role of the renal sinus involvement in RCC had not been investigated.

In 1998, I initiated a study of renal sinus involvement in RCC by totally embedding the interface between the renal sinus and the RCC. The intent of the study was to determine if pT1 and pT2 tumors staged by the 1997 TNM were truly renal limited or if some tumors extended into the renal sinus which by definition is outside of the kidney. The results of a small series of 31 cases of RCC reported in 2000 found that 14 of 31 (45%) cases had invaded the renal sinus fat and/or sinus veins [20]. Most significantly, seven of 14 cases of stage pT1 and pT2 RCC by 1997 TNM criteria were not, in fact, renal limited. They had not only extended into the renal sinus but also into sinus veins.

In 2002, TNM renal sinus fat and renal sinus "muscular" vein involvement were incorporated into pT3a and pT3b, respectively [8]. Sinus invasive disease was further modified in 2009 TNM; "gross" involvement of renal vein or "segmental muscle containing" (sinus) branches were combined with sinus fat invasion into pT3a [9]. These modifications moved extrarenal sinus invasive disease included with renal-limited pT1 and pT2 categories prior to 2002, to the extrarenal pT3 category. This advance should improve stage-related prognostication. It should decrease the slope of the survival curves for stage I and stage II RCC, as illustrated in Fig. 24.2 by eliminating a group of extrarenal disease that contaminated stage groups I and II. It could also contribute to the stage migration that has occurred due to the increased incidence of small incidentally discovered pT1 tumors [21]. More accurate RCC staging relative to the renal sinus could also shift a number of RCCs from the pT2 category into the pT3 category, making pT2 RCC, and particularly pT2b, a less common tumor.

It is important to appreciate that most studies of outcome relative to stage have utilized large archival data bases that include many cases accessioned prior to 2002, often dating back to the 1970s. A significant percentage of the pT1 and pT2 tumors staged by 1997 TNM and earlier formulations and included in the NCDB and other data bases, may not have been renal limited. They are likely under-staged pT3 cases. These cases could account for a substantial fraction of the 15–20% metastatic disease that develops in stage I and II RCC. This is not a criticism of those studies, but simply a reflection that the renal sinus was not sampled since its importance had not yet been appreciated. Evidence in support of this contention was provided by Thompson et al. in 2007 [22]. They reexamined the nephrectomy specimens of 33 cases of stage I RCC by 1997 TNM criteria who died from metastatic RCC. They found that 67% of the RCCs had extended into the renal sinus fat or sinus veins, and were not, therefore, renal limited. They were under-staged pT3 tumors by 2002 and 2009 TNM criteria. Now that the renal sinus invasion has been part of the TNM staging system for over 10 years, outcomes studies should limit their cases to those accessioned after 2002 at the time when renal sinus examination was incorporated into their specimen handling protocol.

The author has personally dissected and histologically sampled the renal sinus–tumor interface of over 500 cases of RCCs. These cases have demonstrated that the renal sinus is the principal site of extrarenal extension for the most common RCC types, and documented the primacy of sinus vein invasion in extrarenal extension, especially for clear cell RCC [23–25]. Table 24.4 provides data on the first 400 cases of RCC examined for sinus involvement; several important points can be made.

It is uncommon for the three most common forms of RCC, clear cell, papillary and chromophobe, to be renal limited when the primary tumor is larger than 7 cm. This is particularly the

Table 24.4 Renal cell carcinomas examined

Tumor	pT1a	pT1b	pT2a	pT2b	pT3	Total
Clear cell	90 (35%)	27 (10%)	4 (1.5%)	2 (0.7%)	135 (52%)	258
Papillary	34 (46%)	20 (27%)	9 (12%)	3 (0.4%)	8 (24%)	74
Chromophobe	9 (39%)	5 (22%)	4 (17%)	1 (0.4%)	4 (17%)	23
Other cancers	16	5	3	1	20	45
Total	149 (37%)	57 (14%)	20 (5%)	7 (1.7%)	167 (42%)	400

case for clear cell RCC where only 2.2% of cases were renal-limited pT2a/b making this a very small stage category (Fig. 24.3). Although papillary RCC and chromophobe cell RCC larger than 7 cm are found to be renal limited more often, it was still relatively uncommon occurring in 12.4 and 17.4% of cases, respectively. As mentioned above, a recent study of size and renal-limited disease found that papillary and chromophobe cell carcinomas are heavily overrepresented in large renal-limited RCCs compared to clear cell [18]. Although the data are not shown in Table 24.4, it is uncommon for RCC to invade the renal capsule without also invading the renal sinus. This occurred in < 2% of 400 cases studied. Conversely, it is very common for RCC to solely demonstrate sinus involvement without capsular invasion. Therefore, although a careful search should be made for peripheral perinephric fat invasion, the renal sinus represents the principal metastatic pathway for RCC and must be the primary focus of gross examination and histologic sections to establish the correct pT stage.

The 2012 ISUP Consensus Conference opinion is that peripheral perinephric fat invasion is best identified grossly with the renal capsule intact and recommended that histological confirmation requires tumor to be in contact with fat, or demonstrate an irregular invasive interface with fat, with or without a desmoplastic response

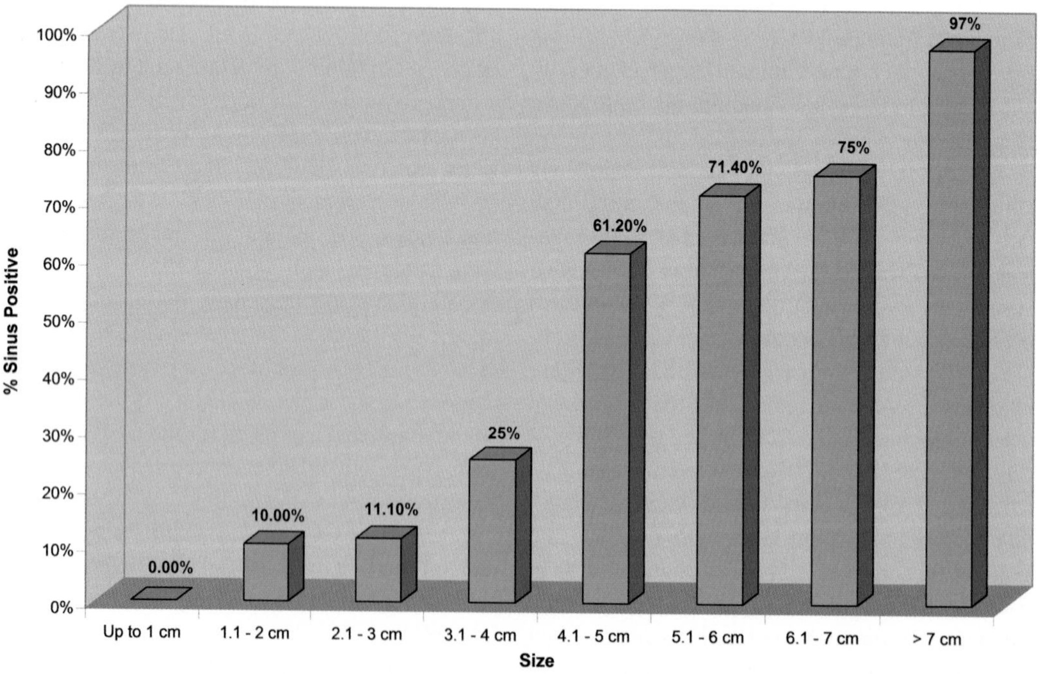

Fig. 24.3 This graph shows the relationship between size and extension into the renal sinus for 120 clear cell RCCs. Notice that the incidence of sinus involvement markedly increases for clear cell RCCs larger than 4 cm, and that only rare clear cell RCCs larger than 7 cm are renal limited

[10]. The number of blocks submitted must be determined by the gross findings and level of suspicion in the individual case. Gross recognition of renal vein invasion or invasion of segmental muscle containing branches within the renal sinus is also part of the current definition of pT3a. Although 78% of the ISUP participants responded that they or their prosectors were familiar with sinus anatomy, and 63% indicated confidence in gross recognition of sinus involvement, this leaves a substantial number of experts who may not be completely comfortable with gross evaluation of renal sinus invasion. If a learning curve is ongoing among experts, gross recognition of sinus invasion may be even less among those with less experience. This places great emphasis on histological assessment for sinus invasion. The ISUP participants agreed (100%) that tumor in contact with fat or tumor within the loose connective tissue outside of the renal parenchyma (75%) qualify for pT3a sinus invasion. Unless there is obvious gross involvement of the sinus, the ISUP recommendation is that at least three blocks of the tumor–sinus interface be submitted.

The 2009 TNM requires "gross" involvement of "muscle containing" veins of the renal sinus for pT3a designation. As demonstrated in Chap. 22, all large sinus veins have smooth muscle and therefore are "muscular veins," although there is often extreme variability in the quantity of muscle. As noted by Dr. Beckwith in Wilm Tumor (WT) and Bonsib in RCC, venous smooth muscle becomes attenuated as tumor expands the vein and tumor will often invade through the wall of sinus veins obliterating their muscularis [21, 23, 25]. The terminology "muscular veins" or "muscle containing" veins, therefore, should probably be eliminated from future TNM stage descriptions. The ISUP participants agreed (100%) that tumor in any endothelial-lined space regardless of size constitutes sinus vein invasion. However, failure to recognize RCC in the sinus as intravenous will not change the stage designation since both fat and vein involvement are designated pT3a.

Main renal vein involvement is usually obvious upon gross examination of the specimen as a large cylindrical protrusion from the hilar region. Although not a staging parameter, uncertainty exists on what constitutes a positive renal vein surgical resection margin since tumor can bulge out of the renal vein beyond the vein margin due to post surgical venous retraction. Does this constitute a positive margin? The surgeon will likely object if called such in a pathology report. The ISUP Consensus Conference participants agreed (75% consensus) that a positive margin requires microscopic confirmation of tumor adherent to the vein wall at the vein margin.

Multifocal Renal Cell Carcinoma and Retrograde Venous Invasion

The incidence of multifocal RCC has been reported to range from 5 to as high as 25%. This wide variability has many causes such as inclusion of familial forms of RCC which are characteristically multifocal, the method of radiological documentation, and the pathologic examination strategy such as thinness of nephrectomy sectioning, use of capsular stripping, or inclusion of adenomas. In a recent retrospective review of 5378 cases from 16 academic centers involved in the Surveillance and Treatment Update Renal Neoplasms (SATURN) project, a multifocal RCC was identified in 5% of cases, a figure that appears more plausible than the higher figure noted above [26, 27]. Multifocal RCC is especially frequent with bilateral RCC which are heavily enriched for familial RCC syndromes, reported to range from 54% in clinical studies to as high as 90% in an autopsy study [27, 28]. Patients with multifocal RCC are more often symptomatic and have higher TNM stages and higher prevalence of tumor necrosis—all poor prognostic features. Compared to patients with a single RCC, patients with multifocal RCCs are at higher risk for recurrent and metastatic disease. The 5- and 10-year cancer specific survival in the SATURN project was 71 and 63.3% with multiple tumors, compared to 84.1 and 77.3% in patients with a single tumor [26].

The incidence of multifocal RCC is known to vary with RCC type, occurring in 11–16% of papillary RCC compared to 2–4% of clear cell RCC. In addition, there is a significant rate of nonconcordance of tumor type in multifocal RCC. Thus, should a biopsy be performed on only one, of two or more renal masses, diagnostic extrapolation to the other mass(es) is unwise. Not only can two types of RCC be present that vary in prognosis, but a benign tumor may coexist with a malignant tumor. These issues aside, multiple primary RCCs at nephrectomy are separately and individually TNM staged. The ISUP Consensus Conference recommendation relating to multifocal tumor sampling is to histologically examine at least the five largest tumors. A challenge when a nephrectomy contains multiple tumor nodules, however, is to distinguish separate independent neoplasms from the recently described invasive behavior of RCC known as retrograde venous invasion.

Retrograde venous invasion (RVI) was first reported by Bonsib and Bhalodia in 2011 [27]. RVI refers to a process which begins when an elongating plug of tumor within a renal sinus vein merges with the venous outflow from a vein, or veins, draining nontumor regions of the kidney (Fig. 24.4). In RVI, the intravenous tumor extends both distally into the main renal vein and proximally back toward the renal parenchyma within the merging veins from the nonneoplastic cortex (Figs. 24.5 and 24.6). Once the intravenous extensions reach the renal parenchyma, additional merging venous tributaries may be involved, resulting in multiple rounded or elongated cortical nodules that can be mistaken for additional primary tumors or so-called satellite nodules. This process occurs in approximately 10% of RCCs and in 22% of pT3a RCC [27]. RVI has only been observed when both renal sinus veins and the main renal vein are occluded. It is particularly common in clear cell RCC, not surprising in light of its remarkable diathesis for venous invasion. However, any tumor that invades sinus veins can demonstrate similar behavior.

Identification of RVI is the easiest on gross examination of the bivalved specimen, especially when the bivalve section is performed through the venous plane (see Chap. 22). Its recognition requires understanding of the normal renal venous outflow. For instance, elongated nodules of tumor located between renal pyramids and rounded

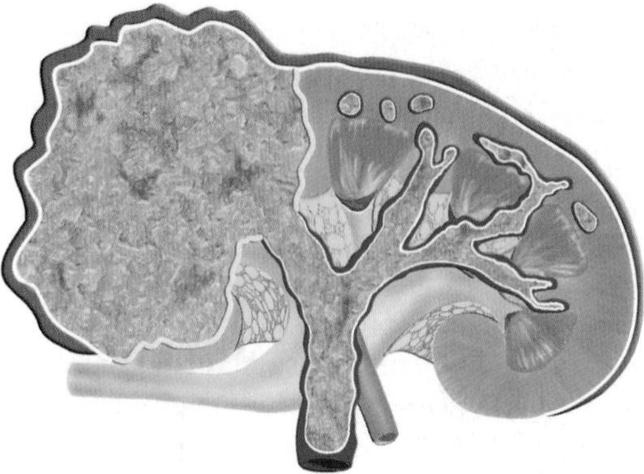

Fig. 24.4 This drawing depicts an example of retrograde cortical venous invasion. The RCC on the *left* has entered the sinus venous system at the *bottom* and extends to the main renal vein. To the *right* veins draining the nonneoplastic cortex merge with the vein draining the RCC. With the main renal vein occluded, the RCC can grow in a retrograde fashion back to the cortex on the *right*. Because of the arborizing venous system, intravenous tumor can be cut in cross and longitudinal planes, imparting an impression of multifocal tumor or "satellite" nodules

nodules arrayed along the corticomedullary junction likely represent RVI within interlobar and arcuate veins, respectively (Figs. 24.5 and 24.6). Histological demonstration of RVI is challenging

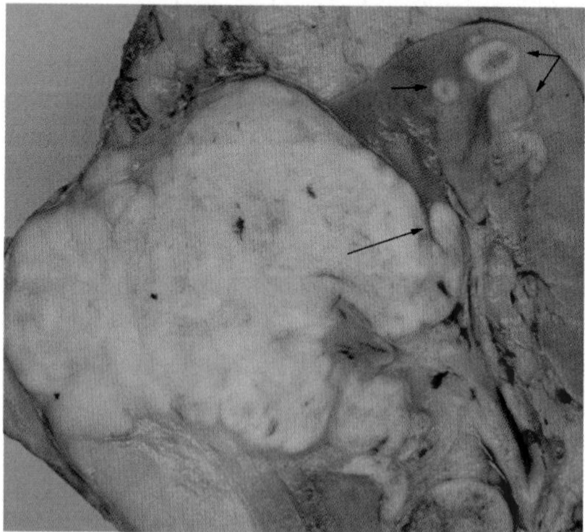

Fig. 24.5 This RCC, unclassified, is demonstrating sinus vein invasion (toward the *bottom* of the image) and retrograde cortical venous invasion. A cylindrical mass of tumor (*long arrow*) is in direct continuity with the primary and extends retrograde into the cortex between two renal pyramids. Cut in cross section are several arcuate veins (*short arrows*) involved by retrograde extension. These are in continuity with the cylindrical intravenous tumor (*long arrow*) visible between the renal pyramids

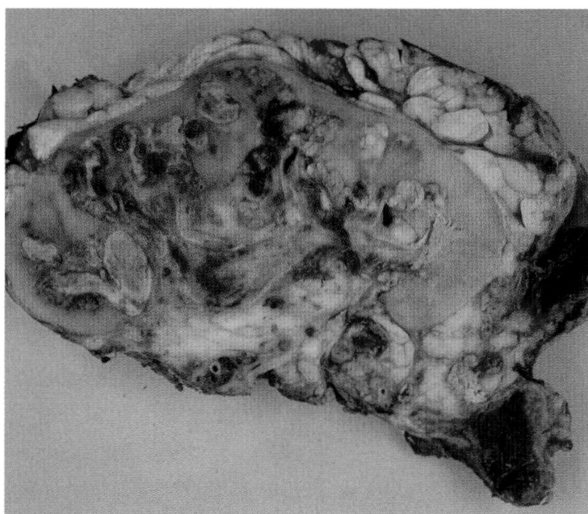

Fig. 24.6 This clear cell RCC is demonstrating extensive sinus vein invasion and retrograde cortical venous invasion. The main tumor is not shown. All of the visible tumor is intravenous, within sinus veins, and within interlobar and arcuate veins that encircle the renal pyramids. To the *lower right,* the adrenal vein in the perinephric fat is involved in a retrograde fashion from the main renal vein

because cortical veins lack smooth muscle media and elastica [27]. Although the venous endothelial lining can be demonstrated in some affected vessels, its presence is often effaced as intravenous tumor enlarges and invades the interstitium. The presence of an adjacent artery is a useful, but nonspecific finding, to support the intravenous origin of a cortical nodule. With extensive RVI, tumor nodules enlarge and can achieve confluence making accurate determination of primary tumor size difficult.

Vena Cava Invasion: pT3b and pT3c

Venous invasion has always been part of regional spread in staging systems and consistently demonstrated to have prognostic importance. The prognostic importance of level of venous invasion, however, has been more controversial, leading to adjustments in definition of the pT3 substages over the past several TNM formulations. Venous invasion has been stratified by cephalad extent since 1997 TNM. The 2009 TNM divides venous invasion into three substages, main renal vein and sinus veins (pT3a), VC below the diaphragm (pT3b), and VC above the diaphragm (pT3c), with the diaphragm representing the cutoff for pT3b and pT3c. An 11-institution consortium established to review venous extension in 1215 patients stratified as proposed by 2009 TNM, recently reported that the level of venous involvement is an independent predictor of survival [28].

The 2009 TNM included a new qualifying feature for pT3c, invasion of the wall of the VC at any level. Thus, tumor in the VC below the diaphragm can represent either pT3b or pT3c dependent upon the absence of, or presence of venous wall invasion, respectively. The latter determination requires evaluation of a caval "thrombus," a resection that can pose staging challenges, especially when submitted not otherwise specified. The specimen can be abundant and gross recognition of vein wall to direct tissue sampling may be difficult. The ISUP Consensus Conference sampling recommendation is to submit at least two blocks of tissue. However, more may be indicated dependent upon the clinical and anatomic features of an individual case.

pT4 and the Adrenal Gland

Extension of tumor beyond Gerota's fascia has been the sole criterion for pT4 designation for decades. The 2009 TNM expanded pT4 to include direct extension into the adrenal gland. Direct adrenal gland extension in continuity with the primary tumor had been included with perinephric fat invasion in the pT3a category for decades. Several groups, however, have shown that direct invasion of the adrenal gland is significantly associated with death from RCC, and that there is no difference in survival between patients with pT4 and pT3a tumors with direct adrenal gland invasion, justifying inclusion in the pT4 category [9, 29]. Adrenal gland involvement can occur by two routes: hematogenous metastasis (M1) or direct extension from the primary tumor (pT4). These are usually easily distinguished grossly.

Lymph Node Involvement: N Stage

Lymph node dissection (LND) represents the most accurate method to document lymph node involvement. However, its role in the treatment of RCC is controversial leading to a progressive decrease in LND over the last two decades. There are currently no universally accepted recommendations on patient selection for LND or even on the extent of the LND if one is performed [30]. In 2008, the European Organization for Research and Treatment of Cancer (EORTC) Genitourinary Group published the results of a 20-year phase three trial of 732 patients [30]. Although this study included a large number of low-risk patients, they found no survival advantage for clinically node negative patients treated with nephrectomy and LND, compared to those treated by nephrectomy alone. Other studies have found, however, a survival advantage in high risk patients with enlarged lymph nodes [31].

The incidence of nodal disease is T-stage specific; thus, most patients with lymph node involvement have metastases elsewhere. A recent large multi-institutional study showed incidences of 1.1, 4.5, and 12.3% for pT1, pT2, and pT3 cases, respectively [32]. Although approximately 7% of RCC patients will have hilar lymph node metastases, paradoxically, para-aortic lymph nodes and supraclavicular lymph nodes will be involved in almost 27 and 21% of the cases, respectively [31]. This apparent conundrum reflects the unpredictability of the normal lymphatic drainage of the kidney as detailed in Chap. 22, which can be further affected once lymphatics are involved and lymphatic obstruction occurs. Nodal disease also selects for certain RCC types, with papillary RCC over represented compared to clear cell. Although patients with nodal disease have in general a poorer prognosis than those without nodal disease, reported 5-year survivals vary greatly and are RCC type dependent, with papillary RCC having an improved survival with nodal disease compared to clear cell of 65% versus 19%, respectively [33].

The TNM has evolved substantially in N-stage definition over time with trending from more complicated to less complicated [7]. In 1978 TNM, the N stage included five groups, N0–N4. This gradually decreased to two groups by 1987 TNM, N0 and N1. The 2002 TNM returned to three groups N0, N1, and N2. The 2009 TNM again simplified the N-category by again eliminating N2; N1 is now defined as one, or more nodes, involved. This conforms to most studies assessing the prognostic impact of nodal disease which show significant survival differences between N0 and N1 disease. Mortality worsens, however, with more nodes involved. A prognostic difference has been noted at four or more positive nodes, a number that differs substantially from the 2009 TNM N0/N1 breakpoint of one lymph node [7]. The extent of lymph dissection is also important since the more nodes are examined, the more positive nodes will be encountered. It has been recommended that at least 12 nodes should be examined, but this is beyond the control of the pathologist [7]. The pathologist's task is simple: submit all apparent nodal tissue grossly identified in the hilar region and from a nodal dissection if submitted. The ISUP Consensus Conference recommends that search for nodal tissue in the peripheral perinephric fat. Microscopic examination of all hilar potentially node-containing tissue is not necessary [10].

Metastases: M Stage

Approximately 30% of RCC patients present with metastatic disease. This includes 10% of cases with lymph node metastases. The most common metastatic sites include bone, liver, lung, brain, and lymph nodes. However, RCC is notorious for its ability to metastasize to almost every organ or anatomic site. There are only two M-stage designations, M0 and MI. The survival for M1 patients is poor, with only 8.2% of patients alive at 5 years (Fig. 24.2) [9].

Additional TNM Descriptors

There are four TNM suffixes employed in conjunction with the pT designation if the context so merits. The suffixes include "m" for

Table 24.5 Additional TNM suffixes

Suffix	Definition
mpT	Multiple primary tumors are present
ypT	During or following chemotherapy, radiation therapy, or both
r1pT	Residual disease when staged after disease free interval r1 = microscopic disease
r2pT	Residual disease when staged after disease free interval r2 = macroscopic disease
apT	Stage determined at autopsy

multiple tumors, "y" for post treatment, "r" for residual tumor, and "a" for autopsy, as defined in Table 24.5. The "r" suffix is employed for both nephrectomies and partial nephrectomies if a positive margin is identified. The r1 versus r2 designation is quite subjective. It requires a judgment as to the likely amount of residual disease, not otherwise defined.

Additional Prognostic Factors

Future TNMs will likely incorporate additional anatomic and nonanatomic data into its prognostic groups. The 2009 TNM recommends documentation of several anatomic data noted below, known to be clinically significant even though not required for staging. Most of these data have long been included in standard pathology reports. The exceptions are data related to lymph node size and extranodal extension, data included in the TNM classification of many cancers of other organ systems:

RCC type*
Fuhrman grade*
Sarcomatoid features*
Histological tumor necrosis*
Size of largest lymph node metastasis
Extranodal extension

The College of American Pathologists "Protocol for the Examination of Specimen From Patients with Invasive Carcinomas of Renal Tubular Origin" recommends in addition to the items above indicated by an asterisk, inclusion of the following data in pathology reports [34]:

Tumor necrosis
Tumor extension into the pelvicalyceal system
Pathologic findings in the nonneoplastic kidney: glomerular disease, tubulointerstitial disease, vascular disease, cysts and adenomas

Conclusion

The 2009 TNM implemented several major changes compared to the 2002 formulation. The introduction of substage in the pT2 category may be of dubious merit since most RCCs larger than 7 cm demonstrate extrarenal extension, especially into the renal sinus, while large renal-limited tumors select for the more indolent RCC types of papillary and chromophobe cell RCC. The complexity of the pT3 category will continue to be problematic because of its numerous combinations of possibilities. The inclusion of invasion of the VC wall does not seem to have been data driven and, therefore, will need further investigation. This may present practical challenges since VC invasion may be missed because of the difficulty in gross recognition. The inclusion of direct adrenal gland extension into pT4 appears to be an important modification.

The derivation of the word "surgery" is from the Greek meaning hand work. Although the nephrectomy represents the surgeon's handiwork, it is the hand work of the surgical pathologist to take the surgeon's product and generate data to forecast the probability of a surgical cure while providing other important prognostic information. Satisfying this critical clinical necessity is straightforward in concept; we must first identify the presence or absence of extrarenal extension as it relates to the staging parameters of TNM 2009. How this is accomplished in the individual case is sometimes less straightforward. The recent ISUP Consensus Conference recommendations provide a very useful framework with many practical guidelines [10]. However, as noted by Dr. Beckwith, "As with all pathological evaluations, there are no universally applicable rules, and individual judgment must be used" [6].

Appendix

Primary tumor (T)			
TX	Primary tumor cannot be assessed		
T0	No evidence of primary tumor		
T1	Tumor 7 cm or less in greatest dimension, limited to the kidney		
T1a	Tumor 4 cm or less in greatest dimension, limited to the kidney		
T1b	Tumor > 4 cm but not more than 7 cm in greatest dimension, limited to the kidney		
T2	Tumor more than 7 cm in greatest dimension, limited to the kidney		
T2a	Tumor > 7 cm but less than 10 cm in greatest dimension, limited to the kidney		
T2b	Tumor > 10 cm in greatest dimension, limited to the kidney		
T3	Tumor extends into the renal vein or perinephric tissues but not into the ipsilateral adrenal gland and not beyond Gerota's fasciab		
T3a	Tumor extends into the renal vein or its segmental (muscle containing) branches or tumor invades perirenal and/or renal sinus fat but not beyond Gerota's fascia		
T3b	Tumor grossly extends into the VC below the diaphragm		
T3c	Tumor extends into the VC above the diaphragm or invades the wall of the VC		
T4	Tumor invades beyond Gerota's fascia, including contiguous extension into the ipsilateral adrenal gland		
Regional lymph nodes (N)			
NX	Regional lymph nodes cannot be assessed		
N0	No regional lymph node metastasis		
N1	Metastasis in regional lymph node(s)		
Distant metastases (M)			
M0	No distant metastasis		
M1	Distant metastasis		
Anatomic stage/prognostic groups			
Stage I	T1	N0	M0
Stage II	T2	N0	M0
Stage III	T1 or T2	N1	M0
	T3	N0 or N1	M0
Stage IV	T4	Any N	M0
	Any T	Any N	M1

Used with permission from [9]

References

1. Wright JR Jr., Albert C. Broders' paradigm shifts involving the prognostication and definition of cancer. Arch Pathol. 2012;136:1437–56.
2. Karakiewicz PI, Suardi N, Capitanio U, Isbarn H, Jeldres C, Perrotte P, et al. Conditional survival predictions after nephrectomy for renal cell carcinoma. J Urol. 2009;182:2607–12.
3. Greene FL, Sobin LH. The staging of cancer: a retrospective and prospective appraisal. CA Cancer J Clin. 2008;58:180–90.
4. Flocks RH, Kadesky MC. Malignant neoplasms of the kidney: an analysis of 353 patients followed for 5 years or more. J Urol. 1958;79:196.
5. Petkovic SD. An anatomical classification of renal tumors in the adult as a basis for prognosis. Urology. 1959;81(5):618–23.
6. Robson CJ, Churchill BM, Anderson W. The results of radical nephrectomy for renal cell carcinoma. J Urol. 1969;101:297–301.
7. Delahunt B. Advances and controversies in grading and staging of renal cell carcinoma. Mod Pathol. 2009;22:S24–S36.
8. Green FL, Page D, Marrow M, Fritz AG, Balch CM, Haller DG, Marrow M. AJCC cancer staging manual. 6th ed. New York: Springer; 2002.
9. Edge SE, Bryd DR, Compton CC, Fritz AG, Greene FL, Trotti A. AJCC cancer staging manual. 7th ed. New York: Springer; 2009. pp. 547–60.

10. Trpkov K, Grignon D, Bonsib S, Amin M, Billis A, Lopez-Beltran A, et al. Handling and staging of renal cell carcinoma: the International Society of Urological Pathology (ISUP) consensus conference recommendations. Am J SurgPathol. 2013;37(10):1505–17.
11. Bell ET. A classification of renal tumors with observation on the frequency of the various types. J Urol. 1937;39:238–42.
12. Thompson RH, Hill JR, Babayev Y, Cronin A, Kaag M, Kundu S, et al. Metastatic renal cell carcinoma risk according to tumor size. J Urol. 2009;182:41–5.
13. Nguyen MM, Gill IS. Effect of renal cancer size on the prevalence of metastases at diagnosis and mortality. J Urol. 2009;181:1020–27.
14. Delahunt b, Kittelson JM, McCredie MRE, Reeve MRE, Stewart JH, Bilous AM. Prognostic importance of tumor size for localized conventional (clear cell) renal cell carcinoma. Assessment of the TNM T1 and T2 tumor categories and comparison of other prognostic parameters. Cancer. 2002;94:658–64.
15. Frank I, Blute ML, Leibovich BC, Cheville JC, Lohse CM, Kwon ED, Zincke H. pT2 classification for renal cell carcinoma. Can its accuracy be improved? J Urol. 2005;173:380–4.
16. Waalkes S, Becker F, Schrader AJ, Janssen M, Wegener G, Merseburger AS, et al. Is there a need to further subclassify pT2 renal cell cancers as implemented by the revised 7th TNM version? Eur Urol. 2011;59:258–63.
17. Novara G, Ficarra V, Antonelli A, Artibani W, Bertini R, Carini M, et al. Validation of the 2009 TNM version in a large multi-institutional cohort of patients treated for renal cell carcinoma: are further improvements needed? Eur Urol. 2010;58:588–95.
18. Rothman J, Egleston B, Wong Y-N, Iffrig K, Lebovitch S, Uzzo RG. Histopathological characteristics of localized renal cell carcinoma correlate with tumor size: a SEER analysis. J Urol. 2009;181:29–34.
19. Beckwith JB. National wilmstumor study: an update for pathologists. Pediatr Devel Pathol. 1998;1:79–88.
20. Bonsib SM, Gibon D, Mhoon M, Greene GF. Renal sinus involvement in renal cell carcinoma. Am J Surg Pathol. 2000;24:451–8.
21. Kane CJ, Mallin K, Ritchey J, Cooperberg MR, Carroll PR. Renal cell cancer stage migration. Analysis of the national cancer data base. Cancer. 2008;113:78–83.
22. Thompson RH, Blute ML, Krambeck AE, Lohse CM, Magera JS, et al. Patients with pT1 renal cell carcinoma who die from disease after nephrectomy may have unrecognized renal sinus fat invasion. Am J Surg Pathol. 2007;31:1089–93.
23. Bonsib SM. The renal sinus is the principal invasive pathway: a prospective study of 100 renal cell carcinomas. Am J Surg Pathol. 2004;28:1594–600.
24. Bonsib SM. T2 clear cell renal cell carcinoma is a rare entity: a study of 120 clear cell renal cell carcinomas. J Urol. 2005;174:1199–202.
25. Bonsib SM. Renal veins and venous extension in clear cell renal cell carcinoma. Mod Pathol. 2007;20:44–53.
26. Siracusano S, Novara G, Antonelli A, Artibani W, Bertini R, Carini M, et al. Prognostic role of tumourmultifocality in renal cell carcinoma. Brit J Urol Int. 2012;110:E443–8.
27. Bonsib SM, Bhalodia A. Retrograde venous invasion in renal cell carcinoma: a complication of sinus vein and main renal vein involvement. Mod Pathol. 2011;24:1578–85.
28. Martínez-Salamanca JI, Huang WC, Mullán I, Bertini R, Bianco FJ, Carballido JA, et al. Prognostic impact of 2009 UICC/AJCC TNM staging system for renal cell carcinoma with venous extension. Eur Urol. 2011;59:120–7.
29. Thompson RH, Cheville JC, Lohse CM, Webster WS, Zincke H, Kwon ED, et al. Reclassification of patients with pT3 and pT4 renal cell carcinoma improves prognostic accuracy. Cancer. 2005;104:53–60.
30. Blom JHM, van Poppel H, Maréchal JM, Jacqmin D, Schröder FH, de Prijck L, Sylvester R. For the EORTC genitourinary tract cancer group. Radical nephrectomy with and without lymph-node dissection: final results of European organization for research and treatment of cancer (EROTC) randomized phase 3 trial 30881. Eur Urol. 2009;55:28–34.
31. Capitanio U, Becker F, Blute ML, Mulders P, Patard JJ, Russo P, et al. Lymph node dissection in renal cell carcinoma. Eur Urol. 2011;60:1212–20.
32. Capitanio U, Jerdres C, Pataard JJ, Perrotte P, Zini L, de La Taille A, et al. Stage-specific effect of nodal metastases on survival in patients with non-metastatic renal cell carcinoma. BJU Int. 2009;103:33–8.
33. Margolis V, Tambolis P, Matin SF, Swanson DA, Wood CG. Analysis of clinicopathologic predictors of oncologic outcome provides insight into the natural history of surgically managed papillary renal cell carcinoma. Cancer. 2008;112:1480–8.
34. Srigley JR, Amin MB, Campbell SC, Chang A, Delahunt B, Grignon DJ, et al. Protocol for the Examination of Specimen From Patients with Invasive Carcinomas of Renal Tubular Origin. College of American Pathologists, Kidney 3.1.0.1, Protocol web posting date: June, 2012.

Surgical Pathology Reporting of Renal Cell Carcinomas

25

Christopher G. Przybycin, Angela Wu and Lakshmi P. Kunju

Introduction

A carefully crafted surgical pathology report for renal cell carcinoma (RCC) provides key information that can direct clinical management and prognosis for a given patient. Chief among the parameters reported are RCC subtype, grade, and tumor stage, all of which are covered at length in other chapters in this volume. The purpose of this chapter is to address remaining features that are important to include in the surgical pathology report.

Additional Tumor Characteristics to Report

Tumor Necrosis

The adverse prognostic significance of tumor necrosis in RCC was first reported by Amtrup et al. in 1974 [1]. Although some subsequent studies have not supported this conclusion [2, 3], a large number of series [4–8] have demonstrated the importance of tumor necrosis as an adverse feature independent of other established parameters. Most recently, Delahunt et al. have proposed a composite grading system for clear cell RCC that incorporates both tumor necrosis and the nucleolar grade recently proposed by the International Society of Urological Pathology (ISUP). This system has superior discriminatory power when compared with ISUP nucleolar grade alone [9]. The importance of necrosis appears to be best established in clear cell RCC and possibly chromophobe RCC, with conflicting data for papillary RCC [6, 7, 9, 10]. It has been suggested that this discrepancy may be due to differences in the mechanism of necrosis among these RCC subtypes.

Because degenerative phenomena are common in RCC (e.g., tumor regression and hyalinization in clear cell RCC, organizing hemorrhage in papillary RCC, a strict histologic definition of tumor necrosis is required for preserving its prognostic importance. Specifically, tumor necrosis consists of "homogeneous clusters of sheets of dead cells, or coalescing groups of cells forming a coagulum, containing nuclear and cytoplasmic debris [7, 9]" (Fig. 25.1).

Recognition of the importance of tumor necrosis was reflected in the recommendations of the 2012 ISUP consensus conference. It was agreed upon by consensus that for clear cell RCC, the presence or absence of tumor necrosis should be included in pathology reports, that assessment should include both macroscopic and

C. G. Przybycin (✉)
Department of Pathology, Cleveland Clinic, Robert J. Tomsich Pathology and Laboratory Medicine Institute, Cleveland, OH, USA
e-mail: przybyc@ccf.org

A. Wu
Department of Pathology, University of Michigan Medical Center, Ann Arbor, MI, USA
e-mail: angelawu@med.umich.edu

L. P. Kunju
Department of Pathology, University of Michigan, Ann Arbor, MI, USA
e-mail: lkunju@med.umich.edu

C. Magi-Galluzzi, C. G. Przybycin (eds.), *Genitourinary Pathology,* DOI 10.1007/978-1-4939-2044-0_25,

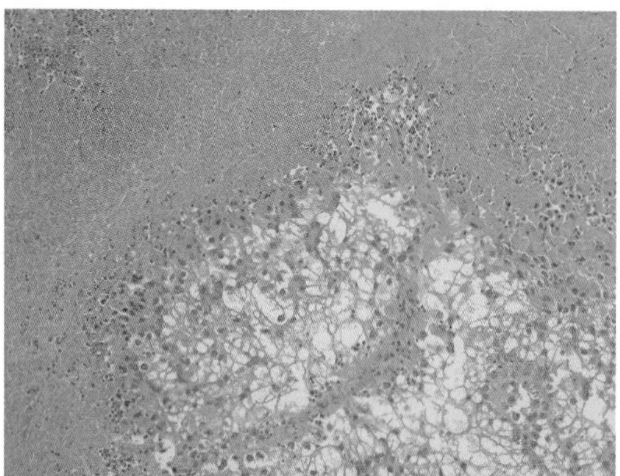

Fig. 25.1 Clear cell carcinoma with coagulative tumor necrosis. True coagulative tumor necrosis, in contrast to hyalinized areas of scarring and regression often seen in clear cell RCC, consists of necrotic "ghost" cells with associated nuclear and cytoplasmic debris

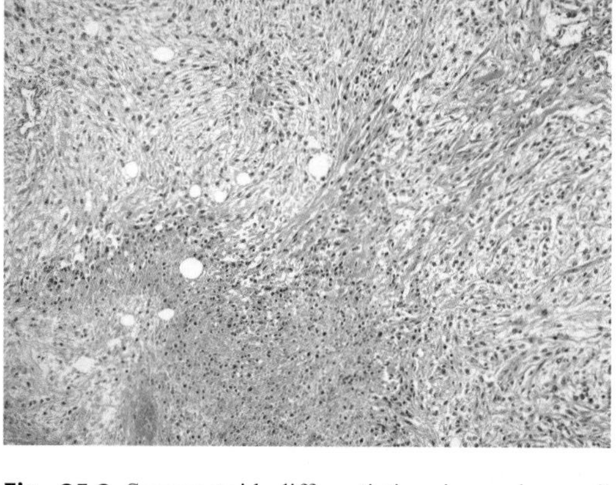

Fig. 25.2 Sarcomatoid differentiation in a clear cell RCC. An area of sarcomatoid differentiation is seen as a malignant spindle cell proliferation that resembles a sarcoma. This example has associated tumor necrosis

microscopic examination, and that the amount of necrosis present should be included as a percentage [11]. In practical terms, however, quantifying necrosis can be a somewhat subjective exercise that is limited by sampling technique and not universally practiced; at our respective institutions, we do not generally submit sections containing only grossly necrotic tumor and do not currently quantitate necrosis, grossly or microscopically.

Sarcomatoid Differentiation

Sarcomatoid differentiation in RCC, recognized as a malignant spindle cell component resembling a sarcoma, is no longer thought to define a distinct subtype of RCC. Rather, it is thought to represent a common pathway of tumor dedifferentiation that can occur in any RCC subtype. Sarcomatoid differentiation in RCC has been demonstrated repeatedly to be associated with aggressive behavior independent of other pathologic parameters; patients with sarcomatoid differentiation have frequent metastases, often at the time of presentation, and short survival (median 6–19 months) [12–14]. In some studies, a higher percentage of sarcomatoid differentiation has been associated with decreased survival [12, 14]. The parent subtype of RCC does not appear to have prognostic significance once sarcomatoid differentiation has occurred [12, 13, 15], although one recent study suggests that patients with metastatic sarcomatoid carcinoma arising in association with clear cell RCC may have a better response to vascular epidermal growth factor (VEGF)-targeted therapy [16].

Grossly, areas of sarcomatoid differentiation are often seen as dense, tan to white fleshy areas with infiltrative borders, often contrasting with the softer character of the associated RCC in which they arose [12].

Microscopically, sarcomatoid differentiation is recognized as a malignant spindle cell component that resembles a sarcoma (Fig. 25.2). The appearance most commonly resembles fibrosarcoma, malignant fibrous histiocytoma, or an unclassified sarcoma. Heterologous differentiation is rare, often taking the form of osteosarcoma, chrondrosarcoma, or rhabdomyosarcoma, and has not been shown to affect outcome in the few instances reported [12, 14, 15].

Because sarcomatoid differentiation is associated with such aggressive behavior, its presence should be mentioned in the surgical pathology report. At the most recent meeting of the ISUP, there was consensus that no minimum amount of sarcomatoid differentiation was necessary to establish a diagnosis of sarcomatoid carcinoma;

thus, any amount of sarcomatoid differentiation should be mentioned in the surgical pathology report [11].

Rhabdoid Differentiation

Rhabdoid differentiation, so named because it describes tumor cells that resemble rhabdomyoblasts, was described in RCC in a series by Gokden et al. in 2000 [17]. The rhabdoid phenotype is most commonly seen in association with clear cell RCC, but has been reported in numerous other subtypes, including papillary, chromophobe, medullary, and acquired cystic disease-associated RCC [18–22]. Cells with rhabdoid differentiation are variably cohesive and contain large, densely eosinophilic intracytoplasmic inclusions and eccentrically located nuclei, often with prominent nucleoli (Fig. 25.3). These hyaline inclusions do not represent muscle differentiation but rather have been shown to be aggregates of cytoskeletal filaments or degraded organelles [17, 21].

Rhabdoid differentiation has been associated with increased tumor grade and stage, as well as frequent metastasis and death of disease in several studies [17, 21, 23]. More recently, it has been shown to be independently associated with poor outcome [24]. Therefore, it should be mentioned when present. This practice was likewise supported by ISUP consensus [11].

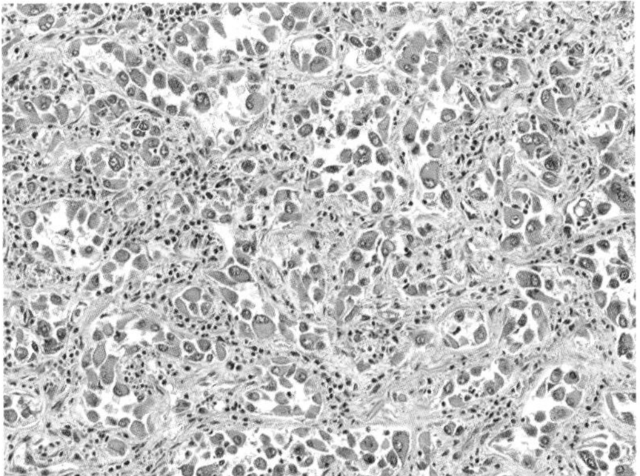

Fig. 25.3 Rhabdoid differentiation in a clear cell RCC. Rhabdoid cells have large eccentric nuclei with vesicular chromatin and prominent nucleoli as well as a densely eosinophilic cytoplasmic inclusion, causing the cells to resemble rhabdomyoblasts

Additional Reporting Considerations

Evaluation of Nonneoplastic Parenchyma in Partial and Radical Nephrectomy Specimens

The second key concern after oncologic control that affects patients with RCC is postsurgical kidney function. This consideration, aided by improvements in surgical techniques over time, is the motivation for the use of nephron-sparing surgery. A significant number of patients (22.4 % of radical nephrectomy patients and 11.6 % of partial nephrectomy patients) without preoperative renal compromise can expect an increase in serum creatinine to greater than 2.0 mg/dL within 10 years of surgery due to surgical loss of nephrons [25]. This problem is compounded in patients with underlying kidney disease (as associated with diabetes mellitus or hypertension) [26].

The pathologist can provide useful information regarding likely future kidney function by sampling and assessing the nonneoplastic renal parenchyma present in a partial or radical nephrectomy specimen. Because mass effect from the tumor can cause local pathologic changes in the kidney parenchyma that are not indicative of global kidney dysfunction, sections for the evaluation of nonneoplastic disease should be taken as far from the tumor as possible. Thus, an evaluation for medical kidney disease is not recommended in partial nephrectomy specimens that contain less than 5 mm of surrounding nonneoplastic renal parenchyma [27].

The medical significance of evaluation of the nonneoplastic renal parenchyma in a nephrectomy specimen is underscored by the lethality of end-stage renal disease, even with dialysis, particularly in older patients. Average 60, 70, and 80-year-old end-stage renal disease patients on dialysis have life expectancies of 4.3, 3.1, and 2.2 years, respectively, indicating that many patients

Fig. 25.4 A sample reporting template for renal tumors

Accession #: ____________________ Name: ____________________

RENAL Neoplasm

Procedure: **Radical nephrectomy**
Partial nephrectomy

Tumor Type: **Renal cell carcinoma:**
Clear cell
Multilocular cystic renal cell carcinoma
Papillary
Chromophobe
Collecting duct
Medullary carcinoma
Mucinous tubular and spindle cell carcinoma
Translocation associated carcinoma:
Tubulocystic renal cell carcinoma
Unclassified
Other:

Rhabdoid Differentiation: **Present: _______ %** **Absent**

Necrosis (microscopic): **Present** **Absent**

ISUP Nucleolar Grade: **/4** **N/A**

Size: _______ **cm**

Extent of Tumor:

- □ **Tumor 4 cm or less in greatest dimension, limited to kidney (T1a)**
- □ **Tumor more than 4 cm but not more than 7 cm in greatest dimension, limited to kidney (T1b)**
- □ **Tumor more than 7 cm but less than or equal to 10 cm in greatest dimension, limited to kidney (T2a)**
- □ **Tumor more than 10 cm, limited to kidney (T2b)**
- □ **Tumor grossly extends into the renal vein or its segmental (muscle containing) branches, or tumor invades perirenal and/or renal sinus fat but not beyond Gerota's facia (T3a)**
- □ **Tumor grossly extends into the vena cava below the diagram (T3b)**
- □ **Tumor grossly extends into the vena cava above the diagram or invades the wall of the vena cava (T3c)**
- □ **Tumor invades beyond Gerota's fascia (including contiguous extension into ipsilateral adrenal gland) (T4)**

Margin Status:

Vascular:	**Pos**	**Neg**	**N/A**
Ureteral:	**Pos**	**Neg**	**N/A**
Parenchymal:	**Pos**	**Neg**	**N/A**
Soft Tissue:	**Pos**	**Neg**	**N/A**

Angiolymphatic Invasion (microscopic): **Present** **Absent**

Lymph Nodes:
- □ **Not assessed (Nx)**
- □ **Negative (N0)**
- □ **Metastasis in regional lymph node(s) (N1)**
  Positive number (/) Site:

Adrenal Gland Involvement:
- □ **Tumor directly invades the adrenal gland (T4)**
- □ **Involved by metastasis (M1)**
- □ **Not involved**
- □ **Not assessed**

Please add a new paragraph after this section that says the following:

- □ **PATHOLOGIC FINDINGS IN NONNEOPLASTIC KIDNEY (check all that apply)**
- □ **Insufficient tissue (partial nephrectomy specimen with <5 mm of adjacent nonneoplastic kidney)**
- □ **Significant pathologic alterations: None identified**
- □ **Glomerular disease (specify type):**
- □ **Tubulointerstitial disease (specify type):**
- □ **Vascular disease (specify type):**
- □ **Other (specify):**

with both end stage renal disease and RCC will more likely die from their renal disease than from their tumors [27].

In a review of 246 nephrectomy specimens, Henriksen and colleagues identified diagnosable medical kidney disease in 24 (10 %) cases, which was not mentioned in 21 (88 %) of the surgical pathology reports. Diagnosable disease included diabetic nephropathy (19 cases, including 12 classifiable as severe diabetic nephropathy), thrombotic microangiopathy (three cases), sickle cell nephropathy (one case), and focal segmental glomerulosclerosis (one case).

Lastly, evaluation of the nonneoplastic kidney parenchyma can provide important clues to the diagnosis of the patient's renal tumor itself, as in the presence of small nests of clear cells in patients with von Hippel–Lindau syndrome and clear cell RCC, oncocytosis in patients with Birt–Hogg–Dubé syndrome as well as oncocytomas, chromophobe RCCs or hybrid tumors, and background end-stage renal disease and acquired cystic kidney disease in patients with acquired cystic-disease-associated RCC. These findings are further discussed elsewhere in this volume in the chapters on familial syndromes associated with renal tumors and newly described diagnostic entities in kidney tumor pathology.

By incorporating the additional parameters discussed in this chapter into the surgical pathology report for tumor nephrectomy specimens, pathologists can more accurately predict patient outcome and play a role in guiding management. The use of a standard RCC reporting template (as in Fig. 25.4, for example) can help to ensure inclusion of relevant data.

References

1. Amtrup F, Hansen JB, Thybo E. Prognosis in renal carcinoma evaluated from histological criteria. Scand J Urol Nephrol. 1974;8(3):198–202.
2. Isbarn H, Patard JJ, Lughezzani G, Rioux-Leclercq N, Crepel M, Cindolo L, et al. Limited prognostic value of tumor necrosis in patients with renal cell carcinoma. Urology. 2010;75(6):1378–84.
3. Minervini A, Di Cristofano C, Gacci M, Serni S, Menicagli M, Lanciotti M, et al. Prognostic role of histological necrosis for nonmetastatic clear cell renal cell carcinoma: correlation with pathological features and molecular markers. J Urol. 2008;180(4):1284–9.
4. Leibovich BC, Blute ML, Cheville JC, Lohse CM, Frank I, Kwon ED, et al. Prediction of progression after radical nephrectomy for patients with clear cell renal cell carcinoma: a stratification tool for prospective clinical trials. Cancer. 2003;97(7):1663–71.
5. Frank I, Blute ML, Cheville JC, Lohse CM, Weaver AL, Zincke H. An outcome prediction model for patients with clear cell renal cell carcinoma treated with radical nephrectomy based on tumor stage, size, grade and necrosis: the SSIGN score. J Urol. 2002;168(6):2395–400.
6. Pichler M, Hutterer GC, Chromecki TF, Jesche J, Kampel-Kettner K, Rehak P, et al. Histologic tumor necrosis is an independent prognostic indicator for clear cell and papillary renal cell carcinoma. Am J Clin Pathol. 2012;137(2):283–9.
7. Sengupta S, Lohse CM, Leibovich BC, Frank I, Thompson RH, Webster WS, et al. Histologic coagulative tumor necrosis as a prognostic indicator of renal cell carcinoma aggressiveness. Cancer. 2005;104(3):511–20.
8. Ficarra V, Martignoni G, Lohse C, Novara G, Pea M, Cavalleri S, et al. External validation of the mayo clinic stage, size, grade and necrosis (SSIGN) score to predict cancer specific survival using a European series of conventional renal cell carcinoma. J Urol. 2006;175(4):1235–9.
9. Delahunt B, McKenney JK, Lohse CM, Leibovich BC, Thompson RH, Boorjian SA, et al. A novel grading system for clear cell renal cell carcinoma incorporating tumor necrosis. Am J Surg Pathol. 2013;37(3):311–22.
10. Przybycin CG, Cronin AM, Darvishian F, Gopalan A, Al-Ahmadie HA, Fine SW, et al. Chromophobe renal cell carcinoma: a clinicopathologic study of 203 tumors in 200 patients with primary resection at a single institution. Am J Surg Pathol. 2011;35(7):962–70.
11. Delahunt B, Cheville JC, Martignoni G, Humphrey PA, Magi-Galluzzi C, McKenney J, et al. The international society of urological pathology (ISUP) grading system for renal cell carcinoma and other prognostic parameters. Am J Surg Pathol. 2013;37(10):1490–504.
12. de Peralta-Venturina M, Moch H, Amin M, Tamboli P, Hailemariam S, Mihatsch M, et al. Sarcomatoid differentiation in renal cell carcinoma: a study of 101 cases. Am J Surg Pathol. 2001;25(3):275–84.
13. Shuch B, Bratslavsky G, Shih J, Vourganti S, Finley D, Castor B, et al. Impact of pathological tumour characteristics in patients with sarcomatoid renal cell carcinoma. BJU Int. 2012;109(11):1600–6.
14. Ro JY, Ayala AG, Sella A, Samuels ML, Swanson DA. Sarcomatoid renal cell carcinoma: clinicopathologic. A study of 42 cases. Cancer. 1987;59(3):516–26.

15. Cheville JC, Lohse CM, Zincke H, Weaver AL, Leibovich BC, Frank I, et al. Sarcomatoid renal cell carcinoma: an examination of underlying histologic subtype and an analysis of associations with patient outcome. Am J Surg Pathol. 2004;28(4):435–41.
16. Golshayan AR, George S, Heng DY, Elson P, Wood LS, Mekhail TM, et al. Metastatic sarcomatoid renal cell carcinoma treated with vascular endothelial growth factor-targeted therapy. J Clin Oncol. 2009;27(2):235–41.
17. Gokden N, Nappi O, Swanson PE, Pfeifer JD, Vollmer RT, Wick MR, et al. Renal cell carcinoma with rhabdoid features. Am J Surg Pathol. 2000;24(10):1329–38.
18. Brcic I, Spajic B, Kruslin B. Chromophobe renal cell carcinoma with rhabdoid differentiation in an adult. Wien klin Wochenschr. 2012;124(11–12):419–21.
19. Cheng JX, Tretiakova M, Gong C, Mandal S, Krausz T, Taxy JB. Renal medullary carcinoma: rhabdoid features and the absence of INI1 expression as markers of aggressive behavior. Mod Pathol. 2008;21(6):647–52.
20. Kuroda N, Tamura M, Hamaguchi N, Mikami S, Pan CC, Brunelli M, et al. Acquired cystic disease-associated renal cell carcinoma with sarcomatoid change and rhabdoid features. Ann Diagn Pathol. 2011;15(6):462–6.
21. Kuroiwa K, Kinoshita Y, Shiratsuchi H, Oshiro Y, Tamiya S, Oda Y, et al. Renal cell carcinoma with rhabdoid features: an aggressive neoplasm. Histopathology. 2002;41(6):538–48.
22. Shannon B, Stan Wisniewski Z, Bentel J, Cohen RJ. Adult rhabdoid renal cell carcinoma. Arch Pathol Lab Med. 2002;126(12):1506–10.
23. Leroy X, Zini L, Buob D, Ballereau C, Villers A, Aubert S. Renal cell carcinoma with rhabdoid features: an aggressive neoplasm with overexpression of p53. Arch Pathol Lab Med. 2007;131(1):102–6.
24. Przybycin CG, McKenney JK, Reynolds JP, Campbell S, Zhou M, Karafa MT, et al. Rhabdoid differentiation is associated with aggressive behavior in renal cell carcinoma: a clinicopathologic analysis of 76 cases with clinical follow-up. Am J Surg Pathol. 2014;38:1260–5.
25. Lau WK, Blute ML, Weaver AL, Torres VE, Zincke H. Matched comparison of radical nephrectomy vs nephron-sparing surgery in patients with unilateral renal cell carcinoma and a normal contralateral kidney. Mayo Clin Proc. 2000;75(12):1236–42.
26. Ito K, Nakashima J, Hanawa Y, Oya M, Ohigashi T, Marumo K, et al. The prediction of renal function 6 years after unilateral nephrectomy using preoperative risk factors. J Urol. 2004;171(1):120–5.
27. Henriksen KJ, Meehan SM, Chang A. Non-neoplastic renal diseases are often unrecognized in adult tumor nephrectomy specimens: a review of 246 cases. Am J Surg Pathol. 2007;31(11):1703–8.

Newly Described Entities in Renal Tumor Pathology

26

Angela Wu, Christopher G. Przybycin and Lakshmi P. Kunju

Introduction

Since the publication of the World Health Organization (WHO) classification of renal cell carcinoma (RCC) subtypes in 2004, several new subtypes of renal epithelial neoplasms have been recognized and most of them included in the recent International Society of Urologic Pathologists (ISUP) Vancouver modification of WHO (2004) Histologic Classification of renal tumors [2]. Several of these entities have important prognostic implications, and all provide insights into the pathogenesis of renal epithelial neoplasia. This chapter provides the key gross and microscopic features of each tumor, as well as ancillary studies helpful in diagnosis, and relevant prognostic information. Newly described tumors with a familial association are described in Chap. 29.

A. Wu (✉) · L. P. Kunju
Department of Pathology, University of Michigan Medical Center, Ann Arbor, MI, USA
e-mail: angelawu@med.umich.edu

L. P. Kunju
e-mail: lkunju@med.umich.edu

C. G. Przybycin
Department of Pathology, Cleveland Clinic, Robert J. Tomsich Pathology and Laboratory Medicine Institute, Cleveland, OH, USA
e-mail: przybyc@ccf.org

Clear Cell Papillary Renal Cell Carcinoma

Clear cell papillary renal cell carcinoma (CCP-RCC, also called clear cell tubulopapillary renal cell carcinoma) is a recently recognized entity [1] that was originally described as a distinctive type of RCC arising in end-stage renal disease (ESRD) [2]. Subsequently, however, these tumors have been described in kidneys not affected by ESRD [3].

This neoplasm has been included in the recent International Society of Urologic Pathologists (ISUP) Vancouver modification of WHO (2004) Histologic Classification of renal tumors [4]. A recent study [5] has reported an incidence of approximately 4% of CCP-RCC (including both sporadic and tumors associated with end-stage renal disease) in 290 consecutive nephrectomies performed for renal cell carcinoma [5].

Gross

CCP-RCCs, which commonly arise in adults and show no sex predilection, are usually small (mean size 2.4 cm, 0.9–4.5 cm), pT1a.). These tumors tend to be well circumscribed with a variable capsule, are frequently Although uncommon, multifocality and bilaterality have been described in some cases and may raise consideration of von Hippel- Lindau (VHL) associated disease.

C. Magi-Galluzzi, C. G. Przybycin (eds.), *Genitourinary Pathology,* DOI 10.1007/978-1-4939-2044-0_26,

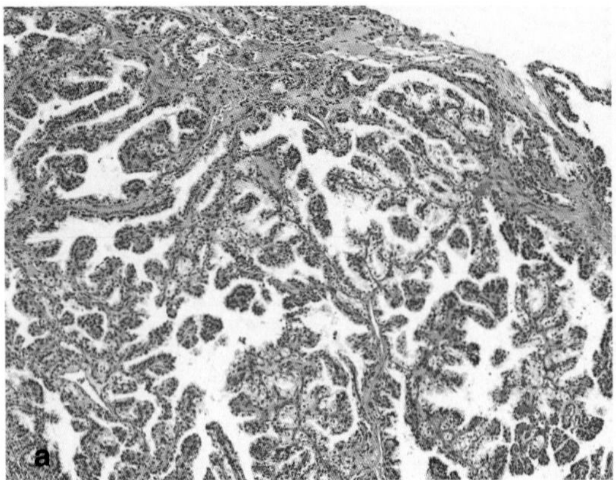

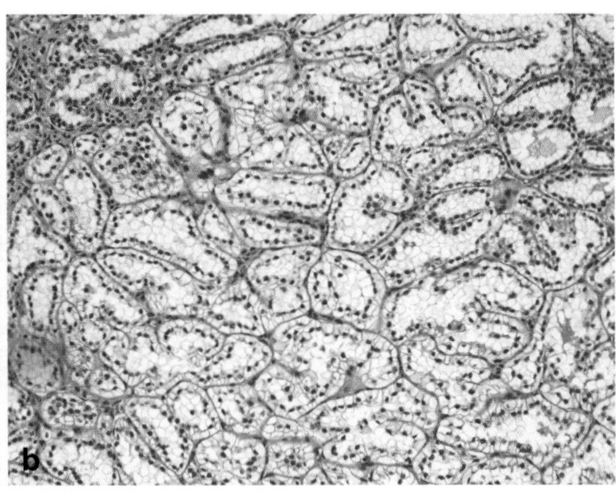

Fig. 26.1 **a** Clear cell papillary RCC showing an aggregate of branching tubules, some cystically dilated and containing small papillary structures. The tubules are lined by cells with clear cytoplasm and low-grade nuclei. **b** Clear cell papillary RCC showing linear arrangement of nuclei away from the basal aspect of the cells, imparting a "piano keys" appearance

Microscopic

CCP-RCCs can have a prominent papillary and/or tubular architecture. The tubules are of varying sizes and can branch and form small cysts (Fig. 26.1a). Occasionally, the tubules can be closely packed, approaching a solid architecture. The tubules may contain eosinophilic secretions. The cells lining the papillae, tubules, and cysts have prominent clear cytoplasm and low-grade nuclei with inconspicuous nucleoli. The most characteristic feature of these tumors is the linear arrangement of nuclei away from the basal aspect of cells; an appearance that resembles secretory endometrium and has been described as "piano keys" (Fig. 26.1b). The delicate sinusoidal/racemose vascular pattern characteristic of classic clear cell type RCC is not observed in these tumors.

Immunoprofile

CCP-RCCs have an unusual immunoprofile which is distinct from both classic clear cell type RCC as well as papillary type RCC. These tumors are diffusely and strongly positive with cytokeratin 7 (CK7) in both the solid and cystic areas and negative with alpha-methylacyl CoA racemase (AMACR). This staining pattern is distinct from both classic clear cell type RCC which are commonly negative with CK7 and papillary type RCC which are typically AMACR positive.

Although diffuse membranous positivity with carbonic anhydrase IX (CA-IX) is well described in clear cell type RCCs, CCP-RCCs have been shown to be positive with CA-IX, showing a characteristic "cup-like" reactivity with the absence of staining on the luminal aspect [6]. These tumors are usually negative or show only focal expression of CD10 and are commonly diffusely positive with high-molecular weight cytokeratin (HMWCK, 34beta E12).

Molecular Profile

So far, these tumors have not been shown to have the von Hippel–Lindau (VHL) gene mutations or 3p deletions commonly observed in classic clear cell type RCCs. They also lack trisomy of chromosome 7 or loss of Y chromosome, cytogenetic changes commonly observed in papillary RCCs (PRCCs) [3, 7]. Recent studies have shown relative overexpression of *VHL* mRNA in CCP-RCCs when compared with clear-cell RCCs. CCP-RCCs have also been shown to express HIF-1α and Glucose-transporter 1 (GLUT-1). The co-expression CAIX, GLUT-1 and HIF-1α in the absence of VHL gene alterations suggest activation of the HIF pathway by non-VHL dependent mechanisms [8]. Low copy number gains of chromosomes 7 and 17 have also been reported in some cases [4].

Prognosis

CCP-RCCs are typically small, biologically indolent tumors. No lymph node or distant metastasis of these tumors has been reported to date in the literature.

Recently a distinct tumorous entity named renal angiomyoadenomatous tumor (RAT) has been described in the literature [9], composed of an intimate mixture of epithelial cells associated with a variably prominent smooth muscle stroma often forming abortive vascular structures. The epithelium, described in these tumors as having a predominant tubular architecture lined by cells with low-grade nuclei and clear cytoplasm, is similar to some of the cases illustrated in the description of CCP-RCC. The epithelial component of RAT is positive with CK7, CA-IX and negative with CD10: an immunoprofile identical to CCP-RCC. The smooth muscle stroma marks with common muscle markers. No VHL mutations have been identified in these tumors. The current perspective is that both CCP-RCC and RAT have orphologic and immunohistochemical similarities and probably represent the spectrum of a single entity [4, 5, 14]

Differential Diagnosis

The most critical differential diagnoses include classic clear cell type RCC and PRCC. Additionally, translocation-associated RCC may enter the differential diagnosis.

Clear cell RCCs, the most common subtype of RCC, are typically golden yellow with a variegated appearance including the presence of hemorrhage and necrosis. These RCCs show a variable cystic appearance ranging from focal to extensively multicystic on gross examination. The tumor cells have clear cytoplasm are arranged in nests, alveoli or solid sheets separated by a characteristic intricate delicate sinusoidal (racemose) vascular network, seen in the vast majority of cases. Some tumors may show prominent areas with granular/eosinophilic cytoplasm, usually associated with a high nuclear grade. While clear cell RCCs may show focal papillary/pseudopapillary areas, a prominent papillary architecture is uncommon as is the characteristic linear arrangement of nuclei seen in CCP-RCC. Most clear cell RCCs are negative with CK7, although focal CK7 expression can be seen in and around cystic areas. Diffuse CK7 expression in the majority of the tumor is not a characteristic of clear cell type RCC [11]. Clear cell RCCs typically show diffuse membranous reactivity with CA-IX [12] and CD10 [7, 13] and commonly lack reactivity to AMACR [14] and HMWCK [15].

CCP-RCC have also been reported in patients with VHL disease [16, 17], an autosomal dominant disorder associated with mutations in the VHL tumor suppressor gene located on short arm of chromosome 3. One recent study [16] reported that these tumors noted in 3 patients with VHL disease had the characteristic morphology and immunoprofile of sporadic CCP-RCC and also lacked 3p deletion. However, another study [17] has reported that the majority of these CCP-RCC-like tumors (12/14) arising in patients with VHL disease lack the characteristic immunoprofile of sporadic CCP- RCC and frequently demonstrate chromosome 3p deletion. Overall, based on the current available data, it appears that that CCP-RCC may occur in VHL disease and should be included in the differential diagnosis when working up cystic and/or bilateral renal tumors with clear cell features in this clinical setting.

PRCCs are the second most common subtype of RCCs and account for 10–15% of all RCCs. These tumors have a unique genotype characterized by trisomy of chromosomes 7 and 17 and loss of chromosome Y. These tumors commonly show a predominant papillary or tubulo-papillary architecture mimicking CCP-RCC; however, they typically lack the homogenous optically clear cytoplasm seen in CCP-RCC. Delahunt and Eble [16] proposed a morphologic subdivision of PRCCs into type 1 and type 2 PRCCs for prognostic purposes. This subdivision is now included in the current WHO classification of renal carcinomas. Type 1 PRCCs, which are more common, are characterized by papillae lined by small cells with low nuclear grade and scant amphophilic cytoplasm arranged in a single layer. They frequently show aggregates of foamy macrophages within fibrovascular cores, cholesterol clefts, and foci of necrosis, all of which are typically absent in CCP-RCC. Although type 1 PRCCs are characteristically positive with AMACR, CK7, and CD10, they are usually negative or only focally positive with CA-IX [1, 11, 17]. Type 2 PRCCs are composed of tumor cells with high Fuhrman nuclear grade, abundant eosinophilic (oncocytic) cytoplasm and pseudostratification of nuclei on papillary cores. Type 2 PRCCs are unlikely to be confused be with the low-grade CCP-RCC.

Translocation-associated RCCs are a rare subtype of RCCs. They are more frequent in pediatric and young adults [1, 17] although a few cases have been described in adults [18]. These tumors typically show prominent papillary and/or solid alveolar growth patterns and are composed of cells with high nuclear grade and clear to granular, eosinophilic cytoplasm. Cells lined exclusively by clear cells are rare. Psammoma bodies are typically present [17]. These carcinomas are usually negative or only focally positive with epithelial markers (CK cocktail, CK7, epithelial membrane antigen, EMA) and vimentin. Transcription factor E3 (TFE3) and transcription factor EB (TFEB) are highly sensitive and specific markers for translocation-associated RCC, which are negative in CCP-RCC. These tumors are described in detail subsequently in this chapter.

Tubulocystic Carcinoma

Tubulocystic carcinoma was originally described in 1956 and classified as low-grade collecting duct carcinoma [19, 20]. Recently, it has become generally accepted that tubulocystic and collecting duct carcinomas are separate tumors from a clinical and molecular perspective, and the current name of tubulocystic carcinoma of the kidney was proposed in 2004 [19, 21]. While some argue that tubulocystic carcinoma is a distinct entity which deserves a separate designation [19], there are some studies that have found compelling evidence of a link between tubulocystic carcinoma and PRCC; first, tubulocystic carcinoma is more often multicentric, similar to papillary carcinoma. Second, tubulocystic carcinoma and papillary carcinoma often occur concurrently and can be intimately admixed. Finally, tubulocystic carcinomas have a similar immunohistochemical and molecular phenotype to PRCC [22]. Whether or not tubulocystic carcinoma is a distinct entity or a tumor closely related to PRCC has not been currently resolved.

Tubulocystic carcinomas are rare; in one study this subtype accounted for <1% of all RCCs [23]. All reported cases have occurred in adults (ranging from 30 to 94), with a male to female ratio of 3–7:1.

Gross

Tubulocystic carcinomas involve the cortex and/or the medulla, and can range from subcentimeter to large (17 cm). They have a distinctive gross appearance similar to "swiss cheese" or "bubble wrap" due to tightly clustered dilated cysts [19, 22, 24, 25].

Microscopy

Microscopically, tubulocystic carcinomas are well circumscribed and composed primarily of variably dilated cysts which are relatively evenly spaced in a fibrotic, hyalinized stroma. No background racemose type vascularity is typically present. The cysts are lined by a single layer of flat to columnar cells with granular oncocytic cytoplasm and nuclei with prominent nucleoli, similar to Fuhrman nuclear grade 3 (Fig. 26.2a). A characteristic feature is the presence of incomplete septae which are free-floating within cystic spaces (Fig. 26.2b). Occasional cysts can be quite dilated up to 1 cm, and prominent hobnailing of the cells can be present. Tumors can occasionally have focal clearing in the cytoplasm of the cells. Very focal cellular stratification and very focal

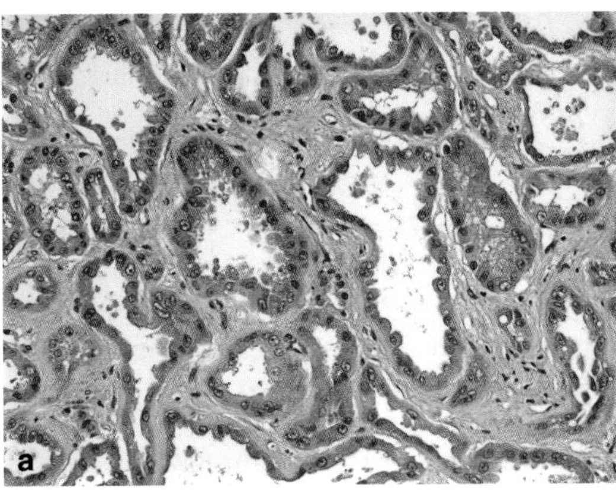

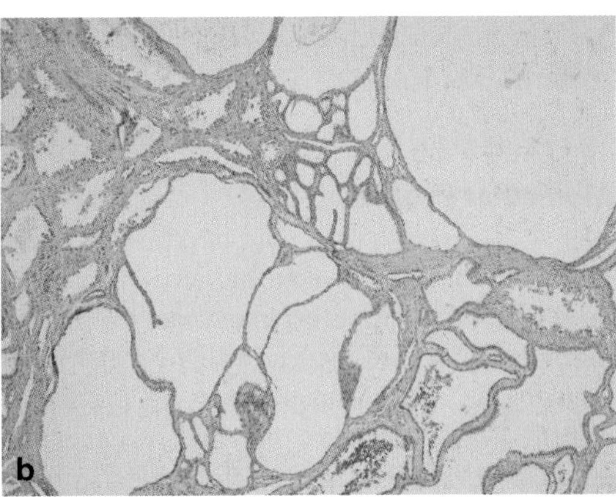

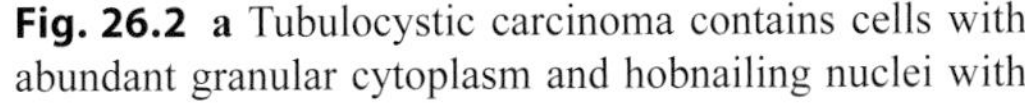

Fig. 26.2 **a** Tubulocystic carcinoma contains cells with abundant granular cytoplasm and hobnailing nuclei with prominent nucleoli. **b** Cystic spaces containing incomplete septae in tubulocystic carcinoma

papillae within the cysts have been described; however, prominent or extensive papillary architecture is not a typical feature and should prompt consideration of an admixed component of PRCC. Increased mitoses, necrosis, and angiolymphatic invasion are not typically present. Desmoplastic stroma and cellular ovarian type stroma are absent [19, 22, 24, 25]. Exceptional cases of tubulocystic carcinoma with poorly differentiated areas, some of which resemble collecting duct carcinoma, have been described [26].

In some studies, tubulocystic carcinomas have been found to be more often multicentric (up to 20% in one series), similar to the rate of multicentricity in PRCC, and higher than the rates of multicentricity seen in other subtypes of RCC [22]. In other series, multicentricity rates in tubulocystic carcinoma were low (6%) [19]. Also, in several series, concurrent or admixed papillary renal neoplasms were common (50% in one larger series); the associated papillary neoplasms included papillary adenomas and type 1 and type 2 PRCCs [22, 25]. In those cases in which the PRCC was intimately admixed with the tubulocystic carcinoma, most had similar cellular morphology in both the tubulocystic and papillary areas [22]. This association with papillary renal neoplasms has not, however, been reported in other series [19].

The appropriate way to classify carcinomas which have both a tubulocystic and papillary component is somewhat controversial; some have recommended classifying such tumors as "renal cell carcinoma, unclassified type, with tubulocystic features" [22]. This would require close communication with the clinical team, however, because some clinicians consider "unclassified type" to necessarily indicate a high-grade aggressive RCC.

Immunoprofile

Tubulocystic carcinomas are typically positive for CK8, CK18, and CK19; most are negative for CK34betaE12, with a few rare cases exhibiting very focal positivity. Tumors are variably positive for CK7, with some series reporting heterogeneous staining for CK7 in most of their cases and others reporting only very focal or weak staining in the majority of their cases. AMACR, CD10, and kidney specific cadherin are frequently strongly positive in tubulocystic carcinomas. PAX-2 is described as being positive in only a subset of cases. Tubulocystic carcinomas are positive for PAX-8, vimentin, and RCC Ma [19, 22–25]. In a few cases in which a papillary RCC component was admixed with the tubulocystic carcinoma and for which immunohistochemical stains were performed, the papillary and tubulocystic component had a similar immunohistochemical profile [22].

Molecular Profile

One study has shown that the gene expression profiles of tubulocystic carcinoma and collecting duct carcinomas are distinct, with the majority of tubulocystic carcinomas showing a statistically significant relative overexpression of vimentin, p53, and AMACR, compared to collecting duct carcinomas [21]. In a few studies, the majority of tubulocystic carcinomas had a molecular profile similar to papillary carcinomas (gains of chromosomes 7 and 17 and loss of chromosome Y). In a few tumors with both a papillary carcinoma and tubulocystic carcinoma component which were analyzed, the molecular profile was found to be similar in both components. Notably, however, there is a subset of tubulocystic carcinomas which does not harbor the characteristic molecular changes of PRCC [22].

Prognosis

The vast majority of reported cases of pure tubulocystic carcinoma presented at low stage (pT1), and the majority of patients were disease-free at the follow-up after resection. However, rare cases of pure tubulocystic carcinomas have been reported to present at high stage (pT3 or with pelvic lymph node metastases), and occasional patients develop either local recurrence or distant metastasis. Interestingly, while all of the described tubulocystic carcinomas have had high nuclear grade features, the majority of tumors had a good prognosis, indicating that Fuhrman nuclear grade may not be predictive of prognosis in this tumor [19, 23–25]. Tubulocystic carcinomas with admixed high-grade PRCC or with poorly differentiated areas may, as expected, have worse prognoses. In one study, a patient with admixed tubulocystic carcinoma and high-grade PRCC developed metastases attributed to the high-grade PRCC [25]. In another study of tubulocystic carcinomas with poorly differentiated areas, two of the three patients had follow up; one had a local recurrence, and the other patient died of distant metastases [26].

Differential Diagnoses

The main items in the differential diagnosis for tubulocystic carcinoma primarily include cystic entities of the kidney, such as benign renal cysts, oncocytoma with prominent cystic change, multilocular cystic RCC, and cystic nephroma/mixed epithelial and stromal tumors (MESTs) of the kidney. On core biopsies (when the entire lesion is not available for examination), it may even be difficult to distinguish tubulocystic carcinoma from dilated nonneoplastic renal tubules. Typically, benign cysts and dilated nonneoplastic tubules are lined by unremarkable attenuated tubular epithelium; hobnailing cells and high nuclear grade features with prominent nucleoli should not be present. The presence of a distinct mass seen grossly or radiographically may also be helpful in distinguishing dilated nonneoplastic tubules from a tubulocystic carcinoma. While tubulocystic carcinomas have high grade, irregular nuclei with chromatin alteration, oncocytomas with prominent cystic change retain relatively round, uniform low-grade appearing nuclei with even chromatin and occasional nucleoli; prominent hobnailing is not typically present, and cystic areas may merge with areas of more conventional nests of oncocytoma. Multilocular cystic RCCs are lined by low-grade cells with optically clear cytoplasm, identical to those seen in low-grade clear cell RCCs; cells with granular eosinophilic cytoplasm, high-grade nuclei, and prominent hobnailing should not be present. Cystic nephromas are composed of multiple cysts with lining epithelium that can range from attenuated to cuboidal or columnar to hobnailing; MESTs, which some believe to be closely related to cystic nephromas, can have similar cysts or may have more variably sized cysts, with some small branching tubules or cysts which can resemble glandular epithelium; ciliated epithelium and epithelium with clear cytoplasm may also be present. In both cystic nephromas and MESTs, the nuclei of the lining epithelium are typically low grade, without prominent nucleoli. In addition, cystic nephromas and MESTs are characterized by intervening cellular spindled "ovarian type" stroma which is estrogen receptor (ER) and progesterone receptor (PR) positive and can occasionally show cellular condensation surrounding the cysts, in contrast to the fibrotic, hyalinized stroma seen in tubulocystic carcinomas. Cystic nephromas and MESTs also often have thick walled or proliferating dilated blood vessels within the stroma, and in addition MESTs can have stromal smooth muscle or adipose tissue. The cysts in cystic nephromas and MESTs can be evenly distributed, as in tubulocystic carcinomas; however, in many cystic nephromas and MESTs, the cysts are clustered, with prominent intervening stroma, which would be unusual in a tubulocystic carcinoma [19, 22].

The characteristic incomplete septae which are free-floating within cystic spaces can be helpful, as these are unusual in the other cystic entities mentioned above. In difficult cases, immunostains may be helpful; tubulocystic carcinomas lack an ER, PR positive stroma and are AMACR positive.

Acquired-Cystic-Disease-Associated Renal Cell Carcinoma

ESRD has been known to be associated with an increased risk of developing RCC, with an overall incidence of renal carcinomas in end-stage kidneys of about 3–7 % [1]. A large clinicopathologic series published in 2006 by Tickoo et al. [2] proposed acquired-cystic-disease-associated renal cell carcinoma (ACD-associated RCC) as a specific subtype of renal cancer arising in end-stage renal disease. These tumors are commonly found incidentally on imaging for surveillance of chronic renal disease.

Acquired cystic kidney disease develops in approximately half of patients undergoing dialysis. While cysts are present in 8 % of all patients beginning dialysis, both the number and size of cysts progressively increase as the duration of dialysis increases (>90 % incidence after 10 years or more of dialysis). The type of dialysis (peritoneal vs. hemodialysis) does not appear to be significant. These patients are at increased risk of developing RCC, with a risk 100 times that of the general population. ACD-associated RCC is becoming a well-recognized subtype of RCC and is diagnosed based on the characteristic histologic appearance and the background cystic disease. These RCCs are the most common subtype of RCC noted in end-stage kidneys and are almost always seen in patients on dialysis. Although more common in end-stage kidneys with ACD, where ACD-associated RCCs account for 46 % of dominant masses, ACD-associated RCCs can also occur in noncystic end-stage kidneys.

It is important to remember that other RCC subtypes can be seen in both acquired cystic and noncystic end-stage kidneys. They include well-documented subtypes such as PRCC, clear cell RCC and chromophobe RCC which account for approximately 40 % of all RCCs arising in end-stage kidneys. Several causes have been proposed for the increased incidence of RCCs in ESRD including depressed cellular and humoral immunity in renal failure, impaired antioxidant defense, chronic infections and inflammation with release of free radicals causing deoxyribonucleic acid (DNA) damage and mutations, use of immunosuppressive medications, and proliferative activity induced by the oxalate crystals [1].

Gross

ACD-associated RCCs are commonly multifocal and bilateral. They can have a thick fibrous capsule and can appear to have arisen in cysts. They are usually well circumscribed and frequently show foci of hemorrhage, necrosis, and calcification. The background kidney can be normal in size or small and scarred. In acquired cystic end-stage kidneys, numerous cortical and medullary cysts are noted, ranging in size from 0.5 to 3 cm. The cysts initially form in the cortex, but in advanced cases medullary cysts can occur.

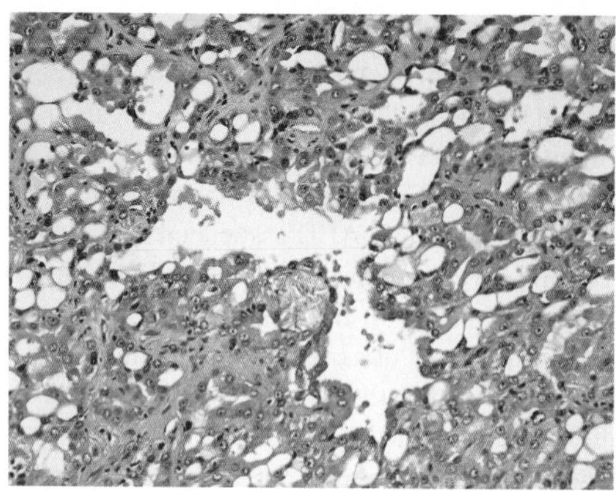

Fig. 26.3 Numerous vacuoles present within acquired cystic disease-associated carcinoma. Associated oxalate crystals are evident

Microscopy

Cells in these RCCs are arranged in a variety of architectural patterns including acinar, papillary, solid, and cystic. The tumor cells are large with abundant eosinophilic/oncocytic cytoplasm and large nuclei with prominent nucleoli, reminiscent of Fuhrman grade 3 nuclei. Frequent cytoplasmic lumina confer the characteristic "cribriform" or "sieve-like" architecture to this tumor. Another characteristic feature seen in the vast majority of these tumors is the presence of abundant intratumoral oxalate crystals [2, 27, 28]. These crystals are seen within the tumor and are not associated with foci of necrosis or inflammation (Fig. 26.3). Focal areas composed of cells with clear cytoplasm are not uncommon; such foci can mimic clear cell RCC. Sarcomatoid and rhabdoid features may be seen in a subset of cases. In the background kidney, especially in the setting of acquired cystic kidney disease, there are numerous cysts lined by a similar population of eosinophilic cells. While these cysts are usually distributed throughout the kidney, occasionally they can be clustered together.

Immunoprofile

Tumor cells are diffusely positive with AMACR and usually negative or only focally positive with CK7. CK AE1/AE3, CD10, and RCC marker are typically positive, and lack of high-molecular weight CK expression has been reported [1, 29, 30]. In our anecdotal, unpublished experience, these tumors are diffusely positive with PAX-8. The cysts in the background kidney are also usually diffusely positive with AMACR and negative or only focally positive with CK7.

Molecular Profile

ACD-associated RCCs lack the characteristic changes seen in clear cell RCCs (VHL gene mutation or 3p deletion) or PRCCs (trisomy of chromosomes 7 and 17 as well as loss of chromosome Y). Comparative genomic hybridization (CGH) and fluorescence in situ hybridization (FISH) studies have shown chromosomal gains on multiple chromosomes including chromosomes 3, 7, 16, 17, and Y. Chromosomal losses are uncommon while frequent gains on chromosomes 3 and Y have been reported [30, 31].

Prognosis

Most tumors are small and have a good prognosis. Metastasis is rare and when present is usually to regional lymph nodes. Rare cases have presented with extrarenal extension, renal vein extension (pT3 disease), and/or sarcomatoid and rhabdoid differentiation [32].

Differential Diagnosis

The most common differential diagnosis of ACD-associated RCC includes PRCC, clear cell RCC, and RCCs with oncocytic cytoplasm.

PRCCs as mentioned previously can be subdivided into type 1 and type 2 PRCCs for prognostic purposes [16]. Type 2 PRCCs may be confused with ACD-associated RCCs as both can have tubulopapillary architecture as well as cells with predominantly oncocytic cytoplasm and high-grade nuclei with prominent nucleoli;

rarely type 1 PRCCs, which tend to show scant basophilic or focally clear cytoplasm with low-grade nuclei, may also be confused with ACD-associated RCC. While PRCCs can be seen in the setting of cystic end-stage kidneys, these tumors lack the characteristic intratumoral oxalate crystals as well as the cytoplasmic lumina imparting a cribriform appearance seen in ACD-associated RCCs. Also, while both tumors express diffuse AMACR expression, the vast majority of PRCCs are diffusely positive with CK7 unlike ACD-associated RCCs.

Classic clear cell RCCs can occasionally cause diagnostic confusion, as ACD-associated RCCs can show foci with clear cell morphology mimicking clear cell RCCs. However, ACD-associated RCCs lack the characteristic delicate sinusoidal "racemose" vasculature characteristically seen in the majority of clear cell RCCs. Although clear cell RCCs can frequently have eosinophilic granular cytoplasm with high-grade nuclei showing prominent nucleoli, clear cell RCCs lack the varied architecture including papillary and cribriform patterns as well as the oxalate crystals frequently seen in ACD-associated RCCs. While both these tumor types are usually negative with CK7, clear cell RCCs are also negative or show only focal AMACR expression. Strong, diffuse, membranous expression with CA-IX is commonly seen in clear cell RCCs. In our experience, CD10 is not very useful in distinguishing these tumors.

RCCs with oncocytic cytoplasm such as chromophobe RCCs or high-grade unclassified type RCCs with oncocytic cytoplasm can rarely enter into the differential diagnosis; careful attention to immunomorphologic features can usually resolve the diagnosis. ACD-associated RCCs lack the plant-like architecture, koilocytic atypia, and diffuse CK7 positivity commonly noted in chromophobe RCCs. Unclassified RCC is a diagnosis of exclusion; these tumors lack the characteristic morphology and oxalate crystals seen in ACD-associated RCCs.

Translocation-Associated Renal Cell Carcinomas

While renal carcinomas associated with Xp11.2 translocations/TFE3 gene fusions have been included in the most recent WHO classification [33], the spectrum of translocation-associated RCCs has greatly expanded. This group of closely related carcinomas is defined by a translocation involving one of the members of the microphthalmia-associated transcription factor (MiTF) family, which codes for basic helix-loop-helix/leucine zipper transcription factors. Members of this family include TFE3, TFEB, TFEC, and MiTF. They share homologous DNA binding and activation domains, and may have functional overlap; MiTF is important in melanogenesis. RCCs which harbor these translocations are collectively referred to as MiTF/TFE family translocation-associated carcinomas and include Xp11.2/TFE3 translocation-associated carcinoma and its purported subtype, melanotic Xp11 translocation tumor, as well as TFEB (t(6;11)) associated carcinoma [34–36].

Xp11.2 Translocation-Associated RCC

Xp11.2/TFE3 translocation-associated RCCs are rare, with reported incidences in large series of adult neoplasms of 1.6–4.2%. This carcinoma constitutes a much higher proportion of RCC in children and young adults; reported incidences in this population range widely (20–76%) depending on the study and the age cutoff. However, given the rarity of RCC in children and young adults, it is likely that the absolute number of Xp11.2 translocation associated carcinomas is higher in adult populations than in pediatric populations [17, 36]. A significant proportion (15%) are associated with a history of chemotherapy [37].

Microscopy

The most characteristic morphology of Xp11.2 translocation-associated carcinomas is architectural heterogeneity; within any given tumor, cells

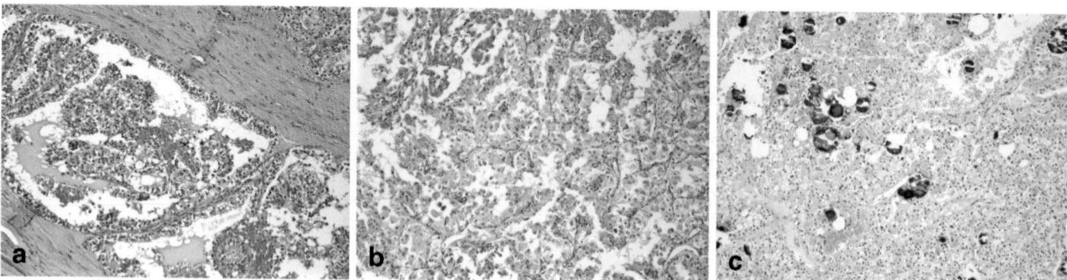

Fig. 26.4 Xp11 translocation-associated carcinoma showing **a** clear cells arranged around true papillae, **b** areas with an alveolar architecture, and **c** numerous psammoma bodies

can be variably arranged in sheets, nests, trabeculae, true papillae, or pseudopapillae. The cells typically have voluminous cytoplasm which can range from eosinophilic and granular to clear and can have bulging cell borders. Within any tumor the nuclear grade can vary, but these are almost uniformly at least focally of high Fuhrman nuclear grade. Clear cells arranged in some areas around true papillae and in other areas in solid sheets and nests with prominent cell borders is a relatively specific morphologic feature seen in many of these tumors (Fig. 26.4a). Many of these tumors exhibit, at least focally, a pseudoalveolar pattern in which cells are arranged in alveoli with central cellular discohesion (Fig. 26.4b). In some areas, the discohesion can lead to the formation of pseudopapillae. Prominent psammoma bodies and scattered xanthoma cells have been described in some tumors (Fig. 26.4c). Different gene fusions may lead to differing morphologic features; those with the ASPL-TFE3 typically are composed of large polygonal cells with abundant cytoplasm and high-grade nuclei arranged in an alveolar or pseudopapillary pattern. Psammoma bodies can be extensive. In contrast, those with the PRCC-TFE3 gene fusion typically have tumor cells with less abundant cytoplasm arranged in nests; psammoma bodies are rare or absent [34, 36, 38, 39]. Recently, newly described Xp11 translocation-associated RCCs have expanded the morphologic spectrum; tumors with a dual population of cells, some with voluminous abundant cytoplasm and prominent cell borders and some with less abundant cytoplasm arranged around hyaline material, similar to that seen in t(6;11) associated RCCs; tumors with pleomorphic neoplastic giant cells; tumors with hobnailing cells arranged in tubules and cysts; tumors with low-grade spindled areas; tumors with prominent cystic change; and tumors resembling infiltrative urothelial carcinoma have been described [18, 40, 41].

Immunohistochemistry

The majority of Xp11.2 translocation-associated carcinomas are either negative for or only very focally positive for epithelial markers such as CK cocktail, CK CAM5.2, CK7, and EMA. The other characteristic immunostain is for the mutant (chimeric) TFE3 protein, which is overexpressed relative to native TFE3; the immunostain utilizes an antibody directed against the C-terminal portion of TFE3, which is preserved across all described gene fusions. Reported sensitivity (82–97.5 %) and specificity (79–99.6 %) for this immunostain vary widely [42–44]. This is likely due to differences in methodology. In addition, the immunostain can be technically challenging, and depending on fixation of the tissue and the methodology of the stain, native TFE3 can pick up the stain; typically Xp11.2 translocation carcinomas exhibit moderate to strong, diffuse nuclear staining that can be appreciated at low power. Therefore, appropriate caution should be used in interpreting this immunostain; comparison with the staining pattern in the adjacent normal kidney is helpful, and it should be interpreted in the context of the overall morphology as well as with any supporting molecular findings [36, 42]. These carcinomas frequently label for PAX-2 and PAX-8. Vimentin is usually negative or only very focally positive. The tumors are typically positive for CD10, RCC, and AMACR

[38, 39, 45, 46]. CA-IX is either negative or only very focally positive, usually around areas of necrosis [46]. One relatively new marker that shows promise is cathepsin-K, a protease whose expression is driven by MiTF in osteoclasts; cytoplasmic expression of cathepsin-K can help distinguish MiTF/TFE RCCs from other RCCs. It has been found to be relatively specific but not particularly sensitive for Xp11 translocation carcinomas. Interestingly, in one study cathepsin-K was found to be positive in RCCs harboring the PRCC-TFE3 gene fusion but not in those harboring ASPSCR1-TFE3 gene fusion, suggesting that expression of this marker may be dependent on the particular gene fusion expressed [47, 48].

Molecular/Genetic Profile

Xp11.2/TFE3 translocation-associated carcinomas most commonly harbor either t(X;17)(p11.2;q25), which leads to a fusion of the transcription factor gene TFE3 with the ASPL gene; or t(X;1)(p11.2;q21), which leads to a fusion of the TFE3 gene with the PRCC gene. Other less commonly described translocations in these RCCs include t(X;1)(p11.2;p34), which leads to the fusion of the TFE3 gene with the PSF gene; inv(X)(p11;q12), which leads to a fusion of the TFE3 gene to the NonO (p54nrb) gene; and t(X;17)(p11.2;q23), which leads to the fusion of the TFE gene to the CLTC gene. RCCs with t(X;3)(p11.2;q23) and t(X;10)(11.2;q23) have been reported; the gene fusion partners are unknown. Such translocations can be diagnosed through FISH analysis or cytogenetic analysis [36]. Reverse transcription polymerase chain reaction (RT-PCR) has also been utilized in the literature, but this is somewhat limited in practice due to the variable gene fusions seen in these tumors.

Prognosis

The prognosis and outcome of these carcinomas is somewhat controversial. In young patients, most series agree that Xp11.2 translocation carcinomas generally present at a higher stage (III/IV) compared to other RCCs [49, 50]. However, some have suggested that despite presenting at higher stage, many have a relatively good prognosis and indolent course [49]; in one series, it was argued that lymph node metastases in the absence of hematogenous disease spread did not necessarily portend a worse prognosis, at least in the short term [49, 51]. Others report poorer outcome (overall and disease free survival) in pediatric patients with TFE3+RCC as compared to those with TFE3-RCC [50]. Complicating these data is the fact that most series have a relatively short follow-up interval, and there have been several case reports of late recurrences occurring as long as 20–30 years after the initial resection [52, 53]. More extensive, long-term follow-up data need to be collected before any definitive conclusions about the prognosis of these RCCs can be made. In adults, Xp11.2 translocation RCCs generally present at higher stage, and the clinical course is more aggressive as compared to other subtypes of RCC, with several deaths due to disease reported [18, 36].

Differential Diagnosis

Because of architectural variation in these tumors, they can, at least focally, mimic other RCC subtypes, such as clear cell RCC and PRCC. Clear cell RCCs can have pseudopapillae, but usually do not have true papillae. Psammomatous calcifications and xanthoma cells are not commonly seen in clear cell RCC. In addition, extensive areas in which cells with voluminous cytoplasm are arranged in sheets without intervening vascular stroma is unusual in clear cell RCC and should prompt consideration of translocation RCC. PRCC can occasionally have true papillae lined by clear cells, but these clear cells are typically in areas of prior hemorrhage, and associated hemosiderin and reactive changes may be seen in close association with the clear cells. Solid nests and sheets of clear cells are not commonly seen in PRCC.

Finally, clear cell PRCC is also often in the differential diagnosis; these carcinomas are typically low grade, in contrast to Xp11 translocation RCC, and cells are arranged in tubules, nests, or sheets, usually without an intervening vascular network. A diagnostic clue to clear cell PRCC, as discussed previously, is the linear arrangement of apically placed nuclei. Clear cell PRCC can

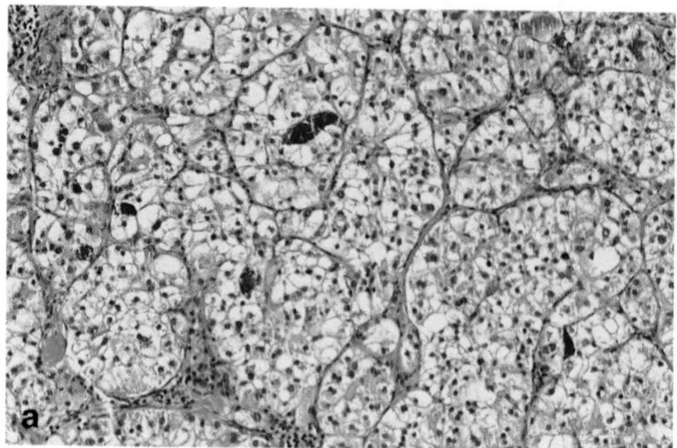

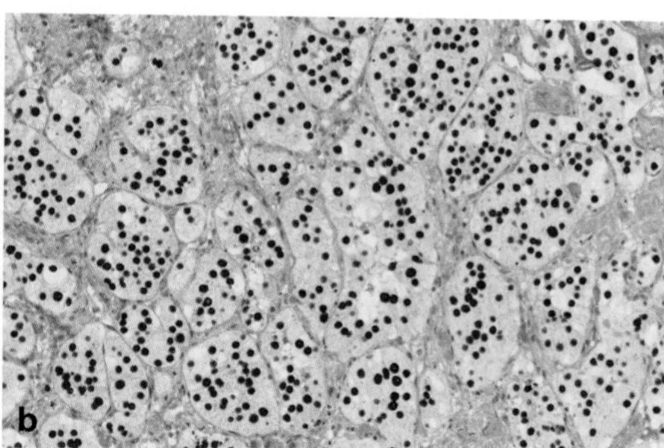

Fig. 26.5 **a** Melanotic Xp11 translocation renal cancer with nests of polygonal cells with finely granular cytoplasm and brown intracytoplasmic pigment. **b** Nuclear immunoexpression of TFE3 in melanotic Xp11 translocation renal cancer

be cystic, which is relatively uncommon in Xp11 translocation RCC, and do not often have psammomatous calcifications.

Occasionally, however, Xp11 translocation RCCs can almost completely mimic either a clear cell or PRCC, and the only clue is the patient's young age. In contrast to Xp11 translocation RCCs, clear cell, papillary, and clear cell PRCCs are usually diffusely strongly positive for epithelial markers CK AE1/3, Cam 5.2, and EMA; positive for vimentin; and negative for cathepsin K and TFE3. In addition, clear cell RCCs are often diffusely strongly positive for CA-IX, and PRCCs may be positive for CK7 (more commonly in type 1 PRCCs). Clear cell PRCCs are typically also diffusely strongly positive for CK7 [54].

Melanotic Xp11 Translocation-Associated Renal Cancer

Melanotic Xp11 translocation-associated renal cancer is a recently described entity for which there are only a handful of small series and case reports; only five definitive cases have been reported. However, given how recently this entity has been described, it is quite possible that some putative cases of primary melanomas or primary epithelioid perivascular epithelioid cell tumors (PEComas) of the kidney do, in fact, represent melanotic Xp11 translocation-associated renal cancer. While the majority of these tumors have been reported in children (ages 11, 12, and 14), a few reports occurred in slightly older patients (ages 18 and 30). All of these tumors by definition harbor a TFE3 translocation. In addition, in all reported cases, melanin pigment is present in at least a subset of the tumor cells [35, 41, 55, 56].

Microscopy

These tumors are composed predominantly of polygonal epithelioid cells with rounded nuclei, only occasional nucleoli, and clear to finely granular cytoplasm arranged in sheets or nests with a background capillary vascular network. Distinctive cellular borders may be present. Focal cellular pleomorphism has been reported in one case. One reported case had a distinctive morphology, composed of areas with cells with abundant clear cytoplasm, resembling clear cell RCC and other areas with nests of cells with granular cytoplasm, small nuclei, and central discohesive and pseudoalveolar patterns. In this case, necrosis was also present. Other unusual features described in one case included stroma with focal perivascular eccentric hyaline sclerosis. Pigment, described predominantly as fine and granular but also focally coarse and refractile and proven in some cases to be melanin pigment through Fontana Masson stains, is present in the cytoplasm of the tumor cells, and ranges from either being present focally to being extensive and throughout the tumor (Fig. 26.5a) [35, 55, 56].

Immunohistochemistry

These tumors typically are negative for epithelial markers (CKs and EMA). They are negative for

S100 and muscle markers such as smooth muscle actin, muscle specific actin, and desmin. In contrast to conventional Xp11 translocation-associated RCCs, they are positive for melanocytic markers HMB45 and Melan A and are negative for renal tubular markers, including RCC, CD10, PAX-2 and PAX-8. All described cases have expressed TFE3 nuclear staining (Fig. 26.5b) [35, 41, 55, 56].

Molecular Profile

In one reported case, the gene fusion partner for TFE3 was PSF, and in the remaining four cases, the partner was not specified (although in two, it was found not to be ASPL). In four cases, the gene fusion was confirmed through FISH for TFE3; in the final case, the gene fusion was confirmed through RT-PCR [35, 41, 55, 56].

Differential Diagnosis

The differential diagnosis is difficult and includes PEComa, primary melanoma, and other carcinomas. PEComa represents probably the most challenging differential diagnosis, as melanotic Xp11 renal cancer can have many features of a PEComa (epithelioid morphology, eccentric hyaline sclerosis of vasculature, positivity for melanocytic markers). Renal PEComas include epithelioid angiomyolipomas (AMLs) and lower-grade oncocytoma-like AMLs. However, most renal PEComas in children arise in the setting of tuberous sclerosis. PEComas may also exhibit spindling, a feature not typically seen in melanotic Xp11 translocation renal cancers; they usually do not exhibit pigmentation, and are usually positive for muscle markers (actin, desmin) and negative for TFE3. Primary renal melanoma is exceedingly rare, and in most cases involves the renal pelvis (possibly due to origin in the urothelium). Most cases of renal melanoma are associated with a disseminated disease from a known primary melanoma. In difficult cases, immunostains may be helpful; most melanomas are S100 positive and should be TFE3 negative. Clear cell RCC is also in the differential; the presence of melanin pigment, the eccentric hyalinization of background stromal capillaries (if present), and the negativity for epithelial markers, negativity for renal tubular markers (CD10, PAX-2/8, RCC) and positivity for melanocytic markers and TFE3 favor a melanotic Xp11 renal cancer over a clear cell RCC [35, 55, 56].

Prognosis

There is some controversy as to whether these melanotic Xp11 renal cancers represent a variant of a primary renal melanoma, PEComa, or carcinoma as they have overlapping immunomorphologic features with these entities. The overall current consensus is that they represent an entity on the spectrum of Xp11 translocation RCCs, with a phenotype that most closely approximates a PEComa [35]. The recent description of extrarenal TFE3+ neoplasms, which are currently classified as PEComas but which are muscle marker negative, occur in young patients, do not have any association with tuberous sclerosis, and seem to have a different pathogenetic mechanism from conventional PEComas which may be another entity that overlaps with melanotic Xp11 renal cancer and conventional Xp11 RCC.

Given the rarity of this tumor and its recent description, its behavior is not well described; however, the majority (three of five) of reported cases presented with high-stage tumors and widely metastatic disease, and one patient has died of disease, suggesting that at least some of these tumors behave aggressively [35, 41, 55, 56].

t(6;11)-Associated RCC

RCCs which harbor a translocation between the gene encoding TFEB on 6p21 and Alpha on 11q12 (t(6;11)-associated RCCs) were first described in 2001; to date, fewer than 30 cases have been described. While the majority of cases have been described in children and adolescents (<20 years), a few cases have been described in adults (30–54 years) [57–61].

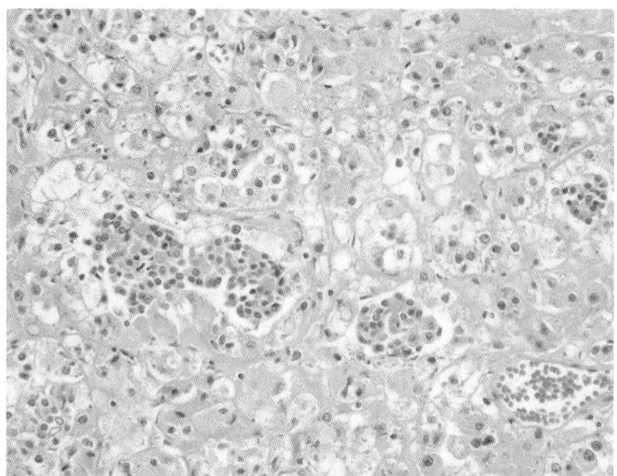

Fig. 26.6 t(6;11) associated RCC with larger polygonal cells and smaller lower-grade cells surrounding basement membrane material in pseudorosettes. (Courtesy of Dr. Victor Reuter, Memorial Sloan-Kettering Cancer Center, New York)

Microscopy

These tumors classically have a solid, nested architecture and have a dual cell population. The majority of the cells resemble those seen in clear cell RCC; they are polygonal with abundant clear to eosinophilic cytoplasm and have rounded nuclei with prominent nucleoli consistent with Fuhrman nuclear grade 3. These cells can be arranged in tubules or nests with a prominent intervening background capillary network or in sheets without any intervening vasculature. The second, smaller population consists of cells having lower grade nuclei with dense chromatin and more scant eosinophilic cytoplasm, arranged in pseudorosettes around hyaline basement membrane material, somewhat reminiscent of Call-Exner bodies (Fig. 26.6). These clusters of smaller cells often are within acini lined by the larger, polygonal cells. Abortive papillae, psammomatous calcifications, and pigmentation have also been described in some tumors. Mitoses are rare, and necrosis is typically absent [57, 59]. Recently, the morphologic spectrum of TFEB translocation RCCs has expanded; a tumor with epithelioid eosinophilic cells, spindling, admixed adipose tissue and dysplastic vessels resembling epithelioid AML; a tumor with a dual cell population with larger polygonal cells with reticulated eosinophilic cytoplasm and prominent cell borders and a second population of smaller cells with perinuclear haloes resembling chromophobe RCC; a tumor with oncocytic cells arranged in true papillae resembling papillary RCC; tumors resembling clear cell RCC with either cystic change or extensive hyalinization and ossification; a tumor with variable morphology, with some areas resembling oncocytoma and some resembling clear cell RCC; and tumors with areas resembling Xp11 RCC have been described [58, 60, 61].

Immunohistochemistry

The most specific immunohistochemical marker is for the overexpressed mutant (chimeric) TFEB protein, which in one series showed moderate to strong nuclear staining in all seven of their molecularly confirmed cases, and was negative in all (1089) other neoplasms tested. Of note, weak (1+) staining for TFEB was noted in a subset of normal lymphocytes [57]. As with the TFE3 immunostain, this immunostain can be technically challenging. Tumors are generally positive for melanocytic markers, HMB45 and Melan A, positive for PAX-8, and positive for vimentin [58]. They are negative for CKs (AE1/3, Cam 5.2, EMA, and CK7), negative for S100, and negative for muscle markers (desmin, myogenin). These tumors are also negative for RCC; CD10 is generally negative, at most being described as very focally positive in a small subset of tumors [57, 61]. These tumors generally show strong diffuse cytoplasmic positivity for cathepsin K and are negative for TFE3 [48, 61].

Molecular Profile

The TFEB gene on 6q21 is, in all cases, fused to the Alpha gene on 11q12, an intron-less gene which does not encode a protein and whose function is unknown. In the literature, the gene fusion has been detected through cytogenetic karyotypic analysis, DNA PCR, RT-PCR, and FISH. Given the constraints of needing fresh tissue for PCR and cytogenetic analysis, and given that the breakpoints in the TFEB and Alpha genes are highly variable, possibly leading to false negative

PCR results, the FISH analysis seems to be the most promising molecular test [58–61].

Prognosis

Given the rarity of these tumors and their recent description, their behavior is not well elucidated; however, the majority appears to behave in an indolent fashion, with most patients disease free after resection. However, at least one patient with a molecularly confirmed case of TFEB translocation tumor has died of disease, indicating that at least a small subset of these tumors behaves aggressively [61].

Differential Diagnosis

The primary differential diagnosis is clear cell RCC, especially in cases in which the tumor is predominantly composed of the large polygonal clear cells and the secondary population of cells with less voluminous cytoplasm and pseudorosette formation around hyaline basement membrane material is inconspicuous or focal. There have been rare cases of t(6;11) RCCs which mimic other subtypes of RCC, such as papillary or chromophobe RCC [58, 60, 61]. Close attention to the dual population of cells and the hyaline basement membrane material, as well as the young age of the patient, can be helpful. Immunohistochemistry can be helpful in difficult cases; clear cell, papillary, and chromophobe RCCs are typically diffusely strongly positive for CKs (AE1/3, CAM5.2) and EMA, in contrast to t(6;11) RCCs. Chromophobe and PRCCs (typically type 1) are positive for CK7. In addition, clear cell and papillary RCCs are positive for CD10 and RCC. The unusual melanocytic marker positive, cathepsin K positive and TFEB positive profile seen in t(6;11) RCCs is also quite helpful in ruling out other RCCs [48, 61]. Finally, there has been one t(6; 11) RCC case which morphologically mimicked an epithelioid AML. AMLs in young patients typically occur in the setting of tuberous sclerosis and, in contrast to t(6;11) RCCs, AMLs are positive for muscle markers and negative for PAX-8, cathepsin K and TFEB.

Thyroid-Like Follicular Carcinoma of the Kidney

Thyroid-like follicular carcinoma of the kidney is a rare renal neoplasm described after publication of the 2004 WHO classification of renal tumors. In 2006, Jung et al. [62] described in a 32-year-old woman a kidney tumor bearing a striking resemblance to follicular carcinoma of the thyroid. Clinical and imaging evaluation of this patient revealed no tumors in the thyroid, and the renal tumor did not express TTF-1 or thyroglobulin. Amin et al. [63] published a series of six similar tumors, the largest series reported to date, for which they proposed the term “Primary Thyroid-Like Follicular Carcinoma of the Kidney.” All six of these patients had no evidence of a primary thyroid tumor upon extensive clinical and radiographic evaluation.

Gross

Thyroid-like follicular carcinomas of the kidney are grossly well-circumscribed tan to brown tumors, ranging in reported cases from 1.9 to 11.8 cm [62–64].

Microscopy

These tumors, often encapsulated, are composed of macrofollicles and microfollicles surrounding

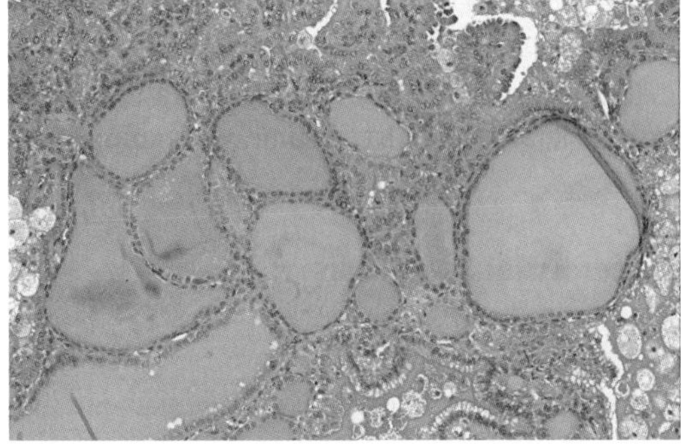

Fig. 26.7 Thyroid-like follicular carcinoma containing cuboidal cells surrounding colloid-like material, resembling a follicular neoplasm of the thyroid gland

inspissated colloid-like material, resembling a follicular neoplasm of the thyroid gland [63–66]. The follicles are lined by bland cuboidal cells with round, regular nuclei, uniform chromatin, and a moderate amount of amphophilic to eosinophilic cytoplasm (Fig. 26.7). Papillary structures and nuclear features of papillary thyroid carcinoma are not present. Significant mitotic activity is not present.

Immunohistochemistry

Primary thyroid-like follicular carcinomas of the kidney by definition lack expression of PAX-8 and thyroglobulin, markers that are expressed in thyroid follicular neoplasms [62–66]. They variably express CK7 and PAX-2, often express vimentin, and typically lack CD10 and RCC antigen [63–66].

Molecular/Genetic Profile

A reliable molecular genetic profile has yet to be described for thyroid-like follicular carcinoma of the kidney. Jung et al. found by CGH analysis of one case multiple genetic alterations, including gain of chromosomes 7q36, 8q24, 12, 16, 17p11-q11, 17q24, 19q, 20q13, 21q22.3, and Xp, and losses of chromosomes 1p36, 3, and 9q21-33[62]. Another case showed chromosomal losses of 1, 3, 7, 9p21, 12, 17, and X by FISH [65]. In the study by Amin et al., CGH analysis of one case detected no abnormalities, and gene expression profiling of three cases demonstrated overexpression of cell cycle regulatory genes, including the mixed lineage leukemia (MLL)/trithorax homolog [63].

Differential Diagnosis

The chief consideration in the differential diagnosis of primary thyroid-like follicular carcinoma of the kidney is a metastasis from a primary thyroid carcinoma. Indeed, this diagnosis should only be accepted once metastatic thyroid carcinoma is ruled out. In most cases of thyroid carcinoma metastatic to the kidney reported in the literature [67–69], a primary tumor was identifiable in the thyroid gland and metastases were widespread. Clinical and radiographic absence of a thyroid mass and metastatic disease to other organs, coupled with lack of TTF-1 and thyroglobulin expression in the kidney tumor, allow for the exclusion of metastatic thyroid carcinoma.

Metastasis from struma ovarii is at least a theoretical, if unlikely, possibility; malignant transformation in struma ovarii is a rare event, and metastases are typically found in the liver, lungs, bones, peritoneum, and omentum [70, 71]. Such a tumor would express TTF-1, and could be excluded in the absence of an ovarian mass.

In addition, some of the more common subtypes of renal epithelial neoplasms (e.g., oncocytoma, clear cell RCC, PRCC, metanephric adenoma) can occasionally contain dilated tubules containing colloid-like material [72, 73]. The finding of areas elsewhere in the tumor more characteristic of these entities would help establish the diagnosis.

Prognosis

Although experience is limited given the rarity of this tumor, these tumors have largely shown indolent behavior, even when metastatic. All of the six patients reported by Amin et al. were alive and well with a mean follow-up of 47 months, including one patient with metastasis to renal hilar lymph nodes [63]. The single patient reported by Sterlacci et al. was alive 5 years after nephrectomy, despite a lung metastasis detected 2 months after primary diagnosis [65].

Aggressive behavior with symptomatic, widely metastatic tumor at presentation has, however, been reported. Dhillon et al. [64] report a case in a 34-year-old woman who presented with intermittent gross hematuria and right flank pain. Computed tomography showed a 6.3 cm right kidney mass and multiple bilateral lung nodules. Biopsy of a lung mass was consistent with thyroid-like follicular carcinoma, and no thyroid nodules were detected by physical examination. After receiving systemic therapy for 1 year, she underwent cytoreductive radical nephrectomy and retroperitoneal lymph node dissection, revealing a primary thyroid-like follicular carcinoma of the kidney with metastases to two retroperitoneal nodes. Follow-up in this case was limited to 3 months, at which time the patient was doing well.

An awareness of the spectrum of described renal neoplasia provides useful prognostic information to patients and may eventually result in therapeutically important distinctions. The number of recognized renal tumors will undoubtedly increase, as there remain tumors that currently defy the classification according to established categories.

References

1. Amin MB, editor. Diagnostic pathology. 1st ed. Manitoba: Amirsys; 2010.
2. Tickoo SK, dePeralta-Venturina MN, Harik LR, Worcester HD, Salama ME, Young AN, et al. Spectrum of epithelial neoplasms in end-stage renal disease: an experience from 66 tumor-bearing kidneys with emphasis on histologic patterns distinct from those in sporadic adult renal neoplasia. Am J Surg Pathol. 2006;30(2):141–53.
3. Gobbo S, Eble JN, Grignon DJ, Martignoni G, MacLennan GT, Shah RB, et al. Clear cell papillary renal cell carcinoma: a distinct histopathologic and molecular genetic entity. Am J Surg Pathol. 2008;32(8):1239–45.
4. Zhou H, Zheng S, Truong LD et al. Clear cell papillary renal cell carcinoma is the fourth most common histologic type of renal cell carcinoma in 290 consecutive nephrectomies for renal cell carcinoma. Hum Pathol 2014; 45(1):59-64.
5. Tickoo SK, Reuter VE. Differential diagnosis of renal tumors with papillary architecture. Adv Anal Pathol 2011;18:120-132.
6. Fine SW, Chen Y, Al-Ahmadie HA, Gopalan A. RVETSK. Immunohistochemical Profile of Clear Cell and Related Renal Cell Cancers, with Emphasis on CK7 and Carbonic Anhydrase-IX (CA-IX) Staining. United States and Canadian Academy of Pathology Annual Meeting; February 2012; Vancouver, BC: Modern Pathology; 2012:204A.
7. Kuroda N, Shiotsu T, Kawada C, Shuin T, Hes O, Michal M, et al. Clear cell papillary renal cell carcinoma and clear cell renal cell carcinoma arising in acquired cystic disease of the kidney: an immunohistochemical and genetic study. Ann Diagn Pathol. 2011;15(4):282–5.
8. Rohan SM, Xiao Y, Liang Y et al. Clear- cell papillary renal cell carcinoma: molecular and immunohistochemical analysis with emphasis on von Hippel Lindau gene and hypoxia-inducible factor pathway-related proteins. Mod Pathol 2011; 24(9): 1207-20.
9. Michal M, Hes O, Nemcova J, Sima R, Kuroda N, Bulimbasic S, et al. Renal angiomyoadenomatous tumor: morphologic, immunohistochemical, and molecular genetic study of a distinct entity. Virchows Arch Int J Pathol. 2009;454(1):89–99.
10. Verine J. Renal angiomyoadenomatous tumor: morphologic, immunohistochemical, and molecular genetic study of a distinct entity. Virchows Arch. 2009;454(4):479–80.
11. Kim MK, Kim S. Immunohistochemical profile of common epithelial neoplasms arising in the kidney. Appl Immunohistochem Mol Morphol. 2002;10(4):332–8.
12. Gupta R, Balzer B, Picken M, Osunkoya AO, Shet T, Alsabeh R, et al. Diagnostic implications of transcription factor Pax 2 protein and transmembrane enzyme complex carbonic anhydrase IX immunoreactivity in adult renal epithelial neoplasms. Am J Surg Pathol. 2009;33(2):241–7.
13. Avery AK, Beckstead J, Renshaw AA, Corless CL. Use of antibodies to RCC and CD10 in the differential diagnosis of renal neoplasms. Am J Surg Pathol. 2000;24(2):203–10.
14. Tretiakova MS, Sahoo S, Takahashi M, Turkyilmaz M, Vogelzang NJ, Lin F, et al. Expression of alpha-methylacyl-CoA racemase in papillary renal cell carcinoma. Am J Surg Pathol. 2004;28(1):69–76.
15. Carvalho JC, Wasco MJ, Kunju LP, Thomas DG, Shah RB. Cluster analysis of immunohistochemical profiles delineates CK7, vimentin, S100A1 and C-kit (CD117) as an optimal panel in the differential diagnosis of renal oncocytoma from its mimics. Histopathology. 2011;58(2):169–79.
16. Delahunt B, Eble JN. Papillary renal cell carcinoma: a clinicopathologic and immunohistochemical study of 105 tumors. Mod Pathol. 1997;10(6):537–44.
17. Wu A, Kunju L, Cheng L, Shah R. Renal cell carcinoma in children and young adults: analysis of clinicopathological, immunohistochemical and molecular characteristics with an emphasis on the spectrum of Xp11.2 translocation-associated and unusual clear cell subtypes. Histopathology. 2008;53:533–44.
18. Argani P, Olgac S, Tickoo S, Goldfischer M, Moch H, Chan D, et al. Xp11 translocation renal cell carcinoma in adults: expanded clinical, pathologic, and genetic spectrum. Am J Surg Pathol. 2007;31:1149–60.
19. Amin MB, MacLennan GT, Gupta R, Grignon D, Paraf F, Vieillefond A, et al. Tubulocystic carcinoma of the kidney: clinicopathologic analysis of 31 cases of a distinctive rare subtype of renal cell carcinoma. Am J Surg Pathol. 2009;33(3):384–92.
20. MacLennan GT, Farrow GM, Bostwick DG. Low-grade collecting duct carcinoma of the kidney: report of 13 cases of low-grade mucinous tubulocystic

renal carcinoma of possible collecting duct origin. Urology. 1997;50(5):679–84.
21. Osunkoya AO, Young AN, Wang W, Netto GJ, Epstein JI. Comparison of gene expression profiles in tubulocystic carcinoma and collecting duct carcinoma of the kidney. Am J Surg Pathol. 2009;33(7):1103–6.
22. Zhou M, Yang XJ, Lopez JI, Shah RB, Hes O, Shen SS, et al. Renal tubulocystic carcinoma is closely related to papillary renal cell carcinoma: implications for pathologic classification. Am J Surg Pathol. 2009;33(12):1840–9.
23. Alexiev BA, Drachenberg CB. Tubulocystic carcinoma of the kidney: a histologic, immunohistochemical, and ultrastructural study. Virchows Arch. 2013;462(5):575–81.
24. Azoulay S, Vieillefond A, Paraf F, Pasquier D, Cussenot O, Callard P, et al. Tubulocystic carcinoma of the kidney: a new entity among renal tumors. Virchows Arch. 2007;451(5):905–9.
25. Yang XJ, Zhou M, Hes O, Shen S, Li R, Lopez J, et al. Tubulocystic carcinoma of the kidney: clinicopathologic and molecular characterization. Am J Surg Pathol. 2008;32(2):177–87.
26. Al-Hussain TO, Cheng L, Zhang S, Epstein JI. Tubulocystic carcinoma of the kidney with poorly differentiated foci: a series of 3 cases with fluorescence in situ hybridization analysis. Hum Pathol. 2013;44(7):1406–11.
27. Kuroda N, Ohe C, Mikami S, Hes O, Michal M, Brunelli M, et al. Review of acquired cystic disease-associated renal cell carcinoma with focus on pathobiological aspects. Histol Histopathol. 2011;26(9):1215–8.
28. Sule N, Yakupoglu U, Shen SS, Krishnan B, Yang G, Lerner S, et al. Calcium oxalate deposition in renal cell carcinoma associated with acquired cystic kidney disease: a comprehensive study. Am J Surg Pathol. 2005;29(4):443–51.
29. Cossu-Rocca P, Eble JN, Zhang S, Martignoni G, Brunelli M, Cheng L. Acquired cystic disease-associated renal tumors: an immunohistochemical and fluorescence in situ hybridization study. Mod Pathol. 2006;19(6):780–7.
30. Pan CC, Chen YJ, Chang LC, Chang YH, Ho DM. Immunohistochemical and molecular genetic profiling of acquired cystic disease-associated renal cell carcinoma. Histopathology. 2009;55(2):145–53.
31. Kuroda N, Yamashita M, Kakehi Y, Hes O, Michal M, Lee GH. Acquired cystic disease-associated renal cell carcinoma: an immunohistochemical and fluorescence in situ hybridization study. Med Mol Morphol. 2011;44(4):228–32.
32. Kuroda N, Tamura M, Hamaguchi N, Mikami S, Pan CC, Brunelli M, et al. Acquired cystic disease-associated renal cell carcinoma with sarcomatoid change and rhabdoid features. Ann Diagn Pathol. 2011;15(6):462–6.
33. Eble J, Suter G, Epstein J, Sesterhenn I, editors. Pathology and genetics of tumours of the urinary system and male genital organs. Lyon: IARC Press; 2004.
34. Argani P, Ladanyi M. Translocation carcinomas of the kidney. Clin Lab Med. 2005;25:363–78.
35. Argani P, Aulmann S, Karanjawala Z, Fraser R, Ladanyi M, Rodriguez M. Melanotic Xp11 translocation renal cancers: a distinctive neoplasm with overlapping features of PEComa, carcinoma, and melanoma. Am J Surg Pathol. 2009;33(4):609–19.
36. Ross H, Argani P. Xp11 translocation renal cell carcinoma. Pathology. 2010;42(4):369–73.
37. Argani P, Lae M, Ballard E, Amin M, Manivel D, Hutchinson B, et al. Translocation carcinomas of the kidney after chemotherapy in childhood. J Clin Oncol. 2006;24(10):1529–34.
38. Argani P, Antonescu C, Couturier J, Fournet J, Sciot R, Debiec-Rychter M, et al. PRCC-TFE3 renal carcinomas: morphologic, immunohistochemical, ultrastructural, and molecular analysis of an entity associated with the t (X;1)(p11.2;q21). Am J Surg Pathol. 2002;26(12):1553–66.
39. Argani P, Antonescu C, Illei P, Lui M, Timmons C, Newbury R, et al. Primary renal neoplasms with the ASPL-TFE3 gene fusion of alveolar soft part sarcoma. Am J Pathol. 2001;159(1):179–92.
40. Suzigan S, Drut R, Faria P, Argani P, De Marzo A, Barbosa R, et al. Xp11 translocation carcinoma of the kidney presenting with multilocular cystic renal cell carcinoma-like features. Int J Surg Pathol. 2007;15(2):199–203.
41. Rao Q, Williamson SR, Zhang S, Eble JN, Grignon DJ, Wang M, et al. TFE3 break-apart FISH has a higher sensitivity for Xp11.2 translocation-associated renal cell carcinoma compared with TFE3 or cathepsin K immunohistochemical staining alone: expanding the morphologic spectrum. Am J Surg Pathol. 2013;37(6):804–15.
42. Argani P, Lal P, Hutchinson B, Lui M, Reuter V, Ladanyi M. Aberrant nuclear immunoreactivity for TFE3 in neoplasms with TFE3 gene fusions. Am J Surg Pathol. 2003;27(6):750–61.
43. Camparo P, Vasiliu V, Molinie B, Couturier J, Dykema K, Petillo D, et al. Renal translocation carcinomas: clinicopathology, immunohistochemical, and gene expression profiling analysis of 31 cases with a review of the literature. Am J Surg Pathol. 2008;32(5):656–70.
44. Klatte T, Streubel B, Wrba F, Remzi M, Krammer B, Martino M, et al. Renal cell carcinoma associated with transcription factor E3 expression and Xp11.2 translocation. Am J Clin Pathol. 2012;137:761–8.
45. Armah H, Parwani A. Xp11.2 translocation renal cell carcinoma. Arch Pathol Lab Med. 2010;134:124–9.
46. Argani P, Hicks J, De Marzo A, Albadine R, Illei P, Ladanyi M, et al. Xp11 translocation renal cell carcinoma: extended immunohistochemical profile emphasizing novel RCC markers. Am J Surg Pathol. 2010;34(9):1295–303.

47. Martignoni G, Gobbo S, Camparo P, Brunelli M, Munari E, Segala D, et al. Differential expression of cathepsin K in neoplasms harboring TFE3 gene fusions. Mod Pathol. 2011;24:1313–9.
48. Martignoni G, Pea M, Gobbo S, Brunelli M, Bonetti F, Segala D, et al. Cathepsin-K immunoreactivity distinguished MiTF-TFE family renal translocation carcinomas from other renal carcinomas. Mod Pathol. 2009;22:1016–22.
49. Geller J, Argani P, Adeniran A, Hampton D, De Marzo A, Hicks J, et al. Translocation renal cell carcinoma: lack of negative impact due to lymph node spread. Cancer. 2008;112(7):1607–16.
50. Rao Q, Guan B, Zhou X-J. Xp11.2 translocation renal cell carcinomas have a poorer prognosis than non-Xp11.2 translocation carcinomas in children and young adults: a meta-analysis. Int J Surg Pathol. 2010;18(6):458–64.
51. Geller J, Dome J. Local lymph node involvement does not predict poor outcome in pediatric renal cell carcinoma. Cancer. 2004;112:1607–16.
52. Dal Cin P, Stas M, Sciot R, De Wever I, Van Damme B, Van den Berghe H. Translocation (X;1) reveals metastasis 31 years after renal cell carcinoma. Cancer Genet Cytogenet. 1998;101:58–61.
53. Rais-Bahrami S, Drabick J, De Marzo A, Hicks J, Ho C, Caroe A, et al. Xp11 translocation renal cell carcinoma: delayed but massive and lethal metastases of a chemotherapy-associated secondary malignancy. Urology. 2007;70(1):e3–6.
54. Ross H, Martignoni G, Argani P. Renal cell carcinoma with clear cell and papillary features. Arch Pathol Lab Med. 2012;136:391–9.
55. Chang I-W, Huang H-Y, Sung M-T. Melanotic Xp11 translocation renal cancer. Am J Surg Pathol. 2009;33:1894–901.
56. Varinot J, Camparo P, Beurtheret S, Barreda E, Comperat E. An adult case of melanotic Xp11 translocation renal cancers: distinct entity or sub-entity? Int J Surg Pathol. 2011;19:285–9.
57. Argani P, Lae M, Hutchinson B, Reuter V, Collins M, Perentesis J, et al. Renal carcinomas with the t(6;11)(p21;q12): clinicopathologic features and demonstration of the specific alpha-TFEB gene fusion by immunohistochemistry, RT-PCR, and DNA PCR. Am J Surgical Pathol. 2005;29:230–40.
58. Argani P, Yonescu R, Morsberger L, Morris K, Netto G, Smith N, et al. Molecular confirmation of t(6;11)(p21;q12) renal cell carcinoma in archival paraffin-embedded material using a break-apart TFEB FISH assay expands its clinicopathologic spectrum. Am J Pathol. 2012;36:1516–26.
59. Argani P, Hawkins A, Griffin C, Goldstein J, Haas M, Beckwith B, et al. A distinctive pediatric renal neoplasm characterized by epithelioid morphology, basement membrane production, focal HMB45 immunoreactivity, and t(6;11)(p21.1;q21) chromosome translocation. Am J Pathol. 2001;158(6):2089–96.
60. Petersson F, Vanecek T, Michal M, Martignoni G, Brunelli M, Halbhuber Z, et al. A distinctive translocation carcinoma of the kidney; "rosette forming," t(6;11), HMB45-positive renal tumor: a histomorphologic, immunohistochemical, ultrastructural, and molecular genetic study of 4 cases. Hum Pathol. 2012;43:726–36.
61. Rao Q, Liu B, Cheng L, Zhu Y, Shi Q-l, Wu B, et al. Renal cell carcinomas with t(6;11)(p21;q12): a clinicopathologic study emphasizing unusual morphology, novel alpha-TFEb gene fusion point, immunobiomarkers, and ultrastructural feature, as well as detection of the gene fusion by fluorescence in situ hybridization. Am J Surg Pathol. 2012;36(9):1327–38.
62. Jung SJ, Chung JI, Park SH, Ayala AG, Ro JY. Thyroid follicular carcinoma-like tumor of kidney: a case report with morphologic, immunohistochemical, and genetic analysis. Am J Surg Pathol. 2006;30(3):411–5.
63. Amin MB, Gupta R, Ondrej H, McKenney JK, Michal M, Young AN, et al. Primary thyroid-like follicular carcinoma of the kidney: report of 6 cases of a histologically distinctive adult renal epithelial neoplasm. Am J Surg Pathol. 2009;33(3):393–400.
64. Dhillon J, Tannir NM, Matin SF, Tamboli P, Czerniak BA, Guo CC. Thyroid-like follicular carcinoma of the kidney with metastases to the lungs and retroperitoneal lymph nodes. Hum Pathol. 2011;42(1):146–50.
65. Sterlacci W, Verdorfer I, Gabriel M, Mikuz G. Thyroid follicular carcinoma-like renal tumor: a case report with morphologic, immunophenotypic, cytogenetic, and scintigraphic studies. Virchows Arch. 2008;452(1):91–5.
66. Alessandrini L, Fassan M, Gardiman MP, Guttilla A, Zattoni F, Galletti TP, et al. Thyroid-like follicular carcinoma of the kidney: report of two cases with detailed immunohistochemical profile and literature review. Virchows Arch. 2012;461(3):345–50.
67. Abe K, Hasegawa T, Onodera S, Oishi Y, Suzuki M. Renal metastasis of thyroid carcinoma. Int J Urol. 2002;9(11):656–8.
68. Garcia-Sanchis L, Lopez-Aznar D, Oltra A, Rivas A, Alonso J, Montalar J, et al. Metastatic follicular thyroid carcinoma to the kidney: a case report. Clin Nucl Med. 1999;24(1):48–50.
69. Falzarano SM, Chute DJ, Magi-Galluzzi C. Metastatic papillary thyroid carcinoma to the kidney: report of two cases mimicking primary renal cell carcinoma and review of the literature. Pathology. 2013;45(1):89–93.
70. Shaco-Levy R, Bean SM, Bentley RC, Robboy SJ. Natural history of biologically malignant struma ovarii: analysis of 27 cases with extraovarian spread. Int J Gynecol Pathol. 2010;29(3):212–27.

71. Robboy SJ, Shaco-Levy R, Peng RY, Snyder MJ, Donahue J, Bentley RC, et al. Malignant struma ovarii: an analysis of 88 cases, including 27 with extraovarian spread. Int J Gynecol Pathol. 2009;28(5):405–22.
72. Ohe C, Kuroda N, Pan CC, Yang XJ, Hes O, Michal M, et al. A unique renal cell carcinoma with features of papillary renal cell carcinoma and thyroid-like carcinoma: a morphological, immunohistochemical and genetic study. Histopathology. 2010;57(3):494–497.
73. Fadare O, Lam S, Rubin C, Renshaw IL, Nerby CL. Papillary renal cell carcinoma with diffuse clear cells and thyroid-like macrofollicular areas. Ann Diagn Pathol. 2010;14(4):284–91.

Clinical and Management Implications Associated with Histologic Subtypes of Renal Cell Carcinomas

27

Maria Carmen Mir, Brian I. Rini and Steven C. Campbell

Introduction

Renal cell carcinoma (RCC) has traditionally been the most lethal of the common urologic cancers and now represents about 2–3% of all adult malignancies. In the USA, RCC accounted for almost 65,000 new cancer diagnoses in 2012, and contributed to approximately 13,570 cancer-related deaths [1]. The incidence of RCC has been gradually increasing over the past several years primarily related to more frequent utilization of cross-sectional imaging. However, an increased prevalence of hypertension and obesity, established risk factors for this cancer, may also be contributing to this trend. One recent study estimated that as many as 40% of RCC cases in the USA are related to obesity, and reported a relative risk of 1.07 for each unit of rising body mass index (BMI) [2]. The relationship between hypertension and RCC is thought to be due to inflammation or metabolic changes in the renal tubules that could increase susceptibility to carcinogens. The other major risk factor for RCC, tobacco use, was recognized several decades ago and is still considered by most authorities to be the strongest predisposing factor.

RCC is primarily a disease of the elderly with peak presentation between 60 and 70 years of age, and a male to female predominance of approximately 3:2 has been documented in many series. Only 2–3% of cases are believed to be familial, with the most common syndrome being von Hippel–Lindau (VHL), which is observed in 1/36,000 individuals in the general population. Other familial RCC syndromes include hereditary papillary RCC, hereditary leiomyomatosis and RCC, Birt–Hogg–Dubé, and tuberous sclerosis, with most presenting with distinctive histologic profiles. However, the vast majority of RCC cases are observed on a sporadic basis. One additional clinical association is noteworthy, namely acquired renal cystic disease in end-stage renal failure. A 5–15-fold increased risk of RCC is noted in this population, with the risk increasing in proportion to the duration of dialysis or other renal replacement therapy. RCC in this population is characterized by a distinct subtype, acquired cystic disease-associated RCC, as well as an increased proportion of papillary histology, although even in this setting clear cell histology still predominates [3].

Most RCC are unilateral and unifocal and most tumors tend to be well encapsulated, but tumor morphology can vary considerably, often correlating with tumor histology. Bilateral involvement can be synchronous or asynchronous

S. C. Campbell (✉) · M. C. Mir
Department of Urology, Cleveland Clinic,
Cleveland, OH, USA
e-mail: Campbes3@ccf.org

M. C. Mir
e-mail: mirmare@yahoo.es

B. I. Rini
Department of Oncology, Cleveland Clinic,
Cleveland, OH, USA
e-mail: Rinib2@ccf.org

C. Magi-Galluzzi, C. G. Przybycin (eds.), *Genitourinary Pathology,* DOI 10.1007/978-1-4939-2044-0_27,

and is found in 2–4% of sporadic RCC, although it is considerably more common in patients with familial forms of RCC. Overall, multicentricity is found in 10–20% of cases, but is more common in association with papillary histology and familial RCC. Infiltrative growth patterns are less common and carry a poor prognosis. These findings are typically associated with grade 4 clear cell tumors, sarcomatoid differentiation, or collecting duct or medullary cell histologies. Differentiation from poorly differentiated urothelial cell carcinomas, adrenocortical carcinomas, sarcomas, lymphoma, or other less common infiltrative neoplasms can be challenging in such cases.

Prognosis for RCC is determined primarily by stage, grade, and histology, but several other factors including tumor size, presence or absence of symptoms, performance status, and various laboratory values have proven to be independent predictive factors in various analyses. Stage migration has occurred over the past 2–3 decades, with more localized tumors being found in the modern era. At present about 60% of patients are diagnosed with localized disease, 20% with locally advanced disease, and 20% with metastatic RCC. Corresponding 5-year overall survival rates for each of these subgroups is approximately 90, 65, and 12%, respectively. Small renal masses (clinically confined and ≤4.0 cm) are now commonly encountered, and most series demonstrate that approximately 20% of such tumors are benign, 60% are relatively indolent, and only 20% harbor potentially aggressive histologic features [4]. Locally advanced RCC can extend into the perinephric or sinus fat, adjacent adrenal gland, hilar or retroperitoneal lymph nodes, or renal vein or inferior vena cava (IVC). Overall, about 10–20% of patients present with lymph node involvement, which is rarely curable for RCC. Ten percent present with venous extension, which if isolated, is potentially curable with a comprehensive surgical approach. Despite the introduction of molecular targeted agents, metastatic RCC remains a lethal disease in the overwhelming majority of cases, although a small percentage (1–2%) of patients with limited and resectable disease can achieve durable disease-free status, and an indolent course is observed in another small subgroup of patients.

Clinical Presentation

Approximately 50–60% of patients with RCC are now diagnosed incidentally, typically during ultrasonography or computed tomography (CT) imaging for the evaluation of unrelated or nonspecific complaints (Table 27.1). This represents a substantial shift from two to three decades previously, when most patients presented symptomatically and the prognosis associated with this cancer was much more dismal. In that era, many patients presented with the “too late triad” of gross hematuria, flank pain, and palpable mass. One other important symptom that can be associated with progressive local growth of the cancer is lower extremity edema, which is derived from obstruction of the IVC by a tumor thrombus. In general, the more aggressive variants of RCC are more likely to present symptomatically [4].

Patients with advanced RCC can also present with symptoms directly related to metastases, with bone pain and neurologic symptoms most commonly observed. RCC is also noteworthy for a wide array of paraneoplastic syndromes, which historically were found in about 10% of cases,

Table 27.1 Distribution of symptoms at presentation for RCC

Asymptomatic (60%)
Symptomatic (40%)
Tumor related
Flank pain
Hematuria
Abdominal mass
Lower extremity edema
Metastasis related
Bone pain
Neurologic symptoms
Persistent cough, hemoptysis
Paraneoplastic syndromes (5–10%)
Hypercalcemia
Hypertension
Polycythemia
Hepatic dysfunction/Stauffer syndrome

but now are somewhat less common. These syndromes can include hypercalcemia related to the production of parathyroid hormone like peptides, hypertension due to dysregulated production of renin, and polycythemia from surplus excretion of erythropoietin. These tumors can also release a variety of cytokines and inflammatory mediators that can lead to constitutional symptoms such as fatigue, malaise, and weight loss, as well hepatic dysfunction, or Stauffer's syndrome, in which hepatic dysfunction is found in the absence of liver metastasis. Hypercalcemia is the most common paraneoplastic syndrome associated with RCC, and typically associated with clear cell RCC. This syndrome is managed medically with furosemide-induced diuresis and bisphosphonates, occasionally supplemented by corticosteroids and calcitonin. All of the other paraneoplastic syndromes associated with RCC are managed primarily through surgical debulking. Virtually, all are associated with a poor prognosis, and are most commonly seen with the aggressive variants of RCC.

Radiographic Evaluation

Cross-sectional imaging, ideally with a dedicated triphasic renal CT scan, plays a primary role in the diagnosis of renal masses, and has changed the landscape of RCC as outlined above. It facilitates proper detection and characterization of renal masses, and provides essential information for clinical staging and surgical planning. In general, any mass that enhances with intravenous (IV) administration of contrast material on CT by more than 15 Hounsfield Units should be considered RCC until proven otherwise. However, within this group of enhancing renal tumors will be a variety of benign neoplasms including oncocytomas and angiomyolipomas. Most angiomyolipomas are readily identified due to distinctive areas with Housefield units (HU) lower than −20, reflecting high fat content, although about 10% are fat poor and impossible to differentiate from RCC based on imaging alone. Avidly enhancing tumors are most commonly clear cell RCC, while hypoenhancing tumors are more likely to correlate with papillary or chromophobe histology [5]. Clear cell RCC also associates with necrosis and retroperitoneal collateral circulation that can be observed on magnetic resonance imaging (MRI). Recent reports demonstrate that papillary RCC are typically hypointense on T2-weighted imaging, whereas clear cell RCC tends to be iso- to hyperintense in this phase. Interestingly, oncocytomas often demonstrate strong contrast enhancement, and can be very difficult to differentiate from RCC based on imaging alone. Other important imaging characteristics such as morphology (well circumscribed vs. infiltrative) and focality (bilaterality and multicentricity) can also provide clues with respect to potential histologic subtypes and familial versus sporadic etiology, as discussed above.

Renal mass biopsy and molecular imaging have been studied in an attempt to provide a more accurate preoperative diagnosis and to allow for more rational and intelligent patient counseling. The main concern has traditionally related to a high incidence of false negative biopsies, but this is much less common in the modern era, representing <1% of cases in most recent series [6]. Nevertheless, differentiation between oncocytoma and the eosinophilic variants of RCC can still be problematic with the limited material provided by a biopsy, and the implications of the diagnosis of "oncocytic neoplasm" have not been adequately defined. Most centers now pursue renal mass biopsy on a utility-based approach, as follows. Young healthy patients who are unwilling to accept the uncertainty of surveillance even if the biopsy is negative, and frail, elderly patients who will be managed conservatively even if the biopsy is positive, should not be exposed to the risk of renal mass biopsy. In contrast, patients who could be considered for a variety of treatment modalities ranging from surgical excision to active surveillance may benefit from further risk stratification. If the biopsy demonstrates a clear cell RCC, surgery would be prioritized, while a diagnosis of oncocytoma or even "oncocytic neoplasm" would encourage a less aggressive approach. Molecular imaging with radioactive antibodies to carbonic anhydrase IX (CA-IX), which is expressed primarily in clear cell RCC, may play a similar role in the future. Renal mass biopsy is also now beginning to play an important role for patients with advanced RCC. Clear cell tumors in particular are most likely to respond to immunotherapy and targeted agents, which can help guide management decisions in this challenging patient population.

Treatment Paradigms

Treatment of RCC has evolved considerably in the last decade, and is best discussed based upon disease categorization, as outlined in Table 27.2. Localized disease includes stages T1-2 tumors without nodal involvement and with a negative metastatic profile. Most smaller tumors (≤4.0 cm) in this group have limited oncologic potential, with 20% benign, and only 20% harboring potentially aggressive features such as high nuclear grade or locally invasive phenotype. Most agree now that radical nephrectomy represents therapeutic overkill for these patients, often leading to chronic kidney disease and its potential adverse sequelae. Partial nephrectomy is considered the reference standard for this population and is typically associated with the local control in 98–99% of cases. Partial nephrectomy should always be prioritized when preservation of renal function is at a premium and for multicentric and familial tumors. Thermal ablation provides local control in about 90% of such patients and often can be administered percutaneously thus minimizing potential morbidity. Active surveillance should be prioritized for patients with limited life expectancy or extensive comorbidities in whom the risk of intervention outweighs the oncologic risk. Most such tumors grow slowly (about 3–4 mm/year) and the risk of metastatic spread within a few years appears to be low (1–2%) presuming sensible patient selection. However, some series contain a subgroup of patients with rapidly growing tumors that appear to have more aggressive tumor biology, underscoring the importance of patient selection and the potential risks of active surveillance. For instance, in the Volpe series [6] eight out of 32 masses (25%) doubled in volume within 12 months, and 11 masses (34%) reached at threshold of 4 cm diameter, most with a rapid doubling time. Infiltrative tumors almost always correlate with aggressive histologic subtypes and should be managed accordingly, even if relatively small. Oncologic potential increases in proportion with tumor size, and most T2 tumors (>7.0 cm) are best managed with radical nephrectomy unless preservation of the renal function is of primary importance.

Table 27.2 Treatment paradigms for RCC

RCC stage	Treatment
Localized RCC	Active surveillance
	Ablative techniques
	Radiofrequency
	Cryotherapy
	Partial nephrectomy
	Radical nephrectomy
Locally advanced RCC	Radical nephrectomy +/− lymph node dissection +/− IVC thrombectomy
	Adjuvant targeted therapy
Metastatic RCC	Cytoreductive nephrectomy
	Metastasectomy with excision of all evidence of tumor, if feasible
	Immunotherapy with high dose IL-2 (for clear cell RCC and good performance status)
	Targeted therapy

RCC renal cell carcinoma, *IVC* inferior vena cava, *IL-2* interleukin 2

Locally advanced RCC is still primarily a surgical disease and complete surgical excision should always be prioritized. Careful preoperative planning and a comprehensive surgical approach are required, often incorporating an extensive retroperitoneal lymph node dissection and/or IVC thrombectomy. Even with resection to R0 status, most such patients are at high risk for disease recurrence and adjuvant systemic therapy trials, currently utilizing targeted agents, should be considered. Neoadjuvant approaches using tyrosine kinase inhibitors (TKIs) have recently been reported for patients with unresectable locally advanced disease related to proximity to vital structures and other complexities. These studies have demonstrated downsizing that can facilitate surgical resection in some patients, but such favorable responses appear to be limited to patients with clear cell histology. In a neoadjuvant sunitinib study, median downsizing for patients with clear cell RCC ($n=22$) was 28 %, and 59 % were able to proceed with surgical resection. In contrast, no substantial responses were observed in patients with nonclear cell histology ($n=8$), and surgical resection was not possible in this subgroup [7]. It is important to emphasize that the neoadjuvant approach remains investigational.

Targeted therapies have revolutionized the management of patients with metastatic RCC, but there is still an important role for surgery in this challenging patient population. Cytoreductive nephrectomy was shown to provide a greater than 6-month prolongation of survival in phase III trials where interferon was the systemic therapy of choice, and most believe that this procedure is still indicated in this era. The precise role of debulking nephrectomy for nonclear cell RCC is less certain as the clinical trials of debulking nephrectomy were limited to the clear cell population. The best candidates are patients with limited metastatic burden, good performance status, and reasonable cardiopulmonary status. A small proportion, certainly <5 %, of patients with metastatic RCC have solitary or oligometastases and can be considered for metastasectomy, which can provide durable cancer-free status in about 30 % of patients in this fortunate category. Beyond this, systemic therapy must be considered [8].

Targeted therapies include bevacizumab which sequesters the vascular endothelial growth factor (VEGF) ligand, TKIs such as sunitinib, sorafenib, pazopanib, and axitinib that target the VEGF receptor, and the mammalian target of rapamycin (mTOR) inhibitors, temsirolimus, and everolimus. These agents provide prolonged progression-free survival when compared to placebo or interferon-alpha, and collectively have extended overall survival for metastatic RCC. As such, they have displaced immunotherapy for the management of patients with metastatic RCC. One exception is high dose IL-2, which is still the only agent that provides a realistic chance (3–5 %) for a durable complete remission. Ideal candidates for high dose IL-2 include patients with excellent performance status and clear cell RCC because the treatment can be rather toxic, and responses have been limited almost exclusively to patients with this histologic subtype.

Each targeted agent now has an established niche for the management of patients with metastatic RCC based on randomized, prospective clinical trials. For instance, sunitinib, pazopanib and a combination of bevacizumab and interferon are now typically chosen for patients with treatment-naïve metastatic RCC, while temsirolimus is often prioritized for patients with poor prognostic features. Axitinib and everolimus are positioned for patients who have failed TKIs, based upon established treatment algorithms. In general, patients with clear cell RCC appear to respond best to targeted therapies based upon the inherent biology of clear cell RCC which results in VEGF overproduction. A reference standard for patients with nonclear cell metastatic RCC is not established at this point in time, and clinical trials are a priority.

Clinical and Management Considerations Related to Histologic Subtype

Clear Cell RCC

Clear cell is the most common histologic type of RCC and its clinical implications are well established, to large extent dictated by its distinctive tumor biology (Table 27.3). Mutation of the VHL tumor suppressor gene is found in over 70–80 % of sporadic clear cell RCC, and in 100 % of patients with clear cell RCC in the setting of VHL. In the latter instance, the mutation is passed on in an autosomal dominant manner, while sporadic clear cell tumors must acquire these mutations spontaneously. Patients with VHL are at risk for vascular tumors of the central nervous system and retina (hemangioblastomas), as well as adrenal gland (pheochromocytoma), in addition to the renal tumors. Clear cell RCC in VHL is more likely to be early onset and multifocal, and most tumors do not acquire a potentially aggressive phenotype in VHL until they reach a size of 3 cm or larger. Nephron-sparing approaches should

Table 27.3 Clinicopathological features according to RCC subtype

	Clear cell carcinoma	Papillary	Chromophobe	Collecting duct	RMC
Incidence	70–80%	10–15%	3–5%	<1%	<1%
Origin	Proximal tubule	Proximal tubule	Cortical portion collecting duct	Medulla	
Familial syndrome association	VHL	Hereditary papillary RCC—type I Hereditary leiomyomatosis RCC—type II	Birt–-Hogg–Dube	None	None
Multifocal	10–15%	30–40%	10–15%	–	–
Necrosis/hemorrhage	+++	++	+/–	+/–	+/–
Venous involvement	+++	++	+/–	+/–	+/–
Lymph node involvement	++	+++	+	+	+
Sarcomatoid features	2–5%	–	1%	–	–
Metastasis at diagnosis	20%	<5%	Rarely	50%	80%
Prognosis	Worse than papillary or chromophobe	According to subtype. Papillary type 2 worse Type 1 favorable	Better prognosis than clear cell	Most unfavorable	
Imaging appearance	Hypervascular	Hypovascular	Hypovascular	Central location, infiltrative, hypovascular	
Other features	Good response to targeted therapy	Unlikely to respond to targeted therapy	Often large tumors yet still confined	Responds to chemotherapy for urothelial carcinoma	

RCC renal cell carcinoma, *RMC* renal medullary carcinoma, *VHL* von Hippel–Lindau

be prioritized in VHL, like most of the familial RCC syndromes, because of the strength of the tumor diathesis, which expresses itself in multicentricity and frequent recurrences with time. In fact, 50% of VHL patients will develop RCC at some point in time, and approximately 85% of patients managed with partial nephrectomy will recur within the same kidney within 10 years of follow-up. Due to improvement in the management of central nervous system lesions in VHL, RCC has become the main cause of death in this syndrome. In sporadic RCC, most data indicate a strong relationship between tumor size and biological aggressiveness, but a similar threshold value has not been established [9]. For instance, for clear cell tumors, each progressive increase of 1 cm is associated with a 25% increased incidence of high-grade tumor (i.e., Furhman grade 3–4).

Loss of function of the VHL protein is the key event in clear cell RCC that leads to increased expression of VEGF and other growth factors. This in turn contributes to the highly vascular nature of these tumors and their enhanced clinical aggressiveness. Correspondingly, clear cell RCC tends to be hypervascular on imaging, and necrosis and hemorrhage are more common than with other histologic subtypes of RCC (Fig. 27.1a–d). Cystic changes are also more common with clear cell RCC, although the factors contributing to this are not well defined. Venous involvement is found most frequently in clear cell RCC, with an incidence of approximately 10%, and this tumor type is most likely to exhibit sarcomatoid differentiation [10]. All these factors contribute to a compromised prognosis for clear cell RCC when compared to the other common histologic types of RCC, namely

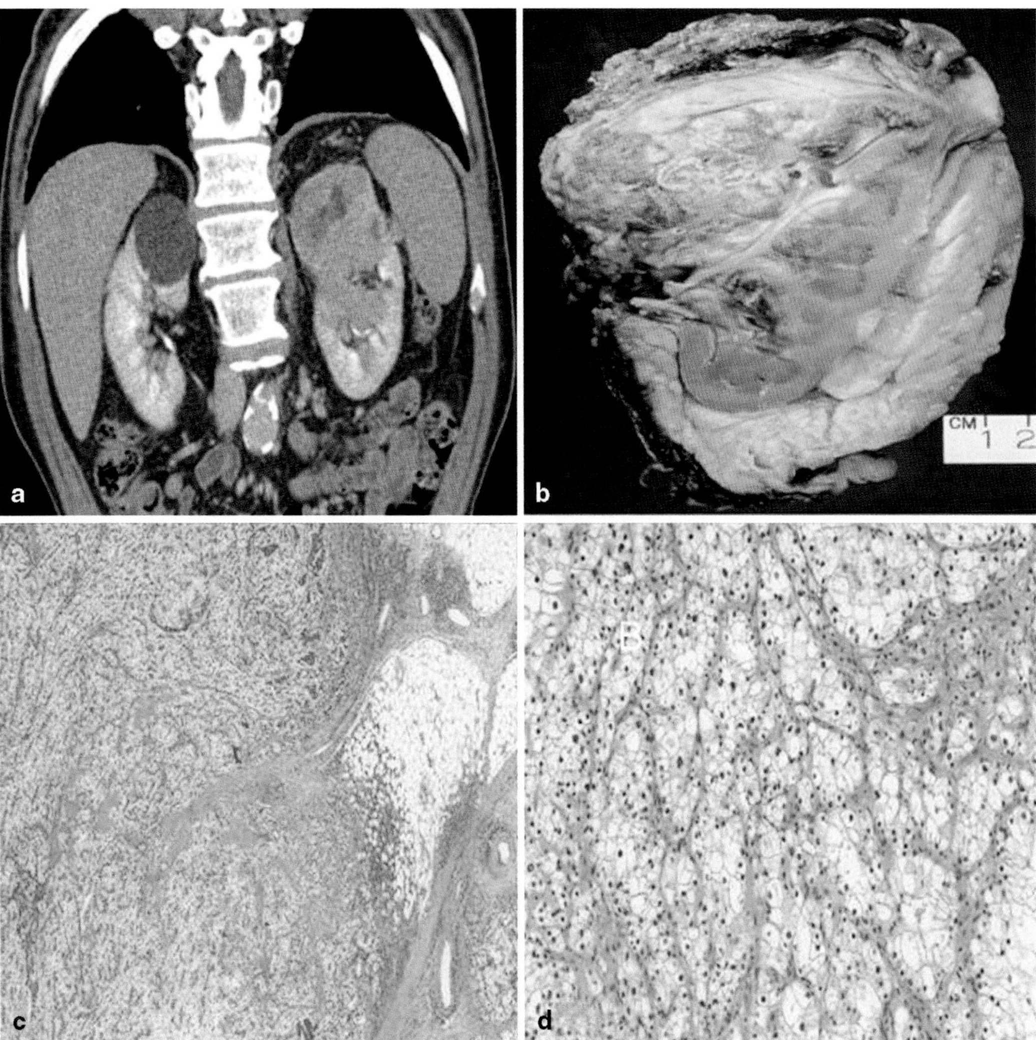

Fig. 27.1 Clear cell RCC. **a.** CT scan showing left upper pole hypervascular RCC with necrosis. **b.** Large variegated yellow-brown tumor that invades into perinephric fat and renal sinus fat. **c.** Tumor cells infiltrating into the perinephric fat, confirming pT3. **d.** High power with clear cell morphology. (Courtesy of Dr. Christopher G. Przybycin, Cleveland, OH)

papillary and chromophobe RCC ($p<0.001$ on multivariable analysis) [11]. One exception is multilocular cystic RCC, which tends to pursue a much more indolent course.

Clear cell RCC is also the most likely to metastasize, as this is seen in about 20% of cases at diagnosis, and recurrence after surgery for organ confined or locally advanced clear cell RCC is also more common than for the other histologic subtypes [12]. Overall, clear cell RCC is overrepresented among patients with metastatic RCC, accounting for about 90% of cases. One paradox is that clear cell RCC is also the most likely to respond to systemic therapies, whether it be immunotherapy with high dose IL-2 or targeted therapies. In reality, most of the novel systemic agents primarily target the VEGF pathway, so it should not be too surprising that the current algorithms for the management of metastatic RCC primarily apply to patients with clear cell histology.

Given all of these considerations, most believe that patients with sporadic clear cell RCC should be treated aggressively whenever possible, independent of disease category. For patients with localized clear cell RCC surgical excision with partial or radical nephrectomy should be prioritized over more conservative options, taking patient age, comorbidities, and the level of renal function into account. For locally advanced clear cell RCC, surgery is prioritized, but enthusiasm for neoadjuvant or adjuvant targeted therapy is higher than for other histologic subtypes. Similarly for patients with metastatic RCC, an aggressive pathway integrating surgery and targeted agents is typically pursued, with adjustments made dependent on performance status, sites and burden of disease, and other relevant factors.

Papillary RCC

Papillary RCC is the second most common histologic subtype of RCC, representing about 10–15% of all cases. A unique feature of papillary RCC is a predilection for multicentricity, which has been reported in 20–40% of patients (Fig. 27.2a–c). Virtually all data about

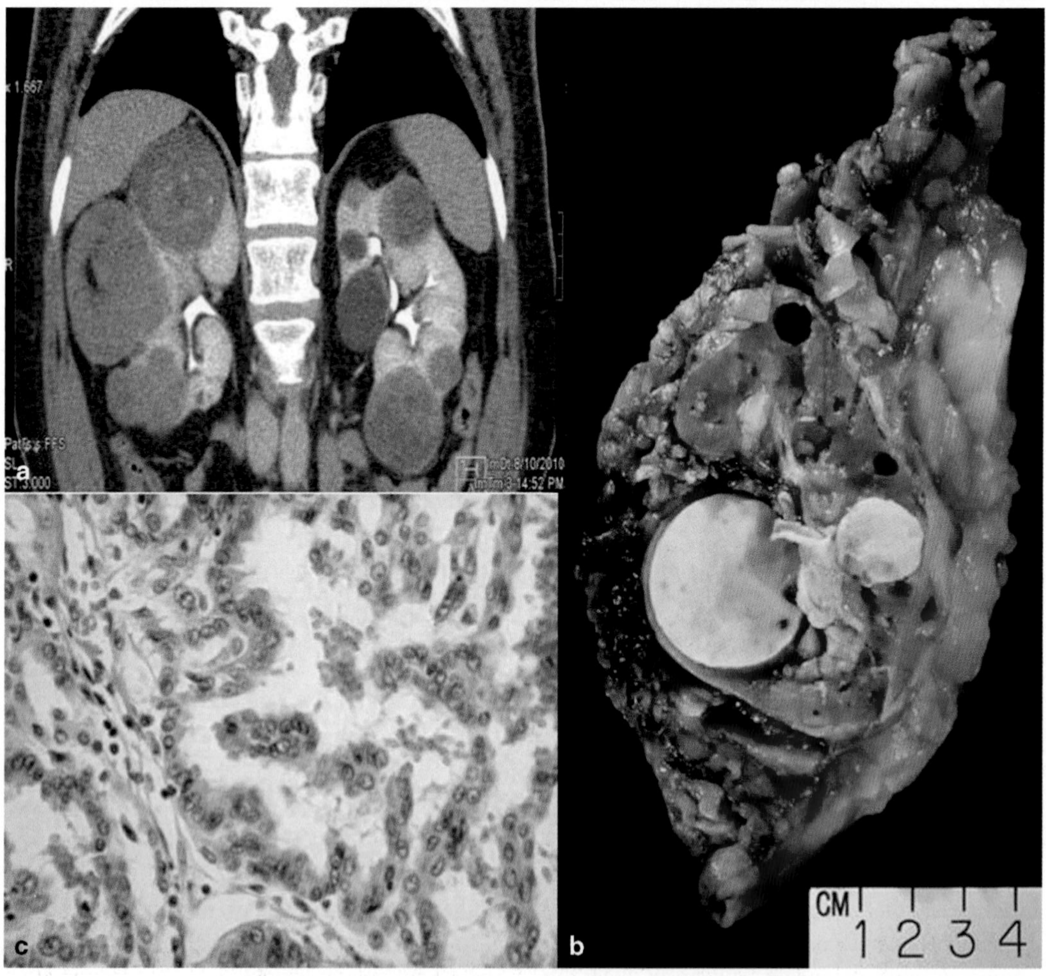

Fig. 27.2 Papillary RCC. **a.** CT scan shows multiple, hypo-enhancing renal tumors. **b.** Gross appearance of three tan, solid, well-demarcated tumors (different patient). **c.** Microscopic appearance of papillary type 1 demonstrating basophillic, uniform cuboidal cells lining complex trabeculae and papillary structures. (Courtesy of Dr. Christopher G. Przybycin, Cleveland, OH)

the incidence and focality of papillary RCC are complicated by controversies about small renal adenomas, which have traditionally been defined as low-grade neoplasms less than 5 mm diameter. These lesions typically exhibit papillary architecture and share in common distinctive cytogenetic features with papillary RCC, namely trisomy of chromosomes 7 and 17. These lesions appear to have very limited biological potential and are relatively common at autopsy. They are often found as satellite lesions associated with papillary RCC and contribute to the increased incidence of multicentricity discussed above.

Most of the older literature about papillary RCC referred to what is now considered type 1 disease, characterized by basophilic cells arranged within papillary architecture, and harboring limited biological potential. The familial form of this neoplasm is hereditary papillary RCC syndrome (HPRCC), in which patients present with early onset, multifocal papillary RCC. This syndrome is somewhat unique in that it is typically not associated with major manifestations in other organ systems, unlike the other familial forms of RCC. It is caused by mutation of the mesenchymal-epithelial transition (MET) proto-oncogene, a hepatocyte growth factor receptor, leading to constitutive activation of the pathway. Autosomal dominant inheritance is observed, in common with all of the familial RCC syndromes. The renal tumors in HPRCC patients are highly penetrant but limited in aggressiveness. It is estimated that an HPRCC patient who lives to age 80 has a nearly 90 % likelihood of developing kidney cancer, and many of these patients harbor over 1000 microscopic papillary tumors per kidney. The clinical management for patients with HPRCC is similar to VHL patients; thus, active surveillance is recommended until the largest tumor reaches the 3 cm threshold, and nephron-sparing approaches should be prioritized [13, 14].

MET is only mutated in a minority of patients with sporadic type 1 papillary RCC, so other genetic alterations must predominate. Nevertheless, a favorable prognosis has been reported in most studies, even after controlling for confounding factors. Hence, many of these tumors can be managed in a conservative manner, particularly when small and organ confined. If advanced age or major comorbidities are a major concern, active surveillance and thermal ablation can be considered. This subtype of RCC is more commonly seen in patients with end-stage renal failure and acquired renal cystic disease.

Type 2 papillary RCC is less prevalent and characterized by eosinophilic staining and increased nuclear and cytologic variability—most are high grade and have increased biological aggressiveness. A familial tumor that, before its description, was likely diagnosed as type 2 papillary RCC is hereditary leiomyomatosis and RCC syndrome (HLRCC), in which patients also develop leiomyomas of the skin and uterus and leiomyosarcomas of the uterus. Mutation of fumarate hydratase is the driver, and most patients develop early onset disease, although multicentricity appears to be less common in this syndrome. Aggressive management is strongly advised for patients with type 2 papillary RCC, whether sporadic or familial, with either radical nephrectomy or partial nephrectomy with wide surgical margins. Many of these tumors are infiltrative rendering the conservative options less appealing. Preservation of renal function is perhaps not as important in this syndrome, and certainly must take a back seat when compared to oncologic concerns.

There are other important clinical correlates for papillary RCC in general that can impact patient management. For instance, venous involvement appears to be less common for patients with papillary RCC than for clear cell RCC; however, the prognostic implications are noteworthy. For patients with venous involvement in the absence of systemic or lymph node metastasis, the 5-year-cancer-specific survival for patients with papillary RCC in one contemporary series was only 35 versus 66 % for similar patients with clear cell RCC. In contrast, patients with nodal involvement from papillary RCC appear to have a better prognosis than similar patients with clear cell

RCC. In one recent series, patients with regional nodal metastases in the absence of other metastases had a 5-year-cancer-specific survival of 65% for papillary histology compared to 19% for clear cell histology [15].

Metastatic disease is less common in papillary RCC, but response to therapy is suboptimal. In the Mayo Clinic series only 4.4% of the patients that developed metastasis from RCC had papillary histology. Choueiri and colleagues reported relatively low response rates for 41 patients with metastatic papillary RCC when treated with sunitinib or sorafenib (only 5% overall and 17% in the sunitinib treated group). Most studies to date concur with this in demonstrating lower response rates to targeted agents for papillary RCC when compared to clear cell RCC.

Hence, novel approaches are being explored, such as the use of foretinib, which targets the tyrosine kinase domain of MET as well as VEGFR2. A multicenter phase II clinical trial of this agent included 74 patients with advanced papillary RCC treated with either a continuous or discontinuous regimen. The overall response rate was 13.5%, with ten partial responses. However, the average response duration was 18.5 months, which is encouraging, and the most durable responses were observed in patients with germ line MET mutations suggesting that patient selection may be feasible. Other candidate approaches for this challenging patient population have included carboplatin and taxol, erlotinib, capecitabine, and temsirolimus. However, response rates have been relatively low, ranging from 1.5 to 26%, and no complete responses have been observed.

Chromophobe RCC

Chromophobe RCC is the third most common subtype of RCC, representing 3–5% of all cases. It is estimated that as many as 5–10% of cases of chromophobe RCC may be familial, associated with the Birt–Hogg–Dubé syndrome (BHD). In addition to early onset, multifocal RCC, these patients also develop benign fibrofolliculomas of the skin and pulmonary cysts that predispose to spontaneous pneumothorax. The product of the BHD gene is folliculin, which is mutated or inactivated in this syndrome. Folliculin interfaces with the mTOR pathway, and experiments with BHD knockout mice have shown a beneficial effect of rapamycin, an mTOR inhibitor. These findings provide a rationale for a better response to mTOR inhibitors for chromophobe RCC patients when compared to patients with papillary RCC, which has been observed in some studies, although this is relative, and clear cell tumors respond best. The renal tumors in BHD include chromophobe RCC but also oncocytomas and hybrid tumors with features of each. In addition, a variety of other RCC subtypes have been reported in BHD, making this syndrome somewhat unique. Most of the other familial RCC syndromes present with only one specific subtype of RCC, e.g., clear cell for VHL. Renal tumors in BHD tend to have limited biological aggressiveness and are in general managed similar to those in VHL, utilizing the 3 cm rule.

Most sporadic chromophobe tumors tend to remain organ confined and have a favorable prognosis, despite growth to extreme size in some cases (Fig. 27.3a–c). Most are hypoenhancing on imaging, and 90% are unifocal. In one recent series, the 5-year-cancer-specific survival for patients with chromophobe RCC was 87% compared to 69% for patients with clear cell RCC [16]. This prognostic advantage for chromophobe RCC holds even after confounding factors are taken into account, based upon the most robust series in the literature. The exception to this rule is the chromophobe tumor with sarcomatoid differentiation, which is found in up to 10–15% of patients in some series. Lymph node involvement and distant metastasis from chromophobe RCC are primarily found in this subset of patients. Interestingly, liver metastasis appears to be more common in these patients than in similar patients with clear cell RCC. Response of patients with metastatic chromophobe RCC to targeted agents or immunotherapy remains poor, and an aggressive surgical approach to render the patient disease-free should be pursued whenever feasible [17].

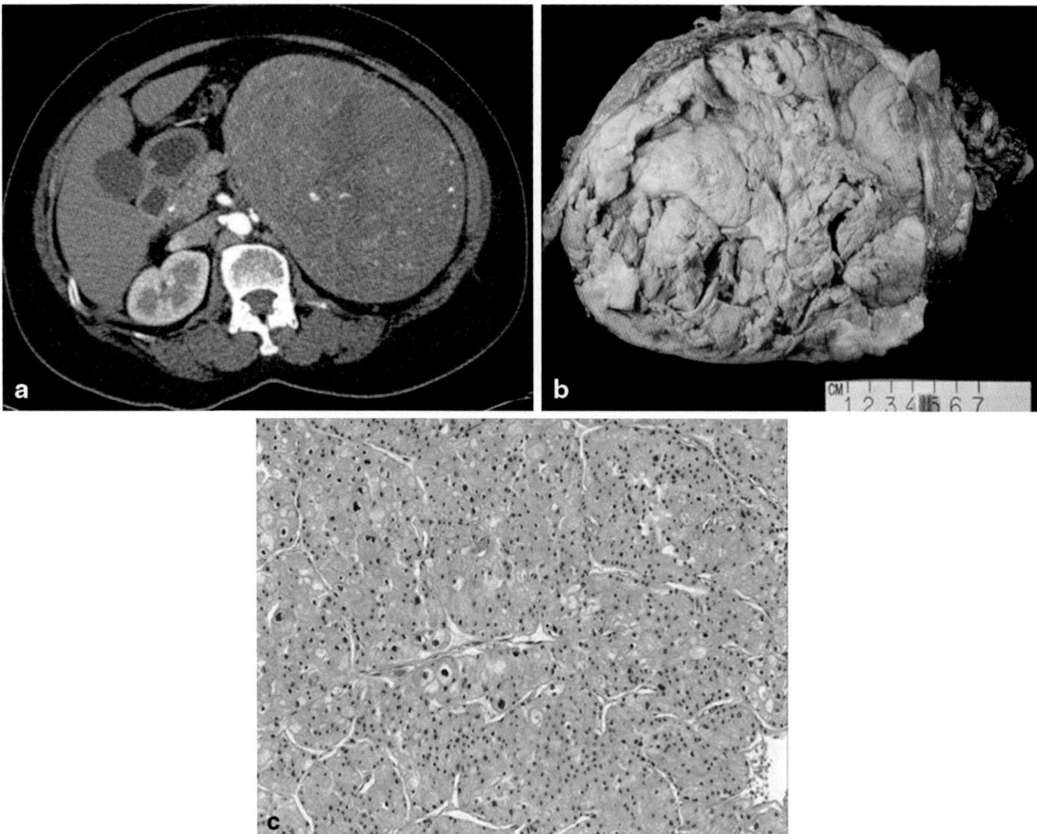

Fig. 27.3 Chromophobe RCC. **a.** CT scan shows a well-circumscribed, large mass. **b.** Macroscopic appearance with large, tan, noninfiltrative tumor. **c.** Chromophobe RCC containing broad nests of tumor cells with prominent cell membranes, irregular nuclear contours, and perinuclear halos. (Courtesy of Dr. Christopher G. Przybycin, Cleveland, OH)

Collecting Duct RCC

Collecting duct RCC is typically included within the list of the most common histologic subtypes of RCC, but it is a somewhat rare neoplasm, accounting for less than 1 % of all cases of RCC. This malignancy has a number of clinical features that distinguish it from the more common histologies of RCC. Collecting duct generally affects younger patients, typically between 30 and 50 years of age. It originates in the medulla, and thus almost all of these tumors are centrally located. It is invariably infiltrative and pursues an aggressive clinical course with a very unfavorable prognosis (Fig. 27.4). Based on imaging and clinical presentation, it can be difficult to differentiate from poorly differentiated urothelial cell carcinoma, and a variety of other infiltrative neoplasms must also be considered in the differential diagnosis. Most patients with collecting duct RCC are symptomatic, with gross hematuria being the most common presenting complaint. In one large series of 81 patients with collecting duct carcinoma, 65 % of patients were symptomatic and 32 % had metastases at diagnosis [18, 19]. Systemic syndromes associated with RCC are frequently found in patients with collecting duct histology, such as increases in erythrocyte sedimentation rate, C-reactive protein, lactate dehydrogenase, and alpha2-globulin. In terms of systemic treatment, collecting duct typically does not respond to immunotherapy or targeted

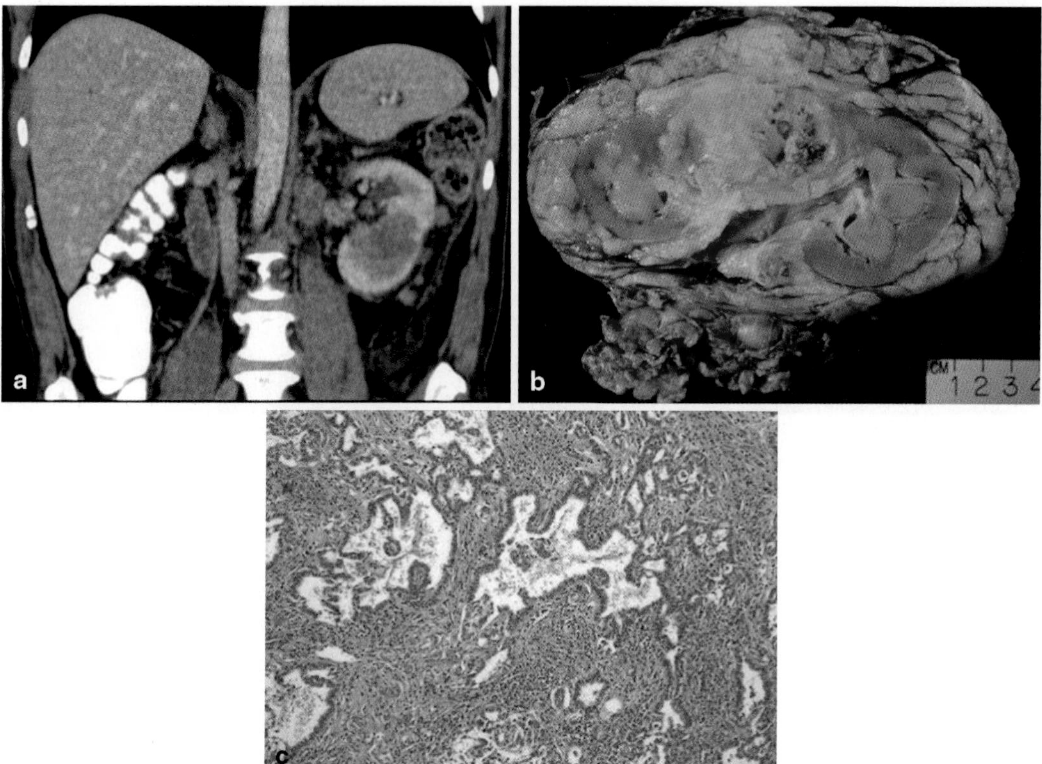

Fig. 27.4 Collecting duct RCC. **a.** CT scan shows a centrally located, infiltrative left renal tumor. **b.** Centrally located tan, partially sclerotic, and hemorrhagic tumor with irregular infiltration into perinephric fat and renal sinus fat. **c.** A high-grade carcinoma growing in irregular tubules and papillary structures separated by a desmoplastic stroma with an accompanying inflammatory infiltrate. (Courtesy of Dr. Christopher G. Przybycin, Cleveland, OH)

therapy. In contrast, it is often treated with cisplatin-based chemotherapy in a manner similar to advanced urothelial cell carcinoma, with which it shares a variety of clinical and morphologic characteristics and unfortunately shares a generally unfavorable outcome.

Renal Medullary Carcinoma

Another rare and highly aggressive version of RCC is renal medullary carcinoma (RMC), which many consider to be a subtype of collecting duct RCC. RMC originates from the renal papillae, and is thus centrally located, and it is highly infiltrative. It is found almost exclusively associated with the sickle cell trait, and thus typically diagnosed in young African-Americans. It is almost always locally advanced and/or metastatic at presentation. RMC does not respond to conventional treatments including targeted treatments, radiotherapy, or immunotherapy. Wide surgical excision with extensive lymph node dissection is probably the only chance for cure, but even with this most patients will develop disseminated disease and die of cancer progression within a few to several months. Mean survival in Davis and coworkers series of 34 patients was only 15 weeks [20].

Sarcomatoid Differentiation

Sarcomatoid differentiation is no longer considered a distinct subtype of RCC, but its prognostic implications have not changed. Sarcomatoid differentiation is most commonly seen in association with clear cell and chromophobe RCC, but all of the malignant variants of RCC can occasionally degenerate in this manner. Sarcomatoid differentiation typically correlates with an infiltrative morphology, locally advanced and/or systemic metastases, and a treatment refractory phenotype. Previous studies have explored a potential role for cytotoxic chemotherapy in the management of these patients. In a phase II study from the Eastern Cooperative Group (ECOG 8802), 38 patients with advanced sarcomatoid RCC were treated with gemcitabine and doxorubicin. Median progression-free survival and overall survival were 3.5 and 8.8 months, respectively, and a 16 % objective response rate was observed. Enthusiasm for this approach has waned with the introduction of targeted agents [21]. Recently, the Cleveland Clinic reported a retrospective series of 43 advanced sarcomatoid RCC patients treated with TKIs or bevacizumab. Partial responses were seen in 19 % of the patients with the majority being in the clear cell subgroup [22]. Patients with limited sarcomatoid features (<20 %) appeared to respond better to targeted therapy [23].

Oncocytoma

Renal oncocytoma represents about 5–15 % of all renal tumors, and presents major challenges in that it is extremely difficult to differentiate from RCC based on clinical presentation and imaging characteristics. Most oncocytomas are discovered incidentally, but some are associated with hematuria, and considerable overlap in clinical features is observed with RCC. The classic imaging characteristics of an oncycotyma, central stellate scar on CT and spoke wheel pattern on angiography, are neither sensitive nor specific enough for the diagnosis, and have been relegated to historical interest alone. Differentiation from the eosinophilic variants of RCC is very difficult on biopsy specimens, limiting the utility of this approach, although molecular profiling may fundamentally alter this perspective in the near future. For the present time, oncocytoma is for the most part a fortunate postoperative diagnosis, given its uniformly benign clinical course, which is observed even when locally invasive features such as extension into the sinus fat are present [24].

Other Histologic Subtypes of RCC

A wide variety of other rare or emerging subtypes of RCC have recently been described and are reviewed in other chapters. Many have distinct clinical/pathologic correlates, such as multiloculated cystic RCC and mucinous tubular and spindle cell carcinoma, which appear to have very favorable prognoses. RCC associated with Xp11.2 translocations/TFE3 gene fusion abnormalities are found mostly in children, and represent 40 % of RCC cases found in the pediatric population. Many of these tumors present with advanced stage, commonly exhibiting nodal involvement, but then follow a relatively indolent course. Comprehensive surgical resection including extensive lymph node dissection is recommended [25]. Unclassified RCC represents 1–3 % of all RCC in most series, incorporating usually high-grade tumors that do not fit neatly into any of the established RCC subtypes and in general has a very poor prognosis, consistent with its often poorly differentiated and treatment refractory phenotype.

References

1. Siegel R, Naishadham D, Jemal A. Cancer statistics, 2013. CA Cancer J Clin. 2013;63(1):11–30.
2. Calle EE, Kaaks R. Overweight, obesity and cancer: epidemiological evidence and proposed mechanisms. Nature reviews. Cancer. 2004;4(8):579–91.
3. Ishikawa I, et al. Renal cell carcinoma detected by screening shows better patient survival than that detected following symptoms in dialysis patients. Ther Apher Dial. 2004;8(6):468–73.
4. Rini BI, Campbell SC, Escudier B. Renal cell carcinoma. Lancet. 2009;373(9669):1119–32.
5. Jinzaki M, et al. Double-phase helical CT of small renal parenchymal neoplasms: correlation with pathologic findings and tumor angiogenesis. J Comput Assist Tomogr. 2000;24(6):835–42.
6. Volpe A, et al. Contemporary management of small renal masses. Eur Urol. 2011;60(3):501–15.

7. Rini BI, et al. The effect of sunitinib on primary renal cell carcinoma and facilitation of subsequent surgery. J Urol. 2012;187(5):1548–54.
8. Hofmann HS, et al. Prognostic factors and survival after pulmonary resection of metastatic renal cell carcinoma. Euro Urol. 2005;48(1):77–81; discussion 81–2.
9. Linehan WM. Molecular targeting of VHL gene pathway in clear cell kidney cancer. J Urol. 2003;170(2 Pt 1):593–4.
10. Rabbani F, et al. Renal vein or inferior vena caval extension in patients with renal cortical tumors: impact of tumor histology. J Urol. 2004;171(3):1057–61.
11. Cheville JC, et al. Comparisons of outcome and prognostic features among histologic subtypes of renal cell carcinoma. Am J Surg Pathol. 2003;27(5):612–24.
12. Umbreit EC, Thompson RH. Metastatic potential of the small renal mass: why can't we agree? Eur Urol. 2011;60(5):983–5; discussion 985–6.
13. Gontero P, et al. Prognostic factors in a prospective series of papillary renal cell carcinoma. BJU Int. 2008;102(6):697–702.
14. Pignot G, et al. Survival analysis of 130 patients with papillary renal cell carcinoma: prognostic utility of type 1 and type 2 subclassification. Urology. 2007;69(2):230–5.
15. Margulis V, et al. Analysis of clinicopathologic predictors of oncologic outcome provides insight into the natural history of surgically managed papillary renal cell carcinoma. Cancer. 2008;112(7):1480–8.
16. Klatte T, et al. Pathobiology and prognosis of chromophobe renal cell carcinoma. Urol Oncol. 2008;26(6):604–9.
17. Baba M, et al. Kidney-targeted Birt-Hogg-Dube gene inactivation in a mouse model: Erk1/2 and Akt-mTOR activation, cell hyperproliferation, and polycystic kidneys. J Natl Cancer Inst. 2008;100(2):140–54.
18. Swartz MA, et al. Renal medullary carcinoma: clinical, pathologic, immunohistochemical, and genetic analysis with pathogenetic implications. Urology. 2002;60(6):1083–9.
19. Tokuda N, et al. Collecting duct (Bellini duct) renal cell carcinoma: a nationwide survey in Japan. J Urol. 2006;176(1):40–3; discussion 43.
20. Davis CJ Jr., Mostofi FK, Sesterhenn IA. Renal medullary carcinoma. The seventh sickle cell nephropathy. Am J Surg Pathol. 1995;19(1):1–11.
21. Nanus DM, et al. Active chemotherapy for sarcomatoid and rapidly progressing renal cell carcinoma. Cancer. 2004;101(7):1545–51.
22. Golshayan AR, et al. Metastatic sarcomatoid renal cell carcinoma treated with vascular endothelial growth factor-targeted therapy. J Clin Oncol. 2009;27(2):235–41.
23. Shuch B, et al. Sarcomatoid renal cell carcinoma: a comprehensive review of the biology and current treatment strategies. Oncologist. 2012;17(1):46–54.
24. Childs MA, et al. Metachronous renal tumours after surgical management of oncocytoma. BJU Int. 2011;108(6):816–9.
25. Argani P, et al. Xp11 translocation renal cell carcinoma (RCC): extended immunohistochemical profile emphasizing novel RCC markers. Am J Surg Pathol. 2010;34(9):1295–303.

28 Independent Predictors of Clinical Outcomes and Prediction Models for Renal Tumor Pathology

Nils Kroeger, Daniel Y. C. Heng and Michael W. Kattan

Introduction

Kidney cancer is a heterogeneous tumor entity, and renal cell carcinoma (RCC) is the most common subtype of kidney cancer. Clinical, pathological, molecular, and genetic analyses of the last decades have proven that RCC by itself comprises additional subcategories all of which display their own propensities and clinical outcome [1]. As a consequence of its heterogeneous biology, it has become apparent that not a single prognostic factor but multiple factors including patient and tumor characteristics need to be applied to make reliable prognostications.

The clinical course of patients having localized and those with metastatic RCC (mRCC) is significantly different. While ~80% of patients with localized disease can be cured by surgery alone, the vast majority of patients with metastatic disease will eventually die from RCC. Consequently, both RCC subgroups have different prognostication systems.

In localized RCC, prognostication is important to individualize follow-up protocols. After surgical treatment only a minority of patients with non-mRCC will experience disease recurrence [2], and thus individualized follow-up is desired, particularly for high-risk patients. The assignment of patients to adjuvant clinical trials is another important issue in the management of patients with localized disease. For this purpose, the definition of high-risk features, which reliably prognosticate disease recurrence, is warranted. In addition, the increase of RCC incidence is mainly caused by localized RCCs and has been paralleled by an increase of surgical treatments [3]. However, this current clinical practice has not led to an improvement of the age adjusted mortality of localized RCC [4]. Therefore, active surveillance (AS) of nonmetastatic small renal masses (SRM) has become a treatment option [5]. One major problem for assignment of patients to either surgical treatment or AS is to prognosticate the potential risk of metastatic spread, and, therefore, it is currently expert consensus that AS is primarily a treatment option in selected patients that are at high risk for surgical complications [6, 7]. Collectively, prognostication of survival outcome and the risk of metastatic spread independent of surgical treatment are of paramount importance in the clinical management of localized RCC.

In mRCC, immunotherapy as a first-line treatment has been supplanted by agents that target the vascular endothelial growth factor (VEGF) and mammalian target of rapamycin (mTOR)

N. Kroeger (✉)
Department of Medical Oncology, Tom Baker Cancer Centre, Calgary, AB, Canada
e-mail: md.nkroeger@gmail.com

Department of Urology, University Medicine Greifswald, Greifswald, Germany

D. Y. C. Heng
Department of Medical Oncology, Tom Baker Cancer Center, Calgary, AB, Canada
e-mail: Daniel.heng@albertahealthservices.ca

M. W. Kattan
Department of Quantitative Health Sciences, Cleveland Clinic, Cleveland, OH, USA
e-mail: kattanm@ccf.edu

C. Magi-Galluzzi, C. G. Przybycin (eds.), *Genitourinary Pathology,* DOI 10.1007/978-1-4939-2044-0_28,

pathways. The change in treatment paradigm has challenged the validity of prognostic and predictive factors because most of them were defined during the immunotherapy era. Thus, much effort has been undertaken to find new markers, improve existing ones, and to develop new prognostication tools. As a result, new prognostic models have successfully been introduced into clinical practice [8–13]. The progress in the development of new targeted agents is paralleled by an increasing armamentarium of molecular and genetic biomarkers which eventually will have the predictive power to provide an individualized cancer therapy, to design new clinical trials and to inform patients accurately on their anticipated course of disease [14].

This chapter describes the current knowledge of prognostic factors and models in localized and mRCC. An introduction to predictive markers of treatment response to targeted therapy agents is given although there is currently no established marker that predicts treatment response to targeted therapy.

Independent Factors in Survival Prognostication and Treatment Response Prediction

Definitions of Prognostication and Prediction in Oncology

In an effort to develop recommendations for the incorporation of biomarkers into clinical trials, a biomarker task force was established by the National Cancer Institute (NCI) [15]. They recently published guidelines and definitions for the future of biomarker research. Prognostic factors can be grossly subdivided into clinical, pathological/anatomic, molecular, and genetic characteristics. According to the biomarker task force guidelines for the development and incorporation of biomarker studies in early clinical trials of novel agents, the following nomenclature is recommended to describe properly biomarkers [15]:

- *Prognostic* factors or prognostic models provide evidence about the overall disease outcome independent of any specific intervention.
- *Predictive* factors/models offer evidence for benefit or toxicity of a specific intervention.
- Depending on their quality, markers are *valid, probably valid, or exploratory*.
- *Surrogate parameters* are variables that are strongly correlated with the end point and thereby capture clinically relevant events and have a clearly defined, easily measurable start and finish [15, 16]. An example would be the progression-free survival (PFS) which is an accepted clinical indicator of overall survival (OS) in certain clinical trial settings [16].

The vast majority of biomarkers for RCC are currently exploratory because validation of their prognostic value is still missing.

Prognostic Factors for Both Localized and Metastatic RCC

Patient-related factors like performance status, obesity, and symptoms at presentation are prognostically relevant for localized and metastatic disease. Performance status, either categorized according to the Eastern Cooperative Oncology Group performance status (ECOG PS) or according to Karnofsky (KPS), has been demonstrated to be of incremental prognostic value for RCC multiple times in various multivariate analyses [9, 17, 18]. The basis for both performance status indicators is the evaluation of patients' functional capacity in daily life activities.

Obesity is a risk factor for the development of RCC [19]. Obesity is a complex disease which is influenced by genetic, nutrition, and lifestyle factors. To the contrary, studies have suggested that the general nutrition status and obesity are predictors of favorable cancer-specific survival (CSS) [20, 21]. From a clinical point of view, obesity increases risk factors like cardiovascular diseases and diabetes mellitus. Furthermore, it is known that obesity induces a permanent inflammatory state with elevated levels of tumor necrosis factor, interleukin (IL)-1, IL-6, IL-1 receptor antagonist, and C-reactive protein (CRP) [22]. Reactive oxygen species, which are permanently increased in obese patients, are able to activate the phosphorinositide-3-kinase-mTOR-pathway [23]. Moreover, insulin-resistance and hyperinsulinemia are typically associated with obesity, and it has been shown that insulin induces cancer progression [24]. In the light of this biological background, it is currently unknown whether obesity is an incremental predictor for improved survival outcome. In fact, none of the studies that have demonstrated an independent influence of body mass index (BMI) and nutrition on CSS had adjusted their multivariate analyses for the ECOG PS or KPS.

Symptomatic presentation of the disease has been reported to be of prognostic value by several authors [25, 26]. Patard et al. [26] assigned patients to three groups (S1–S3) under consideration of the type of symptoms at presentation. S1 symptoms were defined as incidentally discovered tumors in any imaging study that was conducted because of symptoms other than the RCC-related reasons; S2 symptoms were assigned to local symptoms such as lumbar pain or isolated hematuria; and S3 symptoms were defined as systemic symptoms like weight loss, fever, night sweat, etc. In survival outcome prognostication, the symptom classification discriminates three prognostic groups with patients being in group S1 to have the best and S3 the worst prognosis. However, the allocation of patients either as symptomatic or asymptomatic is highly variable between study centers. In one study, the range for assigning patients as symptomatic at presentation varied between study centers from 36.8 to 71 % [27]. This raises concern about the objectivity of this factor for its inclusion into prognostic multivariable models. It is also unknown how well (i.e., accurately) this system predicts.

Prognostic Factors in Localized RCC

Approximately 20 % of RCC patients will experience disease recurrence after surgical treatment, and the metastatic relapse is the most important life limiting factor of this patient population. Therefore, most prognostic factors are assessed for the risk of metastatic relapse after nephrectomy.

In localized RCC, high-risk characteristics for disease recurrence like the tumor size, tumor growth into the adrenal gland, renal sinus invasion, and perinephric fat invasion are included in the T stage. These staging factors are discussed in detail in Chaps. 22 and 24 of this book.

It has been recognized that there are other histological criteria that are powerful tools to prognosticate disease recurrence and survival outcome in localized RCC. All RCC subtypes have a very heterogeneous biological and clinical behavior. In localized RCC, clear cell RCC (ccRCC) has been revealed to be independently associated with worse CSS [28]. Additionally, other studies that have sought to demonstrate a poor prognosis of ccRCC were also mainly comprised of localized RCCs [29]. Collectively, it can be concluded that the ccRCC subtype may be the histological subtype with the worst CSS in localized RCC.

In cancer types like testicular cancer, lymphomicrovascular invasion (MVI) is an important high-risk feature and is consistently reported by pathologists to estimate recurrence and death risks [30, 31]. One study has demonstrated that MVI occurs in at least one out of five patients in RCC and is closely related to CSS and metastatic disease [32]. Recently, an international multicenter study has shown that metastatic relapse can occur even after a long time period of ≥60 months [33]. One of the most important predictors of metastatic relapse was MVI of the primary localized RCC. However, despite the importance of MVI to prognosticate survival and disease recurrence in RCC, it is still not routinely reported by all pathologists worldwide.

Tumor necrosis has frequently been described as a prognostic feature of RCC [34, 35]. The importance of its prognostic value has accumulated in its integration in several prognostication models [34, 35]. It is a particularly important prognostic factor in localized RCC [35]. Thus, any amount of tumor necrosis should lead to a very careful follow-up of patients with primary localized RCC.

RCCs that present with sarcomatoid features are considered to have a more aggressive biological behavior than other tumors [36]. Sarcomatoid differentiation can be present in all RCC subtypes and is not a histologic subtype of RCC on its own [37]. In localized RCC, the description of sarcomatoid features is known to be associated with metastatic relapse [38]. The high risk for disease recurrence and limited treatment options for these tumors underscore the high importance of an accurate pathological reporting of sarcomatoid features in RCCs.

Prognostic Factors in Metastatic RCC

While in localized RCC many tumor-related factors are prognostically relevant, patient-related factors like the time from diagnosis to treatment initiation and serological markers have an important prognostic role in mRCC.

Before targeted therapies became standard of care, cytoreductive nephrectomies and the time from surgery to initiation of a systemic therapy were defined as prognostic characteristics. The combined analyses of two large clinical trials evaluating the influence of cytoreductive nephrectomy on CSS has shown a 31 % risk reduction for death ($p=0.002$) in patients who had a cytoreductive nephrectomy in combination with interferon-α (INF-α) immunotherapy [39]. In the age of targeted therapies, it is currently unknown whether cytoreductive nephrectomy improves the OS. Two large trials, the clinical trial to assess the importance of nephrectomy (CARMENA) trial (NCT00930033) and the European Organisation for Research and Treatment of Cancer (EORTC) trial (NCT01099423), which address this question, are ongoing. Although retrospective studies suggested that cytoreductive nephrectomies are still an important component of mRCC therapy [40], the results of these two prospective randomized trials are anxiously awaited.

Pathological changes of blood parameters may reflect proinflammatory events, high cell turnover or paraneoplastic syndromes. The best investigated blood markers for prognostication of RCC-survival outcome are elevated levels of CRP, alkaline phosphatase (AP), and lactate dehydrogenase (LDH), neutrophilia, thrombocytosis, and low hemoglobin (Hb) levels. Thrombocytosis is particularly associated with diminished survival in mRCC [41]. One study confirmed that high preoperative platelet count is an independent prognosticator for survival [42]. Yet the authors were not able to show an improvement of prognostic models that included tumor-nodes-metastasis (TNM) stage, grade, and ECOG PS after inclusion of thrombocytosis. However, in prognostication of survival outcome of mRCC, thrombocytosis is still a central factor [13].

The immune system has a crucial role in the pathogenesis of mRCC which is underscored due to its responsiveness to immunotherapies in selected patients [43]. All acute phase proteins are correlated with survival outcome [44]. Neutrophil granulocytes are a major component of the inherent immune system and elevated CRP levels can reflect an activation of the immune system in response to the tumor burden of RCC. Subsequently, it has been reported from multivariable examinations that both CRP levels and neutrophilia are important independent prognostic characteristics that are associated with survival outcome in mRCC [9, 45, 46].

Paraneoplastic syndromes caused by RCC can induce both hyperchromasia and anemia. Anemia is one of the most often observed pathological blood abnormalities that are related to RCC. It is correlated with diminished survival outcome [8]. It has become evident that anemia is a substantial factor to prognosticate survival outcome in mRCC [9, 13]. The levels of LDH, AP, and calcium are an expression of a high cell turnover in tumor cells and at metastatic sites. LDH is a prognostic marker in many types of cancer, for example in testicular cancer [30]. In RCC, the independent prognostic value of LDH levels has been demonstrated in different settings and has resulted in its integration into diverse prognostic models [12, 47]. Corrected calcium levels greater than the upper limit of normal were found to be associated with poor prognosis in patients treated with immunotherapies [17, 48]. These findings have been confirmed in the targeted therapy era, and thus high calcium levels continue to be important prognosticators of survival outcome in mRCC [12, 13].

Table 28.1 Independent clinical and pathological characteristics for survival prognostication

Feature	Described association	Reference
Tumor-related characteristics		
Lymph node involvement (N stage)	Survival outcome, RFS	Pantuck [74]
Distant metastases (M stage)	Survival outcome	Zisman et al. [18]
Fuhrman grade	Survival outcome, RFS	Fuhrman [75]
Tumor size	Survival outcome, RFS	Frank et al. [58]
Extension into perinephric fat/renal sinus fat	Survival outcome, RFS	Thompson [76]
Adrenal involvement	Survival outcome	Thompson et al. [76]
Venous involvement	Survival outcome, RFS	Martinez-Salamanca [77]
Metastatic burden	Survival outcome	Flanigan [39], Motzer et al. [48]
Collecting duct invasion	RFS	Klatte et al. [78]
Micro-vascular invasion	Survival outcome, RFS	Kroeger et al. [32]
Sarcomatoid features	Survival outcome, RFS	de Peralta-Venturina et al. [36]
Tumor necrosis	Survival outcome	Sengupta et al. [79]
Patient-related characteristics		
ECOG PS	Survival outcome, PFS, RFS	Zisman et al. [18]
Karnofsky PS	Survival outcome, PFS	Heng et al. [13]
Symptoms at presentation (local/systemic)	Survival outcome, RFS	Patard [80]; Kattan et al. [25]
Nutrition status	Survival outcome	Morgan et al. [20]
Disease free interval	Survival outcome	Motzer et al. [48]
Cytoreductive nephrectomy	Survival outcome	Flanigan and Mickisch et al. [39]
Blood markers		
Thrombocytosis	Survival outcome	Suppiah et al. [41]
Leukocytosis	Survival outcome, PFS	Choueiri et al. [8, 13]
Hypercalcemia	Survival outcome, PFS	Motzer et al. [47, 48]
Elevated alkaline phosphatase	Survival outcome, PFS	Negrier et al. [46]
Elevated CRP	Survival outcome, PFS	Karakiewicz et al. [45]
Elevated blood sedimentation rate	Survival outcome	Ljungberg et al. [44]
Elevated lactatdehydrogenase	Survival outcome, PFS	Motzer et al. [47, 48]
Anemia	Survival outcome	Heng et al. [13]

ECOG PS Eastern Cooperative Oncology Group performance status, *CSS* cancer-specific survival, *RFS* recurrence-free survival, *PFS* progression-free survival, *CRP* C-reactive protein

The survival outcome of metastatic nonclear cell RCC (nccRCC) is generally worse compared to metastatic ccRCC, which is most likely the result of a less effective response to the new targeted agents as compared to ccRCC [49]. However, not all metastatic nccRCC have a worse survival outcome than ccRCC. For example, studies have shown that metastatic chromophobe RCCs have a good prognosis when treated with targeted therapies [50]. The recognition of different RCC histologies needing individual treatments is the first step into the age of individualized cancer therapy in mRCC. In order to accurately prognosticate the clinical outcome of mRCC, it will be one major challenge to identify the genetic, epigenetic, and molecular tumor characteristics of each histological subtype in the near future. A comprehensive summary on prognostic risk factors is shown in Table 28.1.

Clinical Features to Predict Response to Targeted Therapies

In the last 7 years, there has been a fundamental change in the treatment paradigm of mRCC. Therapies targeting key elements of the mTOR and VEGF-pathway have become the international standard of care [51]. Targeted therapies can achieve disease control rates in approximately 80% of patients. However, primary response and duration of response to targeted therapies are very heterogeneous even among tumors with similar histological subtypes and clinicopathological features [52]. Biomarkers are urgently needed to guide clinicians to choose the most effective drug for each individual patient. This may one day be used to prevent unnecessary toxicities and cost incurred to patients who would not benefit from a drug as predicted by a biomarker, and instead allow the selection of a more efficacious drug with fewer side effects on an individual level. None of the numerous clinical, genetic, tissue and blood markers tested during the past years are ready for routine use in clinical practice. External validation of potential biomarkers is still required. The main focus of biomarker studies are molecular and genetic features which will be discussed in a separate chapter. The following paragraphs will focus on some clinical features that may be of predictive value for treatment response to targeted agents.

An interesting clinical biomarker was described by Rini et al. who demonstrated that sunitinib-induced hypertension is associated with a better objective response, PFS, and OS in mRCC. Patients with versus without hypertension had objective response rates of 54.8 versus 8.7%, a PFS 12.5 versus 2.5 months, and OS of 30.9 versus 7.2 months [53]. Since the development of hypertension was not associated with more major adverse events than in patients without hypertension, it may be useful to guide treatment selection in targeted therapies.

The objective of other clinical studies was the influence of the body composition on treatment response to targeted therapies. A study of 475 patients demonstrated that a high BMI is correlated with improved survival with targeted agents (HR 0.67; 95% CI: 0.49–0.91; $p=0.01$) [54]. On the contrary, two other studies did not find a similar association of BMI or body surface area (BSA) with favorable response to targeted therapies. While one of the studies demonstrated a positive impact of high visceral fat area (VFA) and elevated superficial fat area (SFA) on survival, the other study found the complete opposite having used the same measurement methods [55, 56]. In summary, the heterogeneity of these results underscores the importance of external validation.

A recent study of Tran et al. used an interesting 3-step approach for screening, confirmation and validation of blood-biomarkers [57]. In their screening study, they found a blood marker panel comprised of six proteins (IL-6, IL-8, VEGF, Osteopontin, E-selectin, HGF), which could predict survival and response to pazopanib. In the phase II and phase III approval trials of pazopanib, the findings from the training set could be externally validated (Table 28.2). Although this study was well designed and provided external validation of preliminary findings, the study did not demonstrate an improvement on existing prognostic models. Once more, the approach of Tran et al. underscores that survival outcome and treatment response are influenced by a variety of clinical and biological processes, and thus prediction models must include a marker panel rather than one single predictive factor.

Table 28.2 Clinical markers for response to targeted therapies prediction

Clinical markers	Predictive end point	Reference
BMI, BSA	Response to TT	Choueiri et al. [54]
Hypertension	Response to sunitinib	Rini et al. [53]
Blood markers	*Predictive end point*	*Reference*
sVEGF and sVEGFR	OS with bevacizumab, PFS and ORR with sunitinib	Escudier [81], Rini et al. [82]
High IL-6; IL-8, VEGF, osteopontin, E-selectin, HGF	Tumor shrinkage, PFS with pazopanib	Tran et al. [57]
Signature of VEGF, CA-IX, collagen IV, VEGFR-2, TRAIL	PFS with sorafenib	Zurita et al. [83]

VEGF vascular endothelial growth factor, *VEGFR* vascular endothelial growth factor receptor, *IL* interleukin, *HGF* hepatocyte growth factor, *CA-IX* carbonic anhydrase IX,*PFS* progression-free survival, *OS* overall survival, *ORR* objective response rate, *TT* targeted therapy

Integration of Single Factors into Multivariable Prognostic and Predictive Models

During the last decade, several prognostication systems have combined prognostic factors. These models were developed to improve prognostication of recurrence-free survival (RFS) and CSS before or after nephrectomy. While some models were exclusively designed to improve prognostication of patients with localized RCCs, others focused on mRCC or both. There is currently no reliable model that is particularly able to predict treatment response to targeted therapies.

Multivariable Models for Localized and Metastatic RCC

Other models were established for all Union for International Cancer Control (UICC)/American Joint Committee on Cancer (AJCC) stages of patients independent of the RCC subtype. The most studied models are the University of California Los Angeles integrated staging system (UISS) and the Mayo Clinic tumor stage, tumor size, tumor grade, and necrosis (SSIGN) model [18, 58]. Both the UISS [59, 60] and the SSIGN [59] were extensively validated in numerous studies. While the UISS has the advantage that it is simple to use because it integrates standard clinicopathological variables such as the TNM stage, Fuhrman grade, and ECOG PS, the SSIGN model has reached higher accuracies in validation studies [59]. Collectively, both models have proven their applicability in clinical practice and represent useful tools in RCC survival prognostication.

Another model of Karakiewicz et al. has reached concordance indices of 88–89% in the development and validation cohorts, respectively, and they presented the highest accuracies for postoperative survival prognostication. The model includes TNM stage, Fuhrman grade, tumor size, and symptoms at presentation as individual prognostic factors [61]. The practicability of this model has to be evaluated in clinical practice.

Patients want to be informed about their prognosis before treatment decisions are made. Karackiewicz et al. also developed a model for this purpose [62]. The training cohort and validation were comprised of 2474 and 1972 patients and included metastatic and nonmetastatic patients. It has reached impressive concordance indices of 86.8% at 5 years, and 84.2% at 10 years. Thus, this model may present a useful tool to inform patients and their families about their estimated prognosis before invasive treatments are done.

Multivariable Prognostic Models in Localized RCC

Currently, SRM (tumors <4.0 cm) comprise the majority of renal lesions. It has been recognized that between 20 and 30% of them are benign tumors. Moreover, approximately 75–80% of the malignant SRM are indolent and do not behave aggressively in terms of tumor progression and development of metastatic disease [7, 63]. On the other hand, there is a chance that patients having undergone partial or radical nephrectomy will develop chronic kidney disease (CKD) of <60 mL/min per 1.72 m^2 in 20 and 65% of cases, respectively, after 3 years [32]. Furthermore, renal insufficiency of >45 mL/min and <60 mL/min is associated with 20% increased risk of death [64]. Therefore, it has been questioned if the majority of SRMs is overtreated by surgery, causing harm to patients due to the development of CKD. Therefore, physicians have to face two major problems: first, to prognosticate the chance of having a malignant lesion, and second, to prognosticate the likelihood that localized RCC develops metastatic disease with or without surgery. For these two purposes preoperative and postoperative prognostic models were established.

Preoperative Prognostication of Recurrence, Cancer-Specific Survival and Prediction of Tumor-Biology

In an effort to preoperatively distinguish benign versus malignant and indolent versus potentially aggressive lesions in RCC<7.0 cm, Lane et al.

from the Cleveland clinic constructed two nomograms from 862 patients [63]. They used clinical presentation, age, gender, smoking history, and tumor size as components for these nomograms. They reported concordance indices of 0.64 and 0.56 for malignancy and aggressiveness prediction, respectively. Clearly, the effort to predict these two end points preoperatively has to be acknowledged, but these two nomograms need further improvement, e.g., by adding new radiological markers, biopsy results, and genetic serum markers. Another preclinical model including gender, mode of presentation, necrosis, lymphadenopathy, and tumor size by imaging of Raj et al. from the Cleveland clinic was developed based on data of two high-volume centers. The resulting nomogram reached a concordance index of 80 %. In the same cohort, the TNM classification alone had a concordance index of just 71 % (Fig. 28.1) [65].

Two other models from the group of Karackiewicz et al. using preoperative data were developed and validated in order to prognosticate the likelihood of lymph node and distant metastases at nephrectomy [66, 67]. The reported concordance indices were 85.2 % for distant metastases and 78.4 % for lymph node metastases. The only variables in both nomograms were symptoms at diagnosis and tumor size. The prognostication of the likelihood for metastatic disease was based on patient data with synchronous metastases. It is currently uncertain whether tumors presenting with synchronous metastases share the same biological characteristics as tumors developing metastatic disease several years after surgery.

Kutikov et al. from Fox Chase Cancer Center recently reported an interesting comprehensive approach to estimate the risk for kidney cancer death, other cancer death, and noncancer related death under consideration of other mortality risk factors [68]. In a patient cohort of 30,801 patients with localized RCC, the 5-year probability for risk of death from RCC, other cancers, and noncancer mortality were 4, 7, and 11 %, respectively (Fig. 28.2a, b). With regard to AS strategies, the approach of Kutikov et al. is important because it underscores the central role of individualized treatment decisions under consideration of other morbidities, gender, race, and age (Fig. 28.2a, b).

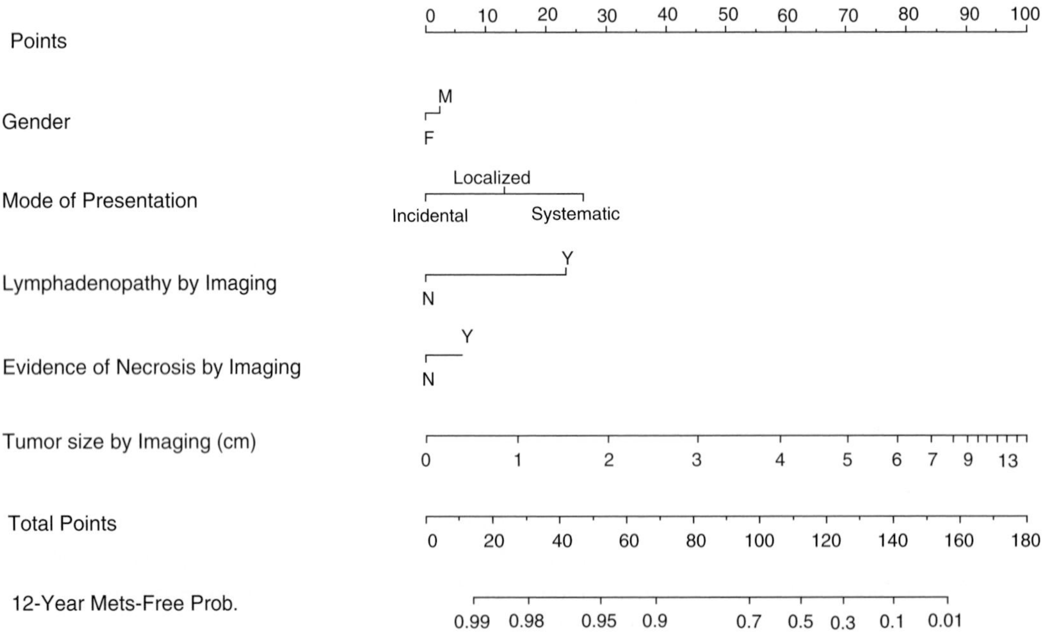

Fig. 28.1 Preoperative prognostic model of Raj et al. [65] predicts the likelihood of postoperative metastatic recurrence. Metastatic recurrence developed in 340/2517 patients with a median follow-up of 4.7 years for patients with recurrence. The nomogram predicts the 12-year probability of metastatic relapse with a concordance index of 0.80 while the TNM classification alone reached only a concordance index of 0.71. (Used with permission from [65])

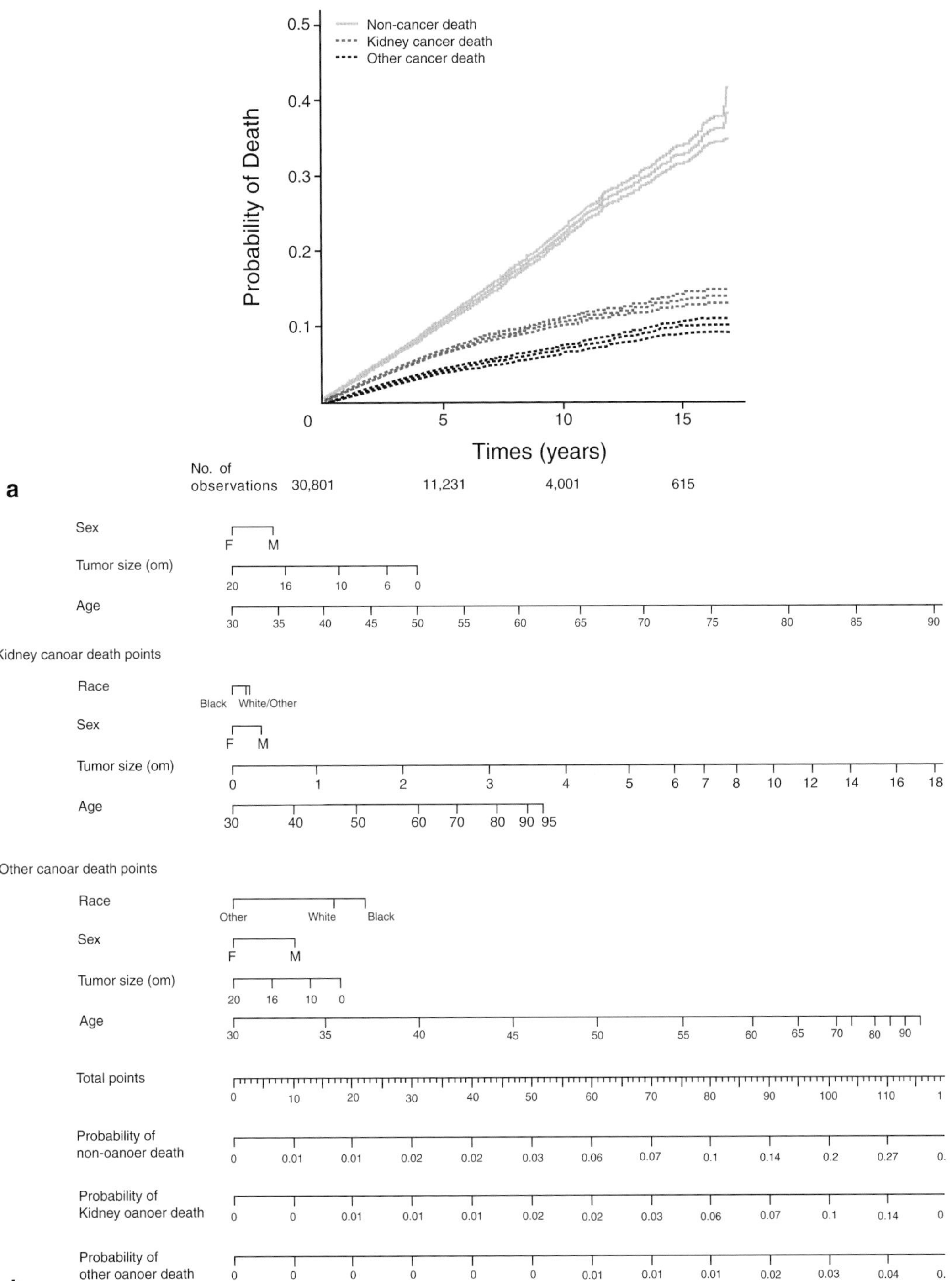

Fig. 28.2 a Cumulative mortality incidence rates and 95% confidence intervals for noncancer-related, kidney-cancer-related, and other cancer-related death. **b** Nomogram that prognosticates the 5-year probability according to competing risk criteria. (Used with permission from [68])

All preoperative nomograms currently available were developed based on patient cohorts who were treated by radical or partial nephrectomy. In the future, it will be one major challenge to integrate clinical, histological, molecular, and genetic features of prospectively collected data of patients managed with AS. A comprehensive overview on preoperative prognostic models in localized RCC is given in Table 28.3.

Recurrence-Free Survival and Cancer-Specific Survival after Nephrectomy

It is important to individualize follow-up protocols and to assign patients at high risk for disease recurrence to clinical trials for adjuvant therapies after surgical treatment of non-mRCC. Several models address this issue (Table 28.3). Most of them are currently based on clinicopathological features only, without consideration of molecular

Table 28.3 Prognostic models in localized RCCs

Preoperative models				
Patient number(Test set; validation cohort)	Endpoint	Follow-up	Concordance index	Reference(year)
296	Recurrence after surgery	48 months (5–129)	65.1%	Yaycioglu (2001) [84]
660	Recurrence after surgery	42 months (2–180)	67.2%	Cindolo (2003) [85]
851	Malignancy and tumor aggressiveness	1.4 years	64.4% (malignancy); 55.7% (aggressiveness)	Lane (2007) [63]
2522; 2136	Lymph node metastases at surgery	n.r.	78.8%	Hutterer (2007) [67]
2517	Recurrence after surgery	4.7 years (patients without evidence of metastatic recurrence)	80%	Raj (2008) [65]
2660; 2716	Visceral metastases at surgery	n.r.	85%	Hutterer (2008) [66]
30801	CSS, OC, NCS	3.8 years (0–203 months)	n.r.	Kutikov (2010) [68]
Postoperative models				
601	RFS	40 months (patients without evidence of metastatic recurrence)	74.0%	Kattan (2001) [25]
1864	RFS to abdominal, thoracic, and bone metastases	6.4 years (0.1–31)	80.5% (abdominal), 82.6% (thoracic), 80.0%(bone)	Frank (2003) [69]
1671	RFS	5.4 years (0–31 years)	81.9%	Leibovich(2003) [35]
701	RFS	32 months (patients without evidence of metastatic recurrence)	82.0%	Sorbellini (2005) [70]
559	RFS solitary, chest, abdominal, bone, brain recurrence	26 months	n.r.	Lam (2005) [86]
170	RFS	7.1 years (0.1–16.9)	90.4%	Klatte (2009) [71]

RFS recurrence-free survival, *n.r.* not reported, *CSS* cancer-specific survival, *OS* overall survival, *NCS* non-kidney cancer survival

or genetic markers. The Leibovich prognostic score from the Mayo Clinic is probably the most often applied prognostic model for localized ccRCC [35]. The model separates three groups with high, intermediate, and low risk for metastatic relapse after nephrectomy by integrating tumor stage, regional lymph node status, tumor size, nuclear grade, and histologic tumor necrosis into a prognostic risk score. Another model of the same institution was constructed with 11 clinicopathological characteristics in order to prognosticate recurrence in specific organ sites. The authors reported excellent concordance indices of 80.5, 82.6, and 80.8 % for the prediction of abdominal, thoracic, and bone metastases, respectively [69]. While these are reasonable concordance indices, there is the question about the practicability of this model in clinical practice since so many variables are necessary for prognostication.

A fundamentally simpler nomogram was presented by Sorbellini et al. [70] from the Memorial Sloan Kettering Cancer Center (MSKCC). This nomogram reached a concordance index of 82.0 % and is based on tumor size, T stage, grade, necrosis, MVI, and presentation of symptoms. The sorbellini nomogram was externally validated in opposite to many other nomograms.

In a proof of principle study Klatte et al. presented a nomogram which combines clinicopathological features and histological markers in order to predict RFS in primary localized RCCs (Fig. 28.2a, b) [71]. The nomogram reached an impressive concordance index of 90.4 %. The model included T stage, ECOG PS, and five histological markers (Ki-67, p53, endothelial VEGFR-1, epithelial VEGFR-1, and epithelial VEGF-D). While Ki-67 and expression of p53 are routinely evaluable markers, distinguishing between epithelial and endothelial VEGF and VEGF-R expression may be challenging in real life practice. However, in biomarker research, it is important to rigorously integrate new biomarkers into existing prognostic tools and to demonstrate the advantages of these markers in order to improve the current practice of prognostication [72]. This model has to be externally validated before it can be used in clinical practice.

Multivariable Prognostication in Metastatic RCC in the Age of Targeted Therapies

Prognostication of survival outcome in mRCC is closely related to the medical treatment of mRCC. As a result of the treatment with targeted agents, median life expectancies of RCC patients have dramatically increased [9, 13]. There are currently at least five prognostic models that were generated in patients treated with targeted therapies [8, 10–13]. The MSKCC or Motzer-criteria comprised of Hb < LLN, LDH > ULN, calcium > ULN, time from diagnosis to treatment > 1 year, and KPS < 80. The Motzer criteria were the standard prognostic tool before targeted agents were introduced into clinical practice. It has proven to have a concordance index of 65.7 % in patients treated with VEGF-inhibitor therapies [9].

Most models derived in the targeted therapy era are based on the MSKCC criteria. The International mRCC Database Consortium (IMDC) or Heng model has been increasingly used in new clinical trials [73]. It separates favorable, intermediate, and poor prognosis patients (Fig. 28.3), and is based on four of five prognostic MSKCC factors (low hemoglobin, corrected calcium, ECOG PS, and time period from diagnosis to treatment). Additionally, the IMDC prognostic model includes platelet count and absolute neutrophil count [9, 13]. The median survival in the favorable, intermediate, and poor prognosis groups are more than 3 years, 26 months, and 9 months, respectively. For comparison, in patients treated with immunotherapies, the median OS was 20, 10, and 4 months in the favorable, intermediate, and poor prognosis groups, respectively [48]. In the training set, the IMDC model has reached a concordance index of 73 % [13]. The external validation study revealed a concordance of 71 % when using all six criteria and 66.4 % when collapsing into three risk groups. The model was more accurately able to reclassify patients by net reclassification improvement compared to other prognostic models [9]. The IMDC was developed independently from the histological RCC subtype and the type of VEGF targeted therapy used. Other models focused on a specific

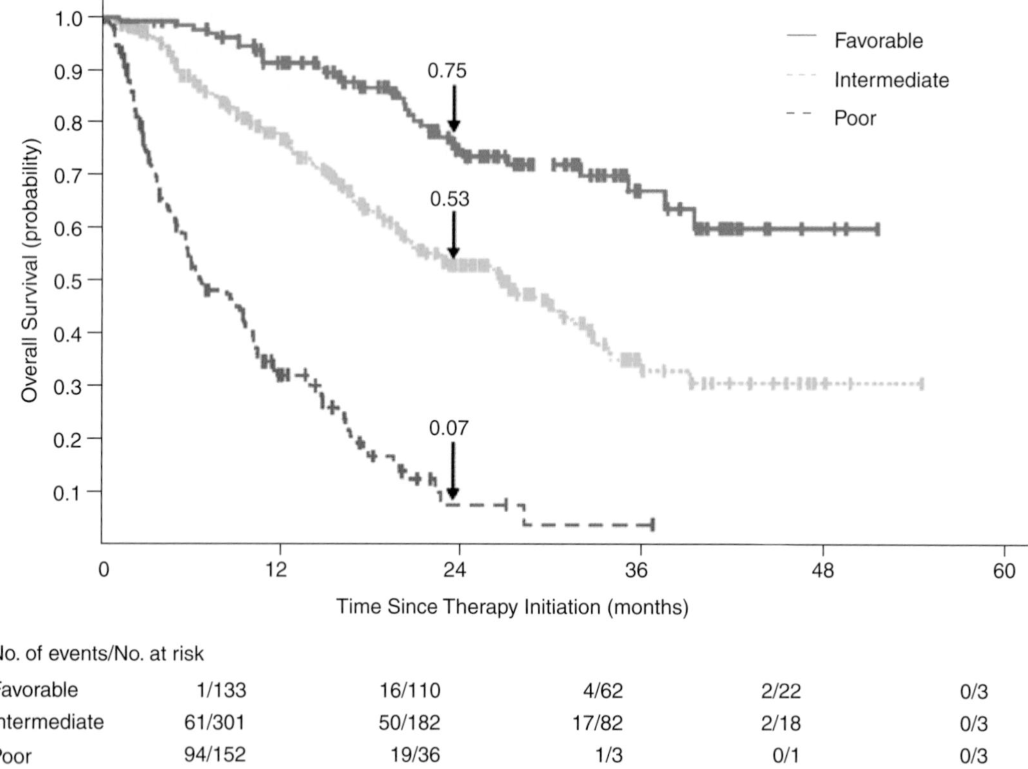

Fig. 28.3 The IMDC (Heng risk criteria) [13] include patient related (time from diagnosis to treatment < 1 year, Karnofsky performance status <80) and blood markers (calcium levels > ULN, Hb<LLN, neutrophilia, thrombocytosis) and segregates mRCC patients into three risk groups with low-, intermediate-, and high-risk for death. The nomogram prognosticates OS in the era of targeted therapies and has reached a concordance index of 0.73 and 0.66 in the development and validation cohorts, respectively. (Used with permission from [13])

type of antiangiogenic therapy such as sunitinib-treated patients only [10–12]. The advantage of the IMDC model is its generalizability, and therefore recently reported clinical trials preferred to use this model [73]. There is currently no model that could predict survival outcome specifically for RCC subtypes such as papillary and chromophobe RCC when treated with targeted therapy. Current investigations evaluate the prognostic applicability of the IMDC prognostic model in the group of nccRCC patients.

The IMDC prognostic model was developed to prognosticate the OS in patients with anti-VEGF therapies. PFS is another important clinical parameter [16]. Recently, the MSKCC group has published a model to prognosticate PFS that consists of ECOG PS, prior nephrectomy, LDH level, platelet count, and more than two metastatic sites in treatment naïve patients [12]. Additionally, the same study reported a prognostic model that included ECOG PS, time from nephrectomy to treatment, LDH level, corrected serum calcium, low hemoglobin levels, and bone metastases for prognostication of the OS. This model needs to be externally validated before it can be introduced into clinical practice. Unfortunately, the authors did not report a concordance index. Table 28.4 displays an overview of prognostic models separated by treatment approaches (immunotherapy vs. targeted therapies).

See Table 28.5 for prognostic models in all UICC stages.

Table 28.4 Prognostic models in metastatic RCCs

mRCC models (developed in patients treated with immunotherapies) patient numbers	Prognostic end point	Treatment	Concordance index	Reference
610	OS/CSS	Nephrectomy, hormones, radiation, chemotherapies	n.r.	Elson (1988) [87]
670	OS	Nephrectomy	n.r.	Motzer (1999) [48]
463	OS	Nephrectomy/IFN	n.r.	Motzer (2002) [17]
251	OS	Nephrectomy and first-line IFN	n.r.	Motzer (2004) [88]
782	OS, PFS, efficacy	Cytokine immunotherapies	n.r.	Négrier (2002) [46]
173	OS	Nephrectomy/IL-2	n.r.	Leibovich (2003) [89]
727	OS	Nephrectomy (ccRCC only)	67%	Leibovich (2005) [90]
352	OS	IFN and IL-2 based immunotherapies	n.r.	Mekhail (2005) [91]
mRCC models (developed in patients treated with targeted therapies) patient numbers	*Prognostic end point*	*Treatment*	*Concordance index*	*Reference*
120	OS	VEGF inhibitors	n.r.	Choueiri (2007) [8]
375	OS	Sunitinib	63%	Motzer (2008) [11]
628; 1028	OS	VEGF inhibitors	73%; 66.5%	Heng (2009;2011) [9, 13]
628	PFS	Bevacizumab	71–75%	Karakiewicz (2011) [10]
375	PFS; OS	Sunitinib vs. IFN	n.r.	Patil (2011) [12]

mRCC metastatic renal cell carcinoma, *RFS* recurrence-free survival, *n.r.* not reported, *OS* overall survival, *PFS* progression-free survival, *CSS* cancer-specific survival, *IFN* interferon, *IL* interleukin, *VEGF* vascular endothelial growth factor, *ccRRC* clear cell renal cell carcinoma

Table 28.5 Prognostic models in all UICC stages

Prognostic models of all tumor stages patient numbers	Prognostic end point	Follow-up	Concordance index (%)	Reference
661	Survival outcome	37 months	82–86	Zisman (2001) [18]
1801	Survival outcome	9.7 (0.1–31)	85	Frank (2002) [58]
318	Survival outcome	28 months (55 months (survivors))	79	Kim (2004) [92]
2530; 1422	Survival outcome	38.8 months (0.1–286)	88–89	Karakiewicz [61]
2530; 3560	Survival outcome	4.2 years (0.1–23.8); 2.7 (0.1–24.9)	87–91	Karakiewicz [93]
818	Survival outcome		73	Parker [94]

Summary

A plethora of prognostic and predictive markers were examined for their independent prognostic association with clinical outcome during the last decade. In the coming years, the biomarker panels will be added to validated prognostic models, such as the UISS or the IMDC prognostic model to further increase prognostic accuracy. These biomarkers will need to have reproducible assays, an assessment of inter- and intrapatient variability in order to obtain reference thresholds, and most importantly external validation [14].

References

1. Rini BI, Campbell SC, Escudier B. Renal cell carcinoma. Lancet. 2009;373(9669):1119–32.
2. Klatte T, Patard JJ, de Martino M, et al. Tumor size does not predict risk of metastatic disease or prognosis of small renal cell carcinomas. J Urol. 2008;179(5):1719–26.
3. Hollingsworth JM, Miller DC, Daignault S, Hollenbeck BK. Rising incidence of small renal masses: a need to reassess treatment effect. J Natl Cancer Inst. 2006;98(18):1331–4.
4. Sun M, Thuret R, Abdollah F, et al. Age-adjusted incidence, mortality, and survival rates of stage-specific renal cell carcinoma in North America: atrend analysis. Eur Urol. 2011;59(1):135–41.
5. Ljungberg B, Cowan NC, Hanbury DC, et al. EAU guidelines on renal cell carcinoma: the 2010 update. Eur Urol. 2010;58(3):398–406.
6. Campbell SC, Novick AC, Belldegrun A, et al. Guideline for management of the clinical T1 renal mass. J Urol. 2009;182(4):1271–9.
7. Van Poppel HB, Becker F, Cadeddu JA, et al. Treatment of localised renal cell carcinoma. Eur Urol. 2011;60(4):662–72.
8. Choueiri TK, Rini B, Garcia JA, et al. Prognostic factors associated with long-term survival in previously untreated metastatic renal cell carcinoma. Ann Oncol. 2007;18(2):249–55.
9. Heng DYC, Xie W, Harshman LC, et al. External validation of the international Metastatic Renal Cell Carcinoma (mRCC) database consortium prognostic model and comparison to four other models in the era of targeted therapy. ASCO Meeting Abstracts. 2011;29(15_suppl):4560.
10. Karakiewicz PI, Sun M, Bellmunt J, Sneller V, Escudier B. Prediction of progression-free survival rates after bevacizumab plus interferon versus interferon alone in patients with metastatic renal cell carcinoma: comparison of a nomogram to the Motzer criteria. Eur Urol. 2011;60(1):48–56.
11. Motzer RJ, Bukowski RM, Figlin RA, et al. Prognostic nomogram for sunitinib in patients with metastatic renal cell carcinoma. Cancer. 2008;113(7):1552–8.
12. Patil S, Figlin RA, Hutson TE, et al. Prognostic factors for progression-free and overall survival with sunitinib targeted therapy and with cytokine as first-line therapy in patients with metastatic renal cell carcinoma. Ann Oncol. 2011;22(2):295–300.
13. Heng DY, Xie W, Regan MM, et al. Prognostic factors for overall survival in patients with metastatic renal cell carcinoma treated with vascular endothelial growth factor-targeted agents: results from a large, multicenter study. J Clin Oncol. 2009;27(34):5794–9.
14. Tang PA, Vickers MM, Heng DY. Clinical and molecular prognostic factors in renal cell carcinoma: what we know so far. Hematol Oncol Clin North Am. 2011;25(4):871–91.
15. Dancey JE, Dobbin KK, Groshen S, et al. Guidelines for the development and incorporation of biomarker studies in early clinical trials of novel agents. Clin Cancer Res. 2010;16(6):1745–55.
16. Hotte SJ, Bjarnason GA, Heng DY, et al. Progression-free survival as a clinical trial endpoint in advanced renal cell carcinoma. Curr Oncol. 2011;18(Suppl2):S11–9.
17. Motzer RJ, Bacik J, Murphy BA, Russo P, Mazumdar M. Interferon-alfa as a comparative treatment for clinical trials of new therapies against advanced renal cell carcinoma. J Clin Oncol. 2002;20(1):289–96.
18. Zisman A, Pantuck AJ, Dorey F, et al. Improved prognostication of renal cell carcinoma using an integrated staging system. J Clin Oncol. 2001;19(6):1649–57.
19. Tang PA, Heng DY, Choueiri TK. Impact of body composition on clinical outcomes in metastatic renal cell cancer. Oncologist. 2011;16(11):1484–6.
20. Morgan TM, Tang D, Stratton KL, et al. Preoperative nutritional status is an important predictor of survival in patients undergoing surgery for renal cell carcinoma. Eur Urol. 2011;59(6):923–8.
21. Waalkes S, Merseburger AS, Kramer MW, et al. Obesity is associated with improved survival in patients with organ-confined clear-cell kidney cancer. Cancer Causes Control. 2010;21(11):1905–10.
22. Ceciliani F, Giordano A, Spagnolo V. The systemic reaction during inflammation: the acute-phase proteins. Protein Pept Lett. 2002;9(3):211–23.
23. Hursting SD, Berger NA. Energy balance, host-related factors, and cancer progression. J Clin Oncol. 2010;28(26):4058–65.
24. Masur K, Vetter C, Hinz A, et al. Diabetogenic glucose and insulin concentrations modulate transcriptom and protein levels involved in tumour cell migration, adhesion and proliferation. Br J Cancer. 2011;104(2):345–52.
25. Kattan MW, Reuter V, Motzer RJ, Katz J, Russo P. A postoperative prognostic nomogram for renal cell carcinoma. J Urol. 2001;166(1):63–7.
26. Patard JJ, Leray E, Rodriguez A, Rioux-Leclercq N, Guille F, Lobel B. Correlation between symptom graduation, tumor characteristics and survival in renal cell carcinoma. Eur Urol. 2003;44(2):226–32.

27. Patard JJ, Dorey FJ, Cindolo L, et al. Symptoms as well as tumor size provide prognostic information on patients with localized renal tumors. J Urol. 2004; 172(6 Pt 1):2167–71.
28. Teloken PE, Thompson RH, Tickoo SK, et al. Prognostic impact of histological subtype on surgically treated localized renal cell carcinoma. J Urol. 2009;182(5):2132–6.
29. Leibovich BC, Lohse CM, Crispen PL, et al. Histological subtype is an independent predictor of outcome for patients with renal cell carcinoma. J Urol. 2010;183(4):1309–15.
30. Krege S, Beyer J, Souchon R, et al. European consensus conference on diagnosis and treatment of germ cell cancer: a report of the second meeting of the European Germ Cell Cancer Consensus group (EGCCCG): part I. Eur Urol. 2008;53(3):478–96.
31. Krege S, Beyer J, Souchon R, et al. European consensus conference on diagnosis and treatment of germ cell cancer: a report of the second meeting of the European Germ Cell Cancer Consensus Group (EGCCCG): part II. Eur Urol. 2008;53(3):497–513.
32. Kroeger N, Rampersaud EN, Patard JJ, et al. Prognostic value of microvascular invasion in predicting the cancer specific survival and risk of metastatic disease in renal cell carcinoma: a multicenter investigation. J Urol. 2012;187(2):418–23.
33. Brookman-May S, May M, Shariat SF, et al. Features associated with recurrence beyond 5 years after nephrectomy and nephron-sparing surgery for renal cell carcinoma: development and internal validation of a risk model (PRELANE score) to predict late recurrence based on a large multicenter database (CORONA/SATURN project). Eur Urol. 2013;64(3):472–7.
34. Klatte T, Remzi M, Zigeuner RE, et al. Development and external validation of a nomogram predicting disease specific survival after nephrectomy for papillary renal cell carcinoma. J Urol. 2010;184(1):53–8.
35. Leibovich BC, Blute ML, Cheville JC, et al. Prediction of progression after radical nephrectomy for patients with clear cell renal cell carcinoma: a stratification tool for prospective clinical trials. Cancer. 2003;97(7):1663–71.
36. de Peralta-Venturina M, Moch H, Amin M, et al. Sarcomatoid differentiation in renal cell carcinoma: a study of 101 cases. Am J Surg Pathol. 2001;25(3):275–84.
37. Lopez-Beltran A, Scarpelli M, Montironi R, Kirkali Z. 2004 WHO classification of the renal tumors of the adults. Eur Urol. 2006;49(5):798–805.
38. Abel EJ, Culp SH, Meissner M, Matin SF, Tamboli P, Wood CG. Identifying the risk of disease progression after surgery for localized renal cell carcinoma. BJU Int. 2010;106(9):1277–83.
39. Flanigan RC, Mickisch G, Sylvester R, Tangen C, VanPoppel H, Crawford ED. Cytoreductive nephrectomy in patients with metastatic renal cancer: a combined analysis. J Urol. 2004;171(3):1071–6.
40. Choueiri TK, Xie W, Kollmannsberger C, et al. The impact of cytoreductive nephrectomy on survival of patients with metastatic renal cell carcinoma receiving vascular endothelial growth factor targeted therapy. J Urol. 2011;185(1):60–6.
41. Suppiah R, Shaheen PE, Elson P, et al. Thrombocytosis as a prognostic factor for survival in patients with metastatic renal cell carcinoma. Cancer. 2006;107(8):1793–800.
42. Karakiewicz PI, Trinh QD, Lam JS, et al. Platelet count and preoperative haemoglobin do not significantly increase the performance of established predictors of renal cell carcinoma-specific mortality. Eur Urol. 2007;52(5):1428–36.
43. Coppin C, Porzsolt F, Awa A, Kumpf J, Coldman A, Wilt T. Immunotherapy for advanced renal cell cancer. Cochrane Database Syst Rev. 2005;1:CD001425.
44. Ljungberg B, Grankvist K, Rasmuson T. Serum acute phase reactants and prognosis in renal cell carcinoma. Cancer. 1995;76(8):1435–9.
45. Karakiewicz PI, Hutterer GC, Trinh QD, et al. C-reactive protein is an informative predictor of renal cell carcinoma-specific mortality: a European study of 313 patients. Cancer. 2007;110(6):1241–7.
46. Negrier S, Escudier B, Gomez F, et al. Prognostic factors of survival and rapid progression in 782 patients with metastatic renal carcinomas treated by cytokines: a report from the GroupeFrancaisd'Immunotherapie. Ann Oncol. 2002;13(9):1460–8.
47. Motzer RJ, Bacik J, Mariani T, Russo P, Mazumdar M, Reuter V. Treatment outcome and survival associated with metastatic renal cell carcinoma of non-clear-cell histology. J Clin Oncol. 2002;20(9):2376–81.
48. Motzer RJ, Mazumdar M, Bacik J, Berg W, Amsterdam A, Ferrara J. Survival and prognostic stratification of 670 patients with advanced renal cell carcinoma. J Clin Oncol. 1999;17(8):2530–40.
49. Gore ME, Szczylik C, Porta C, et al. Safety and efficacy of sunitinib for metastatic renal-cell carcinoma: an expanded-access trial. Lancet Oncol. 2009;10(8):757–63.
50. Choueiri TK, Plantade A, Elson P, et al. Efficacy of sunitinib and sorafenib in metastatic papillary and chromophobe renal cell carcinoma. J Clin Oncol. 2008;26(1):127–31.
51. Patard JJ, Pignot G, Escudier B, et al. ICUD-EAU international consultation on kidney cancer 2010: treatment of metastatic disease. Eur Urol. 2011;60(4):684–90.
52. Harshman LC, Xie W, Bjarnason GA, et al. Conditional survival of patients with metastatic renal-cell carcinoma treated with VEGF-targeted therapy: a population-based study. Lancet Oncol. 2012;13(9):927–35.
53. Rini BI, Cohen DP, Lu DR, et al. Hypertension as a biomarker of efficacy in patients with metastatic renal cell carcinoma treated with sunitinib. J Natl Cancer Inst. 2011;103(9):763–73.

54. Choueiri TK, Xie W, Kollmannsberger CK, et al. The impact of body mass index (BMI) and body surface area (BSA) on treatment outcome to vascular endothelial growth factor (VEGF)-targeted therapy in metastatic renal cell carcinoma: Results from a large international collaboration. ASCO Meeting Abstracts. 2010;28(15_suppl):4524.
55. Ladoire S, Bonnetain F, Gauthier M, et al. Visceral fat area as a new independent predictive factor of survival in patients with metastatic renal cell carcinoma treated with antiangiogenic agents. Oncologist. 2011;16(1):71–81.
56. Steffens S, Grunwald V, Ringe KI, et al. Does obesity influence the prognosis of metastatic renal cell carcinoma in patients treated with vascular endothelial growth factor-targeted therapy? Oncologist. 2011;16(11):1565–71.
57. Tran HT, Liu Y, Zurita AJ, et al. Prognostic or predictive plasma cytokines and angiogenic factors for patients treated with pazopanib for metastatic renal-cell cancer: a retrospective analysis of phase 2 and phase 3 trials. Lancet Oncol. 2012;13(8):827–37.
58. Frank I, Blute ML, Cheville JC, Lohse CM, Weaver AL, Zincke H. An outcome prediction model for patients with clear cell renal cell carcinoma treated with radical nephrectomy based on tumor stage, size, grade and necrosis: the SSIGN score. J Urol. 2002;168(6):2395–400.
59. Ficarra V, Novara G, Galfano A, et al. The 'Stage, Size, Grade and Necrosis' score is more accurate than the University of California Los Angeles integrated staging system for predicting cancer-specific survival in patients with clear cell renal cell carcinoma. BJU Int. 2009;103(2):165–70.
60. Patard JJ, Kim HL, Lam JS, et al. Use of the University of California Los Angeles integrated staging system to predict survival in renal cell carcinoma: an international multicenter study. J Clin Oncol. 2004;22(16):3316–22.
61. Karakiewicz PI, Briganti A, Chun FK, et al. Multi-institutional validation of a new renal cancer-specific survival nomogram. J Clin Oncol. 2007;25(11):1316–22.
62. Karakiewicz PI, Suardi N, Capitanio U, et al. A preoperative prognostic model for patients treated with nephrectomy for renal cell carcinoma. Eur Urol. 2009;55(2):287–95.
63. Lane BR, Babineau D, Kattan MW, et al. A preoperative prognostic nomogram for solid enhancing renal tumors 7 cm or less amenable to partial nephrectomy. J Urol. 2007;178(2):429–34.
64. Go AS, Chertow GM, Fan D, McCulloch CE, Hsu CY. Chronic kidney disease and the risks of death, cardiovascular events, and hospitalization. N Engl J Med. 2004;351(13):1296–305.
65. Raj GV, Thompson RH, Leibovich BC, Blute ML, Russo P, Kattan MW. Preoperative nomogram predicting 12-year probability of metastatic renal cancer. J Urol. 2008;179(6):2146–51; discussion 2151.
66. Hutterer GC, Patard JJ, Jeldres C, et al. Patients with distant metastases from renal cell carcinoma can be accurately identified: external validation of a new nomogram. BJU Int. 2008;101(1):39–43.
67. Hutterer GC, Patard JJ, Perrotte P, et al. Patients with renal cell carcinoma nodal metastases can be accurately identified: external validation of a new nomogram. Int J Cancer. 2007;121(11):2556–61.
68. Kutikov A, Egleston BL, Wong YN, Uzzo RG. Evaluating overall survival and competing risks of death in patients with localized renal cell carcinoma using a comprehensive nomogram. J Clin Oncol. 2010;28(2):311–7.
69. Frank I, Blute ML, Cheville JC, et al. A multifactorial postoperative surveillance model for patients with surgically treated clear cell renal cell carcinoma. J Urol. 2003;170(6 Pt 1):2225–32.
70. Sorbellini M, Kattan MW, Snyder ME, et al. A postoperative prognostic nomogram predicting recurrence for patients with conventional clear cell renal cell carcinoma. J Urol. 2005;173(1):48–51.
71. Klatte T, Seligson DB, LaRochelle J, et al. Molecular signatures of localized clear cell renal cell carcinoma to predict disease-free survival after nephrectomy. Cancer Epidemiol Biomarkers Prev. 2009;18(3):894–900.
72. Kattan MW. Evaluating a marker's contribution to a nomogram: the GEMCaP example. Clin Cancer Res. 2010;16(1):1–3.
73. Rini BI, Escudier B, Tomczak P, et al. Comparative effectiveness of axitinib versus sorafenib in advanced renal cell carcinoma (AXIS): a randomised phase 3 trial. Lancet. 2011;378(9807):1931–9.
74. Pantuck AJ, Zisman A, Dorey F, et al. Renal cell carcinoma with retroperitoneal lymph nodes. Impact on survival and benefits of immunotherapy. Cancer. 2003;97(12):2995–3002.
75. Fuhrman S, Lasky L, Limas C. Prognostic significance of morphologic parameters in renal cell carcinoma. Am J Surg Pathol. 1982;6:655–63.
76. Thompson RH, Leibovich BC, Cheville JC, et al. Should direct ipsilateral adrenal invasion from renal cell carcinoma be classified as pT3a? J Urol. 2005;173(3):918–21.
77. Martinez-Salamanca JI, Huang WC, Millan I, et al. Prognostic impact of the 2009 UICC/AJCC TNM staging system for renal cell carcinoma with venous extension. Eur Urol. 2011;59(1):120–7.
78. Klatte T, Chung J, Leppert JT, et al. Prognostic relevance of capsular involvement and collecting system invasion in stage I and II renal cell carcinoma. BJU Int. 2007;99(4):821–4.
79. Sengupta S, Lohse CM, Leibovich BC, et al. Histologic coagulative tumor necrosis as a prognostic indicator of renal cell carcinoma aggressiveness. Cancer. 2005;104(3):511–20.
80. Patard JJ, Leray E, Cindolo L, et al. Multi-institutional validation of a symptom based classification for renal cell carcinoma. J Urol. 2004;172(3):858–62.

81. Escudier BJ, Ravaud A, Negrier S, et al. Update on AVOREN trial in metastatic renal cell carcinoma (mRCC): efficacy and safety in subgroups of patients (pts) and pharmacokinetic (PK) analysis. ASCO Meeting Abstracts. 2008;26(15_suppl):5025.
82. Rini BI, Michaelson MD, Rosenberg JE, et al. Antitumor activity and biomarker analysis of sunitinib in patients with bevacizumab-refractory metastatic renal cell carcinoma. J Clin Oncol. 2008;26(22):3743–8.
83. Zurita AJ, Jonasch E, Wang X, et al. A cytokine and angiogenic factor (CAF) analysis in plasma for selection of sorafenib therapy in patients with metastatic renal cell carcinoma. Ann Oncol. 2012;23(1):46–52.
84. Yaycioglu O, Roberts WW, Chan T, Epstein JI, Marshall FF, Kavoussi LR. Prognostic assessment of nonmetastatic renal cell carcinoma: a clinically based model. Urology. 2001;58(2):141–5.
85. Cindolo L, de la Taille A, Messina G, et al. A preoperative clinical prognostic model for non-metastatic renal cell carcinoma. BJU Int. 2003;92(9):901–5.
86. Lam JS, Shvarts O, Leppert JT, Pantuck AJ, Figlin RA, Belldegrun AS. Postoperative surveillance protocol for patients with localized and locally advanced renal cell carcinoma based on a validated prognostic nomogram and risk group stratification system. J Urol. 2005;174(2):466–72; discussion 472; quiz 801.
87. Elson PJ, Witte RS, Trump DL. Prognostic factors for survival in patients with recurrent or metastatic renal cell carcinoma. Cancer Res. 1988;48(24 Pt1):7310–3.
88. Motzer RJ, Bacik J, Schwartz LH, et al. Prognostic factors for survival in previously treated patients with metastatic renal cell carcinoma. J Clin Oncol. 2004;22(3):454–63.
89. Leibovich BC, Han KR, Bui MH, et al. Scoring algorithm to predict survival after nephrectomy and immunotherapy in patients with metastatic renal cell carcinoma: a stratification tool for prospective clinical trials. Cancer. 2003;98(12):2566–75.
90. Leibovich BC, Cheville JC, Lohse CM, et al. A scoring algorithm to predict survival for patients with metastatic clear cell renal cell carcinoma: a stratification tool for prospective clinical trials. J Urol. 2005;174(5):1759–63; discussion 1763.
91. Mekhail TM, Abou-Jawde RM, Boumerhi G, et al. Validation and extension of the Memorial Sloan-Kettering prognostic factors model for survival in patients with previously untreated metastatic renal cell carcinoma. J Clin Oncol. 2005;23(4):832–41.
92. Kim HL, Seligson D, Liu X, et al. Using protein expressions to predict survival in clear cell renal carcinoma. Clin Cancer Res. 2004;10(16):5464–71.
93. Karakiewicz PI, Suardi N, Capitanio U, et al. Conditional survival predictions after nephrectomy for renal cell carcinoma. J Urol. 2009;182(6):2607–12.
94. Parker AS, Leibovich BC, Lohse CM, et al. Development and evaluation of BioScore: a biomarker panel to enhance prognostic algorithms for clear cell renal cell carcinoma. Cancer. 2009;115(10):2092–103.

29 Pathology of Inherited Forms of Renal Carcinoma

Maria J. Merino

Introduction

Renal cell carcinoma (RCC) affects more than 58,000 individuals per year in the USA and is responsible for close to 14,000 annual deaths. Kidney cancer has been increasing in recent years, probably due to the intensified use of better imaging techniques. Unfortunately, early detection of these tumors is difficult because there are no reliable screening tests. Known risk factors include tobacco use, hypertension, and use of certain pain medications such as Phenacetin.

While the vast majority of renal tumors occur sporadically, about 5–8 % are found in association with syndromes of a heritable nature. Identification of the genes involved in the hereditary forms of RCC and understanding of the hereditary syndromes have provided significant information about the genes involved in the common or sporadic (nonhereditary) forms of the disease. Recognition of renal cancer in hereditary syndromes is important both clinically and scientifically because it is now recognized that kidney tumors may occur in familial settings more frequently than previously contemplated. Recognition and diagnosis of these tumors is not only important to establish appropriate diagnosis and therapy but also for early detection as well as for genetic counseling of family members.

Author is employee of the US Government.

M. J. Merino (✉)
Department of Pathology, National Cancer Institute, Bethesda, MD, USA
e-mail: mjmerino@mail.nih.gov

Kidney cancer comprises several histologic subtypes, and some of the hereditary types have specific morphological characteristics that correspond to specific molecular and genetic hallmarks, supporting their classification as distinct entities.

Many hereditary syndromes have been associated with renal tumors. The most common include:

- Von Hippel–Lindau (VHL)
- Hereditary papillary renal carcinoma (HPRC)
- Birt–Hogg–Dube (BHD)
- Hereditary leiomyomatosis and renal cell carcinoma (HLRCC)
- Succinate dehydrogenase subunit B (SDHB) deficiency-associated kidney tumors
- Tuberous sclerosis
- Cowden syndrome
- Familial oncocytoma
- Other renal familial syndromes with unknown genetic mutations that are under investigation

Clinically, hereditary tumors are more likely to be multifocal and bilateral and with early or incipient lesions scattered throughout the adjacent renal parenchyma. The most common and perhaps better understood form of hereditary kidney cancer is VHL syndrome, which is associated with clear cell RCC (~75 %). Next in frequency is HPRC syndrome (~10 %), followed by BHD syndrome and tuberous sclerosis. Kidney cancer associated with SDHB deficiency is rare and the incidence of familial renal oncocytoma is not known.

C. Magi-Galluzzi, C. G. Przybycin (eds.), *Genitourinary Pathology,* DOI 10.1007/978-1-4939-2044-0_29,

Von Hippel–Lindau Syndrome

VHL syndrome is an inherited autosomal dominant disorder with an estimated incidence of 1 in 36,000 individuals. The term VHL syndrome was coined in 1964 by Melmon and Rosen, who described a large VHL family and codified the term "von Hippel–Lindau."

Mutations in the *VHL* gene cause VHL syndrome [1]. The *VHL* gene is a tumor suppressor gene that controls cell division and growth. Mutations in this gene prevent production of the VHL protein, which normally targets for degradation of another protein known as hypoxia-inducible factor-1 (HIF1)-α. Lack of regulation of HIF1-α results in the activation of a number of genes involved in glucose uptake and metabolism as well as angiogenesis, leading to the development of tumors. The *VHL* gene is known to be located in 3p25-p26, but changes have been reported in 5q21+(70%) and 14q− (41%). The nondeleted allele of the VHL gene shows somatic mutations or hypermethylation-induced inactivation in 80% of cases.

Individuals affected with VHL are at risk to develop tumors in a number of organs [2]. The most frequent clinical manifestations are:

- Bilateral, multifocal clear cell renal carcinomas
- Central nervous system (CNS) hemangioblastomas (cerebellum, spine)
- Pancreatic neuroendocrine tumors
- Pheochromocytomas (PCCs)
- Retinal angiomas
- Endolymphatic sac tumors
- Epididymal papillary cystadenomas

Renal Cell Carcinoma Associated with VHL

Renal tumors identified in VHL patients are frequently bilateral and multifocal.

Grossly the tumors vary in size (frequently 1–2 cm), and have a characteristic yellow color with areas of hemorrhage. Morphologically, the tumor cells are arranged in solid, tubular, and rarely papillary patterns. They have abundant clear cytoplasm, uniform low grade nuclei and inconspicuous or invisible nucleoli at 100x. (Fig. 29.1). Most of the VHL-related cancers are Furhman nuclear grade 2, especially if the tumor size is 1–3 cm. As the size of the tumor increases, it is not infrequent to find higher nuclear grade as well as eosinophilic changes in the cytoplasm.

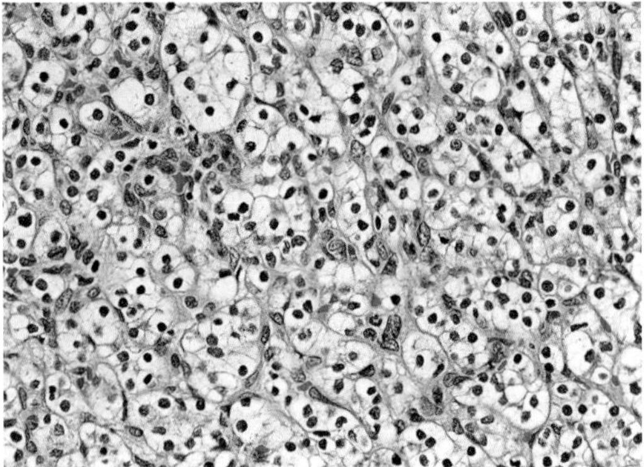

Fig. 29.1 Clear cell RCC, ISUP grade 2. H & E × 100

Cysts are a common element of VHL. They vary in size, and may be lined by rows of clear cells that can have proliferative and papillary growths protruding to the lumen of the cyst. (Fig. 29.2). Not infrequently, the cysts may be associated with areas of prominent fibrosis in which nests of clear cells are trapped.

The adjacent renal parenchyma may show small clusters of clear cells that probably represent the beginning of new lesions. Molecular studies have shown that these smaller lesions

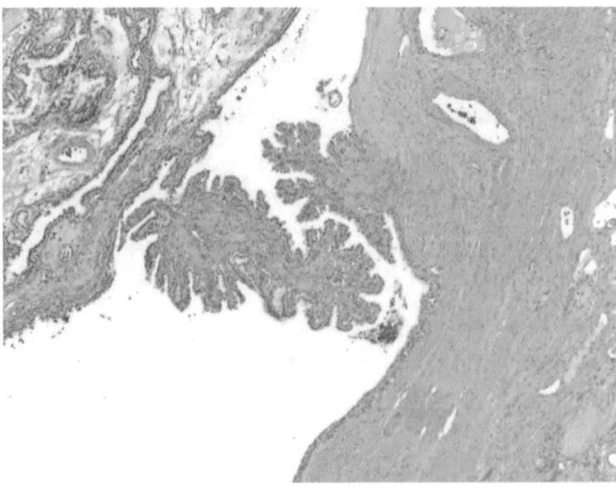

Fig. 29.2 Simple renal cyst with focal papillary formation. H & E × 100

already share similar molecular alterations to the larger tumors.

Treatment of most cases of VHL is surgical, aimed to remove as many tumors as possible before they reach a large size. Metastases in these patients generally occur when tumors are larger than 3 cm. Patients may have long survivals (10–20 years) but metastasis can develop in lung, bone, retroperitoneum, pancreas, and brain. Patients with VHL-associated renal tumors have a better prognosis and longer survivals than those with sporadic RCC. Long-term follow-up of patients with VHL as well as screening of family members is necessary, even if they are children.

Hereditary Papillary RCC

Hereditary papillary renal cell carcinoma (HPRCC) is an autosomal dominant disease with reduced penetrance, characterized by the development of multifocal papillary type I renal cell tumors. Since the original description of the entity by Zbar in 1994 [3], HPRCC has been recognized and established as a new hereditary syndrome.

The disease is caused by mutations in the tyrosine-kinase domain of the *c-MET* proto-oncogene on 7q34 [4]. Activation of the c-Met/hepatocyte growth factor (HGF) signaling pathways is known to be involved in many functions such as cell motility, differentiation, cell proliferation, and invasion [5]. Trisomy of chromosome 7 is thought to be the initiating event along with the loss of a sex chromosome. It is estimated that approximately half the members of affected families will develop tumors by the age of 50 years. Clinically and radiographically, the manifestations are similar to those of VHL, that is, patients present with bilateral and multifocal tumors.

Pathology

Grossly the renal tumors are multifocal and of variable sizes. Unlike VHL, simple cysts are not identified in this syndrome, although some of the tumors may have a cystic appearance. The adjacent renal parenchyma may show smaller lesions, adenomas, and incipient microscopic lesions that probably represent new tumors.

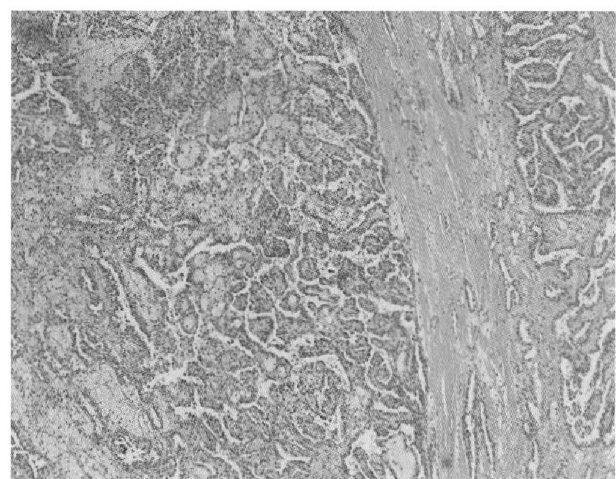

Fig. 29.3 Papillary RCC type I. Notice the pseudocapsule around the tumor and the papillary configuration. × 100 H & E I. H & E × 100

Morphologically, HPRCC tumors show a papillary, tubulopapillary or solid architecture. A fibrous pseudocapsule may surround the tumor nodules (Fig. 29.3). The papillae are short and thin with fibrovascular cores lined by neoplastic cells. These cells have regular small nucleoli with scant amounts of amphophilic cytoplasm. The centers of the papillae are frequently filled by collections of macrophages. In the solid areas, complex papillae may form structures resembling glomeruloid bodies. Marked nuclear atypia and mitotic figures are usually rare. However, cases with large tumors associated with areas of hemorrhage and necrosis have been reported. These tumors follow a more aggressive course and have a tendency to metastasize to lymph nodes and lung. Early or incipient lesions can be found scattered throughout the adjacent renal parenchyma and may have a papillary, solid, or tubular appearance (Fig. 29.4) [6].

Areas of clear cell differentiation have been described in HPRCC tumors but they occur predominantly as changes in the cells bordering the papillae which become larger and similar to the cells seen in clear cell tumors.

HPRCC tumors stain strongly positive for CK7, and are negative for CK20 and Wilm's tumor protein 1 (WT1). Treatment of patients

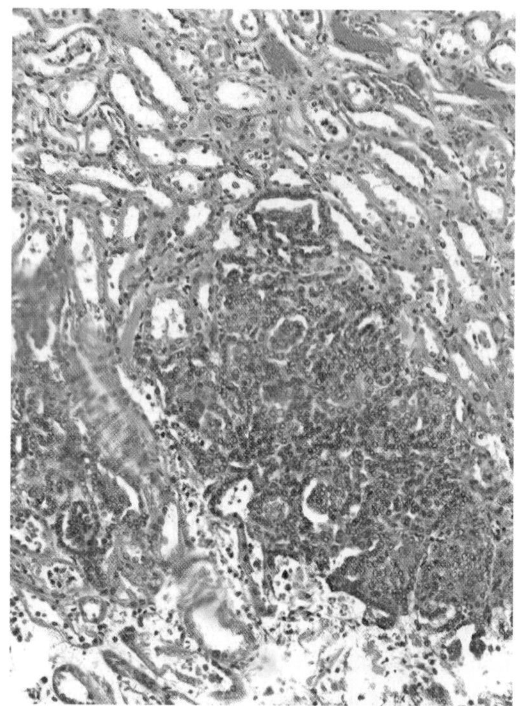

Fig. 29.4 Incipient lesion showing "glomeruloid" structures. × 200 H & E

with HPRCC is similar to VHL consisting of tumor excisions and long-term follow-up. These tumors have metastatic potential, primarily to lymph nodes and lungs. When they occur, the metastases are morphologically similar to the primary tumors. Targeted therapies have shown promising results in the treatment of patients with metastatic disease.

Birt–Hogg–Dubé Syndrome

In 1977, Drs. Birt, Hogg, and Dubé described a familial syndrome characterized by a predisposition to develop multiple small papules on the face and neck [7]. These papules are benign tumors of the hair follicles (fibrofolliculomas). The syndrome has since been redefined, and it is now known that BHD is an autosomal dominant genodermatosis that predisposes to the development of skin fibrofolliculomas as well as spontaneous pneumothorax, lung cysts and renal neoplasms [8]. It is believed that approximately 15–35 % of affected BHD individuals will develop renal tumors, that are morphologically distinct from those occurring in other hereditary syndromes [9].

Clinically, the disease presents with bilateral and multifocal tumors, with a median age of diagnosis of 48 years and a male to female ratio of 2.5:1. Approximately 30 % of the patients present with history of spontaneous pneumothorax and most of these cases have associated lung cysts that are more often found in the lower lobes of the lungs.

BHD patients are at risk to develop chromophobe RCC, oncocytomas, and hybrid tumors. Hybrid tumors and chromophobe RCC are the predominant types. Clear cell RCC can occur as well, but it is uncommon. The size of tumors at presentation is variable. The hybrid tumors average 2.2 cm, the chromophobe RCCs 3.0 cm, and the clear cell RCCs 4.7 cm in diameter. Morphologically, hybrid tumors are characterized by the presence of oncocytoma-like cells and chromophobe cells with granular eosinophilic cytoplasm and small regular pyknotic nuclei surrounded by characteristic perinuclear halos and well-defined cell borders. Cells with clear/pale cytoplasm and crisp borders may be present. Typically, hybrid tumors exhibit nests with an admixture of all these types of cells. These tumors are not encapsulated, blend regularly with the adjacent parenchyma, and may have a central myxohyaline scar (Figs. 29.5 and 29.6) [10]. The percentage of

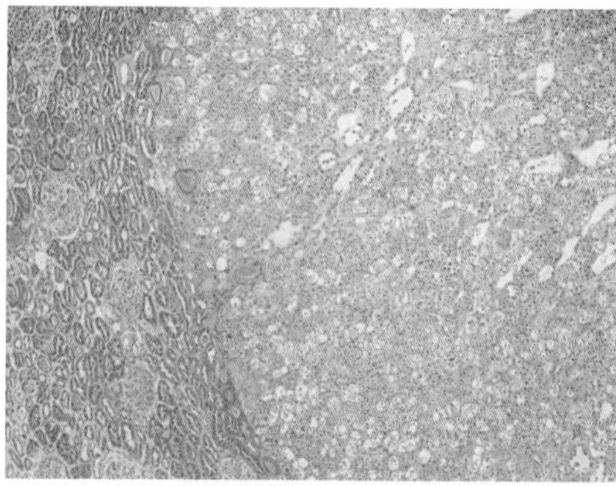

Fig. 29.5 Hybrid tumor. Notice the demarcation from the adjacent renal parenchyma. H & E × 100

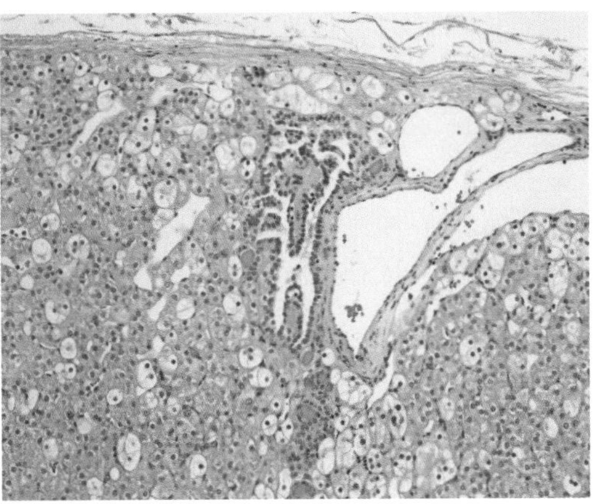

Fig. 29.6 Oncocytic cells mixed with clear and chromophobe type cells. H & E × 150

different cell types in the hybrid tumors has no clinical impact.

Nodules of classic chromophobe RCC can be found growing within some hybrid tumors and may compress the hybrid component to the periphery. These nodules exhibit only one type of chromophobe cells and their homogeneity differentiates them from the hybrid tumor, where the admixture of different types of chromophobe cells confers a more heterogeneous appearance (Fig. 29.7).

IHC demonstrates that Mib-1 proliferation index is low in hybrid tumors, with few nuclei staining for p53. CD117 shows a patchy pattern in the hybrid component in contrast to the diffuse pattern of chromophobe RCC. Nontumoral renal parenchyma shows oncocytosis in about 56% of the cases, consisting of poorly circumscribed lesions as small as a few cells in diameter that tend to expand into adjacent renal tubules. Cells within the areas of oncocytosis have eosinophilic cytoplasm, well-defined borders, large nuclei with stippled heterochromatin, and occasional focal cytoplasmic clearing. Recombination mapping in BHD families has identified the gene on chromosome 17p11.2; the gene product is known as folliculin. The treatment of patients with BHD is similar to that of patients with VHL and HPRCC.

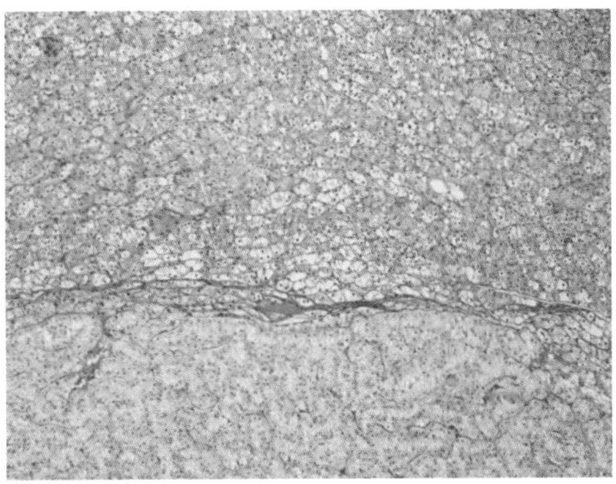

Fig. 29.7 Chromophobe RCC (CMF) arising in association with a hybrid tumor (HYB). H & E × 100

When possible, nephron-sparing surgery is the treatment of choice, depending on the size and location of the tumors. Total nephrectomy may be necessary in some cases [11].

Molecular genetic testing for the family-specific mutation allows for early identification of at-risk family members, improves diagnostic certainty and reduces costly screening procedures in relatives who have not inherited the family-specific disease-causing mutation.

The prognosis of patients with these tumors is better than that of HPRCC and VHL patients, unless clear cell RCC develops.

Hereditary Leiomyomatosis Renal Cell Carcinoma

Hereditary leiomyomatosis and renal cell carcinoma (HLRCC) is an autosomal dominant familial syndrome with incomplete penetrance, characterized by the development of cutaneous and uterine leiomyomas as well as renal tumors. In 2001, Launonen et al. [12] reported on the clinical, histopathologic and, molecular features of a cancer syndrome with predisposition to uterine leiomyomas and papillary renal cancer. Genetic evaluation of families with this disorder found germ line mutations in the gene encoding an enzyme of the Krebs cycle and fumarate hydratase (*FH,* 1q42.3-q43). Mutations of the FH gene were also found in the germ line of some multiple cutaneous leiomyomatosis (MCL) kindreds [13]. It is now believed that MCL and HLRCC are the same disorder. The four original kidney cancer cases reported occurred in young females, had papillary architecture, and presented as unilateral solitary lesions that had metastasized at the time of diagnosis.

HLRCC is the only hereditary syndrome that presents with single unilateral masses that may be cystic in some patients. Three distinct patterns of imaging features have been seen in patients with HLRCC renal tumors. These patterns are characterized as homogeneous and poorly enhancing solid lesions, predominantly cystic with small solid component lesions and heterogenous solid lesions with necrosis. Cystic lesions with smaller, distinctly solid enhancing components and ranging in size from 2.5 to 10 cm are commonly identified [14].

Although the original report described all the tumors as papillary type II, better understanding of the disease has demonstrated a variety of morphologic patterns including tubular, solid, and papillary and mixed. In the papillary tumors, the papillae are thick, with stalks containing vascular structures and abundant collagen [15].

The cells lining the papillae are large, contain abundant eosinophilic cytoplasm and occasionally have nuclei arranged in a pseudostratified manner resembling the rosettes seen in ependymomas (Fig. 29.8). The hallmark of these neoplasms is the presence of large nuclei with prominent orangeophilic nucleoli (Fig. 29.9). These nuclear traits are seen in the majority of the cells, whether lining the papillary or tubular structures. Other nuclear features include marked pleomorphism

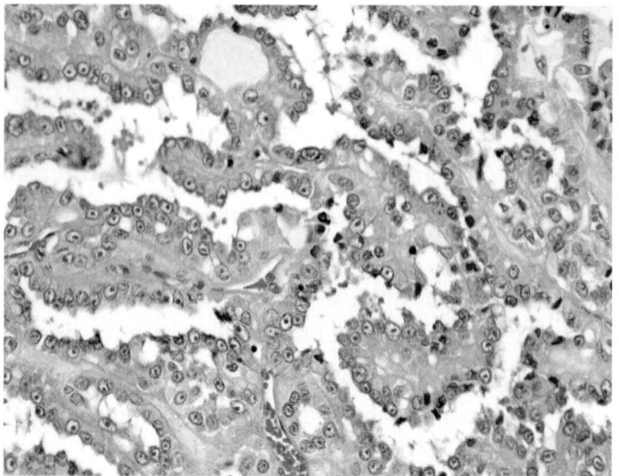

Fig. 29.8 HLRCC with papillary configuration. H & E × 150

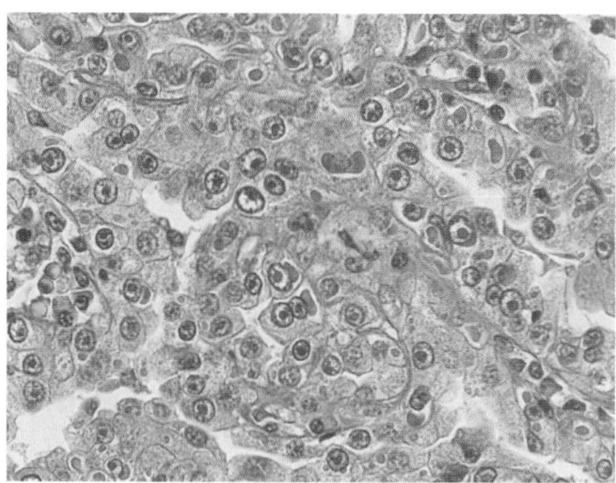

Fig. 29.9 Characteristic prominent nucleoli. H & E × 250

and irregularities of the nuclear membrane. Frequently, the tumors show cystic dilatation in which papillary structures can be identified [16]. Association with areas of clear cell differentiation can occur, but the nuclear changes are present in the clear cells as well. All cases of HLRCC should be considered high grade.

The main differential diagnosis of HLRCC tumors is with collecting duct carcinoma because of the papillary configuration, high grade, and cells with abundant cytoplasm. Collecting Duct Carcinoma (CDC) tumors, however, lack the characteristic nuclear features of HLRCC tumors, have marked desmoplasia, and do not have the same genetic alterations as the tumors associated with the syndrome [17].

HLRCC tumors do not have a specific immunohistochemical marker and are negative for Ulex, CK7, CK20, CD10, C-Kit, high-molecular weight cytokeratin and mucin. Recent studies by Bardella et al. have utilized immunohistochemistry to detect elevated levels of cysteine (2SC), a protein that results from the loss of function of FH. In their study, the presence of this protein in renal tumors corresponded with the identification of losses in the FH gene. This marker may prove of great help to identify patients with either renal or smooth muscle tumors that are part of the HLRCC syndrome [18].

Eighty to 90 % of the affected (with either cutaneous leiomyomas or germ line FH mutation) women have uterine leiomyomas (fibroids). The uterine leiomyomas are usually numerous (1–20 tumors) and large (1.5–10 cm). Most of the affected women had undergone hysterectomy prior to the age of 30 due to severe clinical symptoms caused by the smooth muscle tumors. Histologically, most of the lesions are consistent with atypical leiomyomas and may focally show the same nuclear features seen in the renal tumors [19].

The treatment of the renal cancers depends on the stage of the disease at the time of presentation. Early stage tumors can be treated by surgery. However, most of the patients present with advanced disease due to a distinctive lymphotrophic pattern of spread [20].

Intraperitoneal spread as well as metastasis to lung, liver, and bone are common. These patients fail to respond to interleukin-2 (IL-2)-based therapy and to a variety of chemotherapeutic agents. Recent studies have demonstrated that both HIF-1α and HIF-2α are elevated in these tumors and the elucidation of a VHL-independent HIF-1 prolyl hydroxylases (HPH)-dependent mechanism for HIF elevation may lead to targeting the HIF pathway and the development of new molecularly targeted agents such as bevacizumab/erlotinib. Patients enrolled in protocols and receiving these experimental therapies have shown longer disease-free intervals and longer survivals [21].

HLRCC is the most aggressive and lethal of all the hereditary syndromes associated with kidney cancer. Screening of family members is extremely important for early identification of tumors and for prolonging survivals.

Hereditary Paraganglioma-Pheochromocytoma Syndrome, Succinate-Dehydrogenase-Complex-Related Tumors

Hereditary paraganglioma-pheochromocytoma (PGL/PCC) syndrome is a disease characterized by the presence of PGLs and PCCs Fig. 29.10. PGL syndrome has been classified genetically into four entities, PGL1, PGL2, PGL3, and PGL4. To date, three of these four entities have been associated with germ line mutations in the genes encoding three of the subunits of succinate dehydrogenase (SDH), which has a key function in the Krebs cycle and the respiratory chain. Germ line mutations in SDHB, SDHC, and SDHD have been found in PGL4, PGL3, and PGL1, respectively. The penetrance of the gene is often reported as 77 % by age 50. The average age of onset is approximately the same for SDHB versus non-SDHB-related disease (approximately 36 years).

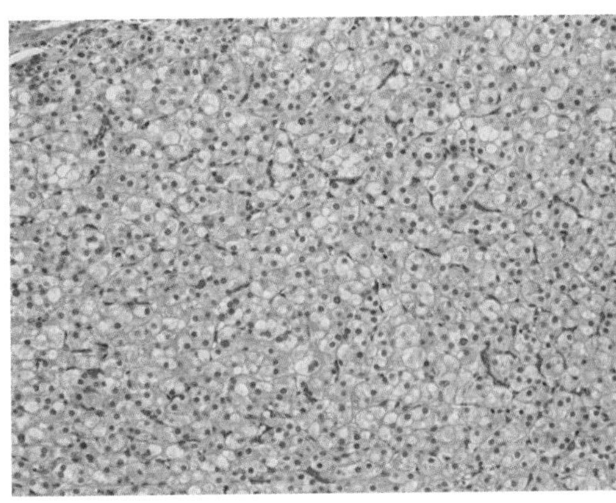

Fig. 29.10 Renal cell carcinoma associated with SDHB mutation. A mixture of clear and eosinophilic cells is present. H & E × 100

Germ line mutations in three genes (*SDHB*, *SDHC* and *SDHD*) are associated with a high risk of head and neck PGLs (HNPGLs) and/or adrenal/extra-adrenal PCCs, and of gastrointestinal stromal tumors (GISTs).

Recently, several reports have confirmed the occurrence of RCC in patients with alterations in these genes and with or without history of PGLs. The gene that codes for SDHB in humans is located on the first chromosome at locus p36.1-p35.

The renal tumors occur predominantly in those cases associated with mutations in the SDHB gene and are often single, solid, and unilateral masses, frequently misdiagnosed as oncocytomas.

Morphologically, the tumors are composed of uniform cells with a mixture of clear and light granular eosinophilic cytoplasm. Many of the cells have a signet ring cell appearance with vacuoles that seem to be filled with amorphous pink material. The nucleus of the cells is large with irregular chromatin distribution. The tumors are not encapsulated and the cells gently blend with the normal renal parenchyma [22]. One tumor has shown spindle cell differentiation and areas of nuclear pleomorphism and necrosis; however, nodules of cells similar to the ones described above were present.

Immunohistochemistry for these tumors is often positive for CAM5.2 and negative for CD10, CD56, CKIT, synaptophysin, chromogranin, CK7, and CK20. SDHB protein immunoexpression is negative in the kidney cancers caused by SDHB mutation, with positive staining in the background kidney parenchyma.

These tumors can metastasize to liver and bone. The treatment of SDHB-related tumors is surgical, and protocols are ongoing for therapy with new molecular targets.

Patients with a family history or diagnosis of SDH-related RCC need long-term follow-up for the high incidence of PGL/PCC and the development of metastasis and recurrences.

Tuberous Sclerosis

Tuberous sclerosis (TS) is an autosomal dominant disease characterized by cortical tubers, giant cell astrocytomas, retinal hamartomas, skin, cardiac, and renal tumors Fig. 29.11. The disease is associated with two predisposing genes, *TSC1* which encodes Hamartin and is located at 9q34 and *TSC2* which encodes Tuberin at 16p13. Most cases of tuberous sclerosis complex (TSC) are first diagnosed through either neurological symptoms (seizures) or dermatologic manifestations (facial angiofibromas, shagreen patches, or periungual fibromas). However, many TSC patients remain asymptomatic and are diagnosed in adulthood when the disease is confirmed in other family members.

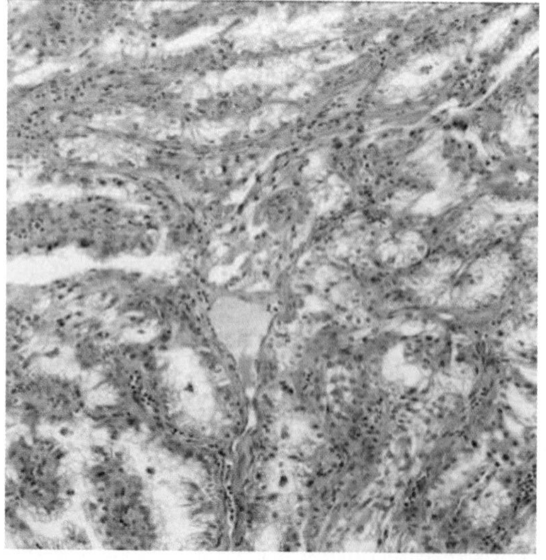

Fig. 29.11 Clear cell carcinoma in a patient with TSC. H & E × 150

Renal pathology is the second most common cause of morbidity and mortality in TSC patients. Angiomyolipomas, cysts, polycystic kidney, and epithelial tumors can occur as part of the syndrome. The most common of the renal lesions are angiomyolipomas, affecting approximately 55–75% of the patients. These are benign tumors of the perivascular epithelioid cell tumor (PEComa) family that often resemble smooth muscle, have variable intracytoplasmic lipid, and commonly involve the wall of medium-caliber vessels. The tumors can be bilateral and occasionally cause intraperitoneal hemorrhage.

Renal epithelial cysts occur in up to 50% of the patients, and are generally asymptomatic, although on occasion they can be associated with hypertension. Polycystic kidney occurs in those cases in which there is a simultaneous mutation in both TSC2 and PKD1 genes.

The overall incidence of renal carcinoma in patients with TSC is approximately 2–3%, but the association of kidney cancer and TSC is not recognized in many instances, so it is possible that the incidence is higher. TSC appears to show pathological heterogeneity. While cases with clear cell carcinomas, chromophobe-like carcinomas andoncocytomas have been reported in association with TSC, distinct subtypes not conforming to established diagnostic categories have also been described [23]. A recent study by Guo et al. identified three major classes of RCC among 57 tumors from 18 patients with tuberous sclerosis: (1) carcinomas resembling renal angiomyoadenomatous tumor (RAT-like) or RCC with smooth muscle stroma (30% of cases), (2) carcinomas resembling sporadic chromophobe type RCC (chromophobe-like, 59% of cases), and (3) a unique granular eosinophilic-macrocystic histology originally described by Schreiner et al. (11 % of cases) [23]. Two of the cases had a mixture of these morphologies. Seventeen of these 18 patients also had histologically confirmed angiomyolipomas (often multiple). The remaining patient had a lesion on the contralateral kidney radiographically suspicious for angiomyolipoma. The study showed a female predominance for these RCCs (M:F = 2.6:1) and a relatively young age at diagnosis (median 43 years) [24].

Cowden Syndrome

Cowden syndrome (CS), or phosphatase and tensin homolog (PTEN) syndrome is inherited as an autosomal dominant condition caused by germ line alterations in the *PTEN* gene. The disease occurs with an estimated incidence of one in 200,000 individuals. A clinical diagnosis is made based on a combination of pathognomonic, (mucocutaneous lesions, acral keratoses, facial papules), major (breast, endometrium, and thyroid cancers) and minor criteria (mental retardation, gastrointestinal (GI) hamartomas). It has been estimated that patients with CS have a >30-fold increased risk of developing kidney cancer. However, the overall incidence of CS-RCC is usually low (4 %). Family history of RCC may or may not be as helpful as in other hereditary syndromes since many patients with CS do not have a history of family members affected with RCC.

Recongnition of CS-RCC may be difficult unless the clinical history is known because unlike many of the other hereditary cancer syndromes such as VHL and HPRCC that are characterized by specific morphology CS-RCC can show different tumor types such as clear cell, papillary, and chromophobe. The tumors can also be bilateral or present as single masses. Molecular studies have confirmed that specific germ line mutations could not be associated with unique histologic types. In a study of Shuch et al., one nonsense mutation in exon 5 (p.R130X) was associated with three tumors in three different individuals that presented with three different histologies—one chromophobe, one papillary type I, and one clear cell [25]. Clinical information will be essential for the suspicion of CS and associated cancers. As with other hereditary syndromes, recognition of the syndrome will lead to early therapy and genetic counseling.

Familial Oncocytoma

In 1998, Weirich et al. reported five families with multiple and bilateral oncocytomas [26]. The tumors had been accidentally found and were consistent with benign oncocytomas. All patients were free of disease after long follow-up. The gene for this condition is not known.

References

1. Latif F, Tory K, Gnarra J, et al. Identification of the von Hippel-Lindau disease tumor suppressor gene. Science. 1993;260:1317–20.
2. Cohen AJ, Li FP, Berg S, et al. Hereditary renal-cell carcinoma associated with a chromosomal translocation. N Engl J Med. 1979;301:592–5.
3. Zbar B, Tory K, Merino MJ, et al. Hereditary papillary renal cell carcinoma. J Urol. 1994;151:561–6.
4. Schmidt L, Duh FM, Chen F, et al. Germline and somatic mutations in the tyrosine kinase domain of the MET proto-oncogene in papillary renal carcinomas. Nat Genet. 1997;16:68–73.
5. Schmidt LS, Nickerson ML, Angeloni D, et al. Early onset hereditary papillary renal carcinoma: germline missense mutations in the tyrosine kinase domain of the met proto oncogene. J Urol. 2004;172:1256–61.
6. Lubensky IA, Schmidt L, Zhuang Z, et al. Hereditary and sporadic papillary renal carcinomas with c-met mutations share a distinct morphological phenotype. Am J Pathol. 1999;155:517–26.
7. Birt AR, Hogg GR, Dube WJ. Hereditary multiple fibrofolliculomas with trichodiscomas and acrochordons. Arch Dermatol. 1977;113:1674–7.
8. Nickerson ML, Warren MB, Toro JR, et al. Mutations in a novel gene lead to kidney tumors, lung wall defects, and benign tumors of the hair follicle in patients with the Birt Hogg-Dube syndrome. Cancer Cell. 2002;2:157–64.
9. Zbar B, Alvord WG, Glenn G, Turner M, Pavlovich CP, Schmidt L, Walther M, Choyke P, Weirich G, Duray P, Gabril F, Greenberg C, Merino MJ, Toro J, Linehan WM. Risk of renal and colonic neoplasms and spontaneous pneumothorax in the Birt-Hogg-Dubé syndrome. Cancer Epidemiol Biomarkers Prev. 2002;11(4):393–400.

10. Pavlovich CP, Walther MM, Eyler RA. Merino MJ. renal tumors in the Birt-Hogg-Dube syndrome. Am J Surg Pathol. 2002;26:1542–52.
11. Boris RS, Benhammou J, Merino M, Pinto PA, Linehan WM, Bratslavsky G. The impact of germline BHD mutation on histological concordance and clinical treatment of patients with bilateral renal masses and known unilateral oncocytoma. J Urol. 2011;185(6):2050–5.
12. Launonen V, Vierimaa O, Kiuru M, et al. Inherited susceptibility to uterine leiomyomas and renal cell cancer. Proc Natl Acad Sci U S A. 2001;98:3387–92.
13. Toro JR, Nickerson ML, Wei MH, Merino MJ, et al. Mutations in the fumarate hydratase gene cause hereditary leiomyomatosis and renal cell cancer in families in North America. Am J Hum Genet. 2003;73(1):95–106.
14. Choyke PL, Glenn GM, Walther MM, Zbar B, Linehan WM. Hereditary renal cancers. Radiology. 2003;226:33–46.
15. Merino MJ, Torres-Cabala C, Pinto P, et al. The morphologic spectrum of kidney tumors in hereditary leiomyomatosis and renal cell carcinoma (HLRCC) syndrome. Am J Surg Pathol. 2007;31:1578–85.
16. Ghosh A, Merino MJ, Linehan MW. Are cysts the precancerous lesion in HLRCC? The morphologic spectrum of premalignant lesions and associated molecular changes in hereditary renal cell carcinoma: their clinical significance. Mod Pathol. 2013;26212A.
17. Kennedy SM, Merino MJ, Linehan WM, Roberts JR, Robertson CN, Neumann RD. Collecting duct carcinoma of the kidney. Hum Pathol. 1990;21:449–56.
18. Bardella C, El-Bahrawy M, Frizzell N, Adam J, Ternette N, Hatipoglu E, Howarth K, O'Flaherty L, Roberts I, Turner G, Taylor J, Giaslakiotis K, Macaulay VM, Harris AL, Chandra A, Lehtonen HJ, Launonen V, Aaltonen LA, Pugh CW, Mihai R, Trudgian D, Kessler B, Baynes JW, Ratcliffe PJ, Tomlinson IP, Pollard PJ. Aberrant succination of proteins in fumarate hydratase-deficient mice and HLRCC patients is a robust biomarker of mutation status. J Pathol. 2011;225(1):4–11.
19. Stewart L, Glenn GM, Stratton P, Goldstein AM, Merino MJ, Tucker MA, Linehan WM, Toro JR. Association of germline mutations in the fumarate hydratase gene and uterine fibroids in women with hereditary leiomyomatosis and renal cell cancer. Arch Dermatol. 2008;144(12):1584–92.
20. Sanz-Ortega J, Vocke C, Stratton P, et al. Morphologic and molecular characteristics of uterine leiomyomas in hereditary leiomyomatosis and renal cancer (HLRCC) syndrome. Am Surg Pathol. 2013;37:74–80.
21. Linehan WM, Bottaro D, Neckers L, Schmidt LS, Srinivasan R. Hereditary kidney cancer: unique opportunity for disease-based therapy. Cancer. 2009;115(10 Suppl):2252–61.
22. Gill AJ, Pachter NS, Chou A, et al. Renal tumors associated with germline SDHB mutation show distinctive morphology. Am J Surg Pathol. 2011;35:1578–85.
23. Schreiner A, Daneshmand S, Bayne A, et al. Distinctive morphology of renal cell carcinomas in tuberous sclerosis. Int J Surg Pathol. 2010;18:409–18.
24. Guo J, Tretiakova MS, Troxell ML, et al. Tuberous sclerosis-associated renal cell carcinoma: aclinicopathologic study of 57 separate carcinomas in 18 patients. Am J Surg Pathol. 2014;38(11):1457–67. doi:10.1097/PAS.0000000000000248.
25. Shuch B, Ricketts CJ, Vocke CD, Komiya T, Middelton LA, Kauffman EC, Merino MJ, Metwalli AR, Dennis P, Linehan WM. Germline PTEN mutation cowden syndrome: an underappreciated form of hereditary kidney cancer. J Urol. 2013;190(6):1990–8.
26. Weirich G, Glenn G, Junker K,Merino MJ, et al. Familial renal oncocytoma: clinicopathological study of 5 families. J Urol. 1998;160:335–4.

The Utility of Immunohistochemistry in the Differential Diagnosis of Renal Cell Carcinomas

30

Ming Zhou and Fang-Ming Deng

Introduction

Renal neoplasms comprise a heterogeneous group of tumors with divergent clinicopathological and molecular characteristics as well as therapeutic options. More than 90 % of the renal neoplasms arise from, or recapitulate the differentiation of, renal tubular epithelia and constitute the vast majority of cases encountered clinically, including malignant clear cell, papillary, and chromophobe renal cell carcinoma (RCC) and benign oncocytoma, and papillary adenoma. Accurate diagnosis and classification are critical for patient management, prognosis and prediction of therapeutic response. Recent emergence of small molecule inhibitors that target different molecular pathways makes accurate histological classification of renal tumors even more imperative. For example, inhibitors of receptor tyrosine kinase pathways and mammalian target of rapamycin (mTOR) pathway are effective for clear cell RCC and show little effect for other RCC subtypes.

Diagnosis and classification of renal tumors are usually straightforward based on gross and microscopic examination of the biopsy and resection specimens. Immunohistochemistry, however, has been increasingly used in the workup of challenging cases [1–5]. Immunohistochemical markers are used to verify histological subtypes, distinguish primary RCCs from other nonrenal cell tumor types that can occur in the kidney, or from the rare metastasis to the kidney. Metastatic RCCs to distant sites often require confirmation of renal origin by immunohistochemistry. Finally, needle biopsies with limited material often require immunohistochemical stains to establish diagnosis and classification [6].

This review discusses the immunophenotypes of major renal tumors and immunohistochemical markers that are commonly used in clinical laboratories. In addition, algorithms incorporating morphology and immunohistochemical profiles in the differential diagnosis of major RCC histological subtypes will also be provided.

Immunohistochemical Markers Commonly Used in the Diagnosis of Renal Tumors

Markers That Support Renal Origin

These markers are expressed in the different parts of the nephron structures and the majority of renal cell neoplasms, but infrequently in nonrenal cell neoplasms. Because of their relative specificity for renal tumors, they are often used to distinguish renal and nonrenal cell neoplasms and to confirm the renal origin of metastatic RCC at distant sites.

M. Zhou (✉) · F.-M. Deng
Department of Pathology, New York University Langone Medical Center, New York, NY, USA
e-mail: Ming.zhou@nyumc.org

F.-M. Deng
e-mail: Dengf01@nyumc.org

C. Magi-Galluzzi, C. G. Przybycin (eds.), *Genitourinary Pathology*, DOI 10.1007/978-1-4939-2044-0_30,

PAX2 and PAX8

Paired-box protein 2 (PAX2) and PAX8 are both nuclear transcription factors mediating embryonic development of the kidney, Müllerian and other organ systems [7, 8]. Their expression in human tissues is similar except PAX8 is also expressed in thyroid follicular cells while PAX2 is not. They are expressed diffusely in normal kidney with higher level in the distal tubules than the proximal tubules (Fig. 30.1a, b) and patchy expression in the urothelium of the collecting system (Fig. 30.1c). They have a similar expression profile and are found in approximately 90 % of all the histological subtypes of renal cell neoplasms (Fig. 30.1d–i), including the newer subtypes such as Xp11.2 translocation RCC and mucinous tubular and spindle cell carcinoma. The expression is also identified in some sarcomatoid RCC cases. PAX2 and PAX8 are therefore considered the most useful markers to confirm a diagnosis of renal cell neoplasms both in the kidney and at distant sites due to their high sensitivity, high percentage of positive tumor cells in positive cases and discrete nuclear staining pattern. These two markers do have some differences. For example, some renal tumors that may be negative or infrequently positive for PAX2, including oncocytoma and chromophobe RCC, are often positive for PAX8. Another diagnostic pitfall is occasional expression of PAX2 and PAX8 in other nonrenal neoplasms, including 10–15 % of pelvic urothelial carcinoma (UC) and tumors derived

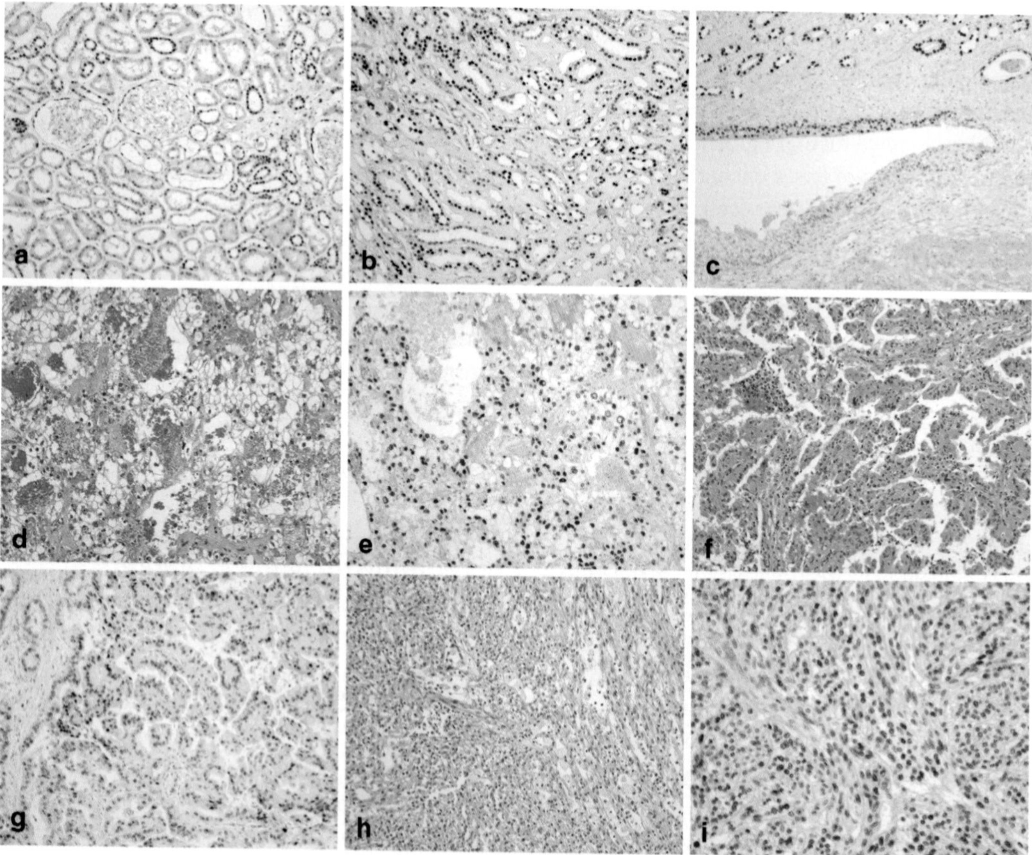

Fig. 30.1 Expression of PAX8 in normal and neoplastic renal tissues. PAX8 is expressed throughout renal tubules, but more intensely in distal tubules and collecting ducts (**a, b**), and urothelium lining the renal papillae (**c**). PAX8 expression tapers and patchy and weak expression are seen in urothelium lining the minor calyx (**c**). PAX8 expression is detected in the majority of renal cell neoplasms, including clear cell RCC (**d, e**), papillary RCC (**f, g**) and mucinous tubular and spindle cell carcinoma (**h, i**)

from the Müllerian and Wolffian duct systems. PAX8 is also expressed in thyroid follicular cells and thyroid neoplasms. However, PAX2 is usually negative in thyroid neoplasms, making it a better marker to use in the distinction between RCC and thyroid carcinoma. Positive staining is also reported in neuroendocrine tumors and B cell lymphoma due to antibody cross-reactivity with other members of the PAX gene family.

RCC Marker

RCC Marker (RCC Ma) is a monoclonal antibody raised against a glycoprotein on the brush border of proximal renal tubules. It is considered a "renal" marker as its expression is found in approximately 80% of renal cell neoplasms, present in almost all low-grade clear cell and papillary RCC (PRCC) [9]. Its expression in other renal tumors is widely variable and the staining is often focal. It is absent in oncocytoma and collecting duct carcinoma. Its main disadvantage is the poor specificity with expression reported in many other nonrenal tumors, including neoplasms of parathyroid, salivary gland, breast, lung, colon, adrenal gland, testicular germ cell tumors, and mesothelioma. Its use to support the renal origin of a poorly differentiated tumor is now largely supplanted by other more sensitive and specific renal markers (i.e., PAX8 and PAX2).

CD10

CD10 is a cell-surface glycoprotein expressed on the proximal renal tubular epithelial cells and podocytes as well as many renal tumors with an expression pattern similar to that of RCC Ma. It has therefore been considered a useful marker to support the renal origin of a poorly differentiated neoplasm. Almost all clear cell and PRCCs are positive for this marker while other types of renal cell neoplasms are negative. Unfortunately, CD10 is even less specific than RCC Ma. Its expression is reported in wide array of nonrenal tumors, including carcinomas of lung, colon, ovary, and urinary bladder, and mesenchymal tumors such as endometrial stromal sarcoma and lymphomas. CD10 has fallen out of favor with the advent of PAX8/PAX2.

Human Kidney Injury Molecule-1 (hKIM-1)

hKIM-1 is a type I transmembrane glycoprotein expressed in injured proximal renal tubules. Its expression is also detected in the majority of clear cell and PRCC [10]. Only rare cases of chromophobe RCC and oncocytoma express this marker. It is therefore a relatively sensitive (80%) and specific (90%) marker for clear cell and PRCC, and metastatic RCCs. However, its expression is also detected in the majority (93.8%) of ovarian clear cell carcinoma, 1/3 of endometrial clear cell carcinoma, and infrequently in colonic adenocarcinoma, limiting its use to narrow clinical circumstances.

Vimentin

Vimentin is found in the majority of RCCs. This stain alone is not a specific renal marker as its expression is found in wide range of neoplasms. Coexpression of vimentin and cytokeratin (CK), however, is limited to RCC and a few other carcinomas including endometrioid carcinoma, thyroid carcinoma, and mesothelioma. Therefore, coexpression of vimentin and CKs suggests RCC as one of the possible diagnoses.

Markers That Are Differentially Expressed in Different RCC Subtypes

Different histological subtypes of RCC are postulated to be derived from, or differentiate towards, different parts of nephron units which have distinct immunoprofiles. Therefore, renal tumors may be classified based on their immunoprofiles that recapitulate those of the normal nephrons. For example, CD10 and RCC Ma are found on the proximal renal tubules as well as in neoplasms that are derived from or recapitulate the proximal renal tubules (clear cell RCC and PRCC). Kidney-specific cadherin (ksp-cadherin), parvalbumin, claudins, and S100A are found on the distal nephrons and corresponding chromophobe RCC and oncocytomas. High-molecular-weight CKs are detected in collecting ducts of Bellini as well as in collecting duct carcinomas. However, morphology-immunophenotype concordance is imperfect. Such discordance occurs as the result of heterogeneity in tumor biology and technicality of immunohistochemistry. Furthermore, most published studies have utilized morphologically straightforward cases but not genetically confirmed difficult cases with ambiguous morphology. It should be emphasized that immunohistochemistry plays a supportive, rather than primary and definitive, role in the histological classification of RCC, and is best applied in the context of differential diagnosis.

Carbonic Anhydrase IX (CA9)

CA9 is a transmembrane protein of the carbonic anhydrase family. It is regulated by hypoxia inducible factor (HIF) and considered a marker for tissue hypoxia. CA9 is not expressed in healthy renal tissue as opposed to other carbonic anhydrase family members. It is instead expressed in most clear cell RCC (CCRCC) through HIF-1α accumulation driven by hypoxia or inactivation of the von Hippel–Lindau (VHL) gene [7, 11]. The staining pattern in CCRCC is circumferential membranous and is usually diffusely positive in most or all tumor cells (Fig. 30.2a). Focal staining is seen in up to one fourth of cases, typically in high-grade cancer (Fig. 30.2b). Its expression is also detected in clear cell tubulopapillary RCC (CCTPRCC), showing a unique "cup-like" pattern with staining decorating the basolateral, but not the apical, portion of cells lining glandular and cystic spaces (Fig. 30.2c). Its expression may also be detected in other high-grade tumors in the kidney including collecting duct carcinoma and pelvic UC (Fig. 30.2d), and can be seen adjacent to tumor necrosis due to ischemia and hypoxia (Fig. 30.2e, f). CA9 is not expressed in chromophobe RCC (ChRCC) and oncocytomas.

CA9 expression is also seen in many nonrenal tumors, including tumors of endometrium, stomach, cervix, breast, lung, liver, neuroendocrine tumors, mesotheliomas, and brain tumors. Therefore, CA9 has limited value in distinguishing renal versus nonrenal carcinomas. It is mainly used to confirm a diagnosis of CCRCC or CCTPRCC.

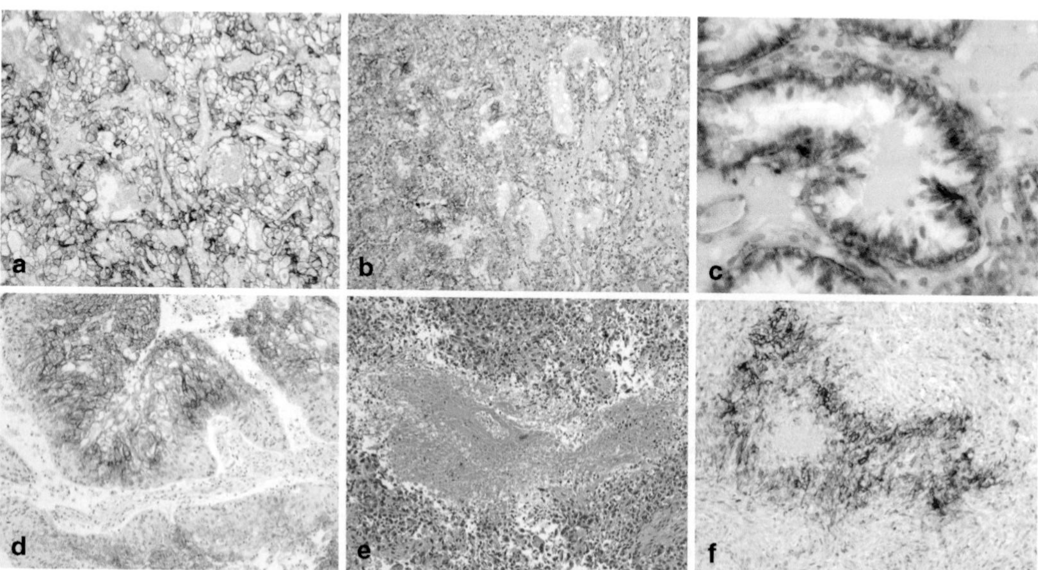

Fig. 30.2 Expression of carbonic anhydrase IX (CA9) in renal cell neoplasms. CA9 expression is diffuse and circumferential membranous in a clear cell RCC (**a**). The staining is focal in a high-grade clear cell RCC (**b**). In CCTPRCC, CA9 stains the basolateral, but not the apical, portion of tumor cells ("cup-like" pattern, **c**). CA9 is expressed in urothelial carcinoma (**d**). It is also expressed in cells surrounding necrosis (**e, f**) in an unclassified renal cell carcinoma

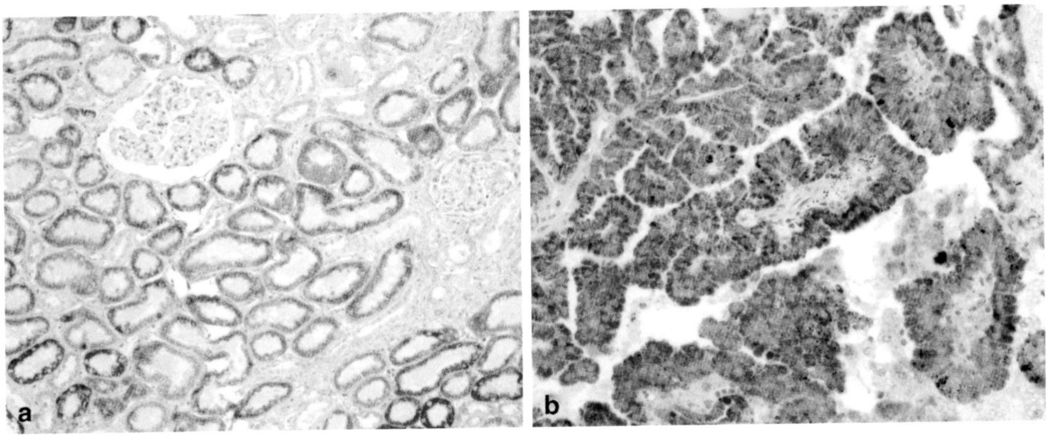

Fig. 30.3 Expression of α-methylacyl coA racemase (AMACR) in normal and neoplastic renal tissues. AMACR expression is detected in proximal renal tubules (**a**) and papillary renal cell carcinoma (**b**) as granular cytoplasmic staining

α-Methylacyl Coenzyme A Racemase

α-Methylacyl coenzyme A racemase (AMACR) is a mitochondrial enzyme involved in the oxidation of branched chain fatty acids and bile acid [12]. In the kidney, it is expressed in the proximal renal tubules (Fig. 30.3a). The majority of PRCC, both type 1 and 2, are positive for AMACR as granular cytoplasmic staining (Fig. 30.3b) [13]. Its expression is also found in mucinous tubular and spindle cell carcinoma, tubulocystic RCC, translocation RCC, but not in CCTPRCC, oncocytomas, and ChRCC. Therefore, positive AMACR staining provides support for a morphological diagnosis of PRCC.

AMACR is found in a wide array of nonrenal tumors, most commonly in prostate adenocarcinoma, rendering it of little use in distinguishing renal from nonrenal tumors.

Parvalbumin

Parvalbumin is a calcium-binding protein involved in intracellular calcium homeostasis. In the kidney, its expression is limited to the distal nephrons from which ChRCC and oncocytomas are postulated to be derived. In support of such a histogenic derivation, parvalbumin expression is detected in these two subtypes of renal cell neoplasms, but is absent in other subtypes [14]. Therefore, parvalbumin immunostains may be used to differentiate oncocytoma and ChRCC from other renal tumors with similar "oncocytic" cytoplasm.

E-Cadherin and Kidney-Specific Cadherin

Epithelial cadherin (E-cadherin) is a calcium-dependent cell–cell adhesion glycoprotein. It is normally expressed in many cell types including renal tubular epithelial cells. Kidney-specific cadherin (ksp-cadherin) is an isoform of E-cadherin whose expression is exclusively found on the basolateral cell membranes of the distal convoluted tubules and collecting ducts (Fig. 30.4a, b) [15]. Both E-cadherin and ksp-cadherin are expressed in almost all ChRCC (Fig. 30.4c) and oncocytomas (Fig. 30.4d), but variably in other subtypes, including collecting duct carcinoma, translocation RCC, mucinous tubular and spindle cell carcinoma, and UC. Their expression in CCRCC and PRCC is, however, uncommon. Therefore, E-cadherin and ksp-cadherin may be used to distinguish ChRCC and oncocytoma from other renal tumors with "oncocytic cytoplasm."

E-cadherin expression is commonly seen in other nonrenal tumors, often with positive staining in a high percentage of tumor cells, including lung, breast, and bladder carcinomas, rendering it unsuitable for differentiating renal from nonrenal tumors.

Claudin 7 and 8

Claudin 7 and 8 are members of a gene family that form tight cell junctions between epithelial cells. In the kidney, they are found primarily in the distal tubules and collecting ducts. Limited

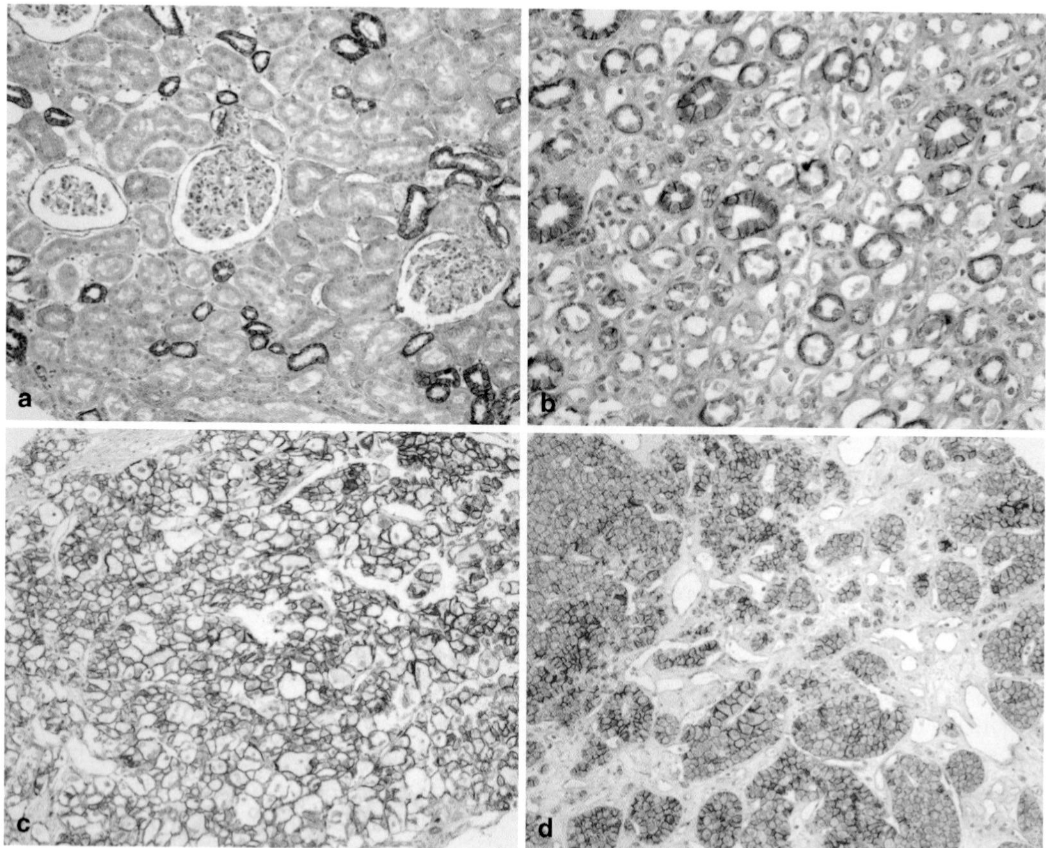

Fig. 30.4 Expression of epithelial cadherin (E-cadherin) in normal and neoplastic renal tissues. E-cadherin is only detected in a few distal convoluted tubules in the cortex (**a**), but is diffusely positive in the thick segments of loop of Henle and collecting ducts (**b**). Chromophobe RCC (**c**) and oncocytoma (**d**) are diffusely positive for E-cadherin

data show that claudin 7 and 8 are expressed in most ChRCC and oncocytomas, but in none or very few of other subtypes. Therefore, claudin 7 and 8 may be used in the differential diagnosis between ChRCC, oncocytomas, and other RCC with oncocytic cytoplasm.

CD117

CD117, or c-Kit, is a receptor tyrosine kinase that, upon binding to its ligands, phosphorylates and activates signal transduction molecules that propagate signals in cells and plays a critical role in cell survival, proliferation, and differentiation. Most ChRCC and oncocytomas are positive for CD117. However, no mutations have been identified in exons 9 and 11 of the c-Kit gene, the presence of which correspond to the therapeutic response to imatinib seen in gastrointestinal stromal tumors. Clear cell and PRCC are in general negative for CD117. Its expression has also been detected in sarcomatoid RCC and pelvic UCs.

S100A1

A member of S100 gene family, S100A1 is a calcium-binding protein whose expression is found in nephrons in the adult kidney. It is expressed in most oncocytomas, but in a significantly lower percentage of ChRCC cases. Such a differential expression pattern may aid in the distinction of these two tumors. Its expression, however, is also found in the majority of CCRCC and PRCC.

TFE3, TFEB, and Cathepsin K

Transcription factor E3 (TFE3) protein is encoded by the TFE3 gene on chromosome Xp11.2, and TFEB protein is encoded by the TFEB gene on chromosome 6p21. Both genes are members of the "microphthalmia transcription factor/transcription factor E (MiTF/TFE)" gene family. RCCs harboring chromosomal translocations involving the respective genes overexpress TFE3 and TFEB proteins which can be detected by immunohistochemistry [16–18]. Although molecular genetic analysis for the chromosomal translocation involving TFE3 and TFEB genes provides the most definitive evidence, immunohistochemical stains for TFE3 and TFEB proteins are sensitive, specific and highly correlate with the TFE3 and TFEB gene status in these tumors. TFE3 is undetectable in normal kidney tissues. TFE3 fusion protein, in contrast, is overexpressed in Xp11 translocation RCC (Fig. 30.5a, b) and is detected in over 95 % of Xp11.2 translocation RCC confirmed molecularly (Fig. 30.5c). However, TFE3 immunostaining can be seen in tumors other than Xp11.2 translocation RCC, including many perivascular epithelioid cell tumors (PEComa) of soft tissue and gynecological tract, a subset of which indeed harbors TFE3 gene alteration, as well as in a possibly related tumor, melanotic Xp11 translocation renal cancer. Rarely TFE3 immunoexpression is also detected in other tumors, including adrenal cortical carcinoma, granular cell tumor, bile duct carcinoma, and high-grade myxofibrosarcoma. The immunohistochemical stain for TFEB protein is both sensitive and specific for RCC associated with TFEB translocation, and is not detectable in other neoplasms. Weak nuclear staining for TFEB is rarely detected in scattered normal lymphocytes. The most significant issue with the immunohistochemical detection of TFE3 and TFEB proteins is that the staining is susceptible to tissue fixation. Inconsistent staining results are often encountered, especially when the staining is performed on an automatic stainer. Some staining protocols call for manual staining.

Cathepsin K is transcriptionally regulated by members of the MiTF/TFE gene family. Its overexpression is seen in all TFEB RCC (Fig. 30.5d) and 60 % of TFE3 RCC, but none of the other RCC subtypes [19, 20]. Its expression in non-renal carcinomas is rare (2.7 %), although very common in mesenchymal tumors (>50 %).

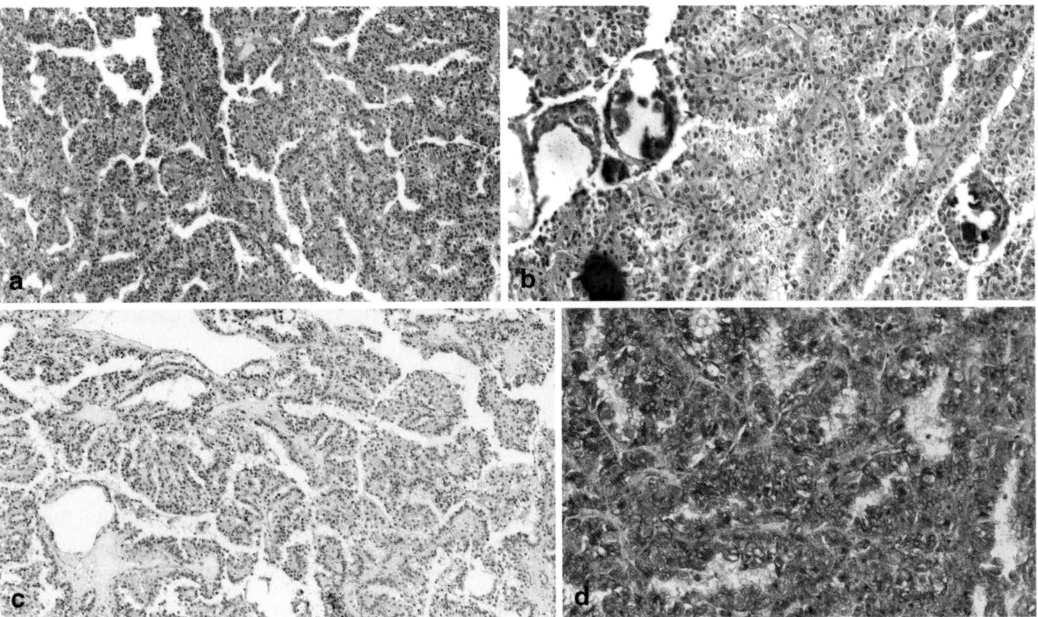

Fig. 30.5 a–d Expression of TFE3 and cathepsin K in a TFE3 translocation renal cell carcinoma (**a**, **b**). TFE3 staining is nuclear (**c**), while cathepsin K is cytoplasmic (**d**). (Courtesy of Dr. Guido Martignoni, University of Verona, Italy)

These findings suggest that cathepsin K may be used as a surrogate marker for TFE3 and TFEB overexpression and is a highly specific marker for translocation RCC.

Markers for Urothelial Lineage Differentiation

Markers for urothelial lineage differentiation, including p63, thrombomodulin, uroplakin III, and GATA 3, are expressed in a high percentage of UC but not in RCC and therefore can be used in the diagnosis of a poorly differentiated carcinoma, where the differential diagnosis is between a UC and RCC [21]. One caveat is that p63 is reported to be expressed in small fraction of collecting duct carcinoma.

Cytokeratins

Different types of CK are expressed in different renal tumors and can be taken advantage of for the purpose of differential diagnosis. For example, CK18, a low molecular weight CK expressed in simple epithelia, is detected while CK20 is virtually absent in all major renal tumors. CK7, a low-molecular-weight CK, is expressed in PRCC (predominantly type 1), CCTPRCC, collecting duct RCC, and UC. High-molecular-weight CKs, detected by antibody clone 34βE12 and CK5/6, in contrast, are expressed in the majority of collecting duct RCC, almost all UCs and significant proportion of CCTPRCC, but uncommonly in other RCC subtypes.

Clinically several CK monoclonal antibody clones are used, including AE1/3, CAM5.2, 34βE12 and CK5/6. AE1/3 is considered a pan-cytokeratin as it detects both low molecular weight (CK7, 8, and 19) and high-molecular-weight (CK10, 14–16) CKs, but it lacks reactivity to CK18, a CK almost ubiquitously present in simple epithelia, including renal tumors. Notably AE1/3 is positive in only one third of CCRCC and one fourth of translocation RCC. If one wishes to confirm the carcinomatous nature of a poorly differentiated tumor in the kidney, a panel of markers, including AE1/3, CAM5.2, and CK18, should be used.

Immunophenotype of Common Renal Tumors

One has to bear in mind that characteristic immunoprofiles are derived from the studies of renal tumors of typical morphology. A poorly differentiated tumor often retains at least partially the characteristic immunoprofile of the renal tumors of the same histological class. However, significant deviation from the "typical" immunoprofile of a particular renal tumor type can occur and may impact the utility of these immunohistochemical markers in the classification of renal tumors. Therefore, while a concordant immunoprofile supports classifying the tumor under study into the subtype with that immunoprofile, a lack of concordance does not invalidate that classification.

Utility of Immunohistochemistry in Morphological Classification of Renal Tumors

With the exception of TFE3 and TFEB, none of the above-mentioned markers are specific for renal tumors. Immunostains should then be used to corroborate, rather than to establish, the morphological classification. One should always carefully examine the hematoxylin and eosin (H&E) morphology of the lesion first to generate a differential diagnosis and then apply appropriate markers. A panel of markers is preferred to include markers that support the favored diagnosis and markers that rule out other diagnoses included in the differential diagnosis.

Renal Tumors with Predominantly Clear Cell Nests and Sheets

Many renal tumors have clear, or pale-staining, cytoplasm as the predominant morphological feature (Table 30.1). Their characteristic morphological features should lead to the correct diagnosis, or at least narrow down the differential diagnosis in most cases. An initial panel of markers, including CK7, CA9, and ksp-cadherin (or CD117), can

Table 30.1 Histological features and immunoprofiles of renal tumors with "pale-staining" or clear cytoplasm

Tumor type	Morphological features	Immunohistochemical profiles				
		CK7	CA9	Ksp-cad	Cathepsin K	HMB45
CCRCC	Nests of clear cells of variable sizes divided by thin "chicken-wire" vascular septa; dilated sinusoid spaces	–	+	–	–	–
CCTPRCC	Low grade clear cells forming long ribbons and lining papillae; nuclei polarized to the apical aspect	+	+ (cup-like pattern)	–	–	–
ChRCC	Pale, finely flocculated cytoplasm; prominent cell borders; "raisinoid" nuclei with halos	+ (diffuse)	–	+	–	–
Pelvic UC	Clear cell change often focal; typical UC can be found	+	+	–	–	–
Translocation RCC	Typically children/young adults; voluminous partially clear, partially eosinophilic cytoplasm; papillae lined with clear cells; psammomatous calcification/hyalinzed fibrovascular cores	– or + (focal and weak)	Variable	Variable	+ (50 %)	–
Epithelioid AML	Fat, smooth muscle and thick vessels may be present; multinucleated tumor cells	–	–	–	+	+
Intrarenal adrenal gland	Finely vacuolated cytoplasm; pale and eosinophilic cells often coexist; liposfuscin pigment	–	–	–	–	–

CCRCC clear cell renal cell carcinoma, *CCTPRCC* clear cell tubulopapillary renal cell carcinoma, *ChRCC* chromophobe renal cell carcinoma, *UC* urothelial carcinoma, *RCC* renal cell carcinoma, *AML* angiomyolipoma

help when working up difficult cases. Additional markers can be performed judiciously based on the differential diagnosis. For example, urothelial markers, including p63, GATA-3, and high-molecular-weight CK (HMWCK) can be stained if UC is suspected. Adrenal cortical markers including inhibin and MelanA can be performed to rule out intrarenal adrenal cortical tissue.

One important clinical question frequently raised by clinicians is whether a poorly differentiated RCC is a CCRCC. The tumor should be extensively sampled to look for areas with classical CCRCC morphology. Such areas may be minute, but if present and possessing a characteristic immunoprofile (CK7 −, CA9 +, ksp-cadherin −, p63 −), support the diagnosis of CCRCC.

Renal Tumors with "Oncocytic" Cytoplasm (Pink Cell Tumor)

Oncocytic cytoplasm can be seen in many renal tumors (Table 30.2) and may pose significant diagnostic challenges. In CCRCC, high-grade tumor cells tend to lose cytoplasmic clarity and acquire oncocytic cytoplasm. The initial panel to work up a challenging tumor with oncocytic cytoplasm should include CK7, CA9, AMACR, and ksp-cadherin (or CD117). Additional markers can be added if other tumors are suspected, including melanocytic markers for oncocytic AML, TFE3, TFEB, and cathepsin K for translocation RCC. One particular diagnostic issue is the distinction between an oncocytoma and ChRCC, an eosinophilic variant. Oncocytomas are characteristically negative or positive in single or small clusters of cells for CK7, and diffusely positive for CD117, ksp-cadherin and E-cadherin. ChRCC, on the other hand, is diffusely positive for CK7, CD117, ksp-cadherin and E-cadherin. Deviation from these characteristic immunoprofiles may justify labeling the tumor as "oncocytic tumor" without further subclassification. For example, an oncocytoma with diffuse CK7 staining is not characteristic and may be labeled as "oncocytic tumor, not otherwise specified," especially when other atypical features, such as diffuse nuclear atypia, are present (Fig. 30.6a–c).

Renal Tumors with Predominantly Papillary Components

Renal tumors with predominantly papillary components are listed in Table 30.3, although focal papillary patterns are seen in many renal tumors, especially in high-grade tumors. The initial panel of markers should include CK7, AMACR, and CA9. A high-grade renal tumor with predominantly papillary architecture should elicit a differential diagnosis of type 2 PRCC, collecting duct carcinoma (CDC), hereditary leiomyomatosis and renal cell cancer (HLRCC) syndrome, and metastatic adenocarcinoma to the kidney. Except for lineage specific markers (CDX-2, TTF-1, etc.), other markers are considerably variable in their expression pattern in these tumors; therefore, they offer little help in classification. Classification of these tumors depends largely on morphology and clinical manifestation.

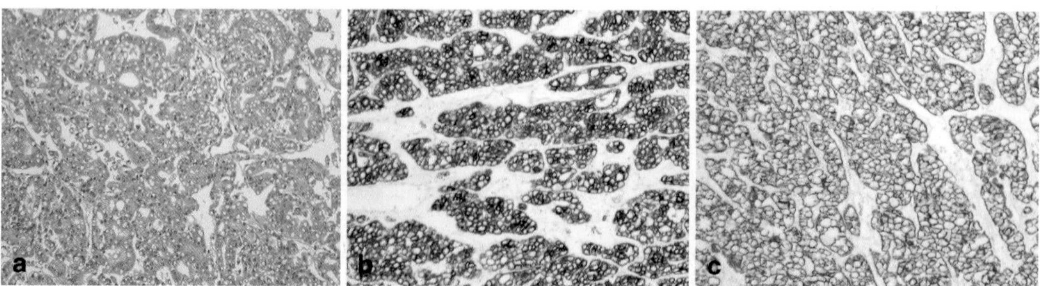

Fig. 30.6 Oncocytic renal tumor. It comprises sheets and cords of oncocytic cells with uniform nuclei (**a**). Tumor cells are diffusely positive for CK7 (**b**) and E-cadherin (**c**)

Table 30.2 Morphological features and immunoprofiles of renal tumors with eosinophilic cytoplasm

Tumor type	Morphological features	Immunohistochemical profiles				
		CK7	CA9	Ksp-cad	AMACR	HMB45
CCRCC with eosinophilic cytoplasm	Nests of clear cells of variable sizes divided by thin "chicken-wire" vascular septa; dilated sinusoid spaces; "pink" area always with higher nuclear grade	–	+	–	–	–
PRCC, oncocytic type	Focal papillae always present; macrophages and hemorrhage	+	–	–	+	–
ChRCC, eosinophilic variant	Intensely eosinophilic cytoplasm; prominent cell borders; "raisinoid" nuclei with halos	+ (patchy to diffuse)	–	+	–	–
Oncocytoma	Nests of oncocytic cells embedded in hyalinized, myxoid stroma; uniform nuclei	+ (in single cells or small clusters)	–	–	–	–
Translocation RCC	Typically children/young adults; voluminous partially clear, partially eosinophilic cytoplasm; papillae lined with clear cells; psammomatous calcification/hyalinzed fibrovascular cores	– or + (focal and weak)	variable	variable	+ (60%)	–
Acquired cystic disease-associated RCC	Intensely eosinophilic cells forming pseudocribriform structures, cysts and papillae; calcium oxalate crystals	–	–	–	+	–
Oncocytic AML	Fat, smooth muscle and thick vessels may be present; multinucleated tumor cells	–	–	–	+	+

CCRCC clear cell renal cell carcinoma, *PRCC* papillary renal cell carcinoma, *ChRCC* chromophobe renal cell carcinoma, *RCC* renal cell carcinoma, *AML* angiomyolipoma, *CK* cytokeratin, *AMACR* α-methylacyl coA racemase, *CA9* carbonic anhydrase IX, *HMB45* human melanoma black 45

Table 30.3 Histological features and immunoprofiles of renal tumors with predominant papillary component

Tumor type	Morphological features	Immunohistochemical profiles				
		CK7	CA9	AMACR	P63	TFE3/TFEB
CCTPRCC	Low grade clear cells forming long ribbons and lining papillae; nuclei polarized to the apical surface	+	+ (cup-like pattern)	–	–	–
PRCC, type 1	Pseudocapsule lined with tumor cells; papillae covered with single layer of tumor cells with scant cytoplasm and low grade nuclei; foamy macrophages, hemorrhage	+	–	+	–	–
PRCC, type 2	Pseudocapsule lined with tumor cells; papillae covered with pseudostratified tumor cells with abundant cytoplasm and high-grade nuclei; foamy macrophages, hemorrhage	+ (usually patchy)	–	+	–	–
Translocation RCC	Typically children/young adults; voluminous partially clear, partially eosinophilic cytoplasm; papillae lined with clear cells; psammomatous calcification/hyalinzed fibrovascular cores	– or + (focal and weak)	Variable	Variable	–	+
Collecting duct RCC	High-grade tumor cells forming multiple patterns; desmoplastic stroma	+	–	Variable	+(15 %)	–
Renal medullary carcinoma	Young patients with sickle cell anemia or trait; high-grade tumor cells forming multiple patterns; desmoplastic stroma	+	–	Variable	–	–
HLRCC syndrome	High-grade tumor cells forming multiple patterns; desmoplastic stroma	+	–	Variable	–	–
Metastatic adenocarcinoma to the kidney	History of primary tumor; widely infiltrative in the renal parenchyma	Variable	Variable	Variable	–	–

CCTPRCC clear cell tubulopapillary renal cell carcinoma, *PRCC* papillary renal cell carcinoma, *RCC* renal cell carcinoma, *CK* cytokeratin, *AMACR* α-methylacyl coA racemase, *CA9* carbonic anhydrase IX, *HLRCC* hereditary leiomyomatosis and renal cell cancer, *TFE3* transcription factor E3

Renal Tumors with Papillae Covered with Clear Cells as Predominant Features

The differential diagnosis includes CCTPRCC, PRCC, and translocation RCC. Characteristic morphological features and immunoprofiles can readily distinguish these three lesions (Fig. 30.7). CCTPCC is a recently described new subtype which behaves in a benign or indolent fashion [22]. Therefore, it is important to distinguish it from CCRCC and PRCC. It has characteristic morphology and immunoprofile (CK7+, CD10−, CA9+ with "cup-like" staining pattern, and AMACR) [22].

Renal Tumors with Tubulopapillary Architecture in Children and Young Adults

If a renal tumor has tubulopapillary architecture in children and young adults, the differential diagnosis should include PRCC, metanephric adenoma and epithelial predominant Wilms' tumor (Table 30.4). With appropriate clinical history and morphology, translocation RCC and metastatic adenocarcinoma may also be considered.

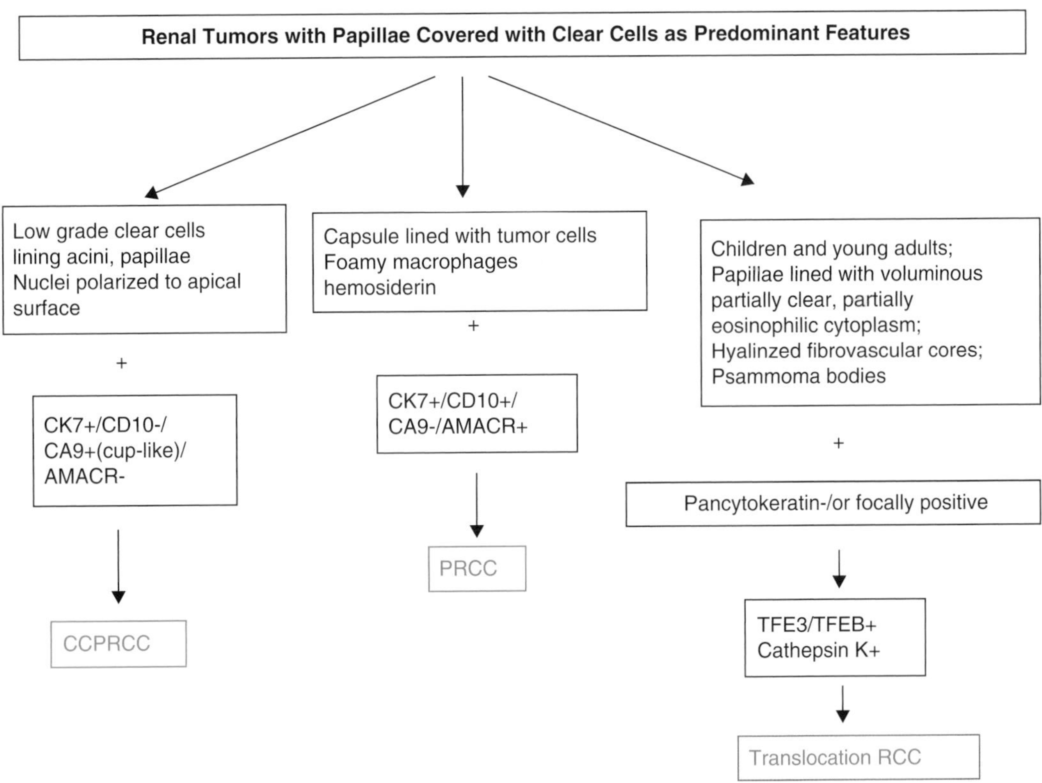

Fig. 30.7 Differential diagnosis of renal tumors with papillae covered with clear cells as predominant features. *AMACR* α-methylacyl coA racemase, *RCC* renal cell carcinoma, *PRCC* papillary renal cell carcinoma, *CCPRCC* clear cell papillary renal cell carcinoma, *TFE3* transcription factor E3

Table 30.4 Histological features and immunoprofiles of renal tumors with tubulopapillary pattern in children and young adults

Tumor type	Morphological features	Immunohistochemical profiles				
		CK7	AMACR	WT-1	CD56	TFE3/TFEB
PRCC	Pseudocapsule lined with tumor cells; foamy macrophages, hemorrhage	+	+	–	–	–
Metanephric adenoma	Lacks tumor capsule; tightly packed primitive tubules and acini; small uniform nuclei; scant cytoplasm	–	–	+	–	–
Epithelial predominant Wilms' tumor	Tumor capsule; overlapping columnar shaped nuclei with fine chromatin and brisk mitosis	– or focal+	–	+	+	–
Translocation RCC	Typically children/young adults; voluminous partially clear, partially eosinophilic cytoplasm; papillae lined with clear cells; psammomatous calcification/hyalinzed fibrovascular cores	– or+(focal and weak)	Variable	–	+	–
Metastatic adenocarcinoma to the kidney	History of primary tumor; widely infiltrative in the renal parenchyma	Variable	Variable	–	–	–

RCC renal cell carcinoma, *CK* cytokeratin, *AMACR* α-methylacyl coA racemase, *PRCC* papillary renal cell carcinoma, *TFE3* transcription factor E3

Renal Tumors with High-Grade Infiltrative Growth Pattern

Renal tumors with multinodular growth and invasive borders (tumor cells infiltrating between renal tubules and glomeruli at the advancing front) are difficult to classify based on morphology alone. There are several critical decision points in the workup of these cases (Fig. 30.8). One has to first rule out a metastasis to the kidney. PAX8 and PAX2 are probably the most useful markers owing to their relatively high sensitivity and specificity. If a tumor is deemed likely to originate in the kidney, UC should always be considered and ruled out as the management for UC and RCC is drastically different. The presence of UC in pelvic mucosa and typical staining pattern (CK7+, CK20+, PAX8−, HMWCK+, p63+) supports a diagnosis of UC.

Use of Immunohistochemical Markers in the Interpretation of Needle Biopsies of Renal Masses

Needle biopsy of renal masses has recently become more popular in the management of patients with renal masses owing to several reasons. The biopsy aims to clarify at least three questions. (1) Is the renal mass a neoplasm? (2) Is it a primary RCC, or metastatic cancer/lymphoma? (3) If a primary RCC, what subtype is it?

The most significant limitation of renal mass needle biopsy is the small quantity of tissue procured which may limit the morphological evaluation of the renal mass lesion. Consequently, immunohistochemistry is often employed to supplement the morphological evaluation. A recent study found that standard morphological evaluation and judicious use of five markers (CD7, CD10,

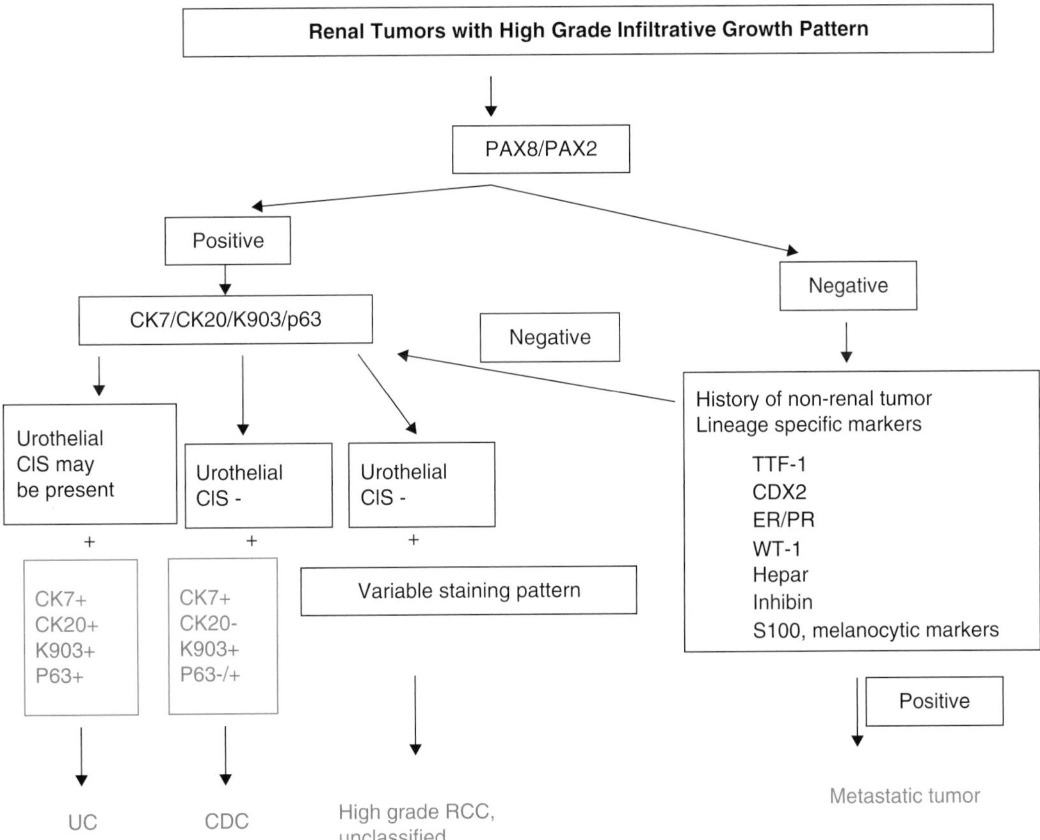

Fig. 30.8 Differential diagnosis of renal tumors with high-grade infiltrative growth pattern. *CDC* collecting duct carcinoma, *RCC* renal cell carcinoma, CIS carcinoma in situ, UC urothelial carcinoma

CA9, AMACR, and CD117) yielded accurate diagnoses in $>90\%$ of cases in an *ex vivo* needle biopsy study after nephrectomy [6]. When using immunohistochemistry to work up a renal mass biopsy, one should use the same, if not more, due diligence as in the workup of nephrectomy specimens. Careful morphological examination should be performed first to generate a list of differential diagnoses. Appropriate markers are then applied and the results are used to corroborate, rather than to establish, the morphological diagnosis.

Prognostic and Predictive Markers

The roles of several genetic pathways, including mTOR and HIF, in renal carcinogenesis and progression have been increasingly elucidated. Key components of these pathways have been investigated for their prognostic and predictive value for targeted therapies. For example, VHL gene, a tumor suppressor gene on chromosome 3p25–26, plays a crucial role in the HIF pathway. In normal cells, VHL targets HIF for proteosome-mediated degradation and therefore keeps HIF at low level. When the *VHL* gene is inactivated by gene mutation or promoter hypermethylation, HIF accumulates and activates downstream target genes, including vascular endothelial growth factor (VEGF) and CA9. Many of these molecules contribute to carcinogenesis in CCRCC. Functional loss of VHL is implicated in hereditary and sporadic CCRCC. However, studies have shown conflicting data on the prognostic value of VHL gene alteration. Loss of function mutation in the VHL gene is correlated with response to anti-VEGF therapy in some studies.

Several studies have found that the level of CA9 expression seems to have prognostic significance, with low expression ($\leq 85\%$ of tumor cells) correlating with worse overall survival in metastatic RCC, and high CA9 expression ($>85\%$) predictive of response to interleukin 2 (IL-2) [23], but final results are awaiting a prospective phase 2 selenium and vitamin E cancer prevention trial (SELECT). In addition, high CA9 expression ($>85\%$) is associated with greater tumor shrinkage in response to sorafenib (a VEGF inhibitor) treatment.

Other molecules that have been investigated for their prognostic and predictive roles in RCC include key components of mTOR pathway, B7 family members that are coregulatory molecules inhibiting T-cell-mediated immunity, insulin-like growth factor II mRNA binding protein 3 (IMP3) which is a member of the insulin-like growth factor II messenger ribonucleic acid (mRNA)-binding protein [24], p53, histone modifying and chromatin remodeling genes [25]. However, the vast majority of published studies are of single-center research and comprise a small number of cases. No marker has so far emerged as being reproducible and consistent across published studies. Therefore, no markers are ready to be recommended in routine clinical use for prognosis and prediction of therapy response. Large, multicenter prospective studies are needed to validate some promising markers. CA9 may be performed at the clinician's request and expression can be quantified as $\leq 85\%$ or $>85\%$.

Summary

Diagnosis and classification of renal cell neoplasms, based primarily on the morphological features, are usually straightforward. Immunohistochemical markers, however, play an important role in several clinical settings, including distinguishing renal from nonrenal tumors, subtyping of renal cell neoplasms and working up renal massneedle biopsy with limited tissue quantity. These markers include those whose expression supports a renal origin (PAX2/PAX8, RCC Ma, CD10, HKIM-1, and vimentin) and those with differential expression in different renal tumor subtypes (CA9, AMACR, parvalbumin, E-cadherin, ksp-cadherin, claudin 7/8, CD117, S100A1, TFE3, TFEB, cathepsin K, markers of urothelial differentiation, and various CKs). Each marker has its utility in a specific diagnostic setting. A panel of markers should be used to corroborate, but not to supplant, the morphological diagnosis and classification. So far, no markers have proven clinical utility in the prediction of clinical outcomes and response to novel targeted therapy.

References

1. Hammerich KH, Ayala GE, Wheeler TM. Application of immunohistochemistry to the genitourinary system (prostate, urinary bladder, testis, and kidney). Arch Pathol Lab Med. 2008;132(3):432–40.
2. Shen SS, Truong LD, Scarpelli M, Lopez-Beltran A. Role of immunohistochemistry in diagnosing renal neoplasms: when is it really useful? Arch Pathol Lab Med. 2012;136(4):410–7.
3. Skinnider BF, Amin MB. An immunohistochemical approach to the differential diagnosis of renal tumors. Semin Diagn Pathol. 2005;22(1):51–68.
4. Truong LD, Shen SS. Immunohistochemical diagnosis of renal neoplasms. Arch Pathol Lab Med. 2011;135(1):92–109.
5. Zhou M, Roma A, Magi-Galluzzi C. The usefulness of immunohistochemical markers in the differential diagnosis of renal neoplasms. Clin Lab Med. 2005;25(2):247–57.
6. Al-Ahmadie HA, Alden D, Fine SW, Gopalan A, Touijer KA, Russo P, et al. Role of immunohistochemistry in the evaluation of needle core biopsies in adult renal cortical tumors: an ex vivo study. Am J Surg Pathol. 2011;35(7):949–61.
7. Gupta R, Balzer B, Picken M, Osunkoya AO, Shet T, Alsabeh R, et al. Diagnostic implications of transcription factor Pax 2 protein and transmembrane enzyme complex carbonic anhydrase IX immunoreactivity in adult renal epithelial neoplasms. Am J Surg Pathol. 2009;33(2):241–7.
8. Ozcan A, de la Roza G, Ro JY, Shen SS, Truong LD. PAX2 and PAX8 expression in primary and metastatic renal tumors: a comprehensive comparison. Arch Pathol Lab Med. 2012;136(12):1541–51.
9. McGregor DK, Khurana KK, Cao C, Tsao CC, Ayala G, Krishnan B, et al. Diagnosing primary and metastatic renal cell carcinoma: the use of the monoclonal antibody 'Renal Cell Carcinoma Marker'. Am J Surg Pathol. 2001;25(12):1485–92.
10. Lin F, Zhang PL, Yang XJ, Shi J, Blasick T, Han WK, et al. Human kidney injury molecule-1 (hKIM-1): a useful immunohistochemical marker for diagnosing renal cell carcinoma and ovarian clear cell carcinoma. Am J Surg Pathol. 2007;31(3):371–81.
11. Ivanov S, Liao SY, Ivanova A, Danilkovitch-Miagkova A, Tarasova N, Weirich G, et al. Expression of hypoxia-inducible cell-surface transmembrane carbonic anhydrases in human cancer. Am J Pathol. 2001;158(3):905–19.
12. Zhou M, Chinnaiyan AM, Kleer CG, Lucas PC, Rubin MA. Alpha-Methylacyl-CoA racemase: a novel tumor marker over-expressed in several human cancers and their precursor lesions. Am J Surg Pathol. 2002;26(7):926–31.
13. Molinie V, Balaton A, Rotman S, Mansouri D, De Pinieux I, Homsi T, et al. Alpha-methyl CoA racemase expression in renal cell carcinomas. Hum Pathol. 2006;37(6):698–703.
14. Young AN, de OliveiraSalles PG, Lim SD, Cohen C, Petros JA, Marshall FF, et al. Beta defensin-1, parvalbumin, and vimentin: a panel of diagnostic immunohistochemical markers for renal tumors derived from gene expression profiling studies using cDNA microarrays. Am J Surg Pathol. 2003;27(2):199–205.
15. Shen SS, Krishna B, Chirala R, Amato RJ, Truong LD. Kidney-specific cadherin, a specific marker for the distal portion of the nephron and related renal neoplasms. Mod Pathol. 2005;18(7):933–40.
16. Argani P, Lae M, Hutchinson B, Reuter VE, Collins MH, Perentesis J, et al. Renal carcinomas with the t(6;11)(p21;q12): clinicopathologic features and demonstration of the specific alpha-TFEB gene fusion by immunohistochemistry, RT-PCR, and DNA PCR. Am J Surg Pathol. 2005;29(2):230–40.
17. Argani P, Lal P, Hutchinson B, Lui MY, Reuter VE, LadanyiM.Aberrant nuclear immunoreactivity for TFE3 in neoplasms with TFE3 gene fusions: a sensitive and specific immunohistochemical assay. Am J Surg Pathol. 2003;27(6):750–61.
18. Camparo P, Vasiliu V, Molinie V, Couturier J, Dykema KJ, Petillo D, et al. Renal translocation carcinomas: clinicopathologic, immunohistochemical, and gene expression profiling analysis of 31 cases with a review of the literature. Am J Surg Pathol. 2008;32(5):656–70.
19. Martignoni G, Bonetti F, Chilosi M, Brunelli M, Segala D, Amin MB, et al. Cathepsin K expression in the spectrum of perivascular epithelioid cell (PEC) lesions of the kidney. Mod Pathol. 2012;25(1):100–11.
20. Martignoni G, Pea M, Gobbo S, Brunelli M, Bonetti F, Segala D, et al. Cathepsin-K immunoreactivity distinguishes MiTF/TFE family renal translocation carcinomas from other renal carcinomas. Mod Pathol. 2009;22(8):1016–22.
21. Albadine R, Schultz L, Illei P, Ertoy D, Hicks J, Sharma R, et al. PAX8 (+)/p63 (−) immunostaining pattern in renal collecting duct carcinoma (CDC): a useful immunoprofile in the differential diagnosis of CDC versus urothelial carcinoma of upper urinary tract. Am J Surg Pathol. 2010;34(7):965–9.
22. Aydin H, Chen L, Cheng L, Vaziri S, He H, Ganapathi R, et al. Clear cell tubulopapillary renal cell carcinoma: a study of 36 distinctive low-grade epithelial tumors of the kidney. Am J Surg Pathol. 2010;34(11):1608–21.
23. Atkins M, Regan M, McDermott D, Mier J, Stanbridge E, YoumansA, et al. Carbonic anhydrase IX expression predicts outcome of interleukin 2 therapy for renal cancer. Clin Cancer Res. 2005;11(10):3714–21.
24. Jiang Z, Chu PG, Woda BA, Rock KL, Liu Q, Hsieh CC, et al. Analysis of RNA-binding protein IMP3 to predict metastasis and prognosis of renal-cell carcinoma: a retrospective study. Lancet Oncol. 2006;7(7):556–64.
25. Hakimi AA, Chen YB, Wren J, Gonen M, Abdel-Wahab O, Heguy A, et al. Clinical and pathologic impact of select chromatin-modulating tumor suppressors in clear cell renal cell carcinoma. Eur Urol. 2013;63(5):848–54.

31

Intraoperative Consultation for Renal Masses: Challenges and Implications for Treatment

Hiroshi Miyamoto and Steven S. Shen

Introduction

Clinical and radiological data provide important clues to the diagnosis of a space-occupying lesion in the kidney. Most of solitary solid renal masses in adults are renal cell carcinomas (RCCs), which usually show typical characteristics on radiological images. In contrast, the majority of cystic renal lesions are benign, although secondary changes such as hemorrhage, fibrosis, or calcifications may make it difficult to clinically distinguish a benign cyst from an extensively cystic RCC. Most urothelial carcinomas of the kidney can be recognized preoperatively, but high-grade invasive urothelial carcinoma can form a large mass, mimicking RCC. Conversely, high-grade RCC, especially collecting duct carcinoma, can simulate urothelial carcinoma. The diagnosis of less common lesions, such as angiomyolipoma and xanthogranulomatous pyelonephritis, can often be made with confidence based on their clinical and radiological findings. In most instances, therefore, urologists are able to plan definitive treatment of a renal mass without a preoperative biopsy. Furthermore, fine needle aspiration and/or needle core biopsy of a renal lesion may not always provide a definitive diagnosis. Thus, the final histopathologic diagnosis is usually made after the definitive procedure has been performed. However, there are circumstances when pathologists play a critical role in selecting an adequate therapeutic procedure during the surgery.

S. S. Shen (✉)
Department of Pathology and Genomic Medicine, Houston Methodist Hospital, Houston, TX, USA
e-mail: stevenshen@houstonmethodist.org

H. Miyamoto
Departments of Pathology and Urology, The Johns Hopkins Medical Institutions, Baltimore, MD, USA
e-mail: hmiyamo1@jhmi.edu

Common Indications for Intraoperative Consultation

- Gross identification of renal mass(es) in the nephrectomy specimen
- Histopathologic diagnosis for renal mass(es) (e.g., benign vs. malignant neoplasm, RCC vs. urothelial carcinoma)
- Surgical margin status during partial nephrectomy
- Histopathologic diagnosis of extrarenal masses or enlarged lymph nodes during nephrectomy

Assessment of Solid Renal Masses

RCCs are typically treated by radical or partial nephrectomy. Large neoplasms are occasionally pretreated with renal artery embolization prior to nephrectomy in an attempt to reduce the vascularity of the tumor and subsequent blood loss during surgery. Following this procedure, an extensive infarct-type necrosis of the tumor is often seen. RCC can also be successfully treated by cryoablation or radiofrequency ablation in highly selective patients. Needle core biopsies for diagnosis of renal masses are increasingly used in recent

C. Magi-Galluzzi, C. G. Przybycin (eds.), *Genitourinary Pathology*, DOI 10.1007/978-1-4939-2044-0_31,

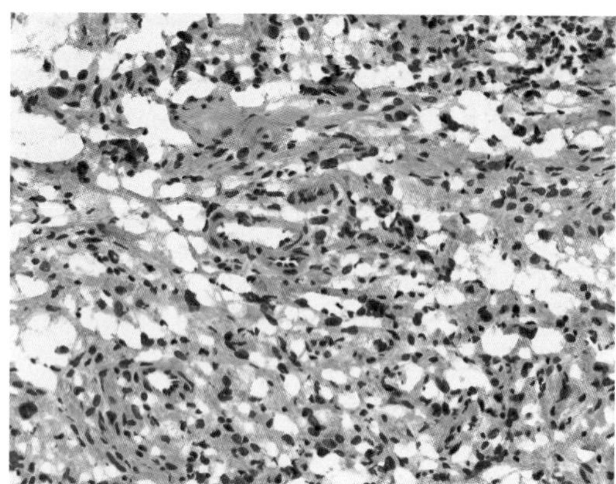

Fig. 31.1 Frozen section of a renal angiomyolipoma mimicking oncocytic renal cell neoplasms. Original magnification × 200

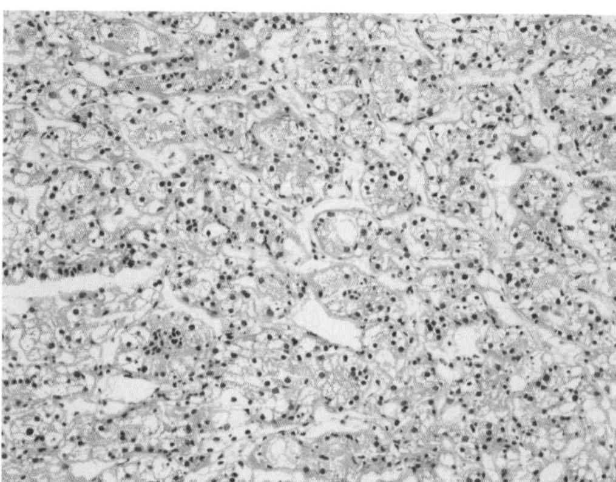

Fig. 31.2 Frozen section of a clear cell renal cell carcinoma which can be mistaken for a chromophobe renal cell carcinoma. Original magnification × 100

years for treatment decision; consequently, specimens are often diagnosed on permanent section.

Angiomyolipoma, one of the most common benign renal neoplasms, is often diagnosed preoperatively by identifying its fatty component on imaging studies, although it can be difficult to distinguish a fat-poor angiomyolipoma from a RCC [1]. Similarly, it may also be difficult to distinguish an angiomyolipoma from clear cell RCC or oncocytic renal neoplasm on frozen section (Fig. 31.1). Only a minority of renal oncocytoma can be recognized by a characteristic central scar that is neither frequent nor specific.

An incisional biopsy of a renal lesion may be submitted for intraoperative consultation when the diagnosis may result in changes in the treatment procedure (e.g., partial nephrectomy for a benign condition vs. radical nephrectomy for a RCC). In this setting, the entire biopsy specimen should be embedded for frozen section assessment (FSA), and multiple levels should be prepared if the diagnosis is in doubt.

During radical nephrectomy, there are usually no immediate management issues at stake. If the surgeon requests an intraoperative consultation, gross examination is often all that is necessary. If the macroscopic findings are equivocal (e.g., cystic RCC vs. complex benign cyst with secondary hemorrhage and fibrosis; see below), it is best to defer the diagnosis to permanent sections instead of performing multiple FSAs to seek for a definitive diagnosis. On frozen section, it can be very difficult to render a definitive histologic diagnosis for a renal neoplasm with prominent clear cells (Fig. 31.2) or papillary growth pattern. Similarly, renal oncocytomas often show characteristic gross findings (i.e., well circumscribed, unencapsulated, mahogany brown, and no necrosis). However, the gross diagnosis of oncocytoma should be provisional. Even when a FSA is performed, clear cell RCC with prominent granular cells and eosinophilic variant of chromophobe RCC can have prominent oncocytic features mimicking oncocytoma.

FSA during radical nephrectomy can be justified in certain situations, including a possibility that the neoplasm is a high-grade urothelial carcinoma forming a mass and thus mimicking a RCC; it is important to make this distinction because the surgeon will proceed with converting the surgical procedure to a nephroureterectomy if a diagnosis of urothelial carcinoma is rendered. Even though the value of an extended lymphadenectomy remains controversial, some surgeons may choose to perform an extended lymph node dissection when the RCC is of high grade or if there are other poor prognostic features, such as a sarcomatoid component. For a RCC, if grading is requested, the surgeon should be informed that there is a possibility of undergrading because of tumor heterogeneity as well as the limitations of FSA that make it difficult to precisely determine the nuclear size and/or presence of prominent nucleoli. Multiple selective sections from different areas of the tumor may be helpful in this setting.

Assessment of Cystic Renal Masses

Up to 15 % of renal tumors are predominantly cystic. Cystic change can easily be recognized on imaging and is often graded using the Bosniak classification that helps to determine malignant risk of renal cysts on the basis of their appearance and enhancement on computed tomography [1]. Treatment varies, and the surgeon may request a FSA to guide the extent of resection particularly when renal parenchymal sparing is of critical importance.

The specimen submitted for FSA is often a wedge biopsy of the cyst wall. The entire specimen should be embedded for FSA. The differential diagnosis includes a simple cyst with superimposing hemorrhage and/or infection, cystic nephroma/mixed stromal and epithelial tumor of the kidney, and RCC with marked cystic change.

Assessment of Surgical Margins During Partial Nephrectomy

Partial nephrectomy recently has become the preferred treatment for all stages of T1a RCCs and some T1b tumors [2, 3]. It provides not only adequate long-term oncologic outcomes, when comparing with radical nephrectomy [2, 4], but also preservation of renal function. This procedure is particularly indicated for patients with: (1) a solitary kidney; (2) bilateral kidney disease; (3) a genetic predisposition to multiple synchronous or metachronous tumors such as von Hippel–Lindau disease, tuberous sclerosis, hereditary papillary renal carcinoma syndrome, and Birt–Hogg–Dubé syndrome; and (4) benign renal tumor such as angiomyolipoma, cystic nephroma, or mixed epithelial and stromal tumor of the kidney.

The partial nephrectomy specimen is often submitted for evaluation of its surgical margins. Two types of specimens are submitted for FSA to assess surgical margins: an entire partial nephrectomy specimen and a biopsy of the tumor bed. In general, a 1-cm margin of normal tissue is optimal for RCC, but narrower yet negative margins do not appear to affect patient outcomes. It has also been shown that positive surgical margins in partial nephrectomy specimens may not be clinically significant, and patients with positive margin do not commonly seem to develop long-term recurrence [5, 6]. Benign neoplasms can be excised with very narrow margins. In a recent study by one of the authors comparing partial nephrectomy cases with ($n=293$) versus without ($n=140$) intraoperative consultation, the FSA was shown to significantly reduce the incidence of positive margins from 17.0 to 4.3 % ($P<0.001$) yet failed to affect recurrence-free survival overall [7]. Nonetheless, this study suggested the usefulness of FSA in select patients because FSA was associated with improved survival in those who had pT1 or exophytic tumors and underwent laparoscopic partial nephrectomy.

Partial nephrectomy specimens should be inked to indicate the renal parenchymal margin and sectioned perpendicular to the margin to determine the relationship of the tumor to the inked margin. When the mass is grossly far (>1 cm) from the resection margin, a section from an area closest to the tumor can be taken. If the mass is closer to the inked margin, we recommend taking one or more perpendicular sections of the tumor including the nearest margin, in case a carcinoma shows microscopic extension beyond the grossly visible lesion. Sections taken perpendicular to the margin also allow the pathologist to measure and report the distance between the carcinoma and the margin.

The following pitfalls may be encountered when evaluating margins of partial nephrectomy specimens:

- Compressed, atrophic renal tubules at the periphery of the tumor may be distorted/crushed and show reactive nuclear atypia and other changes that may suggest the possibility of a low-grade RCC at the surgical margin (Fig. 31.3). However, the presence of glomeruli and mixture of tubules provides evidence

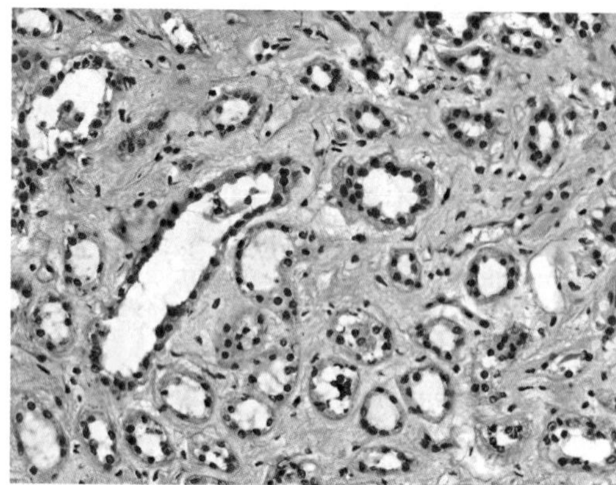

Fig. 31.3 Frozen section of a normal kidney with a mixture of proximal and distal tubules which may mimic an oncocytoma in a small biopsy. Original magnification ×200

for the nonneoplastic nature of these changes. Low-grade RCCs are composed of solid nests, tubules with monotonous population of neoplastic cells.

- It is sometimes difficult to distinguish normal proximal renal tubules from an oncocytoma (Fig. 31.4) or RCC with a tubular growth pattern, especially for a pathologist who has not reviewed the gross specimen. Since the majority of oncocytomas and most of low-grade RCCs are well circumscribed, a correlation between macroscopic and microscopic findings should resolve this problem in most cases.

Assessment of Nephroureterectomy Specimens

The diagnosis of urothelial carcinoma of the kidney is made on the basis of cytologic and histologic findings in addition to clinical and radiological data. For renal pelvic urothelial carcinoma, the choice of treatment is radical nephroureterectomy, which eliminates any potential urothelialneoplasia on the ipsilateral ureter. However, the clinical diagnosis is occasionally inconclusive; for example, it may be difficult to distinguish an urothelial carcinoma close to the medulla of the kidney from variants of RCC that affect the medulla, such as collecting duct carcinoma. In this situation, the surgeon may choose to perform ureteropyeloscopy or proceed with nephrectomy and have the pathologist examine the specimen intraoperatively. Frozen section diagnosis of urothelial carcinoma can be very challenging (Fig. 31.5). Histopathologic features in favor of urothelial carcinoma include papillary tumor involving the pelvocaliceal system, solid nests, squamous differentiation, and marked desmoplastic stromal reaction, but its definitive di-

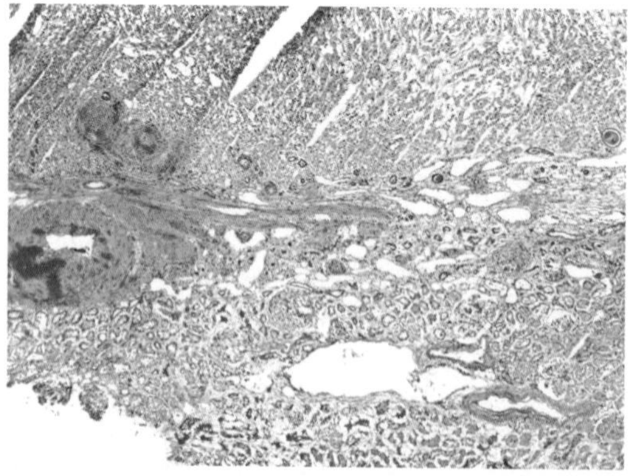

Fig. 31.4 Frozen section of a renal parenchyma with oncocytoma. Renal proximal tubules can be easily interpreted as oncocytoma. Looking for the presence of glomeruli and a mixture of tubules with abundant eosinophilic cytoplasm or scant cytoplasm will be helpful to confirm normal renal tubules. Original magnification ×20

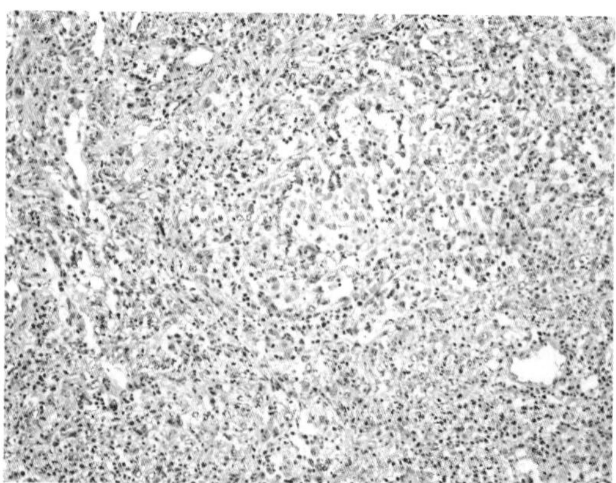

Fig. 31.5 Frozen section of a renal urothelial carcinoma showing diffuse infiltration of tumor cells. A definitive diagnosis of invasive urothelial carcinoma may be difficult on a single frozen section. Original magnification ×100

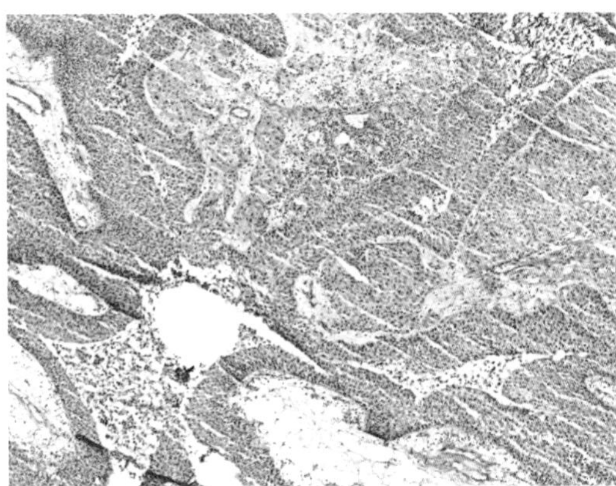

Fig. 31.6 Frozen section taken from the junction of an invasive tumor at the renal pelvis showing invasive urothelial carcinoma along with urothelial carcinoma in situ. Original magnification ×40

agnosis relies on the identification of urothelial carcinoma in situ or papillary urothelial carcinoma in the adjacent pelvocaliceal system or ureteropelvic junction (Fig. 31.6). Therefore, proper sampling of tumor tissue for frozen section is critical for a definitive diagnosis.

The surgeons may also request intraoperative evaluation of the specimen, including FSA of the distal ureteral margin because of synchronous multifocality of in situ and invasive carcinomas.

The nephroureterectomy specimen consists of the kidney, perirenal adipose tissue, Gerota's fascia, the entire ureter, and a cuff of bladder wall. The kidney should be bivalved through the pyelocalyceal system with the help of a probe. If the gross features arecharacteristic of urothelial carcinoma, there is no reason to perform confirmatory FSA of the tumor. If, on the other hand, the nature of the neoplasm is not clear on gross examination, sections should be taken from the periphery of the mass as well as from the calyceal tissue that shows mucosal abnormalities. The latter areas are more likely to show recognizable urothelial carcinoma even if the main mass is a poorly differentiated carcinoma [8].

References

1. Israel GM, Bosniak MA. How I do it: evaluating renal masses. Radiology. 2005;236(2):441–50.
2. Joniau S, Vander Eeckt K, Van Poppel H. The indications for partial nephrectomy in the treatment of renal cell carcinoma. Nat Clin Pract Urol. 2006;3(4):198–205.
3. Crépel M, Jeldres C, Perrotte P, Capitanio U, Isbarn H, Shariat SF, Liberman D, Sun M, Lughezzani G, Arjane P, Widmer H, Graefen M, Montorsi F, Patard JJ, Karakiewicz PI. Nephron-sparing surgery is equally effective to radical nephrectomy for T1BN0M0 renal cell carcinoma: a population-based assessment. Urology. 2010;75(2):271–5.
4. Patard JJ, Shvarts O, Lam JS, Pantuck AJ, Kim HL, Ficarra V, Cindolo L, Han KR, De La Taille A, Tostain J, Artibani W, Abbou CC, Lobel B, Chopin DK, Figlin RA, Mulders PF, Belldegrun AS. Safety and efficacy of partial nephrectomy for all T1 tumors based on an international multicenter experience. J Urol. 2004;171(6):2181–5.
5. Yossepowitch O, Thompson RH, Leibovich BC, Eggener SE, Pettus JA, Kwon ED, Herr HW, Blute ML, Russo P. Positive surgical margins at partial nephrectomy: predictors and oncological outcomes. J Urol. 2008;179(6):2158–63.
6. Bensalah K, Pantuck AJ, Rioux-Leclercq N, Thuret R, Montorsi F, Karakiewicz PI, Mottet N, Zini L, Bertini R, Salomon L, Villers A, Soulie M, Bellec L, Rischmann P, De la Taille A, Avakian R, Crepel M, Ferriere JM, Bernhard JC, Dujardin T, Pouliot F, Rigaud J, Pfister C, Albouy B, Guy L, Joniau S, van-Poppel H, Lebret T, Culty T, Saint F, Zisman A, Raz O, Lang H, Spie R, Wille A, Roigas J, Aguilera A, Rambeaud B, Martinez PL, Nativ O, Farfara R, Richard F, Roupret M, Doehn C, Bastian PJ, Muller SC, Tostain J, Belldegrun AS, Patard JJ. Positive surgical margin appears to have negligible impact on survival of renal cell carcinomas treated by nephron-sparing surgery. Eur Urol. 2010;57(3):466–71.
7. Venigalla S, Wu G, Miyamoto H. The impact of frozen section analysis during partial nephrectomy on surgical margin status and tumor recurrence: a clinicopathologic study of 433 cases. Clin Genitourin Cancer. 2013;11(4):527–36.
8. Perez-Montiel D, Wakely PE Jr., Hes O, Michal M, Suster S. High-grade urothelial carcinoma of the renal pelvis: clinicopathologic study of 108 cases with emphasis on unusual morphologic variants. Mod Pathol. 2006;19(4):494–503.

Genetic and Epigenetic Alterations in Renal Cell Carcinoma

32

Fang-Ming Deng and Ming Zhou

Introduction

Renal cell carcinoma (RCC), a group of heterogeneous tumors arising from the epithelium of the renal tubules, accounts for greater than 90 % of all malignancies in the adult kidney. Classified according to the 2004 World Health Organization criteria, these tumors have unique clinical and pathological features [1]. Cytogenetic and molecular studies have also demonstrated that each histological subtype demonstrates specific genetic changes. Although different histological subtypes of RCC demonstrate unique pathogenesis and genetic alterations, the impact of histological subtypes on prognosis remains controversial [2]. In view of specific genomic and epigenetic alterations associated with a specific RCC subtype, implementation of genetic and epigenetic markers in the management of RCC might become helpful in the future.

Genetic Alterations and Pathogenesis

Clear cell RCC (CCRCC) is the most common subtype, accounting for 60–75 % of RCCs. The most common and characteristic genetic change in CCRCC is an alteration of the short arm of chromosome 3 (−3p, >90 %), followed thereafter by changes in other chromosomal regions, including 5q, 6q, 8p, 9p, 10p, and 14q [3]. Biallelic inactivation, such as by loss of one 3p arm and mutations on the second chromosome 3, is a key event in the tumor development of CCRCC. Additional chromosomal aberrations are often associated with tumor progression. At least three regions harboring several different genes on 3p have been implicated, including the von Hippel–Lindau (*VHL*) gene on 3p25-26, the *FHIT* gene on 3p11-12, and the *RASSF1A*and *DRR1* genes on 3p21-22. VHL functions as a tumor suppressor and plays a critical role in the hypoxia-inducible factor (HIF) pathway. Mutations in the *VHL* gene lead to increased activation of the HIF pathway and its downstream target genes such as vascular endothelial growth factor (*VEGF*), platelet-derived growth factor (*PGDF*), epidermal growth factor (*EGF*), carbonic anhydrase (*CAIX*), *Glut-1*, and erythropoietin. These genes act in concert to promote deregulated epithelial proliferation and angiogenesis and therefore appear to contribute to the pathogenesis of CCRCC. The majority of CCRCCs are sporadic, with less than 5 % occurring in patients with inherited cancer syndromes such as von Hippel–Lindau disease, tuberous sclerosis, and constitutional chromosome 3 translocation syndrome.

Papillary RCC (PRCC) accounts for 10–15 % of RCCs. Gain of chromosomes 7 and 17 and loss of Y chromosome are the most common cytogenetic changes [4]. Additional gain of chromosomes 3, 12, 16, 20, and other chromosomes is often associated with tumor progression.

F.-M. Deng (✉) · M. Zhou
Department of Pathology, New York University Langone Medical Center, New York, NY, USA
e-mail: Dengf01@nyumc.org

M. Zhou
e-mail: Ming.zhou@nyumc.org

C. Magi-Galluzzi, C. G. Przybycin (eds.), *Genitourinary Pathology,* DOI 10.1007/978-1-4939-2044-0_32,

The responsible genes that underlie several hereditary forms of PRCC have been identified including *c-Met* gene mutations (7q31) in hereditary papillary renal cell carcinoma syndrome (HPRCC) and fumarate hydratase (FH) mutations (1q42) in hereditary leiomyomatosis/renal cell carcinoma syndrome (HLRCC). Gain-of-function mutations in *c-MET* result in altered cellular processes related to renal papillary carcinogenesis, although these mutations are uncommon in sporadic PRCC. Fumarate hydratase functions as an enzyme that converts fumarate to malate in the tricarboxylic acid cycle. Recent studies suggest that fumarate hydratase also regulates the stability of hypoxia-inducible factors (HIFs) and may therefore play a role in renal carcinogenesis.

Chromophobe RCC (ChRCC) accounts for 5% of RCC. It frequently has multiple complex chromosomal losses, including Y, 1, 2, 6, 10, 13, 17, and 21 [5]. Renal oncocytoma, a benign tumor that may bear morphological resemblance to chromophobe RCC, is characterized by alterations involving chromosome 11q, partial or complete losses of chromosomes 1 or 14, or a sex chromosome (Y or X). ChRCC and renal oncocytoma share some cytogenetic similarity, although the former typically demonstrates more complex karyotypic alterations than the latter. Patients with Birt–Hogg–Dube syndrome, the gene for which is mapped to 17p11.2, often develop ChRCC, oncocytoma, and hybrid tumors with features of both ChRCC and oncocytoma.

Recently, several distinct RCCs with chromosomal translocations involving the *TFE3* gene at Xp11.2 and *TFEB* gene at 6p21 have been described [6]. The translocation results in overexpression of fusion proteins that harbor the DNA-binding domains from TFE3 and TFEB, and this overexpression has been hypothesized to function in the pathogenesis of this unique class of RCC.

Epigenetic Alterations in RCC

DNA Methylation

DNA methylation, a covalent chemical modification resulting in addition of a methyl group at the carbon 5 position of the cytosine ring in CpG dinucleotides, is one of the most consistent epigenetic changes occurring in human cancer. Morris et al. [7], in a genomewide methylation analysis, found a significant correlation between tumor suppressor gene SCUBE3 DNA methylation and an increased risk of cancer death or relapse in RCC patients. In addition, aberrant promoter methylation of DLEC1 (a tumor suppressor gene at 3p22) is associated with more advanced tumor stage and higher grade [8]. Methylation of microRNA genes miR-9-1 and miR-9-3 is associated with RCC tumor recurrence and decrease in recurrence-free survival time [9].

DNA Hypomethylation

Carbonic anhydrase IX (CAIX) is a transmembrane glycoprotein that may be involved in cell transformation and proliferation. DNA hypomethylation of the CAIX gene has been shown to participate in the activation of its promoter activity in RCC cell lines and clinical tissue samples [10, 11].

Histone Modification and Chromatin Remodeling

Little data on histone modification and prognosis of RCC patients have been published. Ellinger et al. [12] evaluated histone H3 lysine 4 monomethyl (H3K4me1), di-methyl (H3K4me2) and trimethyl (H3K4me3) patterns in renal cell carcinoma (RCC) using a tissue microarray with 193 RCC (including 142 clear cell, 31 papillary, 10 chromophobe, and 10 sarcomatoid RCCs) and 10 oncocytoma specimens. H3K4me3 staining was more intense in papillary RCC, whereas H3K4me1 and H3K4me2 were similar in the diverse RCC subtypes. H3K4me1–3 levels were inversely correlated with Fuhrman grading, pT stage, lymph node involvement, and distant metastasis. Progression-free survival and cancer-specific survival were shorter in patients with low levels of H3K4me1–3 in the univariate analysis, but they did not observe a significant correlation of a single modification in a multivariate model, which also included the established prognostic parameters TNM stage and Fuhrman grade. In comparison, the H3K4me score, which combined staining levels of the H3K4 modifications, was an independent predictor of RCC progression-free survival. Studies from this group also showed that H3 lysine 27(H3K27) methylation levels were inversely correlated with Fuhrman grading and pT stage. Progression-free survival was shorter in patients with lower levels of H3K-27me1 and H3K27me3 in the univariate analysis [13].

Recent studies identified several frequent mutations of histone modifying and chromatin remodeling genes in CCRCC. These include *PBRM1*, a subunit of the PBAF AWI/SNF chromatin remodeling complex [14], ARID1A, a subunit of the BAF AWI/SNF chromatin remodeling complex [15], histodeubiquitinase *BAP1* [16, 17], histone demethylase *KDM5C* [18], and histone methyltransferase *SETD2* [19]. Most mutations of these chromatin modulators discovered in CCRCC are loss of function, implicating major roles for epigenetic regulation of additional functional pathways participating in the development and progression of these diseases. Clinical data have shown these mutations are associated with advanced stage, grade, and tumor invasion [20, 21].

MicroRNA Expression

MicroRNAs (miRNAs), non-coding RNAs regulating gene expression, are frequently aberrantly expressed in human cancers. To date, there are more than 100 publications on microRNA expression and RCC diagnosis, recurrence, and metastasis. Several panels/clusters of miRNAs have been proposed to predict the recurrence and metastatic potentials of RCC. It is interesting to note that as miRNA can be easily detected and quantified in blood, serum assays based on these metastasis-associated miRNAs may be of value. However, further studies in larger patient cohorts are necessary to validate the potential value of microRNA as prognostic biomarkers.

Diagnostic Markers and Applications

Chromosome 3p Alterations

The loss of DNA sequences on chromosome 3p is one of the primary and most frequent events in the pathogenesis of CCRCC [22]. Loss of heterozygosity (LOH) and comparative genetic hybridization (CGH) analyses of CCRCCs have revealed that allelic (interstitial) losses predominantly occur in the chromosome 3p21 region in combination with either 3p25 or 3p13-14, or with both, and these allelic losses are restricted to CCRCC. Chromosome 3p alterations are observed in over 96 % of sporadic and hereditary RCC. Deletion of 3p is the only karyotypic finding in 15 % of non-papillary RCC and in RCC as small as 1 mm. Even the sarcomatoid component of CCRCC retains characteristic 3p alterations. Chromosome 3p alteration is detected in only 8 % of papillary RCC; however, those PRCCs have cytological characteristics of CCRCC. Therefore, loss of 3p is highly specific for CCRCC, and the presence of 3p alteration can provide support for a diagnosis of CCRCC. Detection of 3p changes can be accomplished by conventional cytogenetics, LOH using probes mapped to 3p regions, and CGH.

Quantification of Chromosomes 7, 17

PRCC often demonstrates chromosomal gain, most frequently gain of chromosomes 7 and 17, which are present in 68–75 and 67–80 % of PRCC, respectively [4, 23]. However, trisomy 7 is also a common finding in several other human cancers and in 18–30 % of non-papillary RCC, normal renal cells, and several non-malignant conditions. Therefore, trisomy 7 is, by itself, not specific for PRCC. In contrast, a non-random gain of chromosome 17 is uncommon in other forms of RCC (present in 2.6 % of CCRCC) and other human cancers and, therefore, is a genetic finding fairly specific to PRCC.

Quantification of chromosomes 7 and 17 can be accomplished by cytogenetic study, comparative genomic hybridization (CGH), and fluorescence in situ hybridization (FISH). FISH can be conveniently performed on formalin-fixed, paraffin-embedded tissues using centromeric probes for chromosomes 7 and 17. Brown et al. [24] described a method to isolate intact nuclei from paraffin sections. The majority of the published studies have used tissue sections of 4–8 μm in thickness. To account for the potential nuclear truncation artifact that may affect the chromosomal copy counts on formalin-fixed, paraffin-embedded tissue sections, a normal range is established based on the copy counts of chromosomes 7 and 17 in the adjacent normal kidney tissue.

TFE3, TFEB, and RCC Associated with MITF/TFE Gene Translocation

Some RCCs are associated with chromosomal translocations involving specific genes. RCC associated with Xp11.2 translocation/*TFE3* gene fusion is defined by chromosomal translocation involving the *TFE3* gene on chromosome Xp11.2, resulting in the overexpression of the TFE3 protein, a member of the MITF/TFE transcriptional factor family [6]. The translocation partner genes include *PRCC* on 1q21, *ASPL* on 17q25, *PSL* on 1p34, *NonO* on Xq12, and *CLTC* on 17q23. These carcinomas typically affect children and young adults. Although RCC accounts for less than 5 % of pediatric renal tumors, Xp11.2-associated RCCs make up a significant proportion of these cases. The RCC involving *ASPL-TFE3* translocation characteristically presents at an advanced stage and also with lymph node metastasis. The morphology varies slightly with different chromosomal translocations; however, the most distinctive histological feature is the presence of papillary structures lined with clear cells.

Molecular genetic analysis for the chromosomal translocation involving the *TFE3* gene provides the most definitive evidence. Immunohistochemical stains for the TFE3 protein, on the other hand, offer a simple, sensitive, and specific assay for the Xp11-translocation RCC on formalin-fixed and paraffin-embedded tissues. As it is tightly regulated in normal tissues, TFE3 is undetectable on routine immunohistochemistry even though it is a ubiquitously expressed nuclear transcriptional factor. TFE3 fusion proteins, in contrast, are overexpressed in Xp11 translocation RCC and can therefore be detected by immunohistochemical staining. Argani et al. [25] reported that the TFE3 protein could be detected by immunohistochemistry in 20/21 (95.2 %) of Xp11.2 translocation RCC confirmed molecularly. The only case that was negative for TFE3 was fixed in Bouin's fixative. It is known that TFE3 protein is labile and its antigenicity is affected by fixation, with more intense staining at the periphery of the tissue section. However, TFE3 immunostaining is not entirely specific for the Xp11.2 translocation RCC, as positive staining can be detected in 29 % of perivascular epithelioid cell tumor (PECOMA) of soft tissue and gynecological tract, and rarely in other tumors, including adrenal cortical carcinoma, granular cell tumor, bile duct carcinoma, and high-grade myxofibrosarcoma [26].

Another variant of RCC harbors a t(6;11) (p21;q12) translocation that results in overexpression of TFEB transcriptional factor on 6p21, another member of the MITF/TFE family. Similar to Xp11.2 translocation RCC, RCC associated with TFEB also predominantly affects children and young adults. The characteristic morphology includes a biphasic population of larger and smaller epithelioid cells, with the latter typically clustered around hyaline basement membrane material. The diagnosis can be confirmed by the immunohistochemical stain for TFEB protein, which is both sensitive and specific for RCC associated with TFEB, as it is not detectable in other neoplasms and normal tissues. More recently, Malouf et al. [27] found genomic heterogeneity of translocation RCC (TRCC) that included alterations common with clear cell RCC (e.g., 3p loss) and papillary RCC (e.g., trisomy 7 and/or 17). When compared with young patients (<18 years), adults with TRCC displayed distinct genomic and epigenetic aberrations, exemplified by lower LINE-1 methylation and frequent 17q partial gain, which were consistent with a large-scale dosage effect affecting RCC carcinogenesis.

The results show that besides TFE3/TFEB translocations, TRCC shares alterations commonly present in other RCC histological subtypes, and these are associated with patient outcomes.

Mutations in c-Met, Fumarate Hydratase, and Folliculin Genes

Less than 5% of RCC patients are afflicted with an inherited cancer syndrome. Age of onset in these patients is variable, although most tend to occur at an earlier age. Each of the inherited cancer syndromes predisposes patients to distinct subtypes of RCC [28]. Renal involvement can range from solitary lesions to bilateral and multifocal tumors. Patients may also have characteristic extrarenal manifestations. Family history, early onset, bilateral, and multifocal renal involvement should arouse suspicion for a hereditary renal cancer syndrome. Von Hippel–Lindau disease will be discussed later in this chapter. Three other entities will be mentioned briefly, including hereditary papillary renal cell carcinoma syndrome (HPRCC), hereditary leiomyomatosis/renal cell carcinoma (HLRCC), and Birt–Hogg–Dube syndrome (BHD), and will be covered more extensively in Chap. 29. Molecular assays, including DNA sequencing, are used to detect the germline mutations in these genes in suspected patients, as immunohistochemical assays are not useful in this setting.

HPRCC is caused by mutations in *c-MET* proto-oncogene, which occupies a 110-kb genomic region on 7q31–34 and consists of 20 exons, encoding a protein that belongs to the tyrosine kinase receptor superfamily. Alteration in c-MET function is mostly through germline mis-sense mutations, which are restricted to exons 16–19, the receptor tyrosine kinase domain that is homologous to those in the *c-kit*, and *RET* proto-oncogenes that are linked to other malignancies. In similar fashion, missense mutations within exons 16–19 of *c-MET* lead to constitutive activation of the tyrosine kinase. Such mutations of the *c-Met* gene are infrequent in sporadic PRCC. Besides these germline missense mutations, tumors in HPRCC also demonstrate trisomy 7. Interestingly, although sporadic PRCC is characterized by trisomies in chromosomes 7 and 17, and loss of Y chromosome in men, only trisomy 7 is consistently found in HPRCC tumors.

HLRCC is an autosomal dominant disease. Its gene, *fumarate hydratase (FH)*, is mapped to 1q42.3–43 and contains 10 exons that encode fumarate hydratase (FH), a 511–amino acid enzyme that converts fumarate to malate in the tricarboxylic acid cycle. HLRCC is genetically heterogeneous and up to 50 different mutations have been discovered in this syndrome. The most common germline mutations are missense mutations in *FH*, although truncation and whole-gene deletion have also been observed. Biallelic inactivation has been found in nearly all uterine leiomyomas and papillary RCC. Alterations in *FH* have not been detected in multiple types of sporadic malignant tumors, and no association has been found between the type or site of mutation in *FH* and clinical phenotypes of HLRCC.

Linkage analysis has mapped *BHD* to 17p11. The gene product, folliculin, is conserved across murine, *Drosophila*, and *Caenorhabditiselegans*. In BHD, mutations have been located along the entire length of the coding region of the folliculin gene, with the majority of the mutations predicted to truncate the protein. However, a hotspot mutation consisting of an insertion/deletion of a cytosine in a C8 tract in exon 11 has been identified. Among patients with this hotspot mutation, significantly fewer renal tumors were observed in patients with the C-deletion than those with the C-insertion mutation. No mutations in the folliculin gene have been found in sporadic chromophobe RCC and renal oncocytomas.

Gene Expression Profiles

Recent studies have demonstrated that different RCC subtypes are readily distinguishable with gene expression profiling. Furthermore, unsupervised hierarchical clustering can classify renal tumors according to the appropriate histological subtypes and clinical outcomes. This exceptional discriminatory ability makes gene expression profiling potentially an excellent diagnostic tool; however, DNA-microarray-based tests face many challenges that need to be overcome, including technical, instrumental, computational, and interpretative factors, before the gene expression profiling tests can be reliably applied to aid routine diagnosis and clinical decision making. A major concern about gene expression profiling has been the lack of reproducibility and accuracy. Future work should focus on establishing a set of consensus quality assurance and control criteria for assessing and ensuring data quality, to identify critical factors affecting quality, and to optimize and standardize microarray procedure.

Meanwhile, molecular analysis of a limited number of genes that were chosen based on the molecular pathways involved in the pathogenesis of different RCC subtypes has been shown to be able to accurately classify RCC subtypes. Chen et al. [29] used quantitative RT-PCR to amplify 4 genes (CAIX, AMACR, parvalbumin, and chloride channel KB (CLCNKB)) and found that the mRNA ratios among these genes (i.e., CAIX/AMACR and AMACR/CLCNKB) accurately classified renal tumors into distinct histological subtypes, although some oncocytomas and ChRCC could not be reliably distinguished.

Prognostic/Predictive Markers

VHL Gene Alteration

The alteration of the *VHL* gene as the result of gene mutation, deletion, and methylation in the majority of CCRCC patients, in addition to predicting possible clinical efficacy of agents targeting the VHL pathway, has directed recent efforts to the prognostic significance of the VHL pathway. The status of the *VHL* gene can be examined by direct gene sequencing, loss of heterozygosity (LOH) analysis of 3p25 region, and methylation-specific PCR of the promoter region. One study found that alteration of the *VHL* gene is an independent prognostic factor associated with improved cancer-free survival and cancer-specific survival, especially in high-stage (stage II and III) and high-grade (G3 or higher) CCRCC [30, 31]. However, two other studies found that patients with "loss of function" mutations have a significantly worse prognosis [32, 33]. These studies, however, are limited by the small number of patients, short follow-up time, and low rate of RCC-specific death. In addition, no study has evaluated whether VHL alteration could predict response to cytokine or VEGF-targeted therapy. Currently, the prognostic significance of VHL gene status is best regarded as preliminary, and validation on a large number of prospective patients is required.

Carbonic Anhydrase IX (CAIX)

CAIX is an enzyme that regulates intracellular pH as well as the transfer of CO_2 across the renal tubules. CAIX is regulated by HIF, and its expression reflects the status of the associated HIF and VHL pathways. By immunohistochemistry, CAIX expression is found almost exclusively in the CCRCC subtype of renal tumors. Using a cut-off of CAIX expression in >85% of tumor cells, one study of metastatic RCC found patients with high CAIX expression to have significantly better survival than patients with lower CAIX expression, independent of other known prognostic factors. Such favorable prognosis associated with high CAIX expression, however, is not seen in non-metastatic RCC patients [34]. Although these findings need to be validated in a large prospective study, the lack of a commercially available form of monoclonal antibody used in the published studies may lead to barriers in results comparison. However, the use of CAIX polyclonal antibodies available from several manufacturers may prove useful in future prospective studies on examining the role of CAIX utility. In addition, findings from prior studies have indicated that patients with high CAIX expression are more likely to respond to interleukin-2 therapy, which emphasizes the critical importance of well-designed prospective studies on CAIX expression [35].

Gene Expression Profiling

Gene expression profiling by various array-based techniques provides a high-throughput approach to analyze the expression of tens of thousands of genes simultaneously. Expression of specific groups of genes, or gene expression profiles, can then be correlated with pathological diagnosis, clinical outcomes, or therapeutic response.

A number of gene expression profiling studies have identified a large number of potentially important prognostic markers that can be used to supplement or further refine the staging system and outcome prediction models that are currently in use. Takahashi et al. [36] conducted a study on 29 CCRCC and found that the expression profile of 40 genes clearly segregated tumors into two groups with different 5-year survivals. Vasselli et al. [37] also showed that a panel of 45 genes could stratify 58 uniformly staged metastatic RCCs into two distinct prognostic groups. A very recent comprehensive molecular characterization of CCRCC by The Cancer Genome Atlas research network [21] has shown that aggressive CCRCC demonstrated evidence of metabolic shift, involving downregulation of genes involving TCA cycle, decreased AMPK and PTEN protein level, upregulation of the pentose phosphate pathway and the glutamine transporter gene, increased acetyl-CoA carboxylase protein, and altered promoter methylation of miR-21 and GRB10. Therefore, clinically validated gene expression profiling could be potentially used to identify a subgroup of patients with a distinct prognosis that otherwise would not be distinguished using current staging systems.

It is worthwhile to note that implementation of multiplex biomarkers has not been achieved. Independent replication of microarray-derived predictive gene signatures has also proven to be difficult. One possible explanation is sample selection including interethnic variability. It has also been suggested that intratumoral heterogeneity and sample bias may explain the difficulties in the validation of biomarkers [38].

Cytogenetics

Many cytogenetic and chromosomal abnormalities have been described in RCC, some of which are prognostically relevant. Besides tumor type-specific genetic abnormalities, such as alteration of 3p in CCRCC and gain of chromosomes 7 and 17 in PRCC, additional chromosomal aberrations are often associated with tumor progression. Loss of chromosome 14q correlates with higher stage and nuclear grade and worse clinical outcomes in patients with CCRCC [39]. A high incidence of allelic loss of 9p21 and 9p22-23, revealed by LOH and CGH, has been identified in CCRCC and is associated with advanced pathological stage, high nuclear grade, and poor clinical outcome. Deletions at 9p21 are also associated with tumor progression in PRCC. Similarly, LOH at 9p13 is associated with short survival, independent of grade and stage [40].

While these cytogenetic abnormalities provide insight into the molecular mechanisms in the progression of RCC, they are unlikely to evolve into routine prognostic tests, as karyotypic analysis requires fresh tumor tissue and tissue culture, and LOH and CGH assays are not routinely performed in most laboratories. Candidate genes mapped to these loci, however, can be assayed for their expression and prognostic value using much simpler techniques, such as PCR and immunohistochemistry, after they are identified.

Summary

Tremendous advances have been made in the genetics and epigenetics of RCC. These include the elucidation of characteristic cytogenetic changes, specific gene alterations in RCC subtypes, and identification of new RCC variants. New technology such as gene expression profiling and tissue microarray has made high-throughput identification and validation of molecular diagnostic, prognostic, and therapeutic markers possible. It is hoped that in the future, a classification based on the molecular and genetic characteristics of the different subtypes of RCC will provide not only more accurate pathological classification, but also better prognostic and therapeutic information. In addition, such findings may help design more specific, genetically based therapeutic strategies [41, 42]. Ultimately, molecular markers, coupled with clinical and pathological characteristics, will enable us to predict individual tumor behavior, to stratify patients into more sophisticated risk groups, and to render individualized management and treatment options.

References

1. Eble JN, Sauter G, Epstein JI, Sesterhenn IA. Pathology and genetics, tumors of the urinary system and male genital organs. Vol. 9–88. Lyon: IAPC Press; 2004.
2. Deng FM, Melamed J. Histologic variants of renal cell carcinoma: does tumor type influence outcome? Urol Clin N Am. 2012;39:119–32.
3. Cheng L, Zhang S, MacLennan GT, Lopez-Beltran A, Montironi R. Molecular and cytogenetic insights into the pathogenesis, classification, differential diagnosis, and prognosis of renal epithelial neoplasms. Hum Pathol. 2009;40:10–29.
4. Brunelli M, Eble JN, Zhang S, Martignoni G, Cheng L. Gains of chromosomes 7, 17, 12, 16, and 20 and loss of Y occur early in the evolution of papillary renal cell neoplasia: afluorescent in situ hybridization study. Mod Pathol. 2003;16:1053–9.
5. Brunelli M, Eble JN, Zhang S, Martignoni G, Delahunt B, Cheng L. Eosinophilic and classic chromophobe renal cell carcinomas have similar frequent losses of multiple chromosomes from among chromosomes 1, 2, 6, 10, and 17, and this pattern of genetic abnormality is not present in renal oncocytoma. Mod Pathol. 2005;18:161–9.
6. Argani P, Ladanyi M. Translocation carcinomas of the kidney. Clin Lab Med. 2005;25(2):363–78.
7. Morris MR, Ricketts CJ, Gentle D, McRonald F, Carli N, Khalili H, et al. Genome-wide methylation analysis identifies epigenetically inactivated candidate tumor suppressor genes in renal cell carcinoma. Oncogene. 2011;24:1390–401.
8. Zhang Q, Ying J, Li J, Fan Y, Poon FF, Ng KM, et al. Aberrant promoter methylation DLEC1, a critical 3p22 tumor suppressor for renal cell carcinoma, is associated with more advanced tumor stage. J Urol. 2010;184:731–7.
9. Hildebrandt MA, Gu J, Lin J, Ye J, Tan W, Tamboli P, et al. Has-miR-9 methylation status is associated with cancer development and metastatic recurrence in patients with clear cell renal cell carcinoma. Oncogene. 2010;29:5724–8.
10. Cho M, Uemura H, Kim SC, Kawada Y, Yoshida K, Hirao Y, et al. Hypomethylation of the MN/CA9 promoter and upregulation MN/CA9 expression in human renal cell carcinoma. Br J Cancer. 2001;85:563–7.
11. Grabmaier K, de Weijert M, Uemura H, Schalken J, Oosterwijk E. Renal cell carcinoma-associated G250 methylation and expression: in vivo and in vitro studies. Urology. 2002:60:357–62.
12. Ellinger J, Kahl P, Mertens C, Rogenhofer S, Hauser S, Hartmann W, et al. Prognostic relevance of global histone H3 lysine (H3K4) methylation in renal cell carcinoma. Int J Cancer. 2010;127:2360–6.
13. Rogenhofer S, Kahl P, Mertens C, Hauser S, Hartmann W, Buttner R, et al. Global histone H3 lysine 27 (H3K27) methylation levels and their prognostic relevance in renal cell carcinoma. BJU Int. 2012;109:459–65.
14. Varela I, Taepey P, Raine K, Huang D, Ong CK, Stephens P, et al. Exome sequencing identifies frequent mutation of the SWI/SNF complex gene PBRM1 in renal carcinoma. Nature. 2011;469:539–42.
15. Lichner Z, Scorilas A, White NMA, Girgis AH, Rotstein L, Wiegand KC, et al. The chromatin remodeling gene ARID1a is a new prognostic marker in clear cell renal cell carcinoma. Am J Pathol. 2013;182:1163–70.
16. Guo G, Gui Y, Gao S, Tang A, Hu X, Huang Y, et al. Frequent mutations of gene encoding ubiquitin-mediated proteolysis pathway component in clear cell renal cell carcinoma. Nat Genet. 2012;44:17–9.
17. Pena-Llopis S, Vega-Rubin-de-Celis S, Liao A, Leng N, Pavia-Jimenez A, Wang S, et al. BAP1 loss defines a new class of renal cell carcinoma. Nat Genet. 2012;44:751–9.
18. Dalgliesh GL, Furge K, Greenman C, Chen L, Bignell G, Butler A, et al. Systematic sequencing of renal carcinoma reveals inactivation of histone modifying genes. Nature. 2010;463:360–3.
19. Duns G, van den Berg E, van Duivenbode I, Osinga J, Hollema H, Hofstra RM, et al. Histone methyltransferase SETD2 is a novel tumor suppressor gene in clear cell renal cell carcinoma. Cancer Res. 2010;70:4287–91.
20. Hakimi AA, Chen YB, Wren J, Gonen M, Abdel-Wahab O, Heguy A, et al. Clinical and pathologic impact of select chromatin modulating tumor suppressors in clear cell renal cell carcinoma. Eur Urol. 2013;63:848–54
21. The cancer genome atlas research network. Comprehensive molecular characterization of clear cell renal cell carcinoma. Nature. 2013;499:43–9.
22. Hoglund M, Gisselsson D, Soller M, Hansen GB, Elfving P, Mitelman F. Dissecting karyotypic patterns in renal cell carcinoma: an analysis of the accumulated cytogenetic data. Cancer Genet Cytogenet. 2004;153:1–9.
23. Jones TD, Eble JN, Wang M, MacLennan GT, Delahunt B, Brunelli M, et al. Molecular genetic evidence for the independent origin of multifocal papillary tumors in patients with papillary renal cell carcinomas. Clin Cancer Res. 2005;11:7226–33.
24. Brown JA, Anderl KL, Borell TJ, Qian J, Bostwick DG, Jenkins RB. Simultaneous chromosome 7 and 17 gain and sex chromosome loss provide evidence that renal metanephric adenoma is related to papillary renal cell carcinoma. J Urol. 1997;158:370–4.
25. Argani P, Lal P, Hutchinson B, Lui MY, Reuter VE, Ladanyi M. Aberrant nuclear immunoreactivity for

TFE3 in neoplasms with TFE3 gene fusions: a sensitive and specific immunohistochemical assay. Am J SurgPathol. 2003;27:750–61.
26. Folpe AL, Mentzel T, Lehr HA, Fisher C, Balzer BL, Weiss SW. Perivascular epithelioid cell neoplasms of soft tissue and gynecologic origin: a clinicopathologic study of 26 cases and review of the literature. Am J Surg Pathol. 2005;29(12):1558–75.
27. Malouf GG, Monzon FA, Couturier J, Molinie V, Escudier B, Camparo P, et al. Genomic heterogeneity of translocation renal cell carcinoma. Clin Cancer Res. 2013;19(17):4673–84.
28. Cohen D, Zhou M. Molecular genetics of familial renal cell carcinoma syndromes. Clin Lab Med. 2005;25:259–77.
29. Chen YT, Tu JJ, Kao Y, Zhou XK, Mazumdar M. Messenger RNA expression ratios among four genes predict subtypes of renal cell carcinoma and distinguish oncocytoma from carcinoma. Clin Cancer Res. 2005;11:6558–66.
30. Yao M, Yoshida M, Kishida T, Nakaigawa N, Baba M, Kobayashi K, et al. VHL tumor suppressor gene alterations associated with good prognosis in sporadic clear-cell renal carcinoma. J Natl Cancer Inst. 2002;16:1569–75.
31. Young A, Craven RA, Cohen D, Taylor C, Booth C, Harnden P, et al. Analysis of VHL gene alteration and their relationship to clinical parameters in sporadic conventional renal cell carcinoma. Clin Cancer Res. 2009;15:7582–92.
32. Kondo K, Yao M, Yoshida M, Kishida T, Shuin T, Miura T, et al. Comprehensive mutational analysis of the VHL gene in sporadic renal cell carcinoma: relationship to clinicopathological parameters. Genes Chromosomes Cancer. 2002;34:58–68.
33. Na X, Wu G, Ryan CK, Schoen SR, di'Santagnese PA, Messing EM. Overproduction of vascular endothelial growth factor related to von Hippel-Lindau tumor suppressor gene mutations and hypoxia-inducible factor-1 α expression in renal cell carcinomas. J Urol. 2003;170:588–92.
34. Bui MH, Seligson D, Han KR, Pantuck AJ, Dorey FJ, Huang Y, Horvath S, Leibovich BC, Chopra S, Liao SY, Stanbridge E, Lerman MI, Palotie A, Figlin RA, Belldegrun AS. Carbonic anhydrase IX is an independent predictor of survival in advanced renal clear cell carcinoma: implications for prognosis and therapy. Clin Cancer Res. 2003;9:802–11.
35. Atkins M, Regan M, McDermott D, Mier J, Stanbridge E, Youmans A, Febbo P, Upton M, Lechpammer M, Signoretti S. Carbonic anhydrase IX expression predicts outcome of interleukin 2 therapy for renal cancer. Clin Cancer Res. 2005;15;11:3714–21.
36. Takahashi M, Rhodes DR, Furge KA, Kanayama H, Kagawa S, Haab BB, et al. Gene expression profiling of clear cell renal cell carcinoma: gene identification and prognostic classification. Proc Natl Acad Sci U S A. 2001;98:9754–9.
37. Vasselli JR, Shih JH, Iyengar SR, Maramchie J, Riss J, Worrell R, et al. Predicting survival in patients with metastatic kidney cancer by gene-expression profiling in the primary tumor. Proc Natl Acad Sci U S A. 2003;100:6958–63.
38. Gerlinger M, Rowan AJ, Horswell S, Math M, Larkin J, Endesfelder D, et al. Intratumor heterogeneity and branched evolution revealed by multiregion sequencing. N Engl J Med. 2012;366:883–92.
39. Krorger N, Klatte T, Chamie K, Rao N, Birkhauser FD, Sonn GA, et al. Deletions of chromosomes 3p and 14q molecularly subclassify clear cell renal cell carcinoma. Cancer. 2013;119:1547–54.
40. Klatte T, Rao PN, de Martino M, LaRochelle J, Shuch B, Zomorodian N, et al. Cytogenetic profile predicts prognosis of patients with clear cell renal cell carcinoma. J Clin Oncol. 2009;27:746–53.
41. Linehan WM, Vasselli J, Srinivasan R, Walther MM, Merino M, Choyke P, et al. Genetic basis of cancer of the kidney: disease-specific approaches to therapy. Clin Cancer Res. 2004;10:6282S–9S.
42. Kim W, Kaelin WG Jr. The von Hippel-Lindau tumor suppressor protein: new insights into oxygen sensing and cancer. Curr Opin Genet Dev. 2003;13:55–60.

Role of Needle Biopsy in Renal Masses: Past, Present, and Future

33

Ying-Bei Chen

Introduction

The role of imaging-guided needle biopsies in the clinical management of renal masses has evolved significantly in the past two decades. Advances in modern non-invasive imaging technologies and their popularity have not only contributed to the increasing detection of renal tumors, largely due to many incidentally detected non-symptomatic small renal masses, but also allowed more accurate characterization and a better distinction of renal neoplasms from other benign lesions [1]. Together with advances in intervention techniques and pathologic diagnosis of renal tumors, these progresses have prompted an augmented role of percutaneous renal biopsies in the diagnosis and clinical management of renal masses today. The main focus of this chapter is to review the changes in implications, accuracy, and complications of percutaneous renal needle biopsy and to provide a practical approach for the pathologic diagnosis of renal tumors from core biopsy materials. Fine-needle aspiration (FNA) and random biopsy for renal parenchymal diseases or renal transplants are beyond the scope of this chapter.

Y.-B. Chen (✉)
Department of Pathology, Memorial Sloan Kettering Cancer Center, New York, NY, USA
e-mail: cheny@mskcc.org

Past and Present

Implications

Before the widespread utilization of modern imaging modalities including computerized tomography (CT), magnetic resonance imaging (MRI), and ultrasonography, patients with renal masses often presented with symptoms, and sizes of their renal masses were usually large. In that context, surgical resection (mostly radical nephrectomy) was the standard of care for renal masses, and a preoperative histologic diagnosis was usually not needed. Consequently, the established indications for renal core needle biopsies were mostly clinical scenarios in which a surgical approach might not be necessary, such as when suspicion was high for metastasis, lymphoma, or possibly a benign lesion (e.g., infection) causing the renal mass. Core biopsies were also used to render a pathologic diagnosis in patients who had unresectable tumors or were poor surgical candidates.

In recent years, the large number of renal masses incidentally discovered by imaging modalities, the majority of which are small in size (<4 cm), has posed a new clinical challenge. Advanced CT and MRI imaging technologies often provide more confident characterizations of these small renal masses, with many being categorized as enhancing masses that likely represent true renal neoplasms. While surgical management remains the standard of care for renal cancer, data from multiple nephrectomy series showed that nearly 20% of the surgically resected tumors

C. Magi-Galluzzi, C. G. Przybycin (eds.), *Genitourinary Pathology*, DOI 10.1007/978-1-4939-2044-0_33,

Table 33.1 Indications for renal core biopsy for patients with renal masses

Established indications
Rule out metastasis of extrarenal primary involving kidney
Rule out lymphoma involving kidney
Rule out renal mass caused by a benign condition such as infection
Patients with unresectable tumor
Patients with surgical comorbidities
Emerging indications
Distinguish between benign and malignant tumors for small renal masses
Define the histologic subtypes of primary renal neoplasms for risk assessment and therapy selection
Patients with a renal mass considered for percutaneous ablation

could be benign. This ratio of benign tumors was even higher in masses smaller than 4 cm, and patients with small renal masses in general were at low risk for disease progression and poor outcome [2–5]. Meanwhile, other non-surgical treatment options are emerging for patients with renal masses. Percutaneous radiofrequency ablation and cryoablation have been shown to be effective therapies in appropriate settings [6]; as the majority of small renal masses grow at a slow rate, active surveillance can also be a viable option for some patients [7, 8]. Moreover, considerations of comorbidities and preservation of renal function are other reasons that may prevent some patients from receiving surgical treatment. As a result, whether patients with small renal masses should undergo surgical resection has become a complex management question [9]. To facilitate an informed management decision, percutaneous renal core biopsy offers a helpful approach to define tumor types and provide useful prognostic information.

Currently, while the previously established indications for renal needle biopsy still apply, it is being increasingly used to differentiate between benign and malignant neoplasms for patients with small, incidentally identified renal masses and to provide the histologic subtyping of primary renal neoplasms to allow a better assessment of the risks and benefits of various surgical or non-surgical treatment options. With the advent of systemic targeted therapies for patients with locally advanced or metastatic renal cancer, needle core biopsy has also been increasingly used to guide selection of specific therapeutic regimens (Table 33.1).

Safety

With guidance provided by modern imaging modalities and improved intervention techniques, percutaneous needle biopsy of renal masses is a safe procedure today [10, 11]. The most frequent complication reported has been bleeding, which is usually subclinical and self-limiting. Major bleeding that requires a blood transfusion has been rare and often can be minimized by correcting coagulation abnormalities and controlling hypertension. Hematuria can occur in 5–7 % of cases, but is generally also self-limited. Very rare events such as pseudoaneurysm and arteriovenous fistula formation may cause persistent bleeding and hematuria, but can usually be managed by embolization if needed. Pneumothorax is also rare and can be best avoided using a subcostal approach.

Tumor seeding along the needle track has been a worrisome concern of renal biopsy. However, the risk of seeding has been estimated to be less than 0.01 % [12]. There have been only few such events reported in the literature, suggesting that it is a very rare complication of renal needle biopsy. A recent case report emphasizes the importance of imaging surveillance of the needle tract used by percutaneous biopsy or ablation [13].

Accuracy

The sensitivity and diagnostic accuracy of renal needle biopsy has also been improved significantly in recent years. In core biopsy series published in the last decade, the sensitivity of renal biopsy has ranged from over 70 to 100 %, while the diagnostic accuracy has often been superior to 90 % [10, 11]. The enhanced sensitivity and accuracy are likely consequences of better tumor visualization, improved biopsy technique, increased experience with renal core biopsy interpretation, as well as advances in ancillary studies utilized in pathologic evaluation.

On the other hand, false-negative results can happen because of inappropriate needle placement or obtaining necrotic or scant diagnostic tissue. Therefore, an absence of malignant cells from a biopsy does not necessarily exclude the presence of a malignancy and should be interpreted with caution. In this regard, small masses (≤3 cm) may have higher false-negative rates, due to inaccurate targeting and/or insufficient diagnostic material obtained, which can be reduced by repeat biopsies and a high level of experience in the procedure operator and pathologists [14]. Core biopsies and FNA may have complementary roles as shown in some published series [15, 16]. Performing an onsite FNA assessment of sample adequacy is also likely to help enhance the yield of renal needle biopsies.

Histologic Interpretation and Ancillary Studies

Consistent with the current clinical indications for renal needle biopsies, entities that may be encountered for histologic interpretation include a wide spectrum of neoplastic and non-neoplastic diseases. In addition to renal cell neoplasms, the differential considerations should also comprise various primary renal tumors such as mixed mesenchymal and epithelial tumors, mesenchymal tumors, metanephric tumors, and neuroendocrine tumors, as well as metastatic malignancies to the kidney, tumors arising from adjacent organ sites (e.g., adrenal gland, urinary bladder, and retroperitoneum), primary or secondary lymphomas, and mass-forming benign conditions such as infection. Similar to resection specimens, the interpretation of renal core biopsy relies on a careful examination of both the cytologic and architectural features of sampled tissue. However, renal core biopsies typically only reveal limited diagnostic material, which may make the recognition of architectural patterns incomplete or inconclusive. Given the broad range of histologic features that can be seen in a renal core biopsy, a commonly utilized interpretation approach is to categorize the potential tumors/lesions based on certain cytologic features (e.g., clear vs. eosinophilic) and/or architectural patterns (e.g., papillary) that are discernible even in limited diagnostic material to help narrow down the number of entities considered in the differential diagnosis. While this is a very practical approach, one should be aware of the fact that a limited sampling by core biopsy can be misleading especially when only unusual histologic features are revealed. For difficult or ambiguous cases, ancillary studies such as a selected panel of immunohistochemical stains are often very helpful for establishing a correct diagnosis [17]. The main entities in some of these histologic categories as well as ancillary studies are briefly discussed below. The commonly utilized immunostains for differentiating primary epithelial neoplasms of the kidney are summarized in Table 33.2.

Clear Cell Cytology

Clear cell RCC is the most common type of RCC and comprises approximately 60% of all renal cortical tumors. In a renal core biopsy mainly showing clear cell cytology, clear cell RCC is usually the top consideration among other differential diagnoses. Other tumors or tumor-like lesions that may exhibit clear cell cytology include clear cell papillary RCC, chromophobe RCC, TFE3/TFEB translocation-associated RCC, papillary RCC with focal clear cell areas, adrenal cortical tissue/tumor in an ectopic location or being missampled by the biopsy procedure, angiomyolipoma with abundant clear cells, and foamy histiocyte-rich lesions such as xanthogranulomatous pyelonephritis [18]. The cytoplasm of clear cells in a clear cell RCC or clear cell papillary RCC is typically optically transparent, whereas the clear cytoplasm in a chromophobe RCC tends to show fine granular or fibrillary eosinophilic material. The areas of clear cells in a papillary RCC, more commonly type 1, often also exhibit cytoplasm with focal granular eosinophilia. The clear cells seen in adrenal cortical tissue/tumor have a uniform, vacuolated bubbly appearance, mimicking cells in sebaceous glands (Fig. 33.1a–d).

Clear cell RCC typically comprises solid acini or nests of clear cells separated by delicate,

Table 33.2 Immunohistochemical stains commonly used in the differential diagnosis of primary epithelial tumors of the kidney

	Clear cell RCC	Clear cell papillary RCC	Papillary RCC type 1	Papillary RCC type 2	Chromo-phobe RCC	Renal oncocytoma	MTSCC	Transloca-tion RCC	Meta-nephric adenoma	Collect-ing duct carcinoma	Renal medullary carcinoma	Urothelial carcinoma
Pax8/Pax2	+	+	+	+	+/−	+/−	+	+	+	+/−	+/−	−/+
CA-IX (diffuse, membranous)	+	+[a]	−	−	−	−	−	−/+(focal)	−	−	−	−/+
CD10	+	−	+(often luminal)	+/−	+/−	−	+/−	+	−	−	−	−
CK7	−	+	+	+/−	+/−	−/+	+	−	−/+(focal)	−/+	−/+	+
AMACR	−	−	+	+/−	−	−	+	−	−	−/+	−/+	−/+
CD117	−	−	−	−	+	+	−	−	−	−	−	−
TFE3/TFEB	−	−	−	−	−	−	−	+	−	−	−	−
Cathepsin-K	−	−	−	−	−	−	−	+	−	−	−	−
HMB-45	−	−	−	−	−	−	−	−/+	−	−	−	−
Melan-A	−	−	−	−	−	−	−	−/+	−	−	−	−
INI1 (BAF47)	+	+	+	+	+	+	+	+	+	+	−	+
34βE12 (HMWCK)	−	+/−	−	−	−	−	−	−	−	+/−	−/+	+
p63	−	−	−	−	−	−	−	−	−	−	−	+
GATA3	−	−	−	−	−	−	−	−	−	−	−	+

MTSCC, mucinous tubular and spindle cell carcinoma

[a] The membranous staining of CA-IX in clear cell papillary RCC is often "cup-like," with an absence of labeling along the luminal aspect of the tumor cells.

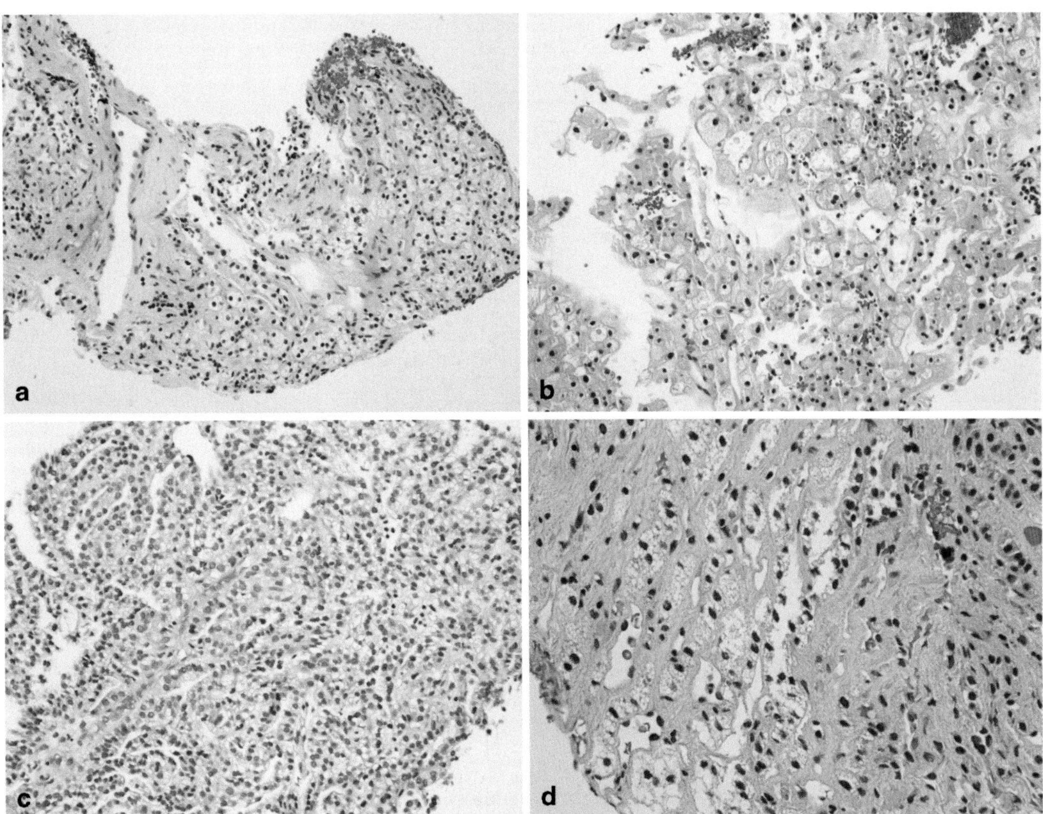

Fig. 33.1 Core biopsies of a clear cell RCC (**a**), chromophobe RCC (**b**), type 1 papillary RCC with clear cells (**c**), and adrenal cortical tissue (**d**). Note the quality of the clear cytoplasm varies in each case

intricately branching fibrovascular septa. Tubular, papillary/pseudopapillary, large alveolar, and solid sheet-like growth patterns can also be seen. Higher nuclear grade often shows a loose association with focal or marked cytoplasmic eosinophilia and certain architectures such as solid sheet-like, pseudopapillary, or large alveolar patterns. Hyalinization is a common finding in these tumors. In extreme examples, rare clusters of clear cells remaining in the hyalinized stroma can be easily missed, whereas the rich vasculature in the stroma can lead to misinterpretation as a vascular lesion. The classical appearance of clear cell RCC, even only present in a focal area, would strongly suggest this diagnosis. Diffuse, membranous staining of carbonic anhydrase IX (CA-IX) in non-necrotic areas is a useful feature to separate clear cell RCC from other primary renal cell neoplasms.

Clear cell papillary RCC is characterized by tumor cells with uniformly clear cytoplasm and low-grade nuclei that are arranged in a linear fashion, away from the basal aspect of the cells. Although this linear arrangement of nuclei may be less apparent in cells with minimal cytoplasm in areas showing collapsed tubular/acinar patterns (Fig. 33.2), an appreciation of such features even in focal areas would be sufficient to trigger a small panel of immunohistochemical studies to help distinguish them from a clear cell or papillary RCC. The clear cell papillary RCC is diffusely positive for CK7, negative for CD10 and AMACR, while showing a cup-shaped membranous staining pattern for CA-IX (absence of staining along the luminal border). Because of its overall indolent behavior, clear cell papillary RCC is an important diagnosis to be recognized on renal core biopsy, as patients may benefit from a more conservative management plan.

Chromophobe RCC is composed of large polygonal cells with prominent cell borders. Besides

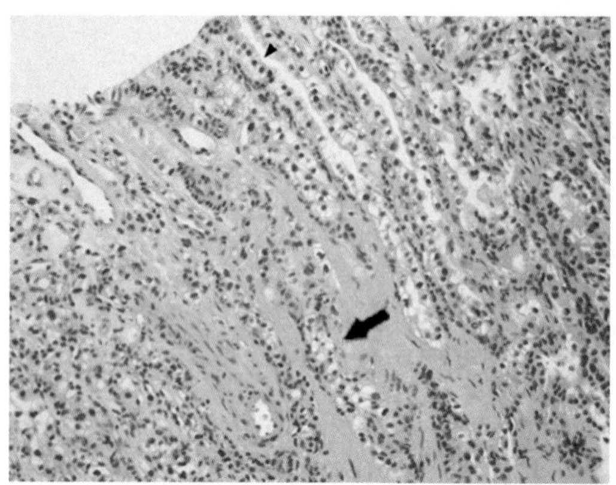

Fig. 33.2 Core biopsy of clear cell papillary RCC showing tubulopapillary growth and low-grade nuclei. Note the apparent linear arrangement of nuclei away from the basal aspect of tumor cells in some areas (*arrowhead*). The feature is difficult to appreciate in the more collapsed area (*arrow*)

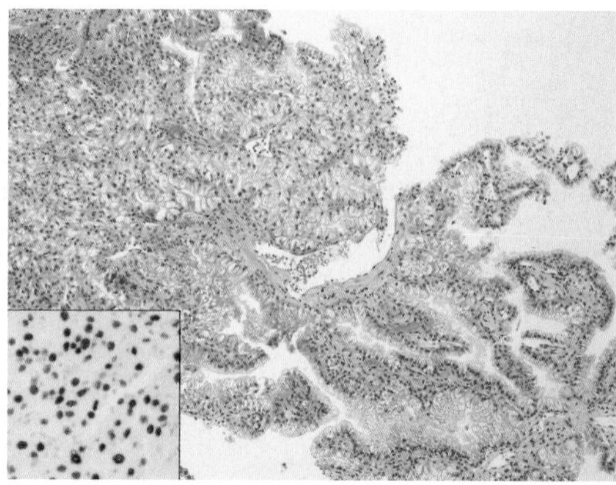

Fig. 33.3 Core biopsy of a TFE3 translocation tumor with intermixed clear and eosinophilic cells in solid nests/alveolar growth pattern. TFE3 immunostain shows diffuse and strong nuclear labeling (*inset*)

the finely granular/reticulated cytoplasm, the wrinkled nuclei and perinuclear halos are helpful features that are distinct from a clear cell RCC. Although a portion of chromophobe RCCs are aggressive, stage by stage, they have a significantly better prognosis than clear cell RCCs.

Papillary RCC typically shows amphophilic or eosinophilic cytoplasm, but focal cytoplasmic clearing is not uncommon, particularly in type 1 papillary RCC. The main differential diagnoses are other tumors with clear cells and papillary or tubulopapillary architecture (see below for further discussion).

MiTF family translocation-associated RCCs are defined by translocations involving MiTF/TFE family genes (*TFE*3 or *TFEB*) and often demonstrate a wide range of histologic features. TFE3 translocation tumors often show abundant clear cytoplasm and high-grade nuclei and display papillary, alveolar, or solid growth. Admixed eosinophilic cells are also common. Psammoma bodies and cytoplasmic hyaline globules are frequently found. Some TFE3 translocation tumors can show lower nuclear grade and less cytoplasm. TFEB translocation tumors typically show biphasic morphology, comprising larger epithelioid cells and smaller cells clustered around basement membrane-like material. Both types of translocation tumors can show significant morphologic overlap with clear cell or other types of RCCs, and their diagnosis on core biopsy relies on immunohistochemical tests for TFE3/TFEB overexpression (Fig. 33.3) or fluorescence in situ hybridization (FISH) assays to confirm *TFE3* or *TFEB* rearrangement. Cathepsin-K expression detected by immunohistochemistry has also been found to be a useful marker for TFEB tumors, TFE3 tumors with *PRCC-TFE3* fusion, as well as alveolar soft part sarcomas [19]. FISH break-apart assays appear to have a higher sensitivity to detect *TFE3/TFEB* translocation than the TFE3/TFEB immunohistochemical staining and have revealed an expanding histologic spectrum for these tumors [20, 21].

Epithelioid angiomyolipoma (AML) of kidney or retroperitoneum can be misclassified as clear cell RCC, particularly if the abnormal vessels and fat are lacking in the biopsy. The clear cytoplasm of AML commonly contains fibrillary or granular material, and there is often a high level of cytologic atypia. The diagnosis of AML is usually supported by immunoreactivity for HMB45 and Melan-A.

Once being included in the differential diagnosis, a few other entities in this histologic category can be readily distinguished from primary renal cell neoplasms. Adrenal cortical tissue or very rarely an adrenal cortical neoplasm arising from ectopic adrenal tissue has distinct cytologic features and also shows dissimilar immunoprofile

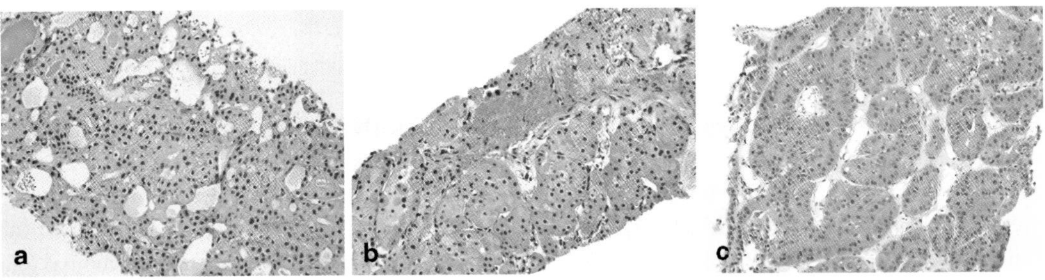

Fig. 33.4 Core biopsies of eosinophilic chromophobe (**a**), a renal oncocytic neoplasm that is favored as oncocytoma (**b**), and a renal oncocytic neoplasm with nuclear pleomorphism and atypia dissimilar to chromophobe RCC, but beyond the typical level of oncocytoma (**c**). Tumor in **c** was resected and proven to be a low-grade RCC, unclassified

when applying immunostaining such as PAX8/2, inhibin, Melan-A, and steroidogenic factor-1 (SF1). Epithelioid histiocytic lesions, xanthogranulomatous pyelonephritis or malacoplakia, lack true nuclear atypia and will be positive for CD68 and negative for epithelial markers. Other uncommon primary renal tumors (e.g., renal cell carcinoma, unclassified) or secondary tumors involving kidney (e.g., clear cell adenocarcinoma) may also show a marked clear cell morphology. These possibilities should be carefully considered based on the clinical context of individual cases after the more common differentials have been excluded.

Eosinophilic Cell Cytology

Many tumors or mass-forming lesions may be composed of eosinophilic cells, but there is a significant overlap of entities in this category with the group of tumors with papillary or tubulopapillary architecture as well as tumors/lesions in other cytologic categories. Therefore, the focus in this section will be mainly on eosinophilic tumors without apparent papillary growth pattern that are not discussed in other categories (Fig. 33.4a–c).

Chromophobe RCC (eosinophilic variant) is predominantly composed of tumor cells with more densely eosinophilic, granular cytoplasm than the "typical" chromophobe RCC. The nuclear membrane irregularity and perinuclear halos should be invariably detected in all cases, although these features are often less prominent when compared to the typical tumors. This increased difficulty in detecting characteristic histologic features of chromophobe RCC makes a distinction from renal oncocytoma quite problematic in the setting of core biopsy. Careful examination of the cytologic features of all available material thus is essential. Instead of the obviously wrinkled nuclei seen in "typical" chromophobe RCCs, the nuclear membrane irregularity is frequently only appreciated in scattered tumor cells. Meanwhile, cells with degenerative atypia or features suggesting processing artifacts should be avoided in this evaluation to prevent an overestimation of the nuclear atypia. The perinuclear halos are also more subtle and often limited to focal areas. Cells with hyperchromatic, bizarre nuclei may be present in some cases. While CK7 staining is diffusely positive in a subset of tumors, a significant portion of eosinophilic variant of chromophobe RCCs exhibit only focal or patchy labeling, indistinguishable from the staining pattern of renal oncocytomas. Hence, CK7 stain should not be used to exclude this diagnosis.

Oncocytoma may show similar architectural patterns as eosinophilic chromophobe RCC on core biopsies. But the nuclear contours in oncocytoma are round, smooth, and rather uniform, except in foci with large, pleomorphic nuclei and degenerative-type atypia. CK7 expression is usually seen in a scattered small number of cells. Because of the limited sampling, it is quite acceptable not committing to a definitive diagnosis of "oncocytoma" on biopsy material; instead a term such as "renal oncocytic neoplasm, favor oncocytoma" is often used in practice.

It is noteworthy that there are also oncocytic tumors with a mixture of features of oncocytoma or eosinophilic variant of chromophobe RCC. Some of them show oncocytoma-like architecture, nuclear shape, and minimal nuclear pleomorphism, but demonstrate small perinuclear clearing. Others may show scattered cells with mild nuclear atypia and nuclear membrane irregularity, but a complete absence of perinuclear halos. Although tumors associated with Birt–Hogg–Dubé syndrome (BHD) or oncocytosis may show similar histologic features, it remains unclear how sporadic tumors with these features should be classified [22]. Overall, these oncocytic tumors are low-grade tumors that behave in an indolent manner.

Succinate dehydrogenase B (SDHB)-associated RCC has recently been described in patients carrying germline SDHB mutations. So far only a small number of cases have been reported in the literature [23, 24]. Some of the reported tumors are composed of cuboidal cells with eosinophilic cytoplasm arranged in solid nests and tubules, with centrally located round nuclei displaying finely granular chromatin and inconspicuous nucleoli. Distinctive cytoplasmic inclusions, which contain either pale eosinophilic fluid-like material or bubbly areas of clearing, are currently considered to be a characteristic feature of these tumors [23]. Cases with high-grade cytologic features and sarcomatoid differentiation are also described. As an emerging entity, more histologic characterization of these tumors is needed. Loss of SDHB protein expression by immunohistochemistry has been suggested to be a characteristic finding in these tumors [23, 25]. Renal tumors associated with germline mutations of other SDH subunits (e.g., *SDHC, SDHD*) also exist, but have not been fully characterized.

Tumors with Papillary or Tubulopapillary Architecture

Papillary architecture identified on renal core biopsies should raise differential diagnostic possibilities of papillary RCC, mucinous tubular and spindle cell carcinoma (MTSCC), hereditary leiomyomatosis and renal cell carcinoma syndrome (HLRCC)-associated RCC, collecting duct carcinoma, renal medullary carcinoma, TFE3/TFEB translocation-associated RCC, clear cell papillary RCC, clear cell RCC with focal papillary architecture, and unclassified RCC [26].

Papillary RCC may show a range of architectural patterns other than papillary. In some cases, tubular, solid, and glomeruloid patterns may be dominant. The papillary fibrovascular cores in some tumors contain foamy macrophages, but are markedly hyalinized or edematous in other tumors. Hemosiderin-laden macrophages and hemosiderin deposition within tumor cells are often seen in papillary RCC. The cytologic features of papillary RCC can be quite variable. The cytoplasm ranges from scant to abundant or from amphophilic to eosinophilic. The current WHO classification divides papillary RCC into two types: type 1 with papillae covered by smaller cells with scant–moderate amphophilic cytoplasm and type 2 with large tumor cells, often higher nuclear-grade, eosinophilic cytoplasm and nuclear pseudostratification (Fig. 33.5a, b). Tumors categorized as type 2 papillary RCC are less defined histologically and molecularly, and some cases demonstrate aggressive clinical behavior. By immunohistochemistry, most papillary

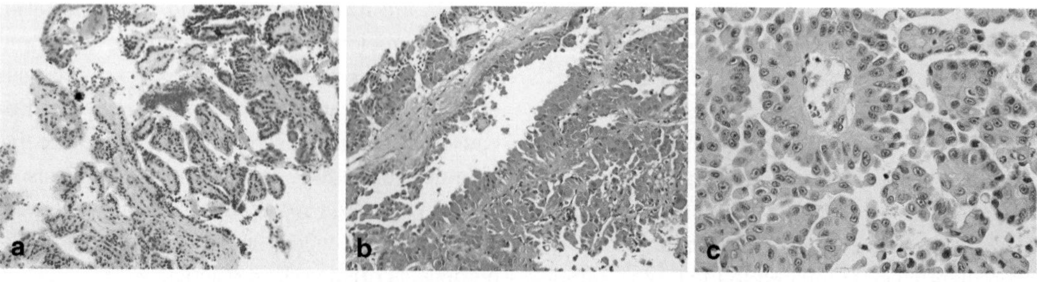

Fig. 33.5 Core biopsies of papillary RCC with type 1 features (**a**) and type 2 features (**b**). In comparison, tumor cells in a papillary area of a HLRCC-associated RCC show prominent nucleoli with perinucleolar halos (**c**)

RCCs show diffuse positivity for CK7, but this reactivity is more often seen in type 1 than type 2 tumors. AMACR shows diffuse cytoplasmic granular staining. The majority of sporadic papillary RCCs are characterized by trisomy of chromosomes 7 and 17 as well as loss of chromosome Y. Copy number gains in 17 and 7 are more often seen in type 1 than type 2 tumors. Absence of trisomy 17 has been associated with poorer prognosis in some studies [27–29].

Metanephric adenoma is in the differential diagnosis for type 1 papillary RCC with predominantly tubular architecture. The tumor cells in metanephric adenoma have uniform nuclei and scant cytoplasm. Nuclear variation and any prominent nucleoli would argue against a diagnosis of this tumor and favor papillary RCC in this differential. Unlike papillary RCC, metanephric adenomas are usually positive for WT1 and CD57 and often negative for AMACR and CK7, but focal CK7 staining may be seen.

Mucinous tubular and spindle cell carcinoma (MTSCC) typically has mucinous stroma, tubular and spindle cell components, and is often in the differential diagnosis for papillary RCC with low-grade spindle cell areas. The tubules in MTSCC tend to have a rigid luminal contour, whereas the elongated tubules in papillary RCC often have an irregular, "shaggy" luminal surface. However, some cases may be extremely difficult to differentiate on needle core biopsies and may require cytogenetic confirmation, if possible. The immunoprofile of MTSCC is very similar to that of papillary RCC. In some cases of MTSCC, there may be an absence of CD10 staining.

HLRCC syndrome-associated RCC are typically very aggressive tumors and have recently been recommended to be recognized as a distinct entity in the International Society of Urologic Pathology (ISUP) Vancouver classification of renal neoplasia [22]. HLRCC is an inherited autosomal dominant disorder in which germline mutations of the *fumarate hydratase* (*FH*) gene confer an increased risk of cutaneous and uterine leiomyomas as well as renal cell carcinoma. Unlike other hereditary RCCs, HLRCC renal tumors may be solitary and unilateral, clinically difficult to distinguish from sporadic tumors. HLRCC tumors were mainly described to be type 2 papillary RCC initially, but a spectrum of architectural patterns is now being recognized [30, 31]. The most characteristic feature of HLRCC renal tumors, as proposed by Merino et al. [30], is the presence of a very prominent inclusion-like eosinophilic nucleolus surrounded by a perinucleolar halo (Fig. 33.5c). However, this feature often is not uniformly present in HLRCC tumors and occasionally is very difficult to distinguish from prominent nucleoli in other high-grade RCCs [31]. An immunohistochemical method for identifying these tumors has been proposed [31, 32]. At present, the diagnosis of HLRCC still relies on germline testing of the *FH* gene, although pathologists can play a very important role in suggesting this possibility.

Collecting duct carcinoma (CDC) is a rare and very aggressive form of RCC that is commonly centered in the renal medulla. It is a high-grade adenocarcinoma, typically displaying tubular and tubulopapillary architectural patterns in a desmoplastic stroma. Other growth patterns (solid, cord-like, sarcomatoid, etc.) can also be seen. A subset of CDCs may show a predominantly papillary architectural pattern. Given this broad spectrum of histologic patterns, the diagnosis of CDC is difficult and often relies on excluding other possibilities in the differential diagnosis. On a renal core biopsy, the possibility of CDC should be raised only after excluding urothelial carcinoma with glandular differentiation and secondary involvement by a metastatic carcinoma. It is difficult to definitively separate CDC from renal medullary carcinoma or unclassified RCC in some cases.

Renal medullary carcinoma (RMC) is another medullary-based high-grade tumor with infiltrative growth pattern. It occurs almost exclusively in young patients with sickle cell trait or rarely sickle cell disease. RMC often shows reticular or cribriform glands, in addition to other patterns such as yolk sac-like, tubular, and solid. Similar to CDC, RMC exhibits desmoplastic or fibrotic stroma and a neutrophil-dominant inflammatory infiltrate. Sickled red blood cells can often be found in the small vessels within and around the tumor. The loss of nuclear expression of INI1

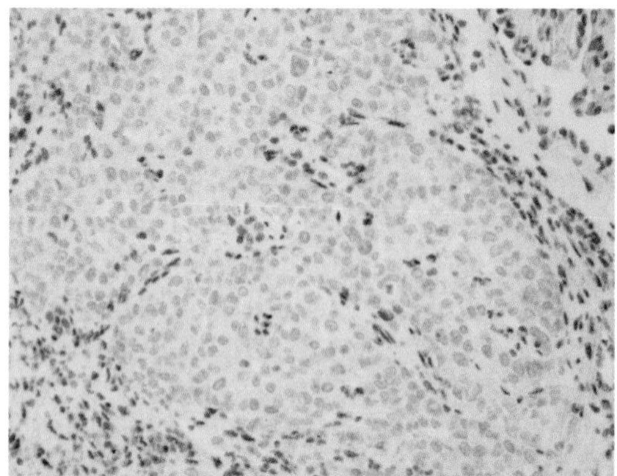

Fig. 33.6 Loss of INI1 (BAF47) nuclear expression in a renal medullary carcinoma. Note the retained INI1 expression in inflammatory, endothelial, and stromal cells

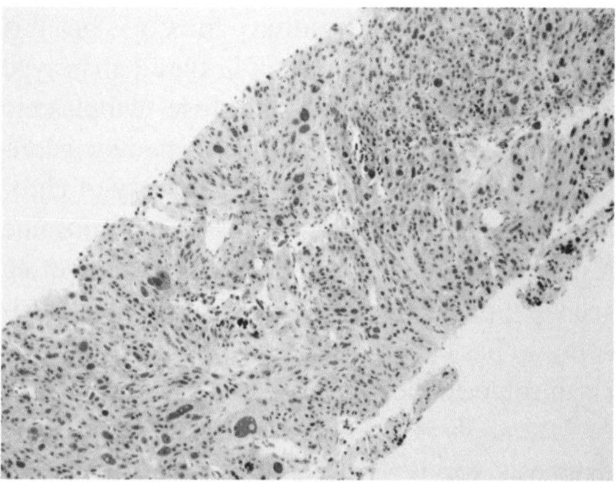

Fig. 33.7 Core biopsy of a metastatic epithelioid leiomyosarcoma involving kidney. There are intermixed large epithelioid cells and spindle cells

(SMARCB1/BAF47) protein by immunohistochemistry is a consistent finding in these tumors (Fig. 33.6) and can be reliably detected in core biopsies. However, it remains controversial whether loss of INI1 is a defining feature of RMC, and the exact molecular mechanism mediating this finding remains unclear.

Tumors with Poorly Differentiated Cell Cytology

When a poorly differentiated tumor encountered on renal needle cores, a broad range of differential possibilities need to be considered, many of which may arise from other organ sites. Among primary kidney tumors, high-grade clear cell RCC, papillary RCC, CDC, unclassified RCC, and epithelioid AML all can have areas showing high-grade cytology, without much clue to suggest their classification. Metastatic carcinoma or sarcoma from other organs involving the kidney, direct extension of urothelial carcinoma, adrenal cortical carcinoma, or tumors of the retroperitoneum are secondary tumors that need to be considered in this setting. Immunohistochemistry plays an essential role in differentiating these poorly differentiated tumors.

Metastatic tumors involving kidney often originate from lung (most common), breast, skin (melanoma), genitourinary, gastrointestinal, and gynecologic tracts, salivary gland, thyroid, pancreas, etc., in addition to high-grade sarcomas arising from soft tissue and bone. In general, morphologic features unusual for distinctive subtypes of renal cell carcinoma or urothelial carcinoma should always raise a suspicion for metastasis. Many metastatic tumors histologically differ from common types of primary renal cell carcinoma, allowing for relatively straightforward recognition. The presence of tumor emboli in vessels also suggests a possibility of metastasis.

Tumors with Spindle Cell Cytology

Low-grade spindle cells are commonly seen in angiomyolipoma, mixed epithelial and spindle cell tumor (MEST), MTSCC, and papillary RCC with low-grade spindle cell component. High-grade spindle cells are seen with sarcomatoid carcinoma component associated with RCC, urothelial carcinoma, or metastatic carcinoma, as well as primary or secondary sarcomas (Fig. 33.7).

Tumors with Neuroendocrine Features

Tumors with neuroendocrine differentiation are only rarely found on renal core biopsies. The differential diagnosis mainly includes primary renal carcinoid tumors, metastatic neuroendocrine tumors, pheochromocytoma from adrenal gland, or paraganglioma arising in the retroperitoneum.

Lymphomas

Lymphoma involving the kidney is most commonly B-cell type. In a few recent series, diffuse large B-cell lymphoma (DLBCL) appears to be the most common subtype of lymphomas [33–35]. Post-transplant lymphoproliferative disorders (PTLD), and very rarely T-cell lymphoma, can also be encountered. In general, the diagnostic criteria and ancillary studies applied to these tumors should be similar to what have been used for lymphomas at other organ sites. If a specific diagnosis cannot be rendered from the limited amount of material in biopsies, more general terms such as "large B-cell lymphoma" or "low-grade B-cell lymphoma" can be utilized.

Future

With the development of nephron-sparing surgery and non-surgical management of renal tumors, the utilization of percutaneous needle biopsy for renal masses will likely further increase in the next decade. In addition to preprocedural uses, needle biopsy may be more widely used as a surveillance tool in patients who have received ablation therapies or choose observation. Furthermore, the need to identify personalized systemic therapies for patients with metastatic disease is expected to drive more biopsy sampling of the primary and metastatic RCC to provide material for biomarker identification. From the pathology point of view, this increasing utilization of core biopsy technique can be translated into enhanced experience of pathologists in interpreting renal core biopsy specimens and opportunities to augment our capability of providing diagnostic and prognostic information that impact on disease management.

While immunohistochemistry currently is the mainstay of the ancillary studies applied to renal core biopsies, other methods such as FISH and a variety of molecular tests have already been utilized in clinical specimens including core biopsies. The rapid advances in these technologies have dramatically improved the accuracy, efficiency, and turn-around time of these assays; these methods are expected to be more closely incorporated into the histologic interpretation of renal core biopsies.

FISH assays are very useful tools in the differential diagnosis of renal epithelial tumors. In addition to *MiTF* translocation-associated RCCs, other novel translocation-associated RCCs are continuously being identified. Particularly, a group of recently identified ALK translocation RCCs may become an emerging entity [22]. FISH tests for chromosomal copy number abnormalities also have the potential to be improved and utilized in clinical practice. Trisomy 7 and 17 test has been commonly used for diagnosing papillary RCC; however, the specificity of this test needs to be further explored in tumors with overlapping features such as MTSCC, HLRCC-associated RCC, and unclassified RCC with papillary areas, in the context of other molecular alterations identified in these cases. Ongoing efforts in molecular characterization of a variety of renal tumors are providing new knowledge for developing enhanced FISH tests for diagnostic purposes.

Array-based SNP or CGH assays are being adapted to clinical use in limited formalin-fixed, paraffin-embedded (FFPE) tissue materials. These assays provide fast and comprehensive assessment of copy number variations and loss of heterozygosity (LOH). Other technologies including next-generation sequencing, miRNA, and methylation analyses are also being developed into clinical tests that can be used in biopsy samples. Meanwhile, the ongoing genomic research efforts in RCC such as The Cancer Genome Atlas (TCGA) program are generating enormous genetic information in subtypes of RCC [36]. These findings will serve as the groundwork for developing diagnostic, prognostic, and prediction markers.

References

1. Zagoria RJ. Imaging of small renal masses: a medical success story. AJR Am J Roentgenol. 2000;175:945–55.
2. Duchene DA, Lotan Y, Cadeddu JA, Sagalowsky AI, Koeneman KS. Histopathology of surgically managed renal tumors: analysis of a contemporary series. Urology. 2003;62:827–30.
3. Remzi M, Ozsoy M, Klingler HC, Susani M, Waldert M, Seitz C, Schmidbauer J, Marberger M. Are small renal tumors harmless? Analysis of histopathological features according to tumors 4 cm or less in diameter. J Urol. 2006;176:896–9.

4. Pahernik S, Ziegler S, Roos F, Melchior SW, Thuroff JW. Small renal tumors: correlation of clinical and pathological features with tumor size. J Urol. 2007;178:414–7.
5. Thompson RH, Kurta JM, Kaag M, Tickoo SK, Kundu S, Katz D, Nogueira L, Reuter VE, Russo P. Tumor size is associated with malignant potential in renal cell carcinoma cases. J Urol. 2009;181:2033–6.
6. Venkatesan AM, Wood BJ, Gervais DA. Percutaneous ablation in the kidney. Radiology. 2011;261:375–91.
7. Chawla SN, Crispen PL, Hanlon AL, Greenberg RE, Chen DY, Uzzo RG. The natural history of observed enhancing renal masses: meta-analysis and review of the world literature. J Urol. 2006;175:425–31.
8. Jewett MA, Mattar K, Basiuk J, Morash CG, Pautler SE, Siemens DR, Tanguay S, Rendon RA, Gleave ME, Drachenberg DE, Chow R, Chung H, Chin JL, Fleshner NE, Evans AJ, Gallie BL, Haider MA, Kachura JR, Kurban G, Fernandes K, Finelli A. Active surveillance of small renal masses: progression patterns of early stage kidney cancer. Eur Urol. 2011;60:39–44.
9. Gill IS, Aron M, Gervais DA, Jewett MA. Clinical practice.Small renal mass. N Engl J Med. 2010;362:624–34.
10. Silverman SG, Gan YU, Mortele KJ, Tuncali K, Cibas ES. Renal masses in the adult patient: the role of percutaneous biopsy. Radiology. 2006;240:6–22.
11. Volpe A, Kachura JR, Geddie WR, Evans AJ, Gharajeh A, Saravanan A, Jewett MA. Techniques, safety and accuracy of sampling of renal tumors by fine needle aspiration and core biopsy. J Urol. 2007;178:379–86.
12. Smith EH. Complications of percutaneous abdominal fine-needle biopsy. Review. Radiology. 1991;178:253–8.
13. Sainani NI, Tatli S, Anthony SG, Shyn PB, Tuncali K, Silverman SG. Successful percutaneous radiologic management of renal cell carcinoma tumor seeding caused by percutaneous biopsy performed before ablation. J Vasc Interv Radiol. 2013;24:1404–8.
14. Rybicki FJ, Shu KM, Cibas ES, Fielding JR, vanSonnenberg E, Silverman SG. Percutaneous biopsy of renal masses: sensitivity and negative predictive value stratified by clinical setting and size of masses. AJR Am J Roentgenol. 2003;180:1281–7.
15. Wood BJ, Khan MA, McGovern F, Harisinghani M, Hahn PF, Mueller PR. Imaging guided biopsy of renal masses: indications, accuracy and impact on clinical management. J Urol. 1999;161:1470–4.
16. Richter F, Kasabian NG, Irwin RJ Jr., Watson RA, Lang EK. Accuracy of diagnosis by guided biopsy of renal mass lesions classified indeterminate by imaging studies. Urology. 2000;55:348–52.
17. Al-Ahmadie HA, Alden D, Fine SW, Gopalan A, Touijer KA, Russo P, Reuter VE, Tickoo SK. Role of immunohistochemistry in the evaluation of needle core biopsies in adult renal cortical tumors: an ex vivo study. Am J Surg Pathol.2011;35:949–61.
18. Reuter VE, Tickoo SK. Differential diagnosis of renal tumours with clear cell histology. Pathology. 2010;42:374–83.
19. Martignoni G, Gobbo S, Camparo P, Brunelli M, Munari E, Segala D, Pea M, Bonetti F, Illei PB, Netto GJ, Ladanyi M, Chilosi M, Argani P. Differential expression of cathepsin K in neoplasms harboring TFE3 gene fusions. Mod Pathol. 2011;24:1313–9.
20. Argani P, Yonescu R, Morsberger L, Morris K, Netto GJ, Smith N, Gonzalez N, Illei PB, Ladanyi M, Griffin CA. Molecular confirmation of t(6;11)(p21;q12) renal cell carcinoma in archival paraffin-embedded material using a break-apart TFEB FISH assay expands its clinicopathologic spectrum. Am J Surg Pathol. 2012;36:1516–26.
21. Rao Q, Williamson SR, Zhang S, Eble JN, Grignon DJ, Wang M, Zhou XJ, Huang W, Tan PH, Maclennan GT, Cheng L. TFE3 break-apart FISH has a higher sensitivity for Xp11.2 translocation-associated renal cell carcinoma compared with TFE3 or cathepsin K immunohistochemical staining alone: expanding the morphologic spectrum. Am J Surg Pathol. 2013;37:804–15.
22. Srigley JR, Delahunt B, Eble JN, Egevad L, Epstein JI, Grignon D, Hes O, Moch H, Montironi R, Tickoo SK, Zhou M, Argani P. The international society of urological pathology (ISUP) Vancouver classification of renal neoplasia. Am J Surg Pathol. 2013;37:1469–89.
23. Gill AJ, Pachter NS, Chou A, Young B, Clarkson A, Tucker KM, Winship IM, Earls P, Benn DE, Robinson BG, Fleming S, Clifton-Bligh RJ. Renal tumors associated with germline SDHB mutation show distinctive morphology. Am J Surg Pathol. 2011;35:1578–85.
24. Papathomas TG, Gaal J, Corssmit EP, Oudijk L, Korpershoek E, Heimdal K, Bayley JP, Morreau H, van Dooren M, Papaspyrou K, Schreiner T, Hansen T, Andresen PA, Restuccia DF, van Kessel I, van Leenders GJ, Kros JM, Looijenga LH, Hofland LJ, Mann W, van Nederveen FH, Mete O, Asa SL, de Krijger RR, Dinjens WN. Non-pheochromocytoma (PCC)/paraganglioma (PGL) tumors in patients with succinate dehydrogenase-related PCC-PGL syndromes: a clinicopathological and molecular analysis. Eur J Endocrinol. 2014;170:1–12.
25. Gill AJ, Benn DE, Chou A, Clarkson A, Muljono A, Meyer-Rochow GY, Richardson AL, Sidhu SB, Robinson BG, Clifton-Bligh RJ. Immunohistochemistry for SDHB triages genetic testing of SDHB, SDHC, and SDHD in paraganglioma-pheochromocytoma syndromes. Hum Pathol. 2010;41:805–14.
26. Tickoo SK, Reuter VE. Differential diagnosis of renal tumors with papillary architecture. Adv Anat Pathol. 2011;18:120–32.
27. Jiang F, Richter J, Schraml P, Bubendorf L, Gasser T, Sauter G, Mihatsch MJ, Moch H. Chromosomal imbalances in papillary renal cell carcinoma: genetic differences between histological subtypes. Am J Pathol. 1998;153:1467–73.

28. Sanders ME, Mick R, Tomaszewski JE, Barr FG. Unique patterns of allelic imbalance distinguish type 1 from type 2 sporadic papillary renal cell carcinoma. Am J Pathol. 2002;161:997–1005.
29. Klatte T, Pantuck AJ, Said JW, Seligson DB, Rao NP, LaRochelle JC, Shuch B, Zisman A, Kabbinavar FF, Belldegrun AS. Cytogenetic and molecular tumor profiling for type 1 and type 2 papillary renal cell carcinoma. Clin Cancer Res. 2009;15:1162–9.
30. Merino MJ, Torres-Cabala C, Pinto P, Linehan WM. The morphologic spectrum of kidney tumors in hereditary leiomyomatosis and renal cell carcinoma (HLRCC) syndrome. Am J SurgPathol. 2007;31:1578–85.
31. Chen YB, Brannon AR, Toubaji A, Dudas ME, Won HH, Al-Ahmadie HA, Fine SW, Gopalan A, Frizzell N, Voss MH, Russo P, Berger MF, Tickoo SK, Reuter VE. Hereditary leiomyomatosis and renal cell carcinoma syndrome-associated renal cancer: recognition of the syndrome by pathologic features and the utility of detecting aberrant succination by immunohistochemistry. Am J Surg Pathol. 2014;38(5):627–37.
32. Bardella C, El-Bahrawy M, Frizzell N, Adam J, Ternette N, Hatipoglu E, Howarth K, O'Flaherty L, Roberts I, Turner G, Taylor J, Giaslakiotis K, Macaulay VM, Harris AL, Chandra A, Lehtonen HJ, Launonen V, Aaltonen LA, Pugh CW, Mihai R, Trudgian D, Kessler B, Baynes JW, Ratcliffe PJ, Tomlinson IP, Pollard PJ. Aberrant succination of proteins in fumaratehydratase-deficient mice and HLRCC patients is a robust biomarker of mutation status. J Pathol. 2011;225:4–11.
33. Schniederjan SD, Osunkoya AO. Lymphoid neoplasms of the urinary tract and male genital organs: a clinicopathological study of 40 cases. Mod Pathol. 2009;22:1057–65.
34. Truong LD, Caraway N, Ngo T, Laucirica R, Katz R, Ramzy I. Renal lymphoma. The diagnostic and therapeutic roles of fine-needle aspiration. Am J Clin Pathol. 2001;115:18–31.
35. Subhawong AP, Subhawong TK, Vandenbussche CJ, Siddiqui MT, Ali SZ. Lymphoproliferative disorders of the kidney on fine-needle aspiration: cytomorphology and radiographic correlates in 33 cases. Acta Cytol. 2013;57:19–25.
36. Cancer Genome Atlas Research Network. Comprehensive molecular characterization of clear cell renal cell carcinoma. Nature.2013;499:43–9.

Part IV

Update on Testicular Tumor Pathology

Anatomy of the Testis and Staging of its Cancers: Implications for Diagnosis

34

Daniel M. Berney and Thomas M. Ulbright

Etymology

The English word "testis" is probably derived from the Latin meaning "witness," which is also the source of the words "testify" and "testimony." The Roman law principle "*Testis unus, testis nullus,*" translated as "one witness means no witness," imputes that the testimony of one witness must be corroborated by a second to be considered valid. The paired nature of the organs in humans, just as witnesses must be paired, likely resulted in use of "testis" for the male gonad.

Embryology

An understanding of the embryology of the testis is key to explaining its cellular morphology and distribution and also its lymphatic drainage and hence the pattern of spread of testicular tumors. Testis-determining factor (TDF), the protein product of the *SRY* gene on the Y chromosome [1], determines the formation of a testis as opposed to an ovary. The germ cells migrate to the genital ridge where proliferating celomic epithelium forms the sex cords and surrounds the germ cells to become the progenitors of the seminiferous tubules. Proliferation and differentiation of intervening mesenchyme gives rise to the Leydig cells. The Sertoli cells secrete anti-Müllerian hormone (AMH; also known as Müllerian-inhibiting substance) causing regression of the Müllerian ducts. Leydig cells produce testosterone, which promotes the development of Wolffian duct structures (if functional androgen receptors are also present). Development of the external genitalia requires testosterone plus androgen receptors plus five-alpha reductase, which converts testosterone to dihydrotestosterone (DHT). Testicular descent from the abdomen to pelvic brim is mediated by insulin-like growth factor, while descent to the scrotum is androgen dependent [2]. The gubernaculum (also called the caudal genital ligament) is undifferentiated mesenchyme attached to the *caudal* end of the testis; its distal portion both proliferates and synthesizes hyaluronic acid causing a "swelling reaction" that guides the testis into the scrotal cavity (Fig. 34.1) [3]. This complicated embryological derivation has a number of important consequences, among which is to help explain a variety of the so-called intersex conditions (also known as disorders of sex development), where undescended testes are associated with female internal genitalia due, for instance, to mutations in the *AMH* gene and leading to defective anti-Müllerian hormone [4]. Another important consequence of an aberrant embryologic process is cryptorchidism, one of

D. M. Berney (✉)
Department of Molecular Oncology, Barts Cancer Institute, Bartshealth NHS Trust and Queen Mary University of London, London, UK
e-mail: d.berney@bartshealth.nhs.uk

T. M. Ulbright
Department of Pathology and Laboratory Medicine, Indiana University School of Medicine, Indianapolis, IN, USA
e-mail: tulbright@iupui.edu

C. Magi-Galluzzi, C. G. Przybycin (eds.), *Genitourinary Pathology,* DOI 10.1007/978-1-4939-2044-0_34,

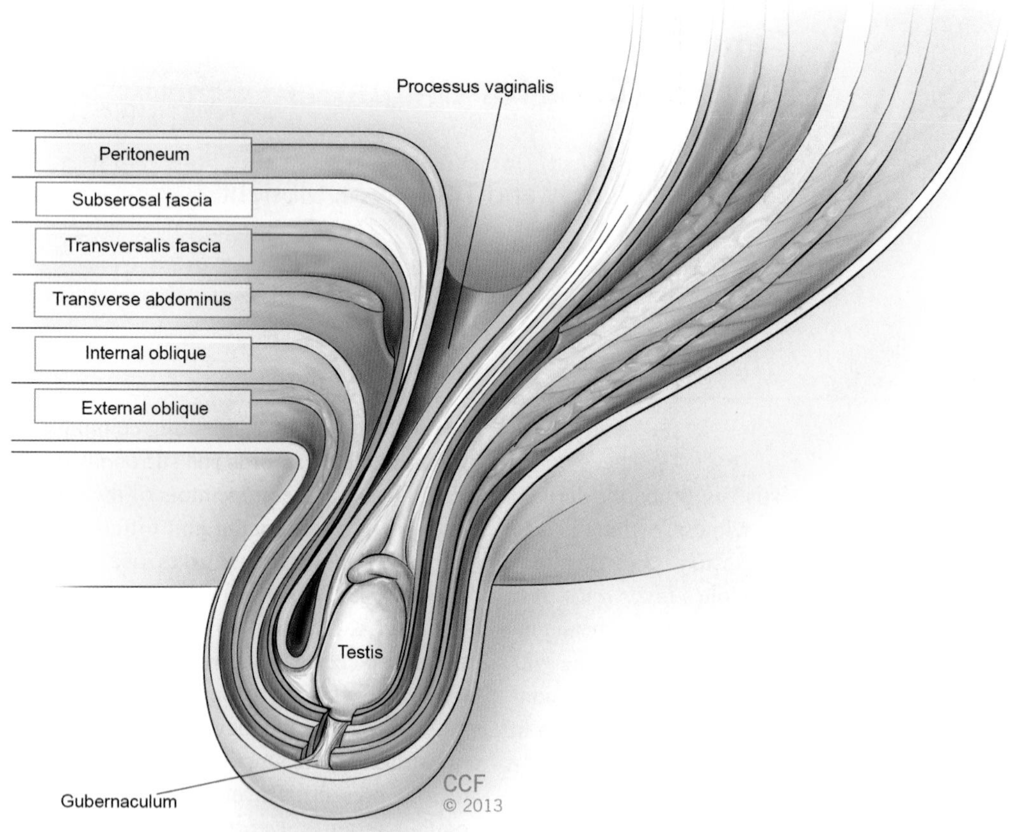

Fig. 34.1 Descent of the testis. (Reprinted with permission, Cleveland Clinic Center for Medical Art & Photography © 2014. All Rights Reserved.)

the relatively few well-recognized risk factors for testicular germ cell tumors, with the degree of aberration showing some correlation with the degree of risk, since there is a higher frequency of tumors in intraabdominal than inguinal testes.

Embryology also explains the metastatic patterns of spread of testicular tumors. The metastatic tumors spread to the retroperitoneal (para-aortic, interaortocaval, paracaval) rather than inguinal lymph nodes as the vascular drainage follows descent from the genital ridge (Fig. 34.2). If there has been previous genital surgery, however, disruption to the drainage pattern may cause spread to the inguinal lymph nodes. Also, if there is failure of testicular descent as in intersex conditions, the lymph node drainage pattern of the testis may also be affected [5], although this is extremely rare.

Testicular Dysgenesis Syndrome

It has been proposed by some that there is a strong causal association between some anatomical abnormalities and germ cell cancers. This has been termed the testicular dysgenesis syndrome (TDS) [6] and should not be confused with the disorder of sex development, gonadal dysgenesis, which is associated with streak morphology and ovarian differentiation. TDS remains a hypothesis, which is disputed by others [7], consisting of four defining conditions: impaired spermatogenesis, undescended testis, hypospadias, and testicular germ cell cancer. It suggests that an underlying genetic predisposition and environment, in utero factors, possibly endocrine, affect the developing fetus. This leads to abnormal Sertoli cell function

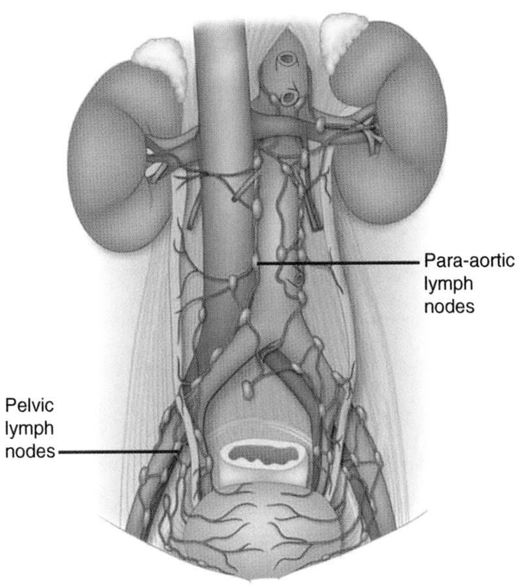

Fig. 34.2 Diagram showing pelvic and para-aortic lymph nodes

and decreased Leydig cell function, with resulting germ cell maldevelopment and androgen deficiency, respectively, and to the four defining features (Fig. 34.3).

Anatomy of the Testis

The adult testis measures approximately $4.5 \times 2.5 \times 3$ cm and weighs 20 g. Degrees of atrophy and testicular development throughout adolescence may be measured with an orchidometer, composed of a series of ovoids.

The testis is largely surrounded by an intrascrotal extension of peritoneal cavity (the processus vaginalis), which becomes the tunica vaginalis. Its visceral layer is apposed to the fibrous capsule of the testis, the tunica albuginea, and its parietal layer lines the most internal aspect of the scrotal wall. A small amount of fluid separates the visceral from the parietal layer. The embryology of testicular descent therefore results in mesothelium covering most of the testicular surface, with the visceral layer reflecting from the testis near the hilum and enveloping the testicular appendages. The testicular parenchyma is composed of seminiferous tubules with their components of various germ cells and Sertoli cells. The interstitium contains Leydig cells, blood and lymphatic vessels, and loose fibrous tissue. The seminiferous tubules connect into the rete testis at the hilum, and these anastomose with the efferent ductules that form the head of the epididymis, with the body and tail forming from convolutions of the Wolffian duct. The epididymis is attached to the posterior surface of the testis and gives rise to the ductus (vas) deferens (Fig. 34.4a–d). The testis is thus surrounded by easily identifiable histological structures: the testicular tunics, epididymis, and spermatic cord. Therefore, for radical orchidectomy cases, margins and tissues are easily identified and there is no need to use ink on macroscopic dissection. Staging is straightforward with appropriate tissue sample selection.

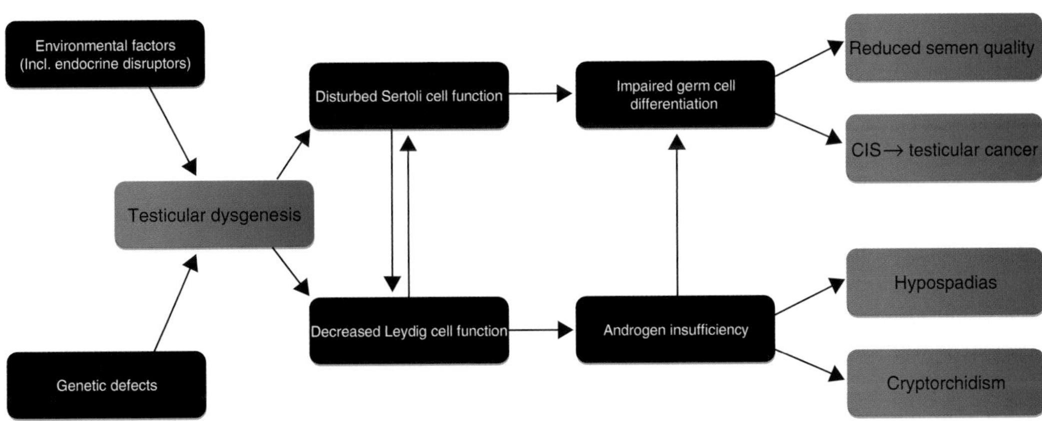

Fig. 34.3 The proposed pathogenesis of testicular dysgenesis syndrome

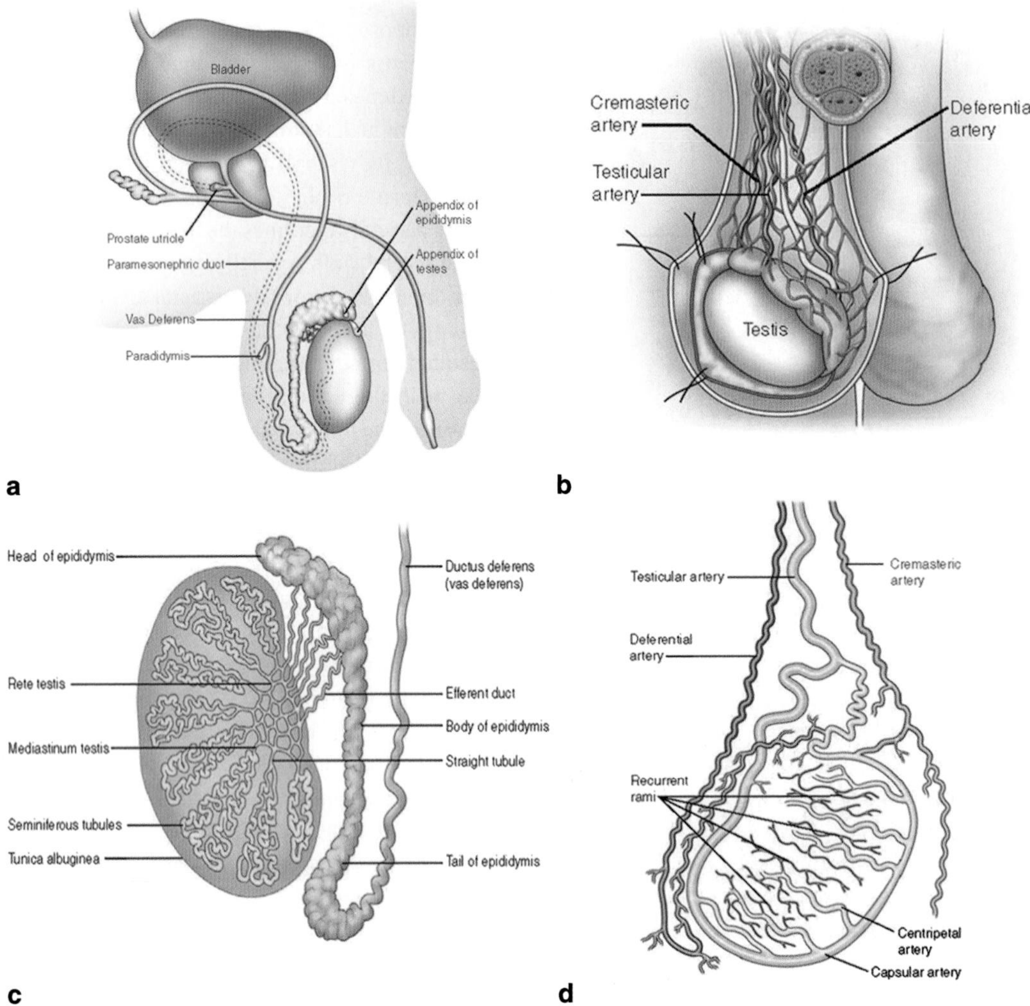

Fig. 34.4 **a** Cross section of the testis and the cord, demonstrating especially, the double-layered nature of the tunica vaginalis and the relationship of the lobules composed of seminiferous tubules to the rete and epididymis. **b** Demonstration of the testicular blood supply. The testicular artery arises directly from the *abdominal aorta* and descends through the *inguinal canal*, while the scrotum and the rest of the external genitalia are supplied by the *internal pudendal artery*. The testis has collateral blood supply from the *cremasteric artery* and the deferential artery. Lymphatic drainage of the testes follows the testicular arteries back to the *para-aortic lymph nodes*. **c** Cross section of the testis demonstrating the relationship of the lobules composed of seminiferous tubules to the rete testis, epididymis, and vas deferens. **d** A demonstration of the rich blood supply to the testis and rich anastomotic network of vessels

In recent years, there has been an increase in partial orchidectomy specimens [8]. This is for a number of reasons. Among them, the increased use of ultrasound has detected more testicular tumors of little clinical significance [9]. These include small sex cord-stromal tumors, Sertoli cell nodules, inflammatory conditions, non-neoplastic cysts, epidermoid cysts, and adenomatoid tumors. In the vast majority of these cases, a partial orchidectomy may be sufficient for cure, permitting better preservation of endocrine function and fertility and improved cosmesis. It is still a relatively infrequent operation, reserved particularly for men who may have already had contralateral orchidectomy or who have poor endocrine function or sperm counts. It is also technically

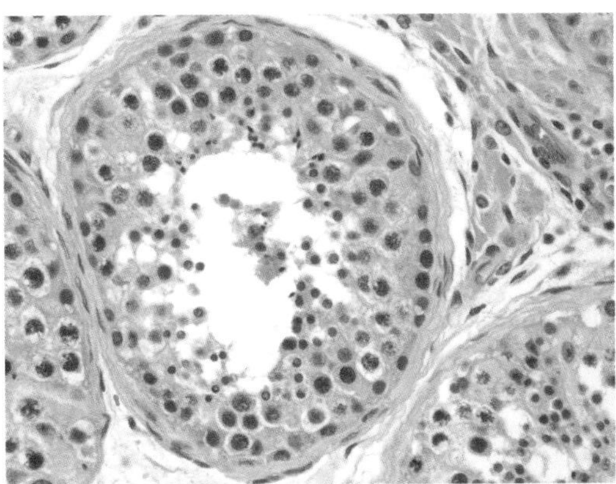

Fig. 34.5 A seminiferous tubule showing the different stages of spermatogenesis

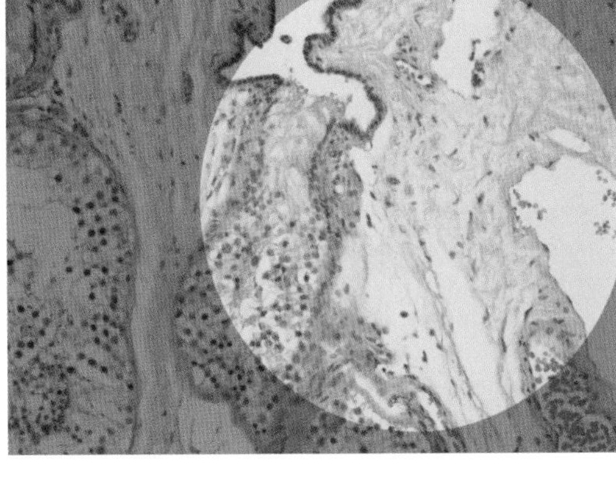

Fig. 34.6 A seminiferous tubule connecting with the distal portion of the rete testis

limited to lesions that are distant from the rete and epididymis.

Partial orchidectomy specimens provide different challenges for the pathologist. They result in an excision specimen partially covered by mesothelium, which, as suggested above, is easily identified, but also having a testicular parenchyma as a surgical margin. On macroscopy, this must be inked so that it can be recognized as a surgical margin.

Microanatomy

Identification of the normal components of the seminiferous tubules is essential both to accurately identify abnormalities, of maturation, and to correctly recognize intratubular germ cell neoplasia. The seminiferous tubules contain germ cells in various stages of development from spermatogonia to spermatozoa along with the Sertoli cells (Fig. 34.5). Each tubule profile may show variable stages of maturation because development tends to occur in waves along the tubules. After the sperm are produced, they travel to the tubuli recti, which are found in the septa radiating out from the mediastinum of the testis (Fig. 34.6). The tubuli recti connect the seminiferous tubules with the rete testis.

Sertoli cells are distinguished by their location just above the basement membrane of the seminiferous tubule and the shape of the nucleus (Fig. 34.7). The Sertoli cell has an ovoid to triangular-shaped nucleus with a neatly punched-out red nucleolus. They form a ring around the basement membrane, between the spermatogonia and the other developing germ cells. The spermatogonia usually hug the basal lamina. They are large round cells with a pale staining round or ovoid nuclei. Dark and light forms, depending on subtle nuclear characteristics, have been noted [10], and the proportions of the different forms have been suggested to affect Leydig cell function.

Primary spermatocytes, which are undergoing the first meiotic division, have a large floccular nucleus, in which the individual condensed

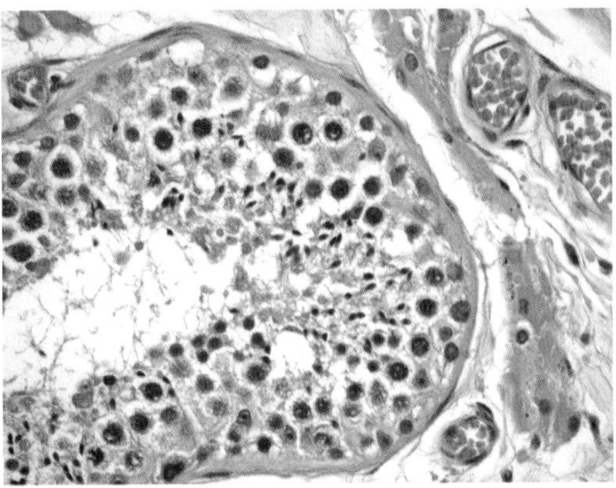

Fig. 34.7 Sertoli cell has an ovoid to triangular-shaped nucleus with a neatly punched-out red nucleolus. Spermatogonia are large round cells with a pale staining round or ovoid nuclei; they usually hug the basal lamina, and primary spermatocytes have a large floccular nucleus

Table 34.1 Johnson scoring of seminiferous tubules for fertility assessments

10—full spermatogenesis
9—slightly impaired spermatogenesis, many late spermatids, disorganized epithelium
8—less than five spermatozoa per tubule, few late spermatids
7—no spermatozoa, no late spermatids, many early spermatids
6—no spermatozoa, no late spermatids, few early spermatids
5—no spermatozoa or spermatids, many spermatocytes
4—no spermatozoa or spermatids, few spermatocytes
3—spermatogonia only
2—no germinal cells, Sertoli cells only
1—no seminiferous epithelium

chromosomes can be sometimes seen forming elongated filamentous structures. Secondary spermatocytes are only rarely identified, as the second meiotic division occurs very rapidly. The early spermatid is small and round with a hyperchromatic nucleus and featureless chromatin. Later the spermatid becomes more conical. It then develops a flagellum and an even denser nucleus to become a spermatozoon (Fig. 34.7).

Relevance to Fertility Assessments

Two relatively new techniques allow the isolation and utilization of a single spermatozoon to fertilize a single egg for implantation in the uterus. These are performed in cases of non-obstructive oligo- or azoospermia and involve extraction of viable spermatozoa directly from the testis. While some practitioners attempt to aspirate spermatozoa with a technique similar to fine-needle aspiration, and then examine the extract for sperm, others use a biopsy technique, possibly more effective, called testicular sperm extraction (TESE). While some of the sample is used for fertilization, the parts of the biopsy not used may be sent for histopathological examination. The most important part of this examination, as far as the andrologists are concerned, is the identification of spermatozoa. When they are present in only small numbers, they can be better identified in histology sections than intraoperatively, and it suggests that a second TESE may be worthwhile if the initial fertility treatment failed. Therefore, the identification of the different meiotic cells in spermatogenesis is of great assistance [11]. Although some who work in this field attempted to "score the tubules" depending on the presence or absence of the developing elements of spermatogenesis (Table 34.1), the most relevant information required is merely the presence of spermatozoa and also the possible presence of intratubular germ cell neoplasia, unclassified (IGCNU).

IGCNU was initially termed "carcinoma in situ," a nomenclature that is still used by some [12]. Nearly the entire array of malignant germ cell tumor elements has been identified in seminiferous tubules; however, the most common by far is intratubular germ cell neoplasia, unclassified. Identification of IGCNU is important because of its virtually uniform eventual progression to an invasive germ cell tumor. In testicular biopsies, it may be found as an incidental finding or at the same time as orchidectomy for germ cell neoplasia in those centers where the contralateral testis is biopsied [13]. However, as there are a number of mimics of germ cell neoplasia, especially classical seminoma, identification of IGCNU may greatly help facilitate a difficult diagnosis where there is a question of germ cell neoplasm versus another process.

Ectopic Tissue and Pseudomalignant Changes

Leydig cells may be present not just in the testicular parenchyma, between the seminiferous tubules, but also in the fibrous capsule of the tunica albuginea, rete testis, paratesticular soft tissue, and occasionally epididymis [14]. They are relatively inconspicuous unless there is a cause of Leydig cell hyperplasia, when they can become more prominent and possibly be mistaken for an invasive Leydig cell tumor. Leydig cells are frequently associated with nerves, which must not be misinterpreted as perineural invasion by a malignant tumor, especially if the testis harbors an otherwise innocuous Leydig cell tumor, which, however, would lack the usual features associated with malignant behavior in this neoplasm.

Therefore, it is important to realize that Leydig cells may be present at "ectopic" locations.

Adrenocortical-like tissue can also be seen in ectopic foci, usually near the rete testis [15] and in the cord. Ectopic foci are generally entirely incidental; however, they become of great importance in the inherited adrenogenital syndrome or "congenital adrenal hyperplasia." In this rare condition, there is gross hyperplasia of these adrenal cells. They often resemble Leydig cells, although they may have more voluminous cytoplasm, more prominent cytoplasmic pigment, lack Reinke crystals, and are associated with fibrosis [16]. While in the initial stages of congenital adrenal hyperplasia the lesions are usually confined to the rete testis, they may expand into the testicular parenchyma where they present as testicular masses. These "tumors" are extremely responsive to high-dose steroid suppression, and the first treatment is always medical, surgery being used only as a last resort due to pain. Unfortunately, cases of bilateral orchidectomy, rendering the patient castrate, for bilateral testicular "tumors" of the adrenogenital syndrome continue to occur; the pathologist needs to be aware of this condition and prevent unnecessary orchidectomy where possible.

Bizarre nuclear change in the epithelium of the epididymal tubules may cause concern for a malignant process. This phenomenon, however, has no clinical significance and appears to be of degenerative nature, entirely analogous to the much more common but similar finding in the seminal vesicles. The nuclei, although enlarged, have dense, smudgy chromatin and sometimes intranuclear cytoplasmic inclusions. Mitotic figures are absent. Along the same lines, complex cribriform arrangements of the glandular epithelium in the epididymal tubules may provoke concern for adenocarcinoma, but this finding is entirely within the spectrum of normal morphology of the epididymis.

Staging of Testis Cancer

The management of testicular tumors, particularly germ cell tumors, differs radically from many other of the genitourinary malignancies. Whereas accurate staging either on imaging or by histology is critical for prostatic adenocarcinomas or urothelial neoplasms, in the complex world of testicular tumors, the tumor type is of supreme importance, although staging of the primary lesion plays a secondary role for the pathologist. This is for a number of reasons. Firstly, the excellent prognosis of most germ cell tumors means that large randomized trials with staging being used to designate treatment are virtually impossible. Outcome data have to be available on thousands of patients to create enough treatment failures to yield significant differences in outcome based on pathological criteria. Secondly, the treating physicians are also likely to utilize non-pathological criteria, such as the levels of serum tumor markers and findings on retroperitoneal imaging, to assist with treatment choices, regardless of pathologic staging of the testicular primary.

The currently recommended staging system for testicular tumors is the AJCC-TNM classification [17], which is summarized in Table 34.2. It should be noted that because tumor markers play such a key role in the management of patients with germ cell tumors and have been shown to have prognostic importance, the degree of elevation of various serum markers is considered in the determination of the stage groups. In fact, any of the T stages can be clinical stage I–III, meaning that the serum markers or imaging not infrequently "trump" the pathological assessment. An even more clinically based system, the International Germ Cell Consensus (IGCC) classification, stratifies patients with non-seminomatous germ cell tumors (NSGCTs) into three risk groups (good, intermediate, and poor prognosis) on the basis of serum markers (measured prior to orchiectomy) and distribution of metastases (Table 34.3).

While the TNM system follows a logical progression of breach of the various pathological boundaries (Fig. 34.8), it remains open to question regarding its prognostic significance. However, as staging by TNM remains an essential element of most urological data sets, it will remain a part of the standard pathological assessment.

Table 34.2 AJCC staging system for testicular cancer. Note that nodes imaging and serology also have a large role in determining the stage

TNM system		Stage grouping
TX—unknown status of testis		Stage 0—Tis, N0, M0, S0
T0—no apparent primary (includes scars)		Stage IA—T1, N0, M0, S0
Tis—intratubular tumor, no invasion		Stage IB—T2-T4, N0, M0, S0
T1—testis and epididymis only; no vascular invasion; may penetrate tunica albuginea but not tunica vaginalis		Stage IS—any T, N0, M0, S1-S3 (post-orchiectomy) Stage IIA—any T, N1, M0, S0-S1
T2—testis and epididymis with vascular invasion or through tunica albuginea to involve tunica vaginalis		Stage IIB—any T, N2, M0, S0-S1 Stage IIC—any T, N3, M0, S0-S1
T3—spermatic cord involvement		Stage IIIA—any T, any N, M1a, S0-S1
T4—scrotum		Stage IIIB—any T, any N, M0-M1a, S2
		Stage IIIC—any T, any N, M0-M1a, S3
		Stage IIIC—any T, any N, M1b, any S
NX—regional lymph nodes cannot be assessed		
N0—no regional lymph node involvement		
N1—node mass or single nodes ≤ 2 cm; no node >2 cm		
N2—node mass >2 cm but <5 cm; or multiple lymph nodes involved >2 cm, but none >5 cm		
N3—node mass >5 cm		
M0—no distant metastases		
M1a—non-regional nodal or lung metastases		
M1b—distant metastasis other than non-regional nodal or lung		
SX—no marker studies available		
S0—marker studies within normal limits		
LDH[a]	HCG (mIU/ml)	AFP (ng/ml)
S1—$<1.5 \times$ N and	<5000 and	<1000
S2—1.5–10 $\times$ N or	5000–50,000 or	1000–10,000
S3—$>10 \times$ N or	$>50,000$ or	$>10,000$

AFP, alpha-fetoprotein; *AJCC,* American joint committee on cancer; *HCG*, human chorionic gonadotropin; *LDH*, lactate dehydrogenase.

[a] LDH levels expressed as elevations above upper limit of normal (N)

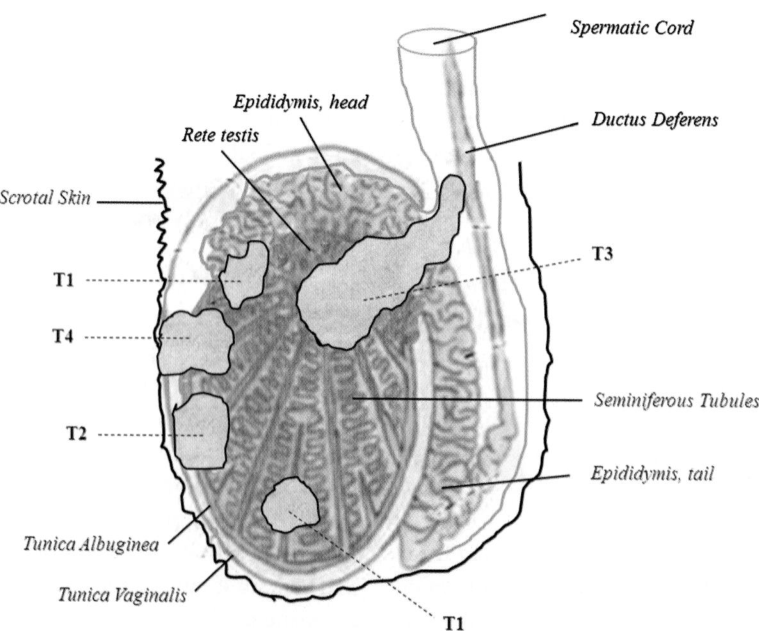

Fig. 34.8 Diagrammatic representation of testicular tumor staging

Table 34.3 International germ cell consensus classification for non-seminomatous germ cell tumors (NSGCTs)

Good prognosis
Testis/retroperitoneal primary site = 0
and
No non-pulmonary visceral metastases = 0
and
AFP good = 0 and HCG good = 0 and LDH good = 0
Max = 0
Intermediate prognosis
Testis/retroperitoneal primary site = 0
and
No non-pulmonary visceral metastases = 0
and
AFP intermediate = 1 or HCG intermediate = 0 or LDH intermediate = 1
Max = 1
Poor prognosis
Mediastinal primary site = 2
or
Non-pulmonary visceral metastases = 2
or
AFP poor = 2 or HCG poor = 2 or LDH poor = 2
Max = 2

Good: AFP < 1000 ng/ml, HCG < 5000 iu/L, LDH < 1.5 x upper limit of normal (N)
Intermediate: AFP 1000–10,000 ng/ml, HCG 5000–50000 iu/L, LDH 1.5–10 × N
Poor: AFP > 10,000 ng/ml, HCG > 50,000 iu/L, LDH > 10 × N

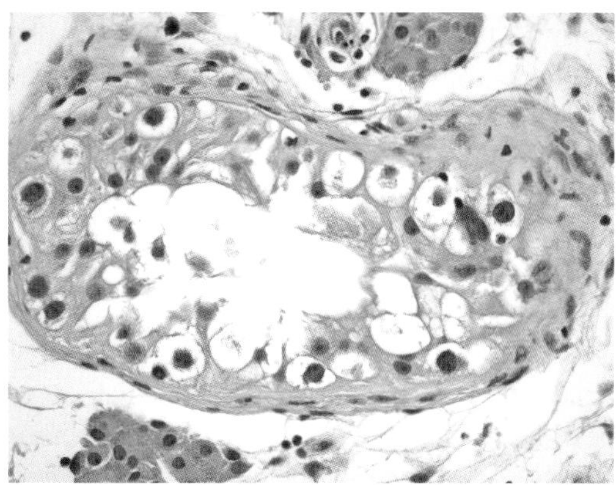

Fig. 34.9 Intratubular germ cell neoplasia, unclassified (IGCNU). IGCNU cells are intermixed with sertoli cells. No normal germ cells are present within the tubule

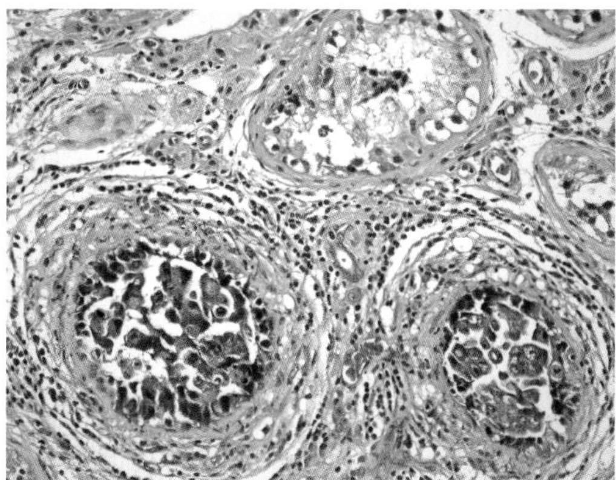

Fig. 34.10 Intratubular embryonal carcinoma coexisting with IGCNU

Tis

In situ germ cell malignancies are confined by the basement membrane surrounding the seminiferous tubules. Any cells present in the testicular stroma are therefore invasive. Most in situ lesions are intratubular germ cell neoplasia, unclassified (IGCNU) (Fig. 34.9), though other forms do exist. Intratubular embryonal carcinoma rarely occurs in isolation, nearly always coexisting with IGCNU and invasive germ cell malignancy (Fig. 34.10). IGCNU may spread in a pagetoid fashion and therefore be present within the rete testis. In these cases, the IGCNU cells are interspersed with the rete tubular epithelium or within the rete lumina. This should still be accounted as Tis unless there is invasion of the rete stroma. Isolated IGCNU is an unusual finding in the testis. It is occasionally found in the contralateral testis after orchidectomy or after chemotherapy. IGCNU cells initially tend to be positioned suprabasally, often in a ring-like fashion at the periphery of the seminiferous tubules, and intermixed with Sertoli cells. Occasionally, the IGCNU cells fill an entire tubule, but this is not a usual finding. The cells have an irregular, often polygonal nucleus, with a variable nucleolus, depending greatly on fixation. The cytoplasm is often vacuolated, though occasionally, normal developing germ cells can be vacuolated, so IGCNU must be diagnosed with caution [18]. Immunohistochemistry can greatly facilitate diagnosis in difficult cases. IGCNU is OCT4 positive, whereas normal germ cells are negative. PLAP and c-KIT may also be useful, but are less sensitive than OCT4 [19], and CD117 may also stain non-neoplastic germ cells. The best alternative choice to OCT4 that is in wide use may be podoplanin.

Gonadoblastoma

This is an unusual form of in situ malignancy which still counts as non-invasive, but it needs to be differentiated in terms of treatment and consequences. Most cases of gonadoblastoma occur in phenotypic females; however, 10 % occur in phenotypic males. In genotypic terms, a Y chromosome is needed to develop gonadoblastoma. It is, therefore, a disease that occurs in intersex conditions. Microscopically, there are rounded nodules of Sertoli cells intermixed with scattered seminoma/IGCNU-like cells as well as some germ cells resembling spermatogonia. Most cases in males are in undescended or maldescended testes. Although adjuvant treatment is not required for gonadoblastoma, removal of the contralateral gonad is indicated, as there is a high incidence of bilaterality and a very high rate of progression to seminoma. The presence of solid areas without interspersed Sertoli cells is indicative of seminoma, although remnant gonadoblastoma may be identified in these cases.

T1 Tumors

These are defined as tumors limited to the testis and epididymis, without vascular invasion and with no invasion of the tunica vaginalis (Fig. 34.8). A number of practical points should be noted. Firstly, the tunica albuginea should not be confused with the tunica vaginalis. On tissue sections, it is the tunica albuginea that is most likely to be seen, and it is very common for germ cell tumors to encroach close to or invade into the inner aspect of this fibrous capsule. However, it requires penetration of its external mesothelial lining for the tumor to no longer be considered a T1 lesion. This is, in fact, a very rare event because of the dense nature of the tunica albuginea. An alternative pathway to tunica vaginalis involvement, while not common, likely is more frequent. A germ cell tumor may invade through the testicular hilum to involve the perihilar structures, including the epididymis and soft tissue that are in continuity with the spermatic cord. Such involvement occurs with some frequency since the tunica albuginea is absent at the hilum. Since the external aspect of these perihilar structures has a layer of mesothelium from the visceral aspect of the tunica vaginalis reflected over them, a tumor may penetrate this external aspect and its mesothelial lining. Sometimes, it may also bridge to the parietal layer of the tunica vaginalis, tethering the testis and hilar structures to it.

Regardless of the mechanism of tunica vaginalis penetration, it is likely best assessed by careful macroscopic inspection. If the visceral layer of the tunica vaginalis has been directly penetrated through the tunica albuginea, it would appear as a roughed focus on the otherwise shiny external aspect of the testis. Such foci should be submitted for microscopic confirmation since many turn out to be a mesothelial reaction caused by rubbing of the enlarged testis against the parietal layer of the tunica vaginalis rather than a focus of tumor penetration. If the tunica vaginalis has been penetrated from a perihilar invasive focus, the parietal layer may no longer slide easily over the tunica albuginea, reflecting its tethering as mentioned above. This is best confirmed by microscopic examination of the parietal layer of the tunica vaginalis.

Invasion of the rete testis and epididymis is also included in T1 tumors; therefore, the tumour may be extensive, yet still qualify as T1 under the current system. Epididymal invasion almost always occurs from extension through the hilum either directly from the testis through the rete or indirectly from perihilar soft tissue that is invaginated between the testis and the epididymis. No differentiation of method has ever been made or examined from the prognostic aspect. It is important not to equate perihilar soft tissue invasion with invasion of the cord (T3).

T2 Tumors

T2 combines two separate criteria: tunica vaginalis penetration (Fig. 34.8), which has been discussed above, and the far more important and common vascular invasion, which is probably one of the few staging-related factors in germ cell cancer that is of interest to the clinician.

Assessment of vascular invasion in testicular tumors remains fraught with false positives due to the difficulty encountered in differentiation of "true" vascular invasion with artifactual invasion, particularly in seminomas. Vascular invasion in non-seminomatous germ cell tumors is easier to identify and most frequently seen in embryonal carcinomas.

In our opinion, strict criteria for the identification of vascular invasion are necessary. The tumor should be preferably in a clump of cells, associated with thrombotic material, and conform to the vessel shape, often adhering to its wall. Once one focus of vascular invasion is seen, it is usually possible to find tumor in adjacent vessels or further cuts of the same vessel.

The main reason for the overreporting of vascular invasion is the very soft nature of some germ cell tumors on cut section, especially seminomas, which smear across sections, causing difficult-to-avoid contamination of the testicular parenchyma. Loose seminoma cells in particular may be scattered throughout a section and smeared over the cut surface or tunica as well as implanted in vascular spaces. This makes identification of vascular invasion in seminomas especially challenging. Interestingly, vascular invasion has been proved to be only a fairly weak poor prognostic factor for seminoma [20], whereas vascular invasion is a strong prognostic factor for relapse in non-seminomas, a fact proven in multiple series over the past 20 years [21–23]. The difficulty in making reliable assessments of vascular invasion in seminomas may account for at least part of this finding.

T3 Tumors

Invasion of the testicular cord has been little examined in prognostic series of testicular tumors, but it has been shown to have an adverse prognostic impact [24]. Differentiating cord invasion from perihilar adipose tissue has only been performed in one study [23], which showed both were poor prognostic factors, but only perihilar invasion remained an independent predictor of distant disease on multivariate analysis. Deposits of tumour may be seen higher up the cord, which are non-contiguous with the testicular primary tumor. If such deposits are limited to the lumina of vessels, as they often are in this location, this finding should not be regarded as T3 disease. If there is invasion of the adjacent soft tissue of the cord (Fig. 34.8), we do consider the case as a T3 tumor, although it could reasonably be argued that they should be considered as soft tissue metastatic deposits rather than as part of the primary T staging.

T4 Tumors

These are defined as showing scrotal invasion (T4) (Fig. 34.8). Although these tumors do occur, they are of great rarity and almost inevitably show metastatic disease at presentation.

Prognostic Factors Not Included in the TNM Staging Classification

There have been a number of recent studies that have challenged the ascendency of TNM and examined other prognostic histopathological markers in testicular tumors. It has become our practice to report most of these routinely to assist clinical decisions after diagnosis.

Percentage of Embryonal Carcinoma

The percentage and volume of embryonal carcinoma are associated with the rate of relapse in stage I NSGCTs [22, 25]. It is recommended that the percentages of the different elements (seminoma, yolk sac tumor, embryonal carcinoma, choriocarcinoma, teratoma) be given in broad estimates after assessment of all the blocks. This should be a practical "eyeball" assessment rather than a tedious non-reproducible exercise. The differences between 40 and 50% embryonal carcinoma are probably of no significance, but a patient whose tumor is composed of 95% teratoma and 5% embryonal carcinoma would be a more appropriate

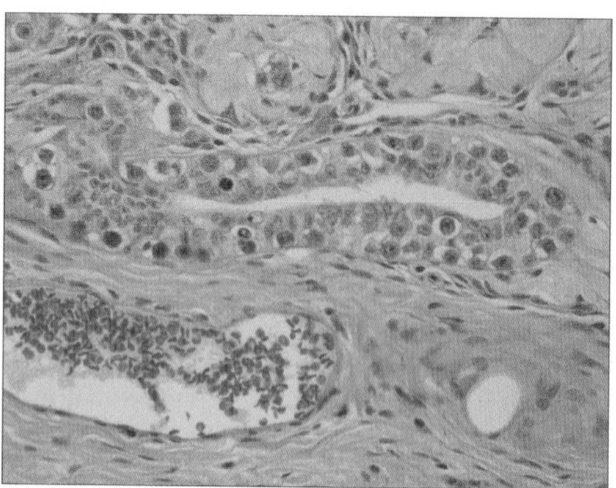

Fig. 34.11 High power of rete testis showing pagetoid invasion of intratubular germ cell neoplasia

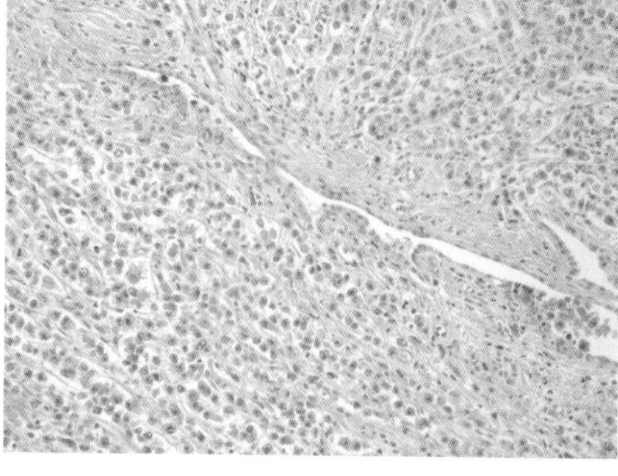

Fig. 34.12 Rete testis surrounded by invasive seminoma. Some loose seminoma cells are also seen in the rete lumen

candidate for surveillance than one having a tumor composed of 95 % embryonal carcinoma.

Size of the Primary Tumour

A number of studies have shown the size of the primary tumor, particularly for seminomas, predicted relapse. One study of patients with seminoma found size greater than 4 cm as a significant independent prognostic factor [20], while another identified a 6-cm cutoff [26]. Another study showed that in non-seminomatous tumors, size was also a prognostic factor, but this was not significant using multivariate analysis [23].

Rete Testis Invasion

As mentioned above, rete testis invasion may be of many types, only some of which are probably of prognostic significance. Pagetoid invasion of the epithelium alone by seminoma-like cells is occasionally seen in association with IGCNU (Fig. 34.11). Also, loose seminoma cells may be seen "floating" within the rete tubules. A number of studies have suggested that rete testis invasion that is interstitial (Fig. 34.12) and not confined to the epithelium is an important prognostic factor in both seminomatous [27, 28] and non-seminomatous germ cell tumors [23]. It should be remembered, however, that size of tumor and rete testis invasion are very closely related. As these are not current parts of the TNM classification, reporting probably depends on discussion with the clinicians, but increasingly, and especially in seminomas, they are being demanded as a pointer to the need for adjuvant treatment for those patients who have clinical stage I disease.

References

1. Sekido R, Lovell-Badge R. Genetic control of testis development. Sex Dev. 2013;7:21–32.
2. Emmen JM, McLuskey A, Adham IM, Engel W, Grootegoed JA, Brinkmann AO. Hormonal control of gubernaculum development during testis descent: gubernaculum outgrowth in vitro requires both insulin-like factor and androgen. Endocrinology. 2000;141:4720–7.
3. Costa WS, Sampaio FJ, Favorito LA, Cardoso LE. Testicular migration: remodeling of connective tissue and muscle cells in human gubernaculum testis. J Urol. 2002;167:2171–6.
4. Giri SK, Berney D, O'Driscoll J, Drumm J, Flood HD, Gupta RK. Choriocarcinoma with teratoma arising from an intra-abdominal testis in patient with persistent Mullerian duct syndrome. Lancet Oncol. 2004;5:451–2.
5. Ismail M, Zaman F, Baithun S, Nargund V, Pati J, Masood J. Inguinal lymph node metastases from a testicular seminoma: a case report and a review of the literature. J Med Case Rep. 2010;4:378.
6. Skakkebaek NE, Rajpert-De Meyts E, Main KM. Testicular dysgenesis syndrome: an increasingly common developmental disorder with environmental aspects. Hum Reprod. 2001;16:972–8.

7. Akre O, Richiardi L. Does a testicular dysgenesis syndrome exist? Hum Reprod. 2009;24:2053–60.
8. Giannarini G, Dieckmann KP, Albers P, Heidenreich A, Pizzocaro G. Organ-sparing surgery for adult testicular tumours: a systematic review of the literature. Eur Urol. 2010;57:780–90.
9. Carmignani L, Gadda F, Gazzano G et al. High incidence of benign testicular neoplasms diagnosed by ultrasound. J Urol. 2003;170:1783–6.
10. Zivkovic D, Bica DT, Hadziselimovic F. Relationship between adult dark spermatogonia and secretory capacity of Leydig cells in cryptorchidism. BJU Int. 2007;100:1147–9. Discussion 1149.
11. Holstein AF, Schulze W, Davidoff M. Understanding spermatogenesis is a prerequisite for treatment. Reprod Biol Endocrinol. 2003;1:107.
12. Joensen UN, Jorgensen N, Skakkebaek NE. Testicular dysgenesis syndrome and carcinoma in situ of the testes. Nat Clin Pract Urol. 2007;4:402–03.
13. Hoei-Hansen CE, Holm M, Rajpert-De Meyts E, Skakkebaek NE. Histological evidence of testicular dysgenesis in contralateral biopsies from 218 patients with testicular germ cell cancer. J Pathol. 2003;200:370–4.
14. Jun SY, Ro JY, Park YW, Kim KR, Ayala AG. Ectopic Leydig cells of testis An immunohistochemical study on tissue microarray. Ann Diagn Pathol. 2008;12:29–32.
15. Paner GP, Kristiansen G, McKenney JK, Amin MB. Rete testis-associated nodular steroid cell nests: description of putative pluripotential testicular hilus steroid cells. Am J Surg Pathol. 2011;35:505–11.
16. Kang MJ, Kim JH, Lee SH, Lee YA, Shin CH, Yang SW. The prevalence of testicular adrenal rest tumors and associated factors in postpubertal patients with congenital adrenal hyperplasia caused by 21-hydroxylase deficiency. Endocr J. 2011;58:501–8.
17. Edge SB, Byrd DR, Compton CC, et al., editors. Testis. AJCC cancer staging manual. 7th ed. New York: Springer; 2010. pp. 469–78.
18. Bruce E, Al-Talib RK, Cook IS, Theaker JM. Vacuolation of seminiferous tubule cells mimicking intratubular germ cell neoplasia (ITGCN). Histopathology. 2006;49:194–6.
19. Looijenga LH, Stoop H, de Leeuw HP, et al. POU5F1 (OCT3/4) identifies cells with pluripotent potential in human germ cell tumors. Cancer Res. 2003;63:2244–50.
20. Warde P, Specht L, Horwich A, et al. Prognostic factors for relapse in stage I seminoma managed by surveillance: a pooled analysis. J Clin Oncol. 2002;20:4448–52.
21. Nicolai N, Miceli R, Artusi R, Piva L, Pizzocaro G, Salvioni R. A simple model for predicting nodal metastasis in patients with clinical stage I nonseminomatous germ cell testicular tumors undergoing retroperitoneal lymph node dissection only. J Urol. 2004;171:172–6.
22. Albers P. Management of stage I testis cancer. Eur Urol. 2007;51:34–43. Discussion 43–34.
23. Yilmaz A, Cheng T, Zhang J, Trpkov K. Testicular hilum and vascular invasion predict advanced clinical stage in nonseminomatous germ cell tumors. Mod Pathol. 2013;26(4):579–86.
24. Ernst DS, Brasher P, Venner PM, et al. Compliance and outcome of patients with stage 1 non-seminomatous germ cell tumors (NSGCT) managed with surveillance programs in seven Canadian centres. Can J Urol. 2005;12:2575–80.
25. Atsu N, Eskicorapci S, Uner A, et al. A novel surveillance protocol for stage I nonseminomatous germ cell testicular tumours. BJU Int. 2003;92:32–5.
26. Parker C, Milosevic M, Panzarella T, et al. The prognostic significance of the tumour infiltrating lymphocyte count in stage I testicular seminoma managed by surveillance. Eur J Cancer. 2002;38:2014–9.
27. Choo R, Thomas G, Woo T, et al. Long-term outcome of postorchiectomy surveillance for Stage I testicular seminoma. Int J Radiat Oncol Biol Phys. 2005;61:736–40.
28. Browne TJ, Richie JP, Gilligan TD, Rubin MA. Intertubular growth in pure seminomas: associations with poor prognostic parameters. Hum Pathol. 2005;36:640–5.

Classification of Testicular Tumors

35

Cristina Magi-Galluzzi and Thomas M. Ulbright

Introduction

Testicular cancers, the great majority of which are of germ cell origin, represent the most common solid malignancy affecting males between the ages of 15 and 35 years, although they account for only 1–1.5 % of all neoplasms in males and 5 % of urological tumors in general. Despite their relative infrequency compared to other malignancies of genitourinary origin, they have a complex morphological spectrum.

Germ Cell Tumors

Testicular germ cell tumors (GCT) represent the most frequent malignancies among men aged 15–45 years [1]; their incidence in Western countries has been increasing for decades, and this trend appears to be ongoing [2]. Germ cell tumors originate most frequently in the testis and the ovaries, but they can also occur in extragonadal sites. Over 90 % of testicular tumors are of germ cell origin. Only approximately 3 % of cases are bilateral at diagnosis.

GCTs are broadly categorized as seminomas or non-seminomatous GCTs (NSGCTs). The peak incidence is in the third decade of life for NSGCTs and in the fourth decade for pure seminoma. The group of NSGCTs includes embryonal carcinoma, yolk sac tumor, teratoma, and choriocarcinoma. Any component of a NSGCT, regardless of how minor, places the case in the NSGCT category, even if otherwise it is all seminoma. The recommended pathological classification (modified from the 2004 version of the World Health Organization [WHO] guide) is shown in Table 35.1 [3, 4]. GCTs may consist of one predominant histologic pattern or represent a mixture of multiple histologic types.

A small metacentric marker chromosome, identified as an isochromosome of the short arm of chromosome 12 [i(12p)], that results in excess DNA from this locus, or other forms of chromosome 12p amplification, have been reported in almost all GCTs analyzed, suggesting that this karyotypic abnormality is characteristic of the whole spectrum of the postpubertal germ cell tumors of the testis [5].

Intratubular Germ Cell Neoplasia

The evolution of the concept of intratubular germ cell neoplasia (also known as testicular intraepithelial neoplasia or carcinoma in situ) indicates that most adult germ cell tumors of

C. Magi-Galluzzi (✉)
Department of Pathology, Cleveland Clinic, Robert J. Tomsich Pathology and Laboratory Medicine Institute, Cleveland, OH, USA
e-mail: magic@ccf.org

T. M. Ulbright
Department of Pathology and Laboratory Medicine, Indiana University School of Medicine, Indianapolis, IN, USA
e-mail: tulbright@iupui.edu

C. Magi-Galluzzi, C. G. Przybycin (eds.), *Genitourinary Pathology,* DOI 10.1007/978-1-4939-2044-0_35,

Table 35.1 Recommended pathological classification of testicular germ cell tumors

Germ cell tumors
Intratubular germ cell neoplasia
Seminoma
Classic
With syncytiotrophoblastic cells
Spermatocytic seminoma (mention if there is sarcomatous component)
Embryonal carcinoma
Yolk sac tumor
Choriocarcinoma
Teratoma (specify if with a secondary malignant component and type)
Tumors with more than one histological type (specify percentage of individual components)
Sex cord/gonadal stromal tumors
Leydig cell tumor
Malignant Leydig cell tumor
Sertoli cell tumor
Large cell calcifying
Sclerosing
Intratubular large cell hyalinizing
Malignant Sertoli cell tumor
Granulosa cell tumor
Juvenile type
Adult type
Thecoma/fibroma group of tumors
Tumors containing germ cell and sex cord/gonadal stromal components
Gonadoblastoma
Unclassified
Miscellaneous tumors of the testis
Carcinoid tumor
Brenner tumor
Tumors of ovarian epithelial types
Others
Metastatic tumors to the testis

the testis evolve from a common neoplastic precursor lesion: intratubular germ cell neoplasia, unclassified type (IGCNU). At 5 years about 50% of patients with a testicular biopsy positive for IGCNU have developed invasive germ cell tumors, and only a small fraction remain free of invasive tumors by 7 years.

Microscopically, IGCNU is characterized by seminiferous tubules showing decreased or absent spermatogenesis. The cells normally lining the tubules are replaced by basally located undifferentiated germ cells. The malignant germ cells have

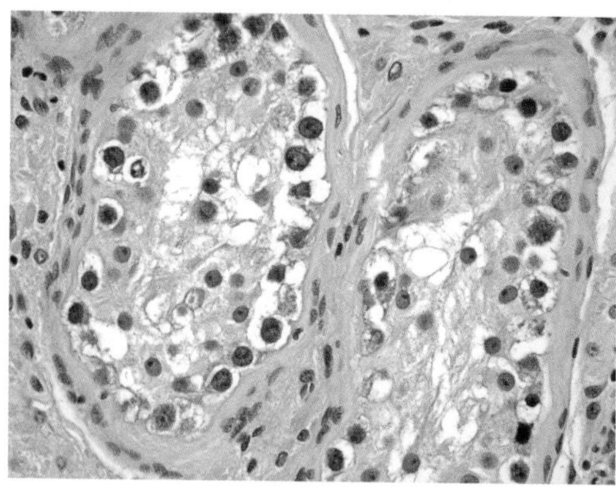

Fig. 35.1 Intratubular germ cell neoplasia, unclassified type (IGCNU). The malignant germ cells have enlarged, polygonal nuclei, coarse chromatin, enlarged single or multiple nucleoli, and clear cytoplasm (40X)

the appearance of seminoma cells with enlarged, polygonal nuclei, coarse chromatin, enlarged single or multiple nucleoli, clear cytoplasm, and distinct cell membranes (Fig. 35.1). IGCNU cells express PLAP, CD117, SALL4, podoplanin, and OCT3/4 (Fig. 35.2a, b) (see Chap. 40).

Seminoma

Seminoma is the most frequent GCT (27–56% of all germ cell neoplasms) and occurs most commonly in young to middle aged men (mean age at diagnosis 40 years) [6]. Grossly, it is typically a diffuse or multinodular soft tan-white mass (Fig. 35.3); focal necrosis may be present. Seminoma cells morphologically and immunophenotypically resemble embryonic germ cells. On microscopic examination, seminoma is characterized by a framework of delicate fibrous septa with associated blood vessels and a sprinkling of lymphocytes (Fig. 35.4). A granulomatous reaction, usually consisting of clusters of epithelioid histiocytes, is present in approximately 50% of cases (Fig. 35.5). The tumor cells have distinct cytoplasmic membranes and polygonal nuclei, which often have "squared-off" nuclear edges, with large nucleoli (Fig. 35.6). Mitoses are variable in number but easily identified. In approximately 10% of cases, syncytiotrophoblastic cells are identified on routine sections, but these cases

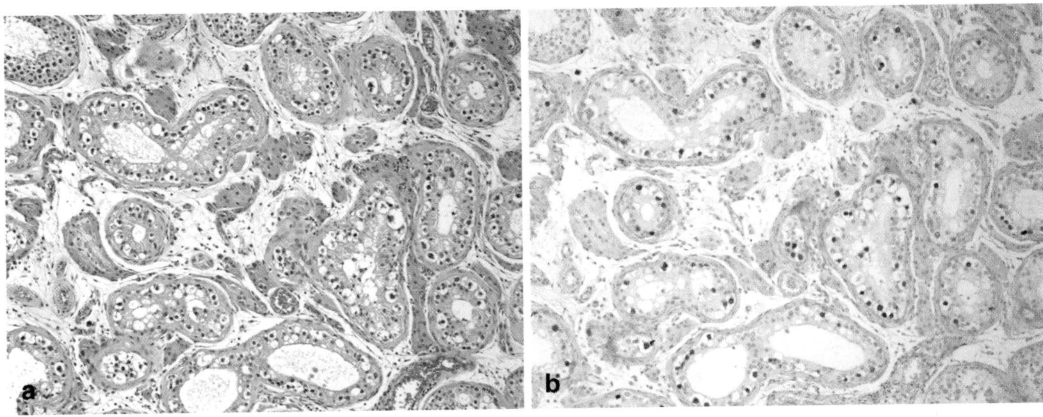

Fig. 35.2 The malignant cells of IGCNU (**a**) are positive for OCT3/4 (**b**) (10X)

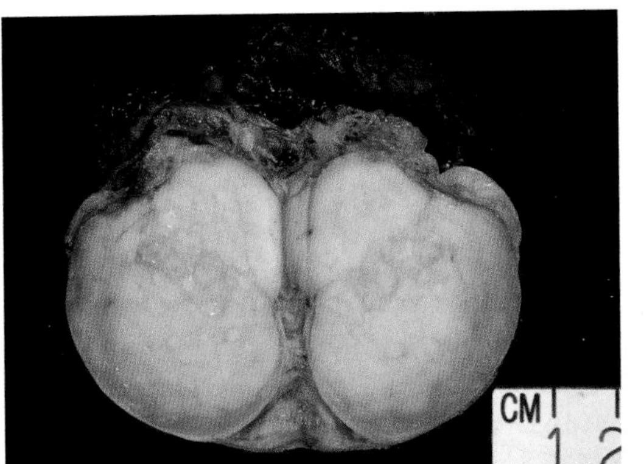

Fig. 35.3 Typical multinodular *tan-white* seminoma

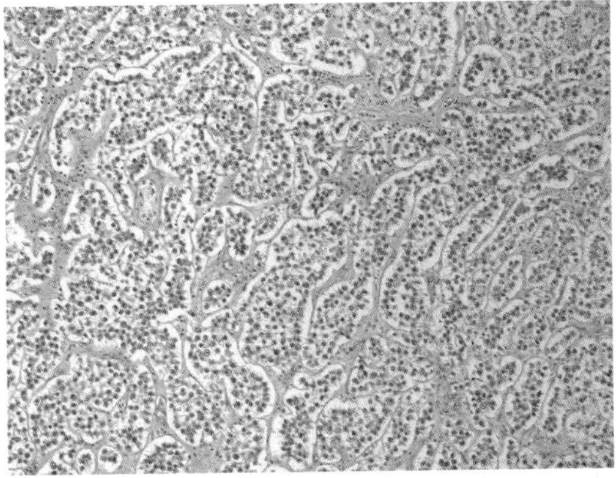

Fig. 35.4 Seminoma composed of uniform cells divided into clusters by delicate fibrous septa associated with mild lymphocytic infiltrate (10X)

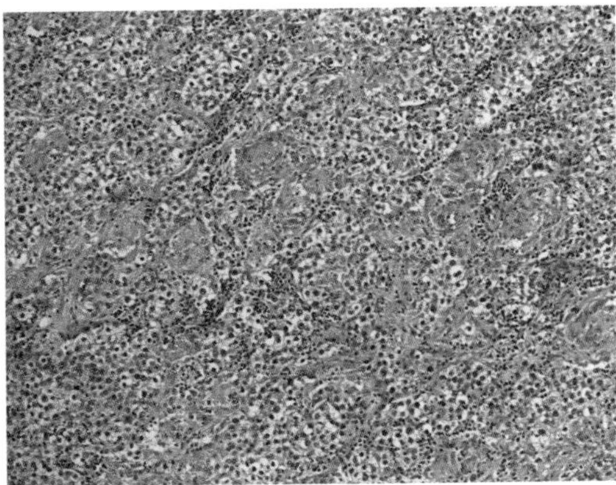

Fig. 35.5 Seminoma with pronounced granulomatous reaction (10X)

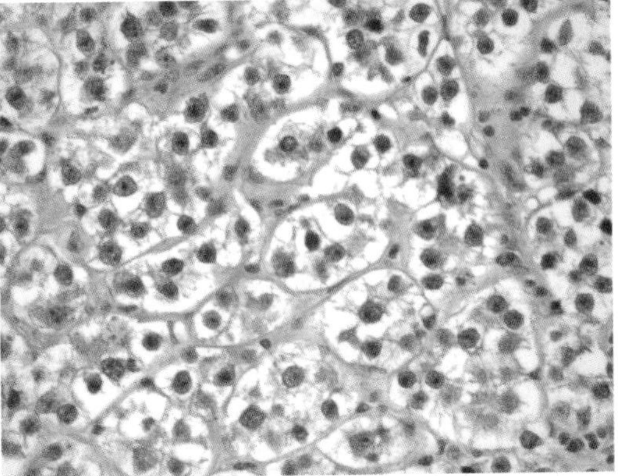

Fig. 35.6 Seminoma cells have distinct cytoplasmic membranes and polygonal nuclei, which often have "squared-off" nuclear edges, with large nucleoli (40X)

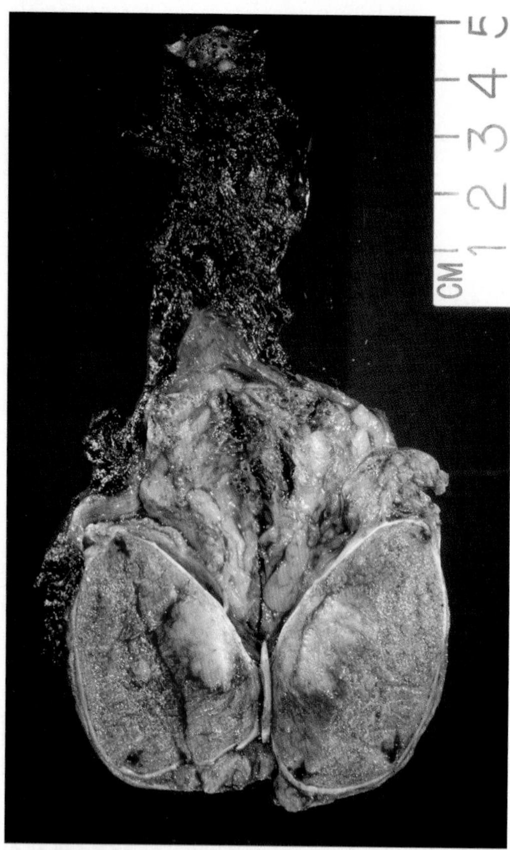

Fig. 35.7 Embryonal carcinoma grossly characterized by a soft gray-pink tumor with peripheral hemorrhage

are still classified as "pure" seminoma. Similar to IGCNU, seminoma cells express PLAP, CD117, SALL4, podoplanin, SOX17, and OCT3/4.

Seminoma, 80 % of which are diagnosed at stage I, is highly sensitive to both radiotherapy and chemotherapy and, therefore, cure is an expected outcome in the majority of cases, even with metastatic disease at presentation [7]. The classical and the syncytiotrophoblastic types of seminoma behave similarly, although the syncytiotrophoblastic subtype is associated with increased serum beta HCG levels. The spermatocytic type is infrequent, occurs in older men, and has a better prognosis since it rarely metastasizes (<1 % of cases) in the absence of sarcomatous transformation, which is very rare. Spermatocytic seminoma and seminoma variants are discussed in Chap. 37.

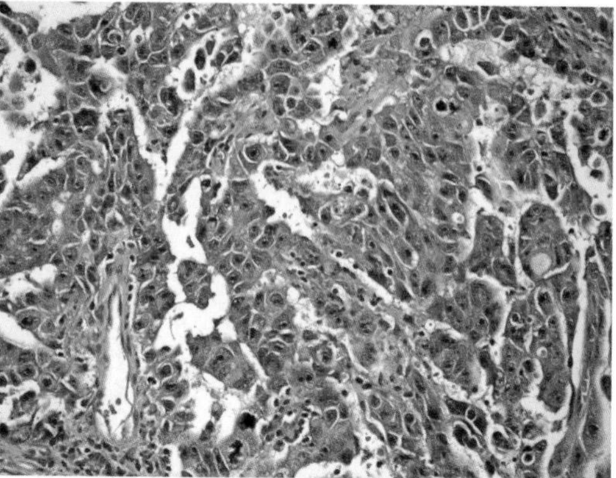

Fig. 35.8 Embryonal carcinoma cells are pleomorphic with abundant cytoplasm and large, irregular nuclei with prominent macronucleoli. The cells border are usually indistinct and the cells tend to crowd with overlapping nuclei (20X)

Embryonal Carcinoma

Although pure embryonal carcinoma comprises approximately 10 % of testicular germ cell tumors, it occurs as a component in more than 80 % of mixed germ cell tumors, mostly in young men, with a peak of incidence around 30 years of age [4, 6]. Grossly, embryonal carcinoma is soft gray-red to tan-yellow with foci of hemorrhage and necrosis (Fig. 35.7). Microscopically it is composed of pleomorphic cells with abundant cytoplasm and large, irregular nuclei with prominent macronucleoli. The cells border are usually indistinct and the cells tend to crowd with overlapping nuclei (Fig. 35.8). Mitotic figures are frequent. The cells can form sheets or acinar, glandular (Fig. 35.9a), papillary (Fig. 35.9b), and tubular structures. Embryonal carcinomas express PLAP, OCT3/4, CD30, SALL4, SOX2, and cytokeratin; EMA and vimentin are usually negative.

Yolk Sac Tumor

Yolk sac tumor is the most common testicular neoplasm in children and occurs in all races: 80 % of pure yolk sac tumors occur in the first 2 years of life. Unlike the germ cell tumors of older patients, those in children have had a steady

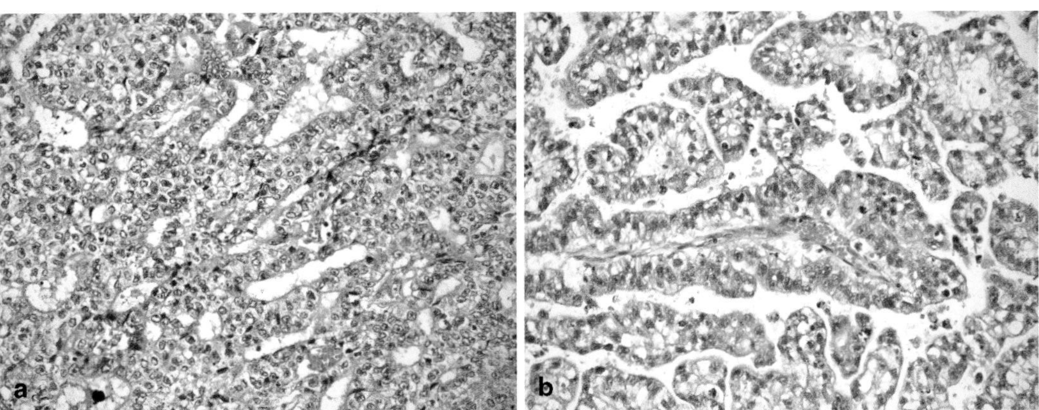

Fig. 35.9 Embryonal carcinoma with glandular (**a**), and papillary (**b**) growth pattern (20X)

incidence over the years and are not associated with IGCNU. Pure yolk sac tumor in adults is uncommon, comprising approximately 1.5% of testicular germ cell tumors; however, yolk sac tumor is found as a component of ~40% of mixed germ cell tumors. The age of incidence in adults corresponds to that of patients with testicular mixed germ cell tumors. Serum alpha fetoprotein (AFP) levels are elevated in 90% of cases.

On gross examination, the tumor is typically solid and soft, white-gray or light yellow with areas of cystic degeneration (Fig. 35.10). Large tumors may show necrosis and hemorrhage. Several microscopic growth patterns have been described, with the microcystic or reticular pattern being the most common one (Fig. 35.11a) [4, 6, 8] and consisting of sheets of prominently vacuolated tumor cells (lipoblast-like) or an anastomosing network of flattened neoplastic cells in a loose stroma. Other patterns include macrocystic, papillary (Fig. 35.11b), glandular, endodermal sinus, solid, myxomatous (Fig. 35.11c), polyvesicular vitelline, hepatoid, enteric, and parietal. Schiller-Duval bodies and eosinophilic hyaline globules are highly characteristic of yolk sac tumor. The former consist of solitary papillae with a central vascular core enveloped by endodermal epithelium. Hyaline globules are non-membrane-bound cytoplasmic and extracellular globules of uncertain composition. Another characteristic finding is bandlike deposits of extracellular basement membrane between tumor cells, so-called parietal differentiation of the tumor.

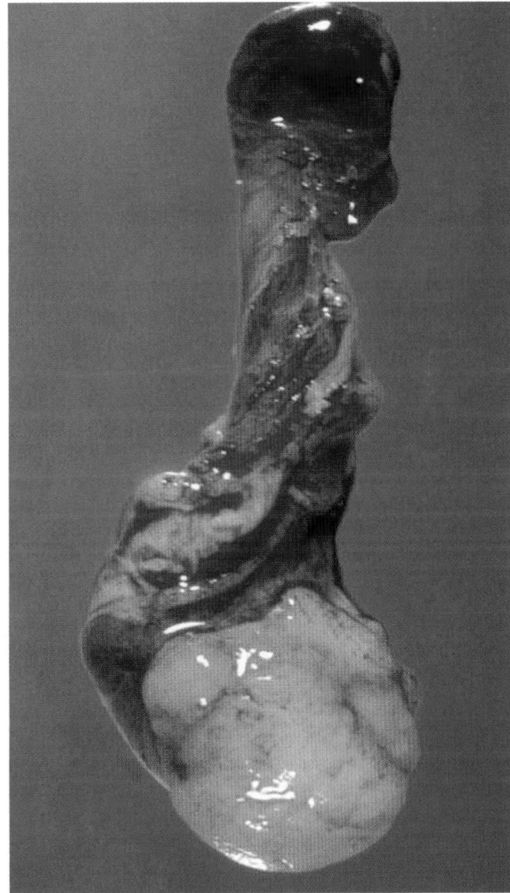

Fig. 35.10 Yolk sac macroscopically characterized by a solid and soft, light gray-yellow tumor

The tumor cells stain for low molecular weight cytokeratin (but not cytokeratin 7), PLAP,

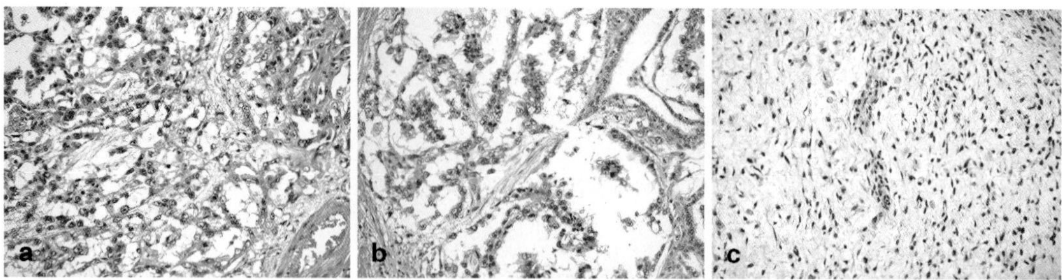

Fig. 35.11 Yolk sac tumor with microcystic or reticular pattern (**a**), papillary pattern (**b**), and myxomatous pattern (**c**) (20X)

glypican 3 and focally for AFP, but are negative for OCT3/4. The solid variant of yolk sac tumor, which may be confused with seminoma, is discussed in Chap. 37.

Choriocarcinoma

Choriocarcinoma is very rare (<1 %) as a pure testicular germ cell tumor; much more often it is admixed with other germ cell tumor elements. It occurs in young patients (mean age 25–30 years) who commonly present with symptoms related to metastatic disease. The patients typically have elevated levels of serum HCG. Grossly, it commonly forms a hemorrhagic and necrotic nodule (Fig. 35.12).

Histologically choriocarcinoma is composed of an admixture of syncytiotrophoblastic, cytotrophoblastic, and intermediate trophoblastic cells (Fig. 35.13a, b). The cytotrophoblastic cells are mononucleated with pale to clear cytoplasm, marked nuclear atypia, and one or two prominent nucleoli. The syncytiotrophoblastic cells are multinucleated with abundant eosinophilic to basophilic cytoplasm; they typically have several, large, irregularly shaped, hyperchromatic nuclei that frequently have a "smudged" appearance (Fig. 35.13a). Intermediate trophoblastic cells have eosinophilic to clear cytoplasm and single

Fig. 35.12 Testis largely replaced by a hemorrhagic nodule of choriocarcinoma

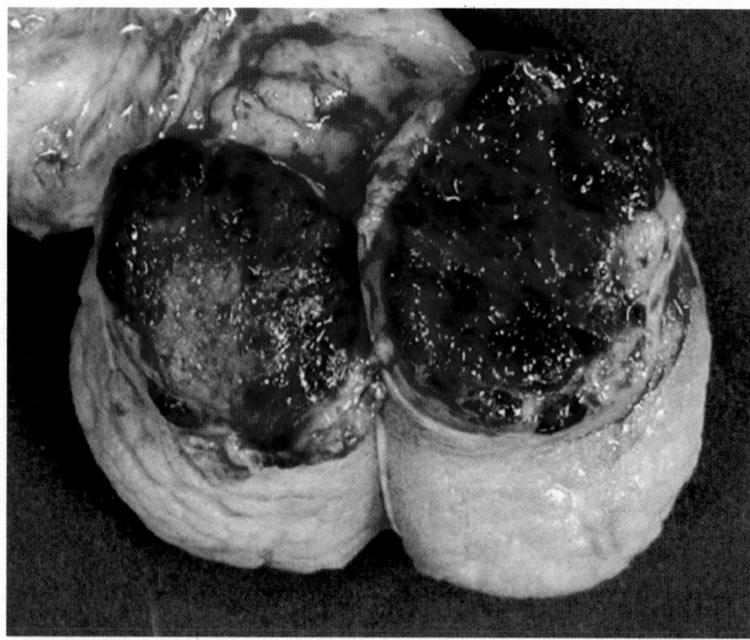

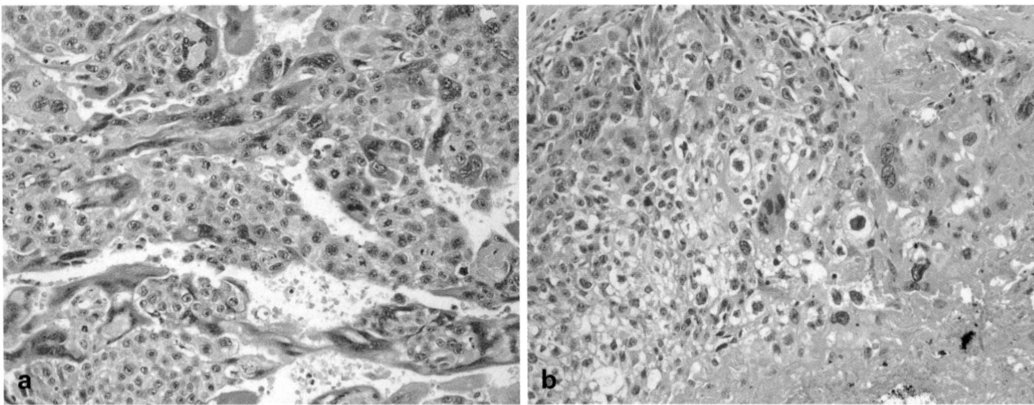

Fig. 35.13 Choriocarcinoma composed of an admixture of syncytiotrophoblastic, cytotrophoblastic (**a**), and intermediate trophoblastic cells in a hemorrhagic background (**b**)

nuclei. The background is extensively hemorrhagic and necrotic [4, 6] (Fig. 35.13b).

The syncytiotrophoblastic cells express HCG, but the cytotrophoblastic ones show weak to no staining. All cell types express cytokeratin, and about half of the cases express EMA and PLAP. Inhibin is also typically positive.

Teratoma

Teratoma occurs in two age groups: in children the incidence ranges from 24 to 36%; in adults pure teratoma accounts for 2.7–7% of testicular germ cell tumors, but a teratomatous component is detected in approximately half of germ cell tumors. Teratoma is the second most common germ cell tumor in young children (first and second year of life), in whom it is invariably benign. On the other hand, almost all tumors occurring at postpubertal ages (young adults) have a malignant potential, even when histologically mature [8]. Most lesions are nodular and firm and have a heterogeneous cut surface with solid and cystic areas (Fig. 35.14). Cartilage, bone, and pigmented areas may be recognizable.

Mature teratoma is composed of well-differentiated somatic tissues resembling those seen at other body sites, including squamous, enteric, and respiratory epithelium, cartilage, and muscular tissue. Immature teratoma, in addition to mature elements, contains incompletely differentiated tissues resembling those of embryonic development including immature neuroectoderm, Wilms tumor-like blastema and stroma and rhabdomyoblastic cells. The teratomas in the postpubertal group commonly show cytologic atypia and disorganized arrangements of elements, whereas those in the prepubertal patients are cytologically bland and frequently organoid. This disparity in morphology reflects their derivation from either IGCNU (postpubertal group) or a non-transformed, benign germ cell (prepubertal group). The presence of immature elements does not alter the behavior of the postpubertal tumors, and it is therefore not considered necessary to make a distinction between mature and immature teratoma. Teratoma with a secondary malignant component is characterized by overgrowth of a malignancy resembling those seen at somatic sites, either a sarcoma, or a carcinoma, or both. A secondary sarcoma (such as primitive neuroectodermal

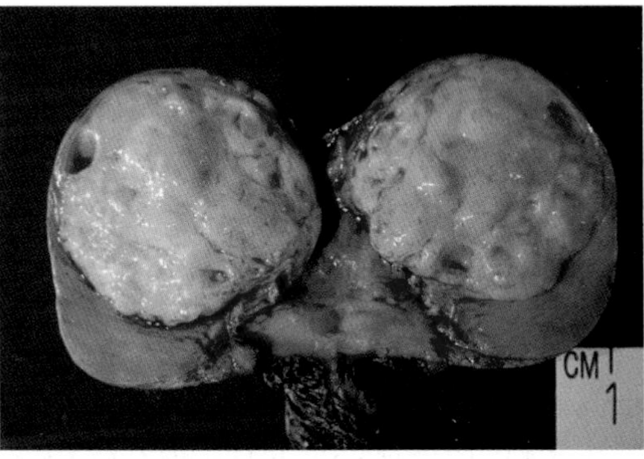

Fig. 35.14 Teratoma with heterogeneous cut surface with solid and cystic areas

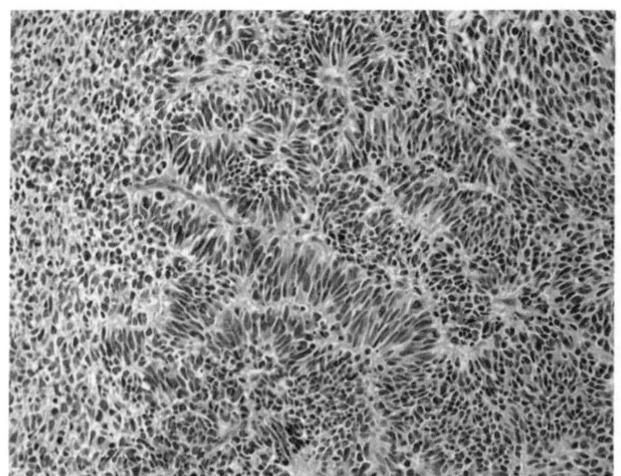

Fig. 35.15 Primitive neuroectodermal tumor (PNET) arising in a teratoma

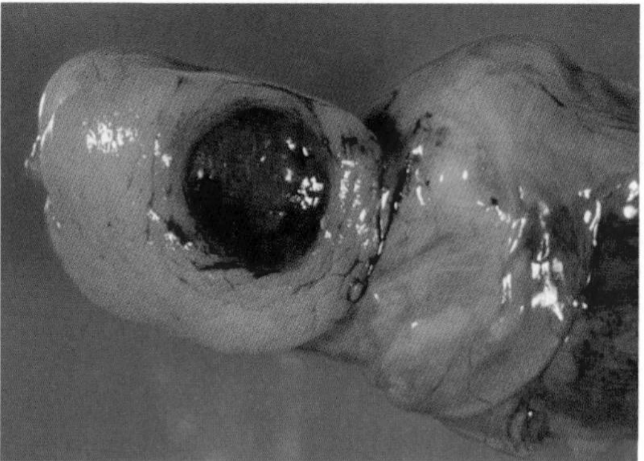

Fig. 35.16 Testis with a well-circumscribed solid tan nodule of Leydig cell tumor

tumor or PNET) arising in a teratoma should be considered when the sarcoma forms a nodule equal to or greater than a 4X objective microscopic field (Fig. 35.15).

Epidermoid cyst, dermoid cyst (mature cystic teratoma), and non-dermoid benign teratoma are discussed in Chap. 37.

Sex Cord/Gonadal Stromal Tumors

Testicular stromal tumors are rare and account for only 2–4 % of adult testicular tumors.

Leydig Cell Tumor

Leydig cell tumors are the most common type of sex cord/gonadal stromal tumor, accounting for 1–3 % of adult testicular neoplasms [9] and 3 % of tumors in infants and children. Approximately 3 % of Leydig cell tumors are bilateral [10]. They exhibit a peak incidence in preadolescent children (3–9 years old) as well as in the older (third to sixth decade) age groups.

Grossly, they are typically well circumscribed, solid, and usually yellow or yellow-tan (Fig. 35.16). Hemorrhage and/or necrosis may be present in 30 % of cases and cause concern for malignancy. Microscopically, the cells are polygonal, with abundant eosinophilic, slightly granular cytoplasm, occasional Reinke crystals (found in approximately 1/3 of cases), and regular nuclei. The most common microscopic pattern is diffuse (Fig. 35.17a), although growth as large tumor nodules, nests, pseudoglandular structures (Fig. 35.17b), and cords may also occur [8]. The cells express vimentin, inhibin, S-100 protein, steroid hormones, calretinin, cytokeratin (focally), and steroidogenic factor-1 [SF-1] [11, 12].

Leydig cell tumors must be distinguished from the multinodular tumor-like and often bilaterally occurring lesions of the adrenogenital syndrome (so-called testicular tumor of the adrenogenital syndrome). The latter usually has a more prominent fibrous stroma, increased cytoplasmic lipofuscin and is positive for synaptophysin and negative for androgen receptor, with Leydig cell tumors having the opposite immunohistochemical pattern [13].

Unusual morphologic features of Leydig cell tumor, such as cyst formation, adipose metaplasia, calcification or ossification and spindle cell pattern, have been described [14, 15]. Cystic spaces may result in confusion with yolk sac tumor; adipose differentiation may be seen in some cases of the testicular tumor of the androgenital syndrome, further complicating the distinction of these two entities.

Malignant Leydig Cell Tumor

Up to 10 % of Leydig cell tumors are malignant. About 15–20 % of the patients with malignant

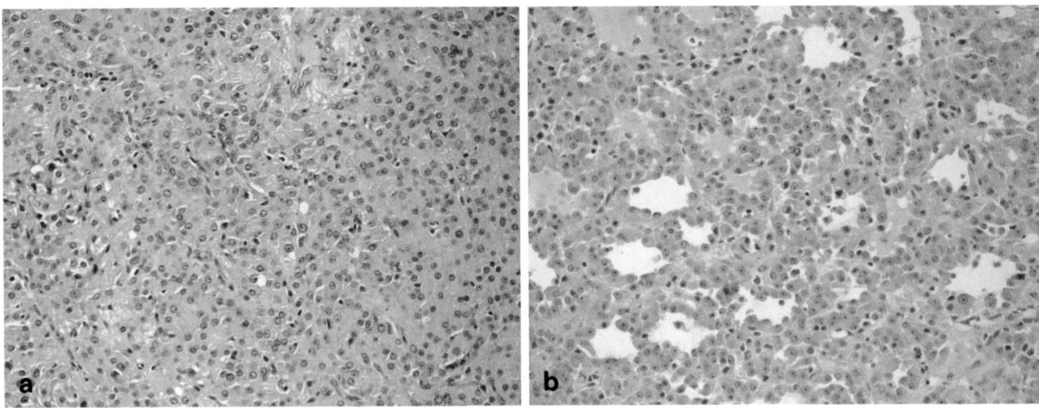

Fig. 35.17 Leydig cell tumor with diffuse (**a**) and pseudoglandular (**b**) pattern of growth (20X)

Leydig cell tumors already present with metastatic disease, particularly in the lymph nodes, lung, and liver. The diagnosis of malignancy is not always easy since there are no absolute histological criteria.

Malignant tumors are associated with the following parameters: large size (>5 cm), nuclear atypia, increased mitotic activity (>3 per 10 high-power field), increased MIB-1 expression (18.6 vs 1.2% in benign), necrosis, lymphovascular invasion, infiltrative margins, extension beyond the testicular parenchyma (invasion into rete testis, epididymis, or tunica), and DNA aneuploidy [16, 17]. In addition, older patients seem to have a greater risk of harboring a tumor of malignant potential. Based on personal experience, there are, however, rare cases that lack all of these features that have nonetheless followed a malignant course. For this reason it is prudent to consider Leydig cell tumors to be neoplasms with a spectrum of biological behavior from those at very low risk to those with highly elevated risk for malignant behavior based on the pathologic findings.

In tumors with histological signs of malignancy, especially in patients of older age, orchidectomy and retroperitoneal lymphadenectomy is recommended. Tumors that have metastasized to lymph nodes, lung, liver, or bone are generally refractory to chemotherapy or radiation and survival is poor [18].

Sertoli Cell Tumor

Sertoli cell tumors account for about 1% of testicular tumors, and the mean age at diagnosis is around 45 years, with rare cases under 20 years of age [19]. Certain subtypes of Sertoli cell tumors (large cell calcifying Sertoli cell tumor, intratubular large cell hyalinizing Sertoli cell neoplasia and Sertoli cell adenoma) may develop in patients with certain clinical conditions (the Carney complex, Peutz-Jeghers syndrome and the androgen insensitivity syndrome, respectively).

Most classic Sertoli tumors are unilateral and unifocal. Grossly the tumors are well circumscribed, yellow, tan or white, with an average diameter of 3.5 cm. Cystic changes may be present. Hemorrhage and necrosis may be seen, particularly in malignant tumors [8]. Microscopically, the cells are eosinophilic to pale with vacuolated cytoplasm. The nuclei are usually regular, sometimes grooved and there may be inclusions. The arrangement of the cells is tubular or solid; a cord-like or retiform pattern is possible (Fig. 35.18). The stroma is typically fine, but in some cases a sclerosing aspect predominates. In many cases a prominent diffuse growth pattern with limited evidence of tubular formation has been reported. The cells express vimentin, cytokeratins, inhibin (40%), and S-100 protein (30%) [19].

Two subtypes of Sertoli cell tumors are currently recognized as distinct variants which differ in apparent malignant potential as well as association with extragonadal disease processes.

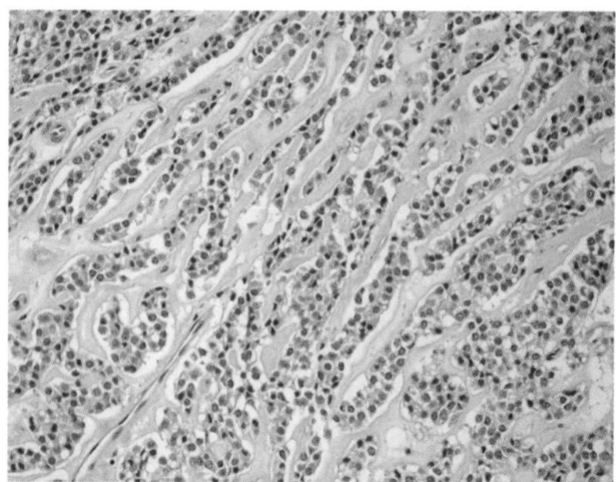

Fig. 35.18 Sertoli cell tumor. The cells are arranged in a cord-like pattern (20X)

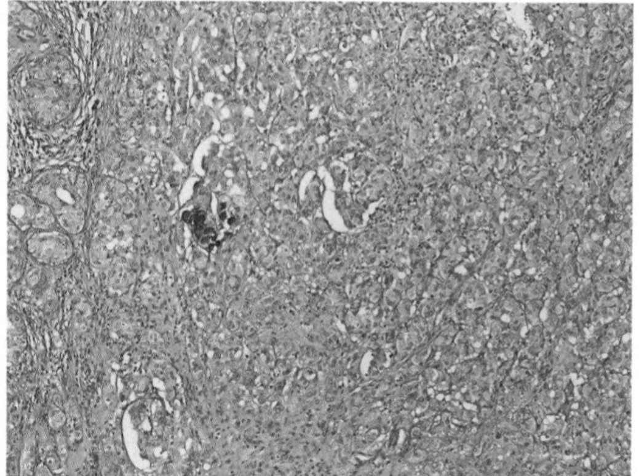

Fig. 35.19 Large-cell calcifying Sertoli cell tumor

Determination of the histological subtype is essential to allow appropriate risk-adapted therapy.

Large-Cell Calcifying Sertoli Cell Tumor

Large-cell calcifying Sertoli cell tumor is diagnosed in younger men (mean age 16 years) and is related to the Carney complex in up to 40 % of the cases and rarely the Peutz-Jeghers syndrome (which is more characteristically associated with intratubular large cell hyalinizing Sertoli cell neoplasia). It occurs predominantly in children and young adults [20]. Macroscopically, the tumors are usually smaller than 4 cm, have well-defined margins, and are yellow-tan. Tumors can be multifocal and bilateral in 20–40 % of cases, almost always in syndromic cases. This variant of Sertoli cell tumor form has a characteristic image on ultrasound study, with brightly echogenic foci due to calcifications.

Microscopically, tumor cells are organized in sheets, nests, cords, ribbons, and trabeculae and there is usually focal solid tubule formation. The cytoplasm of the tumor cells is eosinophilic and the surrounding stroma can be myxoid to collagenous with frequent neutrophilic infiltration [21]. Prominent foci of calcification with large laminated calcified nodules are a frequent finding and are considered to be one of the diagnostic criteria (Fig. 35.19).

Malignant tumors are more likely to be unilateral and solitary. A strong association with malignant behavior has been reported with size larger than 4 cm, extratesticular growth, necrosis, high-grade cytologic atypia, vascular invasion, and a mitotic rate of more than three mitoses for ten high-power fields. All malignant cases exhibited at least two of the above-mentioned features [22]. There are some hints that discrimination between an early and late onset type may define a different risk for metastatic disease (5.5 % compared with 23 %) [23]. In the malignant cases the prognosis is very poor and it is difficult to select the best treatment because of the limited experience with this type of tumor.

Since tumors occurring in younger patients with genetic syndromes and/or endocrine abnormalities have a low malignant potential and rarely give rise to distant metastases, in cases suspicious for large cell calcifying Sertoli tumors, partial orchiectomy is recommended over total orchiectomy, especially if bilateral and multifocal [20, 24].

Intratubular large cell hyalinizing Sertoli cell neoplasia and large cell calcifying Sertoli cell tumor are also discussed in Chap. 37.

Sclerosing Sertoli Cell Tumor

Forty-two cases of sclerosing Sertoli cell tumor have been reported [25, 26]. Grossly the tumor is a hard, well circumscribed, white to tan nodule. Histologically the tumor is characterized by solid and hollow, simple and anastomosing tubules, large irregular aggregates, and thin cords of Sertoli cells in a prominent collagenous background [27] (Fig. 35.20). The tumor cells are of medium

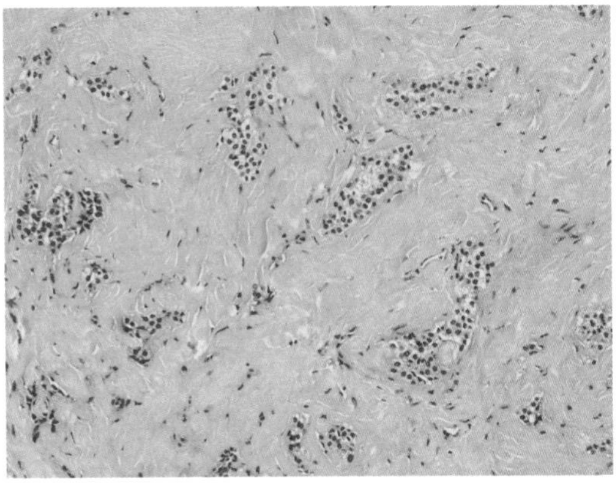

Fig. 35.20 Sclerosing Sertoli cell tumor composed of thin cords of Sertoli cells in a prominent collagenous background

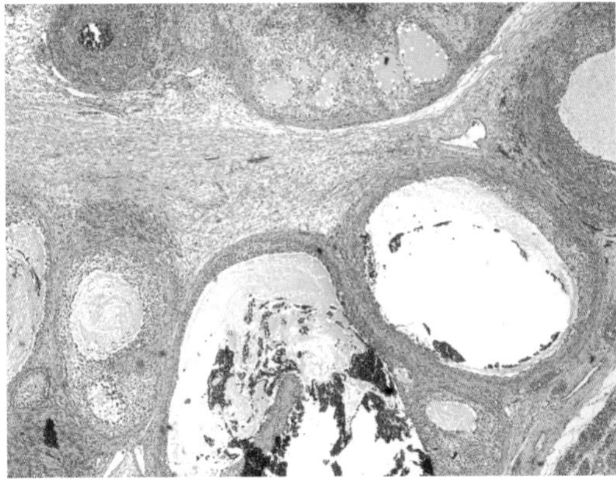

Fig. 35.21 Low-power magnification of juvenile type granulosa cell tumor with mixed epithelial and stromal pattern and cyst formation (4X)

size and have pale cytoplasm, which sometimes contained large lipid vacuoles; the round nuclei vary from small and dark to vesicular. Only one case of sclerosing Sertoli cell tumor with a malignant course has been reported [26], and this tumor, unlike the others, exhibited invasive growth and lymphovascular involvement.

Malignant Sertoli Cell Tumor

The rate of malignant tumors ranges between 10 and 22 %, and fewer than 50 cases have been reported [22, 28]. Features of a malignant Sertoli tumor are large size (>5 cm), moderate to severe nuclear atypia, increased mitotic activity (>5 per 10 HPF), necrosis, and vascular invasion [8]. A diffuse growth pattern is more likely to be seen in malignant tumors.

Granulosa Cell Tumors

Granulosa cell tumor is a sex cord/stromal neoplasm that more commonly arises in the ovaries. Approximately 80 cases have been reported in the testis, 30 of the adult type, and 50 of the juvenile type [29]. Malignant tumors represent around 20 % of the adult cases. They are usually >7 cm diameter. Vascular invasion and necrosis are features suggestive of a malignant clinical course. The behavior of the juvenile type has been uniformly benign, in contrast to the ovarian counterpart.

Juvenile Type Granulosa Cell Tumor

The juvenile type granulosa cell tumor mostly involves infants (typically in the first few months of life) and has a benign course. It is the most frequent congenital tumor of the testis and represents 6.6 % of all prepubertal testicular neoplasms. These tumors are white-yellow and lobulated, vary greatly in size, and may replace most of the testis. A partially cystic appearance is characteristic. The microscopic appearance ranges from predominantly epithelial to predominantly stromal, although a mixed pattern with some degree of follicle formation is the most common [8] (Fig. 35.21). A lobular pattern at low magnification is typical. The nuclei usually lack the nuclear grooves characteristic of the ovarian adult granulosa cell tumor. Juvenile granulosa cell tumors in males are always benign, and simple orchiectomy suffices for cure.

Juvenile granulosa cell tumor is also discussed in Chap. 37.

Adult Type Granulosa Cell Tumor

With the adult type, the average age at presentation is 44 years. The typical morphology is of a homogeneous, yellow-grey tumor, with elongated cells with grooves in diffuse, microfollicular, and

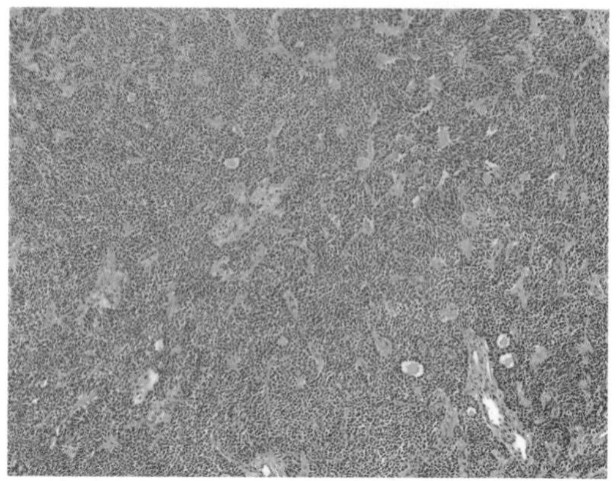

Fig. 35.22 Low-power magnification of adult type granulosa cell tumor

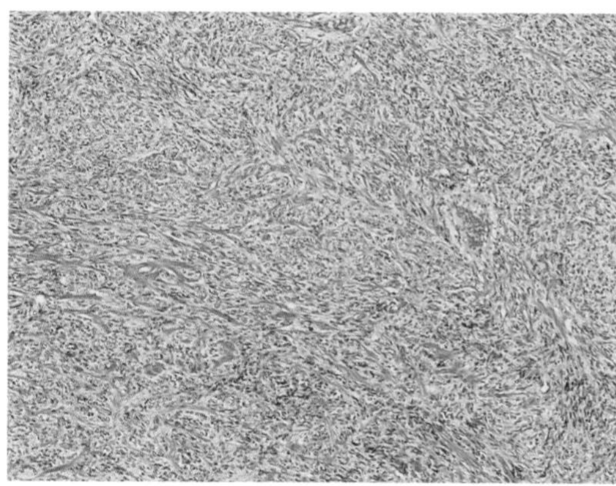

Fig. 35.23 Low-power magnification of testicular fibrothecoma

Call-Exner body arrangements (Fig. 35.22). The tumor cells express CD99, calretinin, inhibin, and may express smooth muscle actin. Keratin stains, placental alkaline phosphatase, and CD117 are negative, excluding embryonal carcinoma and seminoma. AFP, which is positive in yolk sac tumor, is negative in granulosa cell tumors [29].

Similarly to the ovarian counterpart, approximately 20% of testicular adult type granulosa cell tumors have been reported to be malignant [30, 31]. Tumor size larger than 5 cm has been suggested as a feature associated with malignancy in the testis [32]. However, there are no established discriminating criteria at present to predict which tumors will follow an aggressive course.

Fibrothecoma

Thecomas are benign stromal tumors arising from ovarian theca cells and constitute 1% of all ovarian tumors. Ovarian stromal tumors are classified into either thecoma or fibroma, and frequently grouped together as "fibrothecoma."

Testicular fibrothecoma is a rare intratesticular spindle cell neoplasm [33]. It presents most commonly in the third and fourth decades of life as a painless testicular mass, or rarely with scrotal pain. It ranges from 0.5 to 7.6 cm in diameter and appears as a tan-white, well-circumscribed, although not encapsulated, firm nodule [34]. Macroscopically, fibrothecomas typically about the tunica albuginea; occasionally they may be centered on the rete testis. Hemorrhage or necrosis is not present. Microscopically, the tumor is mildly to markedly cellular with bland spindle cells arranged in a randomly interweaving or storiform pattern (Fig. 35.23). Small dilated blood vessels are frequently present. Various degrees of collagen deposition can be seen, either in bands or investing individual cells, and may form acellular plaques within the tumor. Tumor cells show variable immunoreactivity for inhibin, calretinin, melan-A, pan keratin, smooth muscle actin, and vimentin [33, 34]. Although testicular fibrothecoma may show worrisome features including minimal invasion into the surrounding stroma, elevated mitotic rates, and high cellularity, their behavior appears to be uniformly benign [34].

Thecoma is an extremely rare tumor in the testis and only two cases have been reported to date, one of them in the context of the Gorlin syndrome. This tumor arose from the tunica albuginea of the testis and was composed predominantly by spindle cells with occasional luteinization [35].

Tumors Containing Germ Cell and Sex Cord/Gonadal Stromal Cells

Gonadoblastoma

Gonadoblastoma is a rare gonadal neoplasm that occurs mostly in individuals who are phenotypic females and have an underlying gonadal

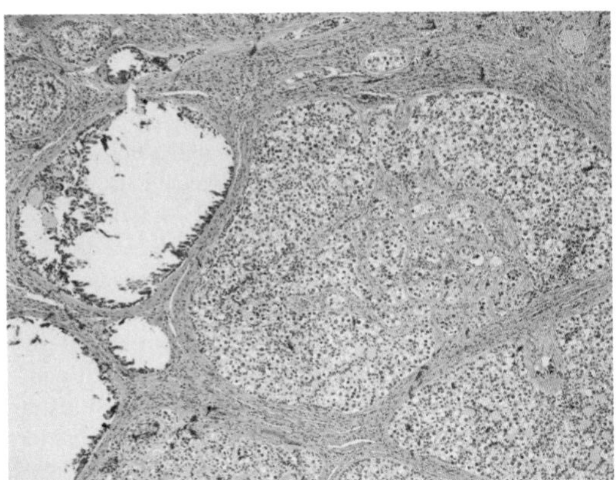

Fig. 35.24 Low-power magnification of gonadoblastoma

disorder (gonadal dysgenesis with ambiguous genitalia). Many patients have genetic conditions that result in deficient Sertoli cell development. Bilateral tumors are present in 40% of cases. Gonadoblastoma is composed of nests of germ cells and immature cells of Sertoli or granulosa type; cells resembling Leydig and lutein cells are usually present as well in the intervening stroma (Fig. 35.24). The germ cells often vary in appearance, with some having the morphological and immunophenotypic features of IGCNU, others having features of germ cells with delayed maturation, and still others appearing normal. The prognosis is correlated with the invasive growth of the germ cell component.

Miscellaneous Tumors of the Testis

Carcinoid Tumor

Testicular carcinoid tumors are very rare and account for less than 1% of all testicular neoplasms [36]. These tumors may be classified into three distinct groups, most commonly: primary testicular carcinoid (first), carcinoid differentiation within a mature teratoma (second), and metastases from an extra-testicular source (third).

Recently 29 testicular carcinoid cases were reported in a multi-institution study: 19 were pure carcinoid tumors, 3 were associated with cystic teratoma, 2 with cysts lacking epithelial lining, 4 with epidermoid cyst, and 1 with dermoid cyst [37]. Patients ranged in age from 12 to 65 years (mean 36); mean size was 2.5 cm. Two patients had carcinoid syndrome including diarrhea, hot flashes, and palpitations. Intratubular germ cell neoplasia, unclassified type was not present in any of the cases.

Most primary carcinoid tumors of the testis have a benign clinical course even if associated with epidermoid/dermoid cysts, or histologically mature teratoma. However, lesions with the morphology of atypical carcinoid can occasionally exhibit metastatic spread [37].

Metastatic Tumors to the Testis

Metastatic carcinomas to the testis may simulate primary testicular neoplasms. Prostate is the most common primary site, followed by kidney, colon, urinary tract (bladder and renal pelvis), lung, and esophagus [38]. Findings useful in accurate diagnosis include the occasional lack of a distinct mass on gross examination, bilaterality (although this is unusual), conspicuous intertubular growth, and prominent intralymphatic spread. The occurrence of conspicuous intrarete or intratubular growth in some cases (especially prostate carcinoma) may cause confusion with primary rete testis adenocarcinomas or germ cell tumors, respectively [38].

References

1. Rosen A, Jayram G, Drazer M, Eggener SE. Global trends in testicular cancer incidence and mortality. Eur Urol. 2011;60(2):374–9.
2. Bray F, Ferlay J, Devesa SS, McGlynn KA, Moller H. Interpreting the international trends in testicular seminoma and nonseminoma incidence. Nature clinical practice Urology. 2006;3(10):532–43.
3. Albers P, Albrecht W, Algaba F, Bokemeyer C, Cohn-Cedermark G, Fizazi K, et al. Guidelines on Testicular Cancer 2010. http://www.uroweb.org/gls/pdf/10_Testicular_Cancer.pdf.
4. Woodward PJ, Heidenreich A, Looijenga LHJ, McLeod DG, Moller H, Manivel JC, et al. In: Eble JE, Sauter G, Epstein JI, Sesterhenn IA, editors. Germ cell tumours. Pathology and genetics of tumours of the urinary system and male genital organs. Lyon: IARC Press; 2004.
5 Gibas Z, Prout GR, Pontes JE, Sandberg AA. Chromosome changes in germ cell tumors of the testis. Cancer Genet Cytogenet. 1986;19(3–4):245–52.

6. Cheville JC. Classification and pathology of testicular germ cell and sex cord-stromal tumors. Urol Clin North Am. 1999;26(3):595–609.
7. Boujelbene N, Cosinschi A, Boujelbene N, Khanfir K, Bhagwati S, Herrmann E, et al. Pure seminoma: a review and update. Radiat Oncol. 2011;6:90.
8. Young RH. Testicular tumors—some new and a few perennial problems. Arch Pathol Lab Med. 2008;132(4):548–64.
9. Cruceyra Betriu G, Tejido Sanchez A, Duarte Ojeda JM, Garcia De La Torre JP, De La Morena Gallego JM, Martinez Silva V, et al. Leydig cell tumor: report of 8 cases and review of the literature. Actas Urol Esp. 2002;26(1):36–40. Tumor de celulas de leydig: presentacion de ocho casos y revision de la literatura.
10. Kim I, Young RH, Scully RE. Leydig cell tumors of the testis. A clinicopathological analysis of 40 cases and review of the literature. Am J Surg Pathol. 1985;9(3):177–92.
11. Sesterhenn IA, Cheville JC, Woodward PJ, Damjanov I, Jacobsen GK, Nistal M, et al. Sex cord/gonadal stromal tumors. In: Eble JN, Sauter G, Epstein JI, Sesterhenn IA, editors. Tumors of the urinary system and male genital organs. Lyon: IARC press; 2004. pp 250–8.
12. Sangoi AR, McKenney JK, Brooks JD, Higgins JP. Evaluation of SF-1 expression in testicular germ cell tumors: a tissue microarray study of 127 cases. Appl Immunohistochem Mol Morphol. 2013;21(4):318–21.
13 Wang Z, Yang S, Shi H, Du H, Xue L, Wang L, et al. Histopathological and immunophenotypic features of testicular tumour of the adrenogenital syndrome. Histopathology. 2011;58(7):1013–8.
14. Ulbright TM, Srigley JR, Hatzianastassiou DK, Young RH. Leydig cell tumors of the testis with unusual features: adipose differentiation, calcification with ossification, and spindle-shaped tumor cells. Am J Surg Pathol. 2002;26(11):1424–33.
15 Billings SD, Roth LM, Ulbright TM. Microcystic Leydig cell tumors mimicking yolk sac tumor: a report of four cases. Am J Surg Pathol. 1999;23(5):546–51.
16. Cheville JC, Sebo TJ, Lager DJ, Bostwick DG, Farrow GM. Leydig cell tumor of the testis: a clinicopathologic, DNA content, and MIB-1 comparison of nonmetastasizing and metastasizing tumors. Am J Surg Pathol. 1998;22(11):1361–7.
17. McCluggage WG, Shanks JH, Arthur K, Banerjee SS. Cellular proliferation and nuclear ploidy assessments augment established prognostic factors in predicting malignancy in testicular Leydig cell tumours. Histopathology. 1998;33(4):361–8.
18. Mosharafa AA, Foster RS, Bihrle R, Koch MO, Ulbright TM, Einhorn LH, et al. Does retroperitoneal lymph node dissection have a curative role for patients with sex cord-stromal testicular tumors? Cancer. 2003;98(4):753–7.
19. Young RH, Koelliker DD, Scully RE. Sertoli cell tumors of the testis, not otherwise specified: a clinicopathologic analysis of 60 cases. Am J Surg Pathol. 1998;22(6):709–21.
20. Kaluzny A, Matuszewski M, Wojtylak S, Krajka K, Cichy W, Plawski A, et al. Organ-sparing surgery of the bilateral testicular large cell calcifying sertoli cell tumor in patient with atypical Peutz-Jeghers syndrome. Int Urol Nephrol. 2012;44(4):1045–8.
21. Gourgari E, Saloustros E, Stratakis CA. Large-cell calcifying Sertoli cell tumors of the testes in pediatrics. Curr Opin Pediatr. 2012;24(4):518–22.
22. Kratzer SS, Ulbright TM, Talerman A, Srigley JR, Roth LM, Wahle GR, et al. Large cell calcifying Sertoli cell tumor of the testis: contrasting features of six malignant and six benign tumors and a review of the literature. Am J Surg Pathol. 1997;21(11):1271–80.
23. Giglio M, Medica M, De Rose AF, Germinale F, Ravetti JL, Carmignani G. Testicular sertoli cell tumours and relative sub-types. Analysis of clinical and prognostic features. Urol Int. 2003;70(3):205–10.
24. Ulbright TM, Amin MB, Young RH. Intratubular large cell hyalinizing sertoli cell neoplasia of the testis: a report of 8 cases of a distinctive lesion of the Peutz-Jeghers syndrome. Am J Surg Pathol. 2007;31(6):827–35.
25. Calcagno C. Sclerosing sertoli cell tumor of the testis. Urologia. 2007;74(1):37–9.
26. Kum JB, Idrees MT, Ulbright TM. Sclerosing sertoli cell tumor of the testis: a study of 20 cases. Mod Pathol. 2012;24(suppl 2):222A.
27. Zukerberg LR, Young RH, Scully RE. Sclerosing sertoli cell tumor of the testis. A report of 10 cases. Am J Surg Pathol. 1991;15(9):829–34.
28. Henley JD, Young RH, Ulbright TM. Malignant sertoli cell tumors of the testis: a study of 13 examples of a neoplasm frequently misinterpreted as seminoma. Am J Surg Pathol. 2002;26(5):541–50.
29. Miliaras D, Anagnostou E, Moysides I. Adult type granulosa cell tumor: a very rare case of sex-cord tumor of the testis with review of the literature. Case Rep Pathol. 2013;2013:932086.
30. Colecchia M, Mikuz G, Algaba F. Rare tumors of the testis and mesothelial proliferation in the tunica vaginalis. Tumori. 2012;98(2):270–3.
31. Hammerich KH, Hille S, Ayala GE, Wheeler TM, Engers R, Ackermann R, et al. Malignant advanced granulosa cell tumor of the adult testis: case report and review of the literature. Hum Pathol. 2008;39(5):701–9.
32. Hanson JA, Ambaye AB. Adult testicular granulosa cell tumor: a review of the literature for clinicopathologic predictors of malignancy. Arch Pathol Lab Med. 2011;135(1):143–6.
33. Frias-Kletecka MC, MacLennan GT. Benign soft tissue tumors of the testis. J Urol. 2009;182(1):312–3.
34. Zhang M, Kao CS, Ulbright TM, Epstein JI. Testicular fibrothecoma: a morphologic and immunohistochemical study of 16 cases. Am J Surg Pathol. 2013;37(8):1208–14.

35. Ueda M, Kanematsu A, Nishiyama H, Yoshimura K, Watanabe K, Yorifuji T, et al. Testicular thecoma in an 11-year-old boy with nevoid basal-cell carcinoma syndrome (Gorlin syndrome). J Pediatr Surg. 2010;45(3):E1–3.
36. Neely D, Gray S. Primary carcinoid tumour of the testis. Ulster Med J. 2011;80(2):79–81.
37. Wang WP, Guo C, Berney DM, Ulbright TM, Hansel DE, Shen R, et al. Primary carcinoid tumors of the testis: a clinicopathologic study of 29 cases. Am J Surg Pathol. 2010;34(4):519–24.
38. Ulbright TM, Young RH. Metastatic carcinoma to the testis: a clinicopathologic analysis of 26 nonincidental cases with emphasis on deceptive features. Am J Surg Pathol. 2008;32(11):1683–93.

36 Testicular Cancer Reporting on Radical Orchiectomy and Retroperitoneal Lymph Node Dissection After Treatment

Daniel M. Berney

Introduction

Testicular germ cell tumors show unmatched chemo- and radiosensitivity when compared to other solid tumors. This has led to treatment strategies which differ markedly from other primary neoplasms. The resection of residual tumor foci after treatment has become extremely common over the past 20 years. This can be because the primary tumor was unresected before medical treatment was instituted: more usual in cases of widely disseminated disease. Secondly, there may be disease detectable on imaging in the retroperitoneum or other organs after resection of the primary tumor and subsequent treatment.

The most common sites for metastasis for a germ cell tumor, as might be expected, considering its embryological descent from the retroperitoneum, are the retroperitoneal lymph nodes. Thus, retroperitoneal lymph node dissection (RPLND) has become an established therapy for residual disease.

Germ cell tumors after therapy may show a variety of unusual changes and morphologies. Some of these changes are seen within weeks of treatment but other relapse changes may not become apparent for many years after primary therapy. These changes may radically change the second line therapy administered, and different diagnoses may result in further surgery, varied chemotherapeutic regimens, radiotherapy, or surveillance. Therefore, an understanding of germ cell tumors after treatment is essential, if correct therapy is to be administered.

Macroscopic Assessment

Testicular Specimens After Chemotherapy

The macroscopic assessment of the testis after chemotherapy does not vary from standard protocols used in diagnostic cases. However, the changes seen after chemotherapy may be subtle. Even sizeable tumors may regress or even completely disappear after chemotherapy, depending on the length of time between administration of chemotherapy and excision. The testis often has lost its typical yellow golden parenchyma and become fibrotic with dull and tan areas. Sometimes areas of hemorrhage are seen. It is important to sample carefully all the different areas, as well as any normal parenchyma so that intratubular germ cell neoplasia, unclassified type (IGCNU) can be diagnosed.

Retroperitoneal Lymph Nodes

Clinical Considerations

RPLNDs may either occur as primary resections, at the same time as the diagnostic tumor is removed, or after therapy. Prior to therapy, the changes in RPLNDs mirror those of the primary

D. M. Berney (✉)
Dept of Molecular Oncology, Barts Cancer Inst., Bartshealth NHS Trust and Queen Mary University of London, Charterhouse Sq, London EC1M 7BQ, UK
e-mail: d.berney@bartshealth.nhs.uk

C. Magi-Galluzzi, C. G. Przybycin (eds.), *Genitourinary Pathology,* DOI 10.1007/978-1-4939-2044-0_36,

tumor. The practice of primary prophylactic RPLND is performed in some centers, but is not universal. Although it can prevent later recurrence, the morbidity of the surgery is such that the vast majority of patients are cured with less invasive techniques: either radiotherapy to involved lymph nodes or chemotherapy.

Primary RPLNDs may be carried out for rare non-germ cell primary testicular tumors such as malignant Sertoli cell tumors [1]. The reasoning here is that these tumors do not respond to adjuvant treatments, and therefore, prophylactic resection remains the only hope of long-term control and survival. However, these tumors are too rare for any formal study.

The vast majority of RPLNDs are performed after orchidectomy and chemo-/radiotherapy on residual masses. Paradoxically, during chemotherapy some masses may enlarge: this is thought to be due to maturation of malignant elements such as embryonal carcinoma to teratoma, and be a good prognostic indicator [2]. Surgery may also be guided by the serum markers: A high alpha fetoprotein (AFP) or beta human chorionic gonadotropin (β-HCG) will likely indicate residual yolk sac tumor or trophoblast, respectively, and indicate the need for further chemotherapy prior to excision.

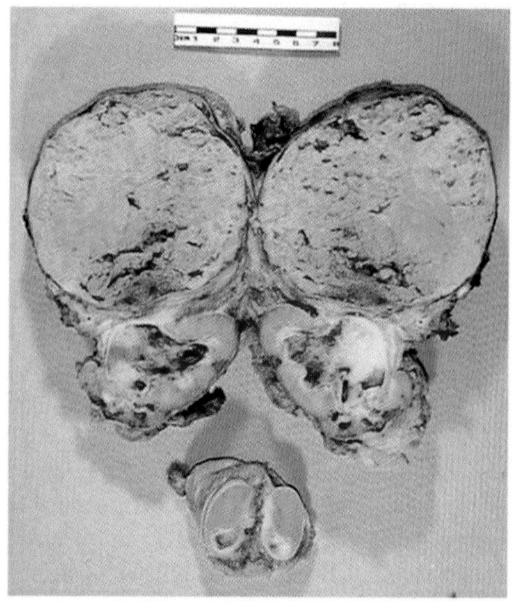

Fig. 36.1 A large necrotic metastasis which has necessitated a nephrectomy after chemotherapy. The testis is also seen *below* with a much smaller mass showing teratoma

Macroscopic Examination

Retroperitoneal lymph node excision specimens may vary from the excision of large masses which may be attached to adjacent organs, especially the kidneys (Fig. 36.1) to the excision of small lymph nodes embedded in adipose tissue, showing no macroscopic abnormality.

The techniques used therefore have to vary according to circumstance. Margin positivity for tumor is rare in RPLNDs but it is a poor prognostic factor [3]. Therefore, we recommend inking any specimens with enlarged lymph nodes. Sampling of the enlarged nodes should be extensive: at least 1 block/cm, as small tumor foci can be missed in large necrotic foci.

It is also very important to have adequate clinical history and the reason for the RPLND. This should include the serum markers, as fairly small tumor deposits can produce substantial amounts of β-HCG and AFP.

Metastatectomies for germ cell tumor in other organs are also increasing in frequency. Lung and liver metastases may all be resected, especially if the clinicians believe that they consist of mature teratoma. Again, close inspection, inking of margins, and generous blocking are good practice.

Microscopy of Postchemotherapy Germ Cell Tumors

In most cases the microscopic examination of most RPLNDs is relatively straightforward, as the vast majority will show either necrosis or teratoma. Below we describe the varied findings in RPLNDs.

Necrosis

Necrosis is the most frequent RPLND finding. The necrotic areas are often surrounded by a prominent infiltrate of foamy macrophages, scattered hemosiderin, and an active fibroblastic

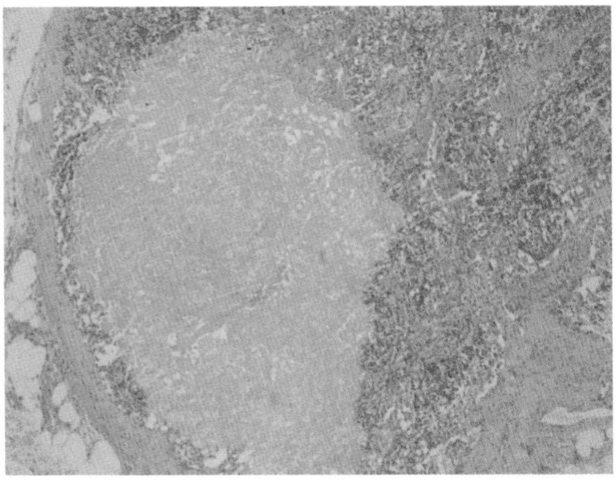

Fig. 36.2 Postchemotherapy necrosis within a lymph node. Ghost outlines of the malignant tumor are seen

proliferation. Within the necrotic foci, pyknotic nuclei in the ghost-like outlines of tumor cells may be seen, often surrounding vessels (Fig. 36.2). These foci often retain their immunophenotype (Fig. 36.3). These semideposits or unviable deposits should not be considered evidence of persistent germ cell tumor. Only cells with intact nuclei and well-preserved chromatin pattern and cytoplasm should be considered as viable.

Mature Teratoma

This is the second most frequent finding at RPLND. The presence of teratoma is often expected on macroscopy as the lymph nodes are often multicystic (Fig. 36.4) and filled with clear

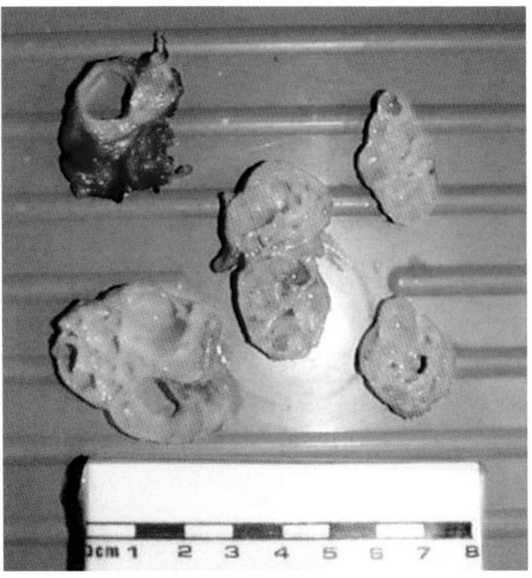

Fig. 36.4 Macroscopic appearance of postchemotherapy retroperitoneal lymph nodes showing extreme cystic change. The lymph nodes are involved by teratoma

or brown fluid. On close inspection some solid areas can have the glistening surface of cartilage.

Microscopically, the tumor shows a typical mixed organoid pattern with epithelial and stroma elements, as seen in testicular teratoma (Fig. 36.5).

Persistent teratoma often shows significant cytological atypia in both mesenchymal and epithelial components. In the absence of stromal invasion or overgrowth, with preservation of a typical organoid appearance by the teratoma the

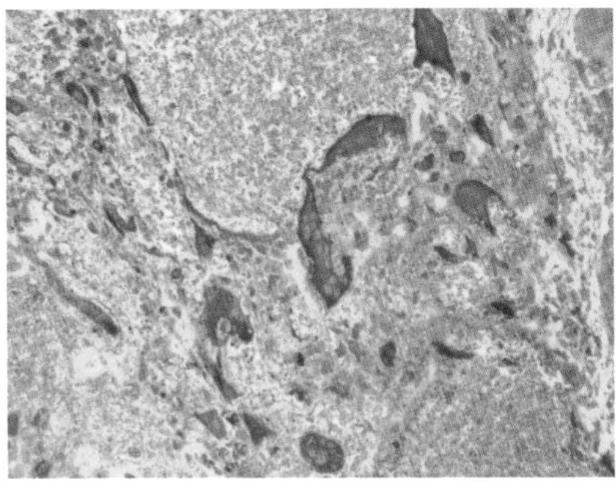

Fig. 36.3 Immunohistochemistry for β-HCG on this necrotic postchemotherapy metastasis can still highlight syncytiotrophoblastic cells

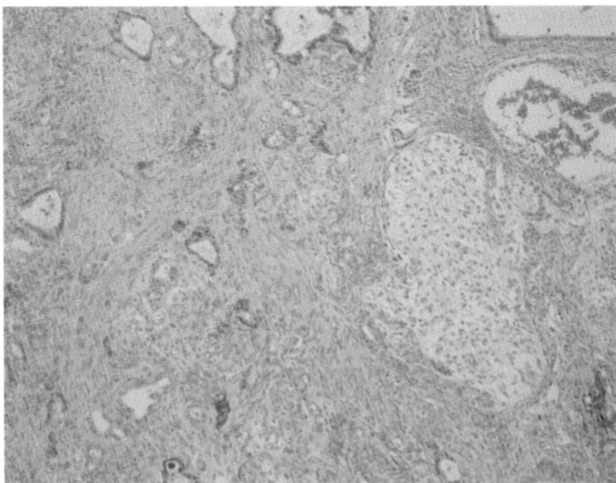

Fig. 36.5 Microscopic features of a solid area from a postchemotherapy teratoma. Note the organoid arrangement of components with many epithelial and stromal elements

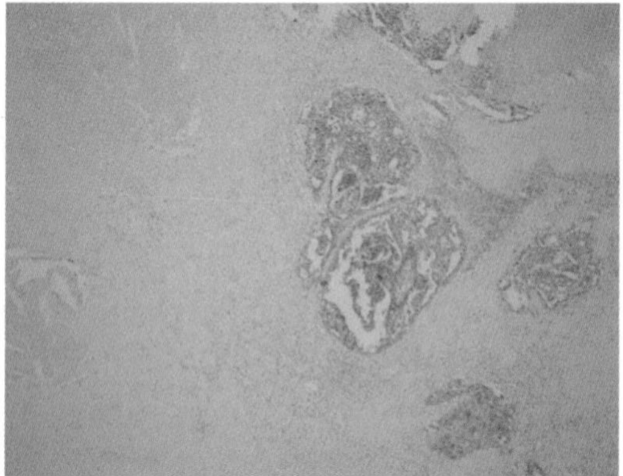

Fig. 36.6 Residual embryonal carcinoma after chemotherapy, which is here surrounded by substantial necrosis

presence of cytologic atypia has no adverse significance and can be ignored [4].

Residual "Malignant" Germ Cell Tumor

This is a relatively unusual finding and is often suspected due to raised serum markers. Most cases will only have small amounts of tumor present, as cases where the serum markers are very high will not be considered for resection.

Embryonal carcinoma is similar in appearance to that seen in the testis (Fig. 36.6), though it should be noted that CD30 is often negative in these tumors after chemotherapy [5]. OCT3/4 is positive, however, and morphology should be sufficient to differentiate embryonal carcinoma from seminoma.

Seminoma in RPLNDs is unusual: often seminoma is highly infiltrative in the retroperitoneum, and resection is surgically challenging, and imaging often shows tumor wrapped around major vessels. In any chemo- or radioresistant seminoma it is worth taking a second look at the tumor to exclude the possibility of a malignant Sertoli cell tumor that has been erroneously diagnosed.

Yolk sac tumor has a protean nature, and in late recurrences, it tends to show even more unusual patterns, especially the glandular form which may resemble an adenocarcinoma and lead to misdiagnosis (Fig. 36.7). As long as the pathologist is aware of a high serum AFP, this should not occur; however, the morphological appearances may be misleading and immunohistochemistry for AFP may be patchy, though glipican-3 now provides a more sensitive immunomarker [6]. The glandular type of yolk sac tumor appears to be particularly resistant to chemotherapy while the hepatoid form is more common in metastases (Fig. 36.8).

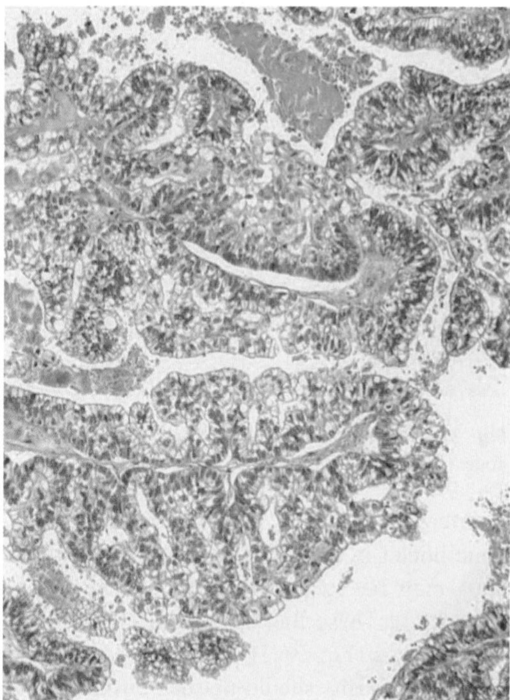

Fig 36.7 Glandular type yolk sac tumor. This is usually seen in late recurrences and is usually chemoresistant

Choriocarcinomas may be difficult to diagnose without knowledge of the serum markers. They may lack a well-defined biphasic pattern and mainly consist of mononucleated trophoblast

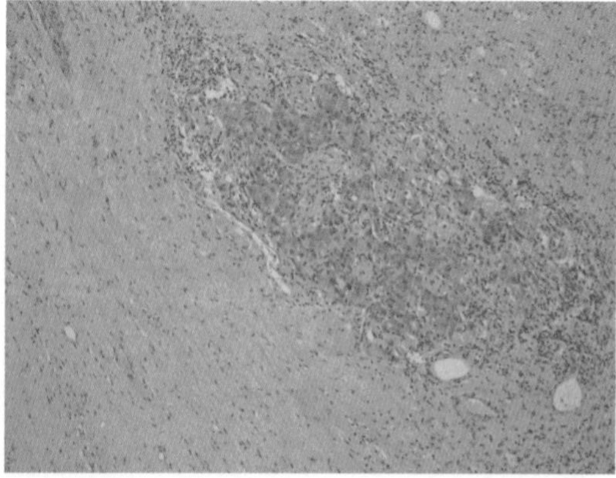

Fig. 36.8 A small amount of hepatoid type yolk sac tumor in the edge of a largely necrotic postchemotherapy germ cell tumor

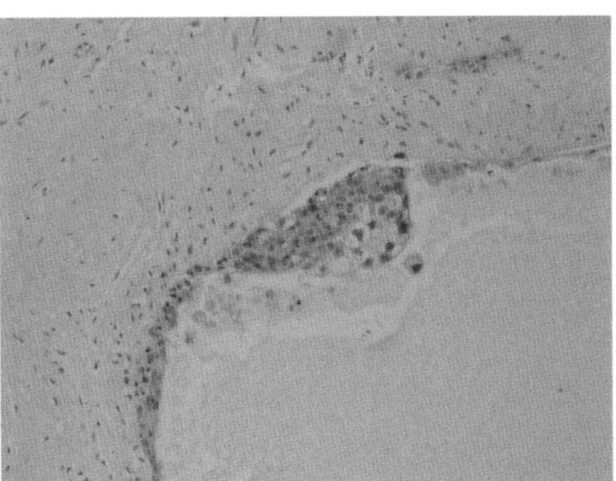

Fig. 36.9 A cyst lined by atypical partially viable cells, which were positive for β-HCG. This represents cystic trophoblastic disease

cells alone. As they frequently metastasize to unusual sites, they may be seen by non-genito-urinary pathologists, and if a history is not available, misdiagnosis is not infrequent. We have seen choriocarcinoma misdiagnosed as squamous cell carcinoma on a number of occasions.

Cystic trophoblastic tumor is an entity unique to germ cell oncology thought to be derived from postchemotherapy metastatic choriocarcinoma [7]. Cysts are lined with semiviable cells (Fig. 36.9) with partially smudged nuclei and degenerate chromatin. Small papillary ingrowths may occur as well as cells apparently free floating in the cyst fluid. Syncytiotrophoblastic cells may also be seen. These appearances are not considered a reason for additional chemotherapy.

The volume of residual malignant germ cell tumor has also been used by some to predict the need for further therapy [3]. It has been suggested that patients with very small volumes of nonteratoma on RPLND may escape further salvage therapy; therefore, quantification of the residual tumor may be important.

Somatic Transformations

A number of case series analyses since the mid-1980s have sought to understand the behavior of germ cell tumors that undergo transformation to a malignant non-germ cell phenotype, usually after platinum-based chemotherapy. Sarcomas (leiomyosarcoma, rhabdomyosarcoma, liposarcoma, chondrosarcoma), primitive neuroectodermal tissue (neuroblastoma, neuroepithelioma), nephroblastoma, mesothelioma, adenocarcinoma, and even non-Hodgkin's lymphoma and leukemia have all been described [8–13]. Their pathogenesis is disputed. Some suggest there is differentiation of totipotent (embryonal) cells which subsequently become malignant. Selection for chemoresistant malignant cells following chemotherapy is also possible, and the third hypothesis suggests that chemotherapy may be inducing malignant transformation of the germ cell tumor. Somatic malignant transformations are usually diagnosed on follow-up imaging which show an enlarging mass or masses in spite of falling or negative germ cell tumor markers. Therefore, a high index of suspicion is necessary and simple follow-up with serial AFP and β-HCG is probably insufficient. Chemotherapy appears largely ineffective in treating these tumors. RPLND is the preferred mode of treatment, therefore with clearance of as many metastases as possible.

Transformation Versus Immature Teratoma

It can be challenging to differentiate a teratoma with widespread immaturity from a somatic transformation. Teratomas tend to preserve their organoid arrangement with mixed epithelial and stromal elements. Atypical mesenchymal elements that overgrow the surrounding germ cell tumor and exceed >0.5–1 low-power field (×4 objective) are suspicious for transformation. The presence of atypical mitoses within the transforming area has also been used [12].

Sarcomatous Transformations

In the most recent published series the tumors included embryonal rhabdomyosarcoma ($n=29$), angiosarcoma ($n=6$), leiomyosarcoma ($n=4$), undifferentiated sarcoma ($n=3$), and single examples of myxoid liposarcoma, malignant peripheral nerve sheath tumor, malignant "triton" tumor, and epithelioid hemangioendothelioma [13]. It also confirmed the poor outcome of sarcomatous transformation compared with recurrent germ cell tumor.

Primitive Neuroectodermal Transformation

Primitive neuroectodermal transformation is one of the more frequent transformations seen (Fig. 36.10). The morphological type of PNET is variable and is predictive of behavior. Eighty percent are synaptophysin positive and one third is positive for chromogranin. They are also positive for CD99, demonstrating the MIC-2 protein characteristic of Ewing's sarcoma and PNET. When primary transformation is seen in the testis, the outcome is generally favorable, but when seen in metastases, surgical resection is the mainstay of therapy and outcome is generally poor, though long-term survival is reported [14].

Adenocarcinomatous Transformation

This is an exceptionally rare phenomenon but has been well reported, and has a poor outcome (Fig. 36.11). It should be differentiated from intestinal type recurrent yolk sac tumor, and thus the serum AFP should be within normal limits [10, 15]. Fluorescence in situ hybridization (FISH) for chromosome 12p (Fig. 36.12) can prove multiple copies of 12p and thus help facilitate the diagnosis of a transformed germ cell tumor.

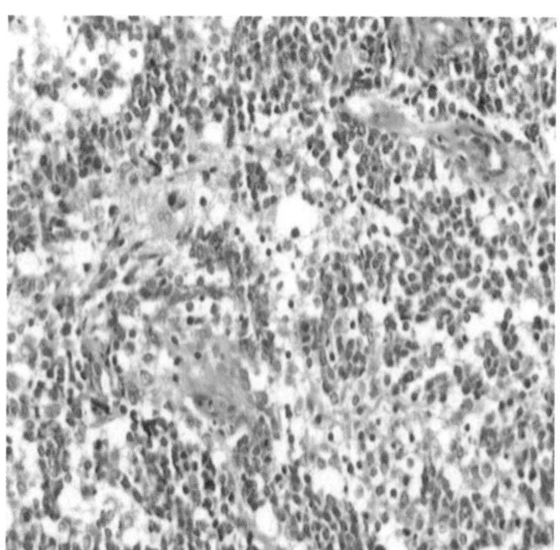

Fig. 36.10 Pure neuroectodermal tissue, representing transformation of a germ cell tumor to a primitive neuroectodermal tumor

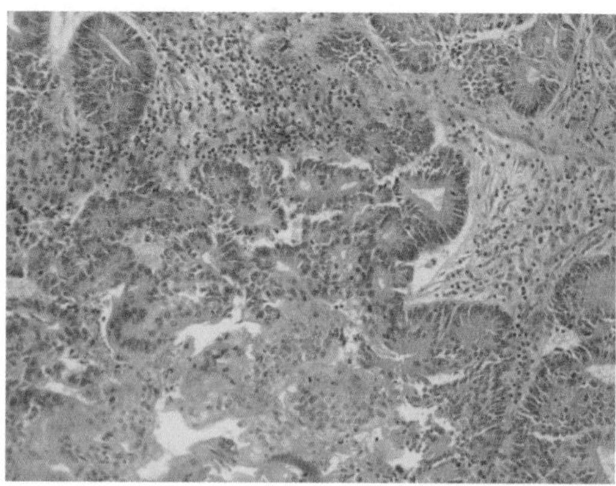

Fig. 36.11 Somatic transformation of a germ cell tumor to adenocarcinoma

Nephroblastomatous Transformation

This is, once again, a rare transformation. Nephroblastomas arise often within a mature teratoma, usually at metastatic sites. The dif-

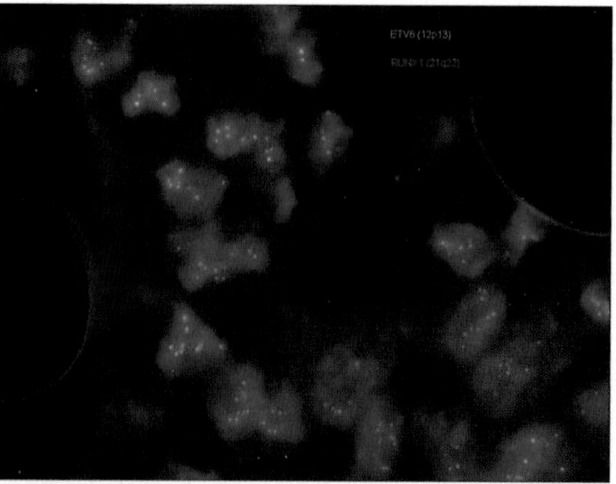

Fig. 36.12 In difficult cases, proof of isochromosome 12p can help to establish a germ cell origin of a somatic transformation. This was an adenocarcinoma arising in the testis which showed multiple copies of i12p

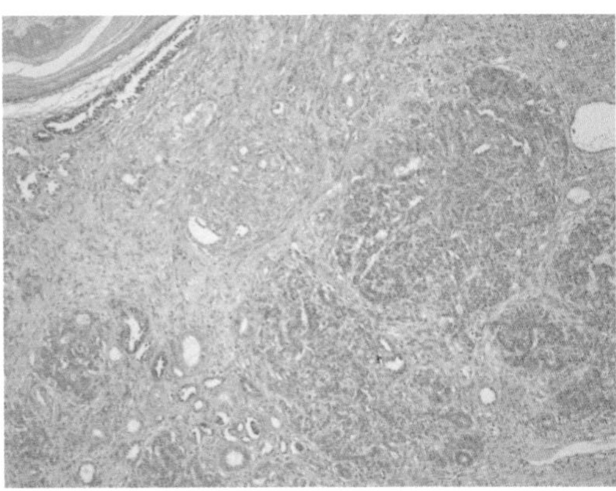

Fig. 36.13 Nephroblastomatous transformation of a germ cell tumor showing blastema, glomeruloid structures, and in the *top left*, squamoid areas

ferentiation from other forms of transformation, especially PNET, is important, as they have a better prognosis and long-term cure is usual (Fig. 36.13). Morphologically, they show a typical triphasic pattern of epithelium, blastema, and stroma. Immunohistochemically, they do not stain with neuroendocrine markers and are negative for CD99 [12, 16].

References

1. Mosharafa AA, et al. Does retroperitoneal lymph node dissection have a curative role for patients with sex cord-stromal testicular tumors? Cancer. 2003;98(4):753–7.
2. Stella M, et al. Retroperitoneal vascular surgery for the treatment of giant growing teratoma syndrome. Urology. 2012;79(2):365–70.
3. Berney DM, et al. Prediction of relapse after lymph node dissection for germ cell tumours: can salvage chemotherapy be avoided? Br J Cancer. 2001;84(3):340–3.
4. Ulbright TM. Germ cell tumors of the gonads: a selective review emphasizing problems in differential diagnosis, newly appreciated, and controversial issues. Mod Pathol. 2005;18(Suppl 2):S61–79
5. Berney DM, et al. Loss of CD30 expression in metastatic embryonal carcinoma: the effects of chemotherapy? Histopathology. 2001;39(4):382–5.
6. Zynger DL, et al. Glypican 3: a novel marker in testicular germ cell tumors. Am J Surg Pathol. 2006;30(12):1570–5.
7. Ulbright TM, et al. Cystic trophoblastic tumor: a nonaggressive lesion in postchemotherapy resections of patients with testicular germ cell tumors. Am J Surg Pathol. 2004;28(9):1212–6.
8. Spiess PE, et al. Malignant transformation of testicular teratoma: a chemoresistant phenotype. Urol Oncol. 2008;26(6):595–9.
9. Oldenburg J, Wahlqvist R, Fossa SD. Late relapse of germ cell tumors. World J Urol. 2009;27(4):493–500.
10. Michael H, et al. The pathology of late recurrence of testicular germ cell tumors. Am J Surg Pathol. 2000;24(2):257–73.
11. Ulbright TM, Berney DM. Testicular and paratesticular tumors. In: Mills SE, editor. Sternberg's diagnostic surgical pathology. Philadelphia: Lippincott, Williams and Wilkins; 2009.
12. Rajab R, Berney DM. Ten testicular trapdoors. Histopathology. 2008;53(6):728–39.
13. Malagon HD, et al. Germ cell tumors with sarcomatous components: a clinicopathologic and immunohistochemical study of 46 cases. Am J Surg Pathol. 2007;31(9):1356–62.
14. Ganjoo KN, et al. Germ cell tumor associated primitive neuroectodermal tumors. J Urol. 2001;165(5):1514–6.
15. Game X, et al. Dedifferentiation of mature teratomas secondary to testicular cancer: report of 2 cases. Prog Urol. 2001;11(1):73–6; discussion 76–7.
16. Colecchia M, et al. Teratoma with somatic-type malignant components in germ cell tumors of the testis: a clinicopathologic analysis of 40 cases with outcome correlation. Int J Surg Pathol. 19(3):321–7.

37 Difficult or Newly Described Morphologic Entities in Testicular Neoplasia

Daniel M. Berney and Thomas M. Ulbright

Introduction

The range of morphology in testicular tumors is unparalleled in any other male genitourinary organ. Germ cell tumors are the most protean of any of the neoplastic lesions, and there are also many other tumors primary to the testis that may mimic them. This unique diversity, coupled with the relative uncommonness of most testicular neoplasms, means that they remain unfamiliar to many general pathologists, and consequent diagnostic errors are relatively frequent [1]. Spermatocytic seminoma may be encountered only a few times in a working life, so that differentiating it from other testicular neoplasms remains an extra challenge. We present some unusual variants of testicular tumors, and discuss the pitfalls leading to diagnostic misinterpretation.

D. M. Berney (✉)
Department of Molecular Oncology, Barts Cancer Institute, Bartshealth NHS Trust and Queen Mary University of London, London, UK
e-mail: d.berney@bartshealth.nhs.uk

T. M. Ulbright
Department of Pathology and Laboratory Medicine, Indiana University School of Medicine, Indianapolis, IN, USA
e-mail: tulbright@iupui.edu

Seminoma Variants

Seminoma may be both the easiest and most difficult of diagnoses. It is the most common tumor of the testis, and, therefore, might be thought to be the most familiar. The classic appearances of seminoma are well known. Broad fibrous bands and an associated lymphoplasmacytic infiltrate are readily identified at low power. At higher power, the cytology is characteristic with polygonal cells possessing clear cytoplasm, well defined cellular borders, and very characteristic nuclei with a frequent box-like contour. The large nucleoli are frequently rather ill defined. Outside this classic appearance there are many variants, however, which may be misdiagnosed as nonseminoma or even nonneoplastic conditions:

1. **The inflammatory infiltrate is variable:** The extreme variation that may be seen in seminoma is a cause for diagnostic misinterpretation. Although rare, occasional seminomas may lack a lymphoplasmacytic infiltrate, leading to diagnostic confusion. This seems to be more commonly the case when the tumor has an unusual architecture including microcystic and tubular patterns [2], further complicating the interpretation. However, a more common problem is when the inflammatory infiltrate overwhelms the tumor cells, so that rare seminoma cells are studded in a dense inflammatory infiltrate (Fig. 37.1). The pale cytoplasm of the seminoma cells may make

C. Magi-Galluzzi, C. G. Przybycin (eds.), *Genitourinary Pathology*, DOI 10.1007/978-1-4939-2044-0_37,

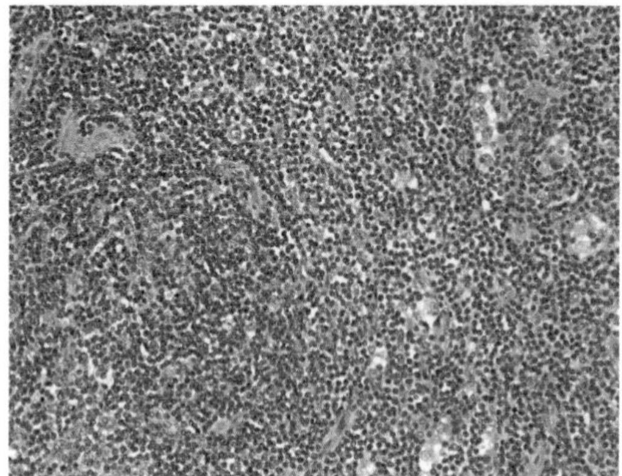

Fig. 37.1 Seminoma with marked lymphoplasmacytic infiltrate overwhelming the tumor cells

the neoplastic cells stand out like stars on a winter's night, in a similar way that macrophages stand out in a Burkitt lymphoma. As a consequence, any testicular lesion that at first glance appears inflammatory must be examined with care to discern scattered seminoma cells. Granulomatous inflammation may also be present and may overwhelm the tumor. These cases should be treated with caution and a careful hunt made for typical seminoma cells. If there is any reason for suspicion, a sensitive immunostain, such as OCT4, may be employed to identify underlying neoplastic cells. Tuberculosis, sarcoidosis, leprosy, and other even rarer granulomatous infections may affect the testis, but ruling out seminoma is vital. Therefore, in all inflammatory rich processes involving the testis the question should be asked, "Am I missing a seminoma?"

2. **Intertubular seminoma:**
   Seminoma cells usually form a solid sheet and displace the seminiferous tubules. However, the cells may also show an "intertubular" pattern of spread [3] where single cells infiltrate in an insidious pattern between the seminiferous tubules (Fig. 37.2a). Thus, the overall architecture of the testis is preserved and, at low power, no neoplasm may be apparent. This pattern is usually mixed with more solid appearing seminoma, but rarely in early stage disease; where there is plentiful intratubular germ cell neoplasia, unclassified type (IGCNU), intertubular foci may be missed. Clues to the presence of intertubular seminoma include an association with inflammation in the stroma and a rather more plentiful parenchyma between the seminiferous tubules. Immunostains for OCT4 may be helpful in identifying neoplastic cells (Fig. 37.2b).
3. **Tubular and signet ring seminoma:**
   Morphological variants of seminoma cells themselves have been described relatively recently [2]. Occasionally a seminoma may mimic a nonseminoma, especially a glandular pattern yolk sac tumor (Fig. 37.3) or embryonal carcinoma, because of a tubular morphology. Cytology will usually differentiate between the two as the cells retain the classic

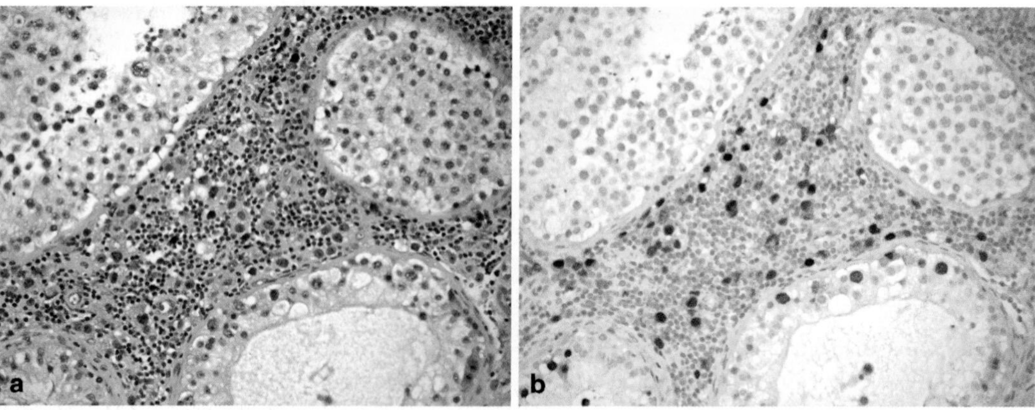

Fig. 37.2 Intertubular seminoma with single cells infiltrating between seminiferous tubules (**a**). OCT4 stains the neoplastic cells within the marked inflammatory infiltrate (**b**) and also intratubular germ cell neoplasia (IGCNU)

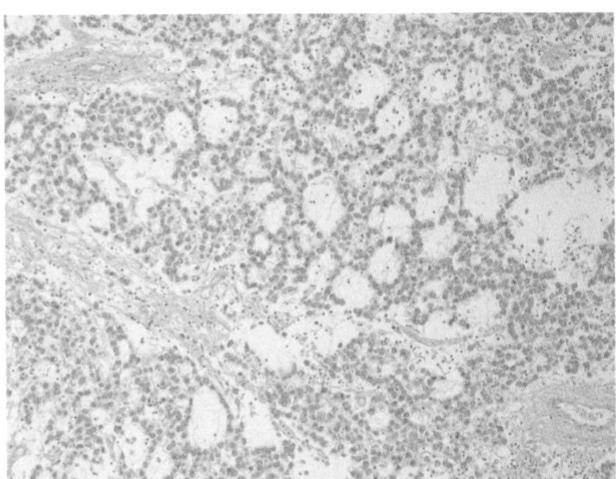

Fig. 37.3 A tubular seminoma showing classic seminoma nuclear morphology in spite of a pattern reminiscent of nonseminomatous germ cell tumor types

cytomorphology of seminoma rather than the more variable nuclear morphology of yolk sac tumor or showing the more extreme nuclear overlapping, irregular contours and larger size of embryonal carcinoma. In ambiguous cases, immunochemistry for OCT4 (positive in seminoma, negative in yolk sac tumor), CD30 (negative in seminoma, positive in embryonal carcinoma) and CD117 or podoplanin (positive in seminoma, negative in embryonal carcinoma) is helpful. Signet ring morphology in seminoma has also been described. This may mimic a metastasis, but the foci of signet ring morphology have always been mixed with more typical areas, making this a less challenging diagnosis.

4. **Anaplastic seminoma:**
Anaplastic seminoma is a term we do not recommend. Occasional seminomas have unusual features in terms of nuclear morphology, mitotic rate, or inflammatory infiltrate. The excellent prognosis of seminoma, however, means that a study involving many thousands of patients and standardized care would be necessary to identify, with certainty, such an entity and to prove its legitimacy by virtue of a more aggressive behavior than typical seminomas. Furthermore, it would be necessary to show that it could be reproducibly diagnosed, and neither of these requirements has been accomplished.

Spermatocytic Seminoma

Spermatocytic seminoma, as its pathogenesis and etiology are entirely separate from other germ cell tumors, should really be regarded as quite different from usual seminoma and needs to be considered apart. Unfortunately, it may be misdiagnosed as seminoma, and therefore inappropriate treatment could be instituted [4].

Patients with spermatocytic seminoma are older than most patients with testicular germ cell tumors, averaging 50–60 years of age. It is also more frequently bilateral than other germ cell tumors. Spermatocytic seminoma has never been described as originating in any site other than the testis and shows no special association with cryptorchidism; the presence of spermatogenesis is apparently necessary for its development, differentiating it from other germ cell tumors that may occur in extragonadal sites, particular those along the midline [5]. These features suggest that while other germ cell tumors arise from primordial germ cells (which may be misplaced), meiotic activity is necessary for the pathogenesis of spermatocytic seminomas. Molecular data also support the separate pathogenesis of these tumors [6] and implicate the primary spermatocyte as the cell of origin.

Spermatocytic seminomas typically show enormous cellular polymorphism. Three cellular populations occur: small lymphocyte-like degenerate cells, intermediate cells which have round nuclei with granular chromatin and variably prominent nucleoli, and giant cells which may be mononucleated or multinucleated, also with prominent nucleoli (Fig. 37.4). Some may also have a "spireme" chromatin pattern similar to that of meiotic phase spermatocytes. Mitoses, including atypical forms, and apoptosis are prominent. Intratubular growth of spermatocytic seminoma is common but there is no IGCNU.

An "anaplastic" variant of spermatocytic seminoma has been described which consists mostly of intermediate cells [7]. However, this terminology appears inappropriate to us and, as the behavior of this variant is identical to the usual type of spermatocytic seminoma, we believe that there merely needs to be an awareness of the variabil-

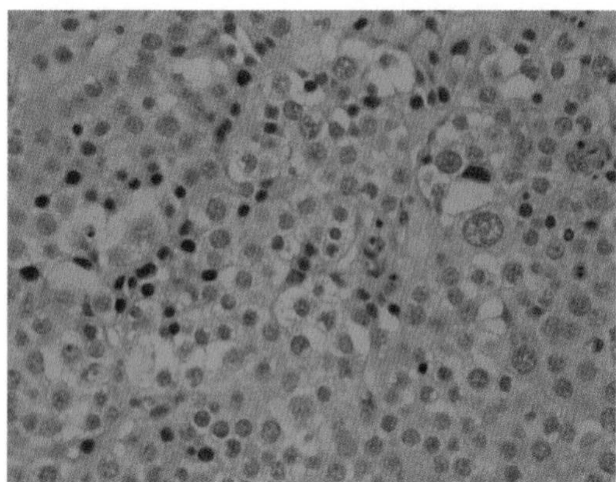

Fig. 37.4 High power of a spermatocytic seminoma. One larger cell is seen, and there is more cellular size variation than usually seen in a classical seminoma

ity of the morphologic picture. Immunostains are negative for OCT4 but CD117 positivity is rather common. More recently, spermatocytic seminomas have been found to stain for the general germ cell tumor marker, SALL4 [8].

Despite its "malignant" appearance, spermatocytic seminoma metastasizes only exceedingly rarely. There are only two well-documented cases of metastasis. In the personal experience of one of the authors, who has also seen a case of spermatocytic seminoma metastasizing as a single lung nodule, this may be an "embolic" process. Adequate treatment, therefore, consists of orchiectomy alone without adjuvant treatment, since the potential mortality of further therapy exceeds the risk of tumor-related death.

Sarcomatous transformation is a rare complication of spermatocytic seminoma [9]. The sarcomatous component is often intermingled with usual type spermatocytic seminoma and can have an undifferentiated, spindle cell appearance or exhibit rhabdomyosarcomatous differentiation [10]. These tumors behave aggressively with about 50 % of the patients developing metastatic disease and dying of the tumor. The disseminated tumor consists only of the sarcomatous component.

Unusual Variants of Nonseminomatous Germ Cell Tumors

Solid Variant Yolk Sac Tumor

The varied patterns of yolk sac tumor can make the diagnosis challenging in rare cases. Some rare variants are seen mainly after treatment and will be discussed elsewhere; however, the solid variant of yolk sac tumor is seen in primary lesions and may be misdiagnosed.

Solid variant yolk sac tumor is rare in its pure form, and is usually intermingled with other yolk sac tumor patterns and germ cell tumor elements such as embryonal carcinoma or teratoma. However, when pure, the solid variant shows more than a passing resemblance to seminoma (Fig. 37.5), thus leading to potential diagnostic confusion and the danger of mistreatment [11].

Points of distinction include the lack in solid yolk sac tumor of the typical fibrous septa and lymphocytic infiltrate of seminoma, and the greater variation in nuclear size of most cases, with many examples showing cells with small nuclei and others with large nuclei, unlike seminoma where the nuclei are more uniformly large. Schiller–Duval bodies are not seen in the solid variant, but hyaline globules and bands of intercellular basement membrane can be very helpful as they do not occur in seminoma. The importance of knowing the serum markers is also

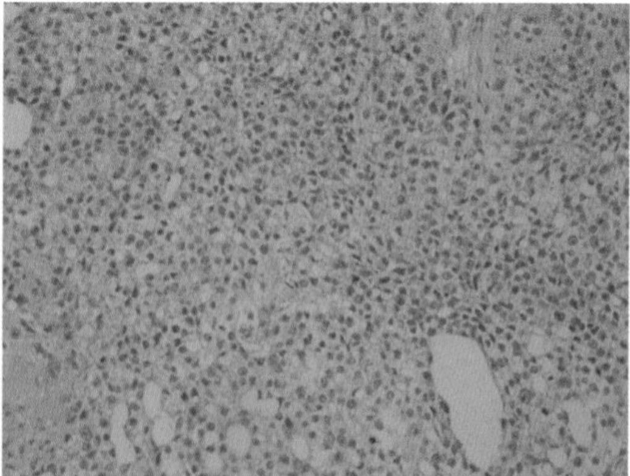

Fig. 37.5 Solid variant yolk sac tumor showing a mixture of large and also smaller cells, not seen in seminoma. Focal microcysts are also seen

emphasized: knowledge of a raised alpha-fetoprotein (AFP) should always lead one to suspect yolk sac tumor. Immunohistochemistry for AFP can be patchy in all yolk sac tumors and is even more apt to be negative in the solid pattern. For this reason glypican-3 is now a preferable immunochemical marker because of its greater sensitivity and consistent negativity in seminoma [12]. Another very helpful feature is negative reactivity for OCT4, contrasting with the seminoma. It is important to be aware that CD117 is frequently positive, potentially reinforcing confusion with the seminoma.

Teratoma

In the vast majority of postpubertal cases, teratoma is mixed with other elements, including embryonal carcinoma, trophoblast, seminoma, and yolk sac tumor. However, some cases of teratoma may cause diagnostic problems that may be difficult to resolve. Recent advances have also suggested some novel variants, which appear to have a separate pathogenesis and natural history.

Teratomas in postpubertal males, despite the lack of apparent malignant appearance in many cases, are capable of metastasis. In this they contrast significantly with the great majority of ovarian teratomas [13]. They may show immature elements, which are discussed below. They are almost inevitably associated with scarring of the surrounding testicular parenchyma with loss of normal spermatogenesis. Such scarring may be due to regression of other germ cell tumor components, thus explaining how, in spite of their indolent appearance, they are frequently accompanied by metastasis. The usual occurrence of IGCNU in the surrounding seminiferous tubules reinforces the close relationship of most postpubertal teratomas with the nonteratomatous germ cell tumors.

Immaturity in Teratomas

Immaturity is often seen in testicular germ cell tumors with a substantiatial amount of teratoma. Such foci typically form embryonic-type neuroectodermal elements, but other embryonic-type tissues (rhabdomyoblasts, nephrogenic blastema, and tubules) also qualify. As expected, such foci have a primitive appearance with active proliferation and apoptotic cells. It is also common for mature teratomatous elements to show atypical features, but these are not truly of embryonic type and therefore not considered "immature." For instance, glandular-lined cysts may show stratification, atypical nuclei and mitoses; squamous epithelium may show dysplasia, and the stromal elements may show changes that in another situation would lead to a diagnosis of sarcoma [4]. Cartilage may show atypia, which in different contexts would lead to a presumption of chondrosarcoma. These atypical features reflect the derivation of postpubertal teratomas from other forms of germ cell tumors. Despite these changes, they do not affect the overall prognosis of the patient, and high threshold should be set for transformation to somatic-type malignancies in the primary testicular germ cell tumor, typically requiring overgrowth of a pure population of malignant-appearing mesenchymal or embryonic tissues to the exclusion of other elements and occupying at least a 4× low power microscopic field. For carcinomatous transformation an overtly invasive growth pattern is required. Because scattered embryonic-type elements do not confer a worse outcome, and given that pure "mature" postpubertal teratomas may be associated with metastases of either teratoma or nonteratomatous forms of germ cell tumor, the most recent WHO classification excluded immature teratoma as a diagnostic entity.

Primitive Neuroectodermal Tumor

Some teratomas contain substantial overgrowth of primitive neuroectodermal tissue, and this should be separately recognized as primitive neuroectodermal tumor (PNET). Most typically, PNET has morphology akin to PNETs of the central nervous system as most commonly seen in children. Many form primitive tubules resembling medulloepithelioma. In rare tumors, it eclipses all other elements, resulting in a pure PNET.

The prognostic implications of PNET limited to the testis are less worrisome than might be imagined. The small published series suggest that even in its pure form, most men are cured of their disease. However, they behave in a worse manner than teratomas without PNET [14]. This situation contrasts with finding PNET in metastases, which will be discussed separately.

When confronted with one of these cases, we suggest that the amount of PNET be accounted for in percentage form and mentioned specifically. Although, at present, standard germ cell tumor protocols generally apply, many oncologists recommend staging retroperitoneal lymphadenectomy for clinical stage I patients with a PNET component in their tumor rather than followup on a surveillance protocol.

Epidermoid Cyst

So called epidermoid cysts of the testis are composed of laminated keratin, usually in a well circumscribed nodule, most often 1–3 cm in diameter. Occasionally, the cyst may rupture leading to a less well circumscribed appearance.

Microscopically they have a typical appearance of concentric laminated keratin surrounded by a simple keratinizing squamous epithelium, although giant cell reactions may be seen if the cyst has ruptured. They have a different pathogenesis from most testicular teratomas [15] and lack the key cytogenetic abnormality that characterizes the usual forms of postpubertal testicular germ cell tumors, including teratomas: the presence of amplification of a portion of the short arm of chromosome 12, most commonly in the form of an isochromosome (i[12p]) [16].

Systematic blocking is necessary to exclude other germ cell elements. The background testis typically shows normal spermatogenesis and uniformly lacks IGCNU. They may be treated conservatively with preservation of the testis, but it is important that the surrounding parenchyma is sampled adequately to ensure the absence of IGCNU.

Dermoid Cysts and Nondermoid Benign Teratomas

Similar to epidermoid cysts, dermoid cysts within the testis are rare but benign entities of unknown pathogenesis where there are skin appendigeal elements present as well as the squamous epithelial component that characterizes epidermoid cyst. These are arranged in an organoid, skin-like fashion [17]. Importantly and more diagnostically challenging is a small subset of teratomas that, like dermoid cysts, also appear to have a benign clinical course but that lack the skin-like morphology, instead consisting of various mature elements, including bone, cartilage, smooth muscle, respiratory-type mucosa and others. It is vital to distinguish these apparently benign neoplasms from the usual postpubertal teratoma, which is capable of metastasis. Unlike its malignant relative, dermoid cysts/benign teratomas are not associated with surrounding IGCNU, which is almost inevitably present around teratomas capable of malignant spread. Other features supportive of a benign lesion include lack of the tubular atrophy, sclerosis, impaired spermatogenesis, microlithiasis and interstitial fibrosis that are commonly found with most postpubertal germ cell tumors, including the usual teratomas [4]. Instead there are unremarkable seminiferous tubules with intact spermatogenesis. Additionally, these lesions lack the common cytologic atypia seen in usual testicular teratoma. Further evidence to differentiate these entities comes from recent i(12p) data, showing that both dermoid cysts and benign teratomas lack the typical i(12p) chromosomal abnormalities seen in teratomas capable of metastasis [18]. They also tend to occur in a younger age group than other nonseminomatous germ cell tumors, and it has been suggested that at least some are in fact prepubertal teratomas that have persisted into the postpubertal age. This supposition does correlate with the known indolent clinical behavior of prepubertal teratomas of the testis [19].

Practically, it is difficult to know whether these patients can be spared the repeated imaging studies required of patients with usual testicular teratomas, but certainly followup can be conservative and reassurance of the patient seems reasonable from the available data.

Regression in Germ Cell Tumors

Spontaneous regression is relatively frequent in testicular germ cell tumors compared to most other malignant neoplasms. The most common scenario is a patient who presents with a germ cell tumor in a typical metastatic distribution for a testicular primary, most commonly the retroperitoneal lymph nodes, but who lacks clinical evidence of a testicular tumor. Sometimes, but not always, meticulous clinical palpation or skilful testicular ultrasound will disclose subtle testicular abnormalities. Absence of testicular anomalies may lead to a presumption of an extratesticular primary lesion. If orchiectomy is performed, it typically shows distinct areas of scarring in association with widespread tubular atrophy and sclerosis and frequent microlithiasis (Fig. 37.6). A lymphoplasmacytic infiltrate and "ghost" tubules in the scarred area are also common, as are prominent numbers of small blood vessels. Less common are large, coarse calcifications within expanded tubular profiles within the scarred foci. The surrounding testis shows IGCNU in about one-half of the cases [20]. We consider IGCNU and large, coarse intratubular calcifications in a scarred testis as diagnostic of a regressed (burnt-out) germ cell tumor. The latter feature corresponds to residual dystrophic calcification that developed in completely necrotic intratubular embryonal carcinoma, a lesion that commonly undergoes comedo-type necrosis. Unfortunately both of these features are absent in up to half of the cases, so pathologists must be aware of the constellation of findings that accompany germ cell tumor regression

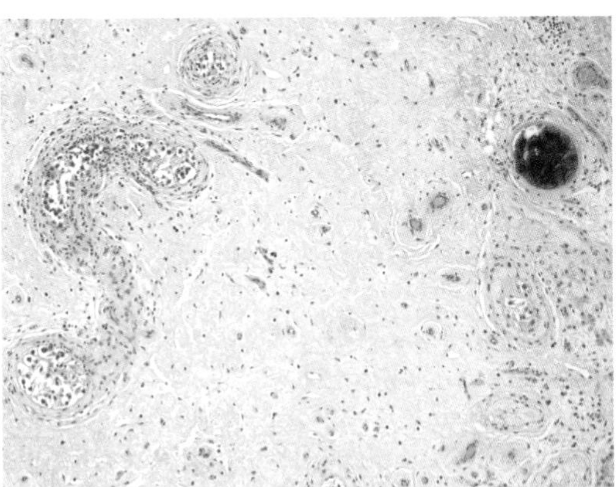

Fig. 37.6 Regressed germ cell tumor. Testicular parenchyma with distinct areas of scarring in association with tubular atrophy, sclerosis, and microlithiasis (*right*); the seminiferous tubules on the *left* show intratubular germ cell neoplasia (IGCNU)

Sex Cord–Stromal Tumors

The sex cord–stromal tumors form almost as heterogenous a group of tumors as the germ cell tumors. They are usually benign and therefore of less clinical significance than the germ cell tumors. However, there are some tumors that are associated with specific clinical conditions. Additionally, there are some tumors that mimic germ cell or other malignancies and may be misdiagnosed. Lastly, some tumors have features that may indicate malignancy and should prompt further clinical action apart from orchiectomy.

Syndrome Associated Sex Cord–Stromal Tumors

Intratubular Large Cell Hyalinizing Sertoli Cell Neoplasia

This distinctive lesion is characteristic of patients with the Peutz-Jeghers syndrome [21]. Gynecomastia is a frequent presenting feature, and there is typically bilateral testicular involvement by ultrasonographically detected, small, multifocal nodules. Microscopic examination shows expanded seminiferous tubules with large Sertoli cells with vacuolated to eosinophilic cytoplasm admixed with globular deposits of basement membrane and sometimes occasional flecks of calcification (Fig. 37.7). These testicular lesions in Peutz-Jeghers patients show a low frequency of invasive tumors and no reported case with metastasis. They therefore appear to show

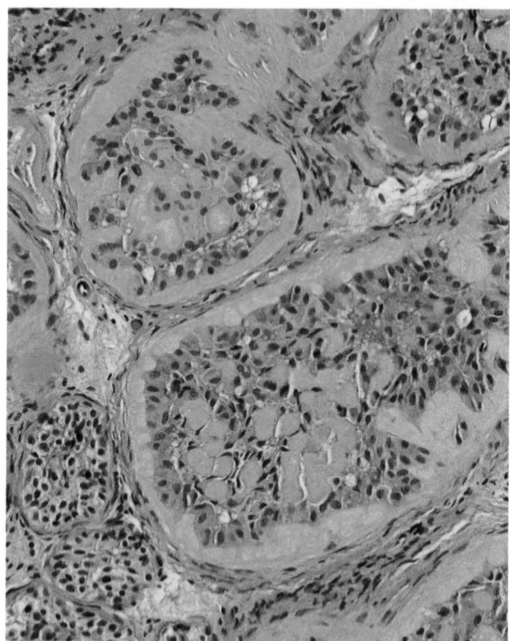

Fig. 37.7 Intratubular large cell hyalinizing Sertoli cell neoplasia shows proliferation of large Sertoli cells with abundant eosinophilic cytoplasm in expanded seminiferous tubules with prominent peritubular and intratubular basement membrane deposits

distinct features compared with sporadic large cell calcifying Sertoli cell tumor (see below). Orchiectomy is necessary only when there is evidence of invasion or to control hormonal manifestations.

Large Cell Calcifying Sertoli Cell Tumor

A substantial proportion of patients with this neoplasm have the Carney complex, although sporadic cases are likely more common based on our experience. The clinical profiles of these two groups tend to be different. Those with the Carney complex, an autosomal dominant disorder with a risk for cardiac, endocrine, cutaneous, and neural tumors, as well as a variety of pigmented lesions of the skin and mucosae, develop multifocal and bilateral testicular tumors, with many examples likely undetected because of their small size and indolent growth. Fortunately, in the Carney complex associated tumors malignant behavior is rare, although it has been reported [22]. This contrasts with the nonsyndrome-associated large cell calcifying Sertoli cell tumors, which are more frequently clinically malignant and further contrast with the other group by being larger, unilateral, and single.

As its name implies, a characteristic feature of these tumors is calcification that may vary from minor to massive and may take the form of psammoma bodies, mulberry-like shapes, irregular, coarse aggregates, or trabecular bone. The tumor cells are characteristically arranged in solid nests, tubules, and cords and typically have abundant eosinophilic cytoplasm and round nuclei with fine chromatin and a distinct nucleolus. A common and helpful clue to the diagnosis is a neutrophilic stromal infiltrate, but it is not always seen.

Juvenile Granulosa Cell Tumors

Juvenile granulosa cell tumors are neonatal testicular tumors and usually present as cystic, painless, testicular masses. They are diagnosed mostly in the first 6 months [23]. They may occur in undescended testes of infants with intersex conditions and can be associated with chromosomal abnormalities, especially of the Y chromosome, and mosaicism.

Macroscopically, there is usually an admixture of solid and cystic areas filled with viscid fluid. On microscopy, there are round, follicle-like structures lined by cells with pale eosinophilic cytoplasm and hyperchromatic, round nuclei with nucleoli (Fig. 37.8). Grooves are not conspicuous and mitoses may be abundant. These are frequently arranged in lobular groupings in a fibromatous stroma.

Easily Misdiagnosed Tumors

Malignant Sertoli Cell Tumors Which Resemble Seminoma

Sertoli cells tumors are responsible for about 1 % of testicular tumors and have an extremely varied morphology. As a result, their relative rarity may present diagnostic difficulty. A recent series described a number of Sertoli cell tumors that mimicked seminoma [24], and personal experience,

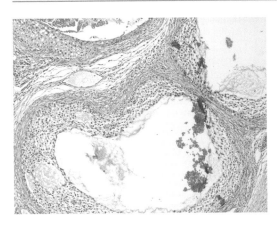

Fig. 37.8 Juvenile granulosa cell tumor characterized by follicle-like structures lined by cells with pale eosinophilic cytoplasm

again, suggests that this tumor is more common than initially realized.

In the series of Henley et al., there were clear cells in sheets associated with inflammatory cells that caused a low power appearance very similar to seminoma. In some cases, the nature of the tumor was uncovered after an initial misdiagnosis of seminoma when it was reviewed after failure of adjuvant radiotherapy and the patient subsequently developed metastatic disease in the radiated field, a very rare event in cases of true seminoma.

Differentiation of the two entities relies on a constellation of factors. Microscopic features more in favor of Sertoli cell tumor include any tubular or spindle cell areas and, at higher power, a much blander cytology than seminomas, with less frequent mitotic figures and a more mixed acute and chronic inflammatory cell infiltrate (Fig. 37.9a, b). Immunohistochemistry may be extremely helpful in these cases, especially OCT4, which is positive in seminoma and negative in sex cord–stromal tumors. Markers of sex cord–stromal differentiation may be variable.

Testicular Tumors of the Adrenogenital Syndrome (Testicular Adrenal Rest Tumors)

The presence of a craggy testicular mass with highly suspicious imaging appearances is often the cue for an orchidectomy. The presence of bilateral masses might be thought even more alarming. However, this admittedly rare entity can result in the unnecessary castration of the patient for a hyperplastic lesion that can be treated medically in the vast majority of cases.

Congenital adrenal hyperplasia includes several *autosomal recessive diseases* resulting from *mutations* of *genes* for *enzymes* mediating the biochemical steps of production of *cortisol* from *cholesterol* by the *adrenal glands*. Most cases are secondary to 21-hydroxylase deficiency [25]. The exact nature of the hyperplastic cells is unknown. To the endocrinologist, they are highly sensitive to ACTH and behave like adrenocortical

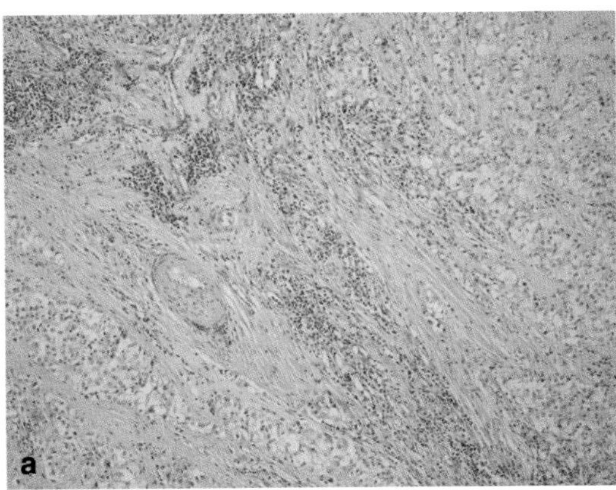

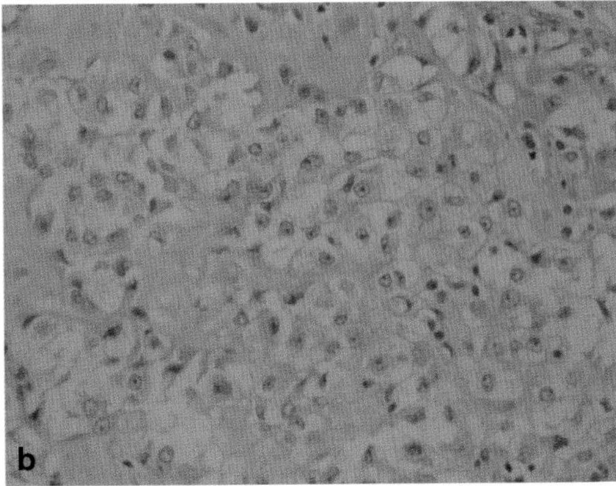

Fig. 37.9 Low (**a**) and high (**b**) power of a malignant Sertoli cell tumor. At low power fibrous bands and an inflammatory infiltrate are seen. At higher power the cells are regular with punched out nucleoli, eosinophils and a lack of mitotic activity

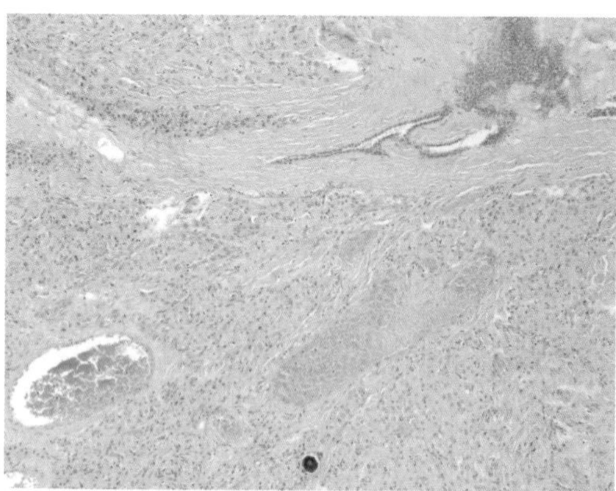

Fig. 37.10 Testicular tumor of the adrenogenital syndrome showing large cells with voluminous cytoplasm and associated fibrosis surrounding the rete testis

cells. To the pathologist their appearance is very analogous to Leydig cells, as they possess highly eosinophilic cytoplasm rather than the foamy cytoplasm of cells from the zona fasciculata of the adrenal gland. It has been noted that the cytoplasm appears more voluminous than in typical Leydig cells and they are associated with characteristic prominent fibrous bands (Fig. 37.10). Reinke crystals are not seen and cytoplasmic lipofuscin tends to be more prominent that in Leydig cell tumors. In early cases the nodules are close to the rete, but gradually the hyperplastic cells expand into the testicular parenchyma and may replace the seminiferous tubules. Immunhistochemical staining for synaptophysin, CD56 and androgen receptor (AR) may assist in the distinction from Leydig cell tumor, as the "tumors" of the adrenogenital syndrome are frequently positive for the first two markers and negative for AR, whereas, Leydig cell tumors tend to have the opposite pattern of reactivity [26, 27].

References

1. Delaney RJ, et al. The continued value of central histopathological review of testicular tumours. Histopathology. 2005;47(2):166–9.
2. Ulbright TM, Young RH. Seminoma with tubular, microcystic, and related patterns: a study of 28 cases of unusual morphologic variants that often cause confusion with yolk sac tumor. Am J Surg Pathol. 2005;29(4):500–5.
3. Henley JD, et al. Seminomas with exclusive intertubular growth: a report of 12 clinically and grossly inconspicuous tumors. Am J Surg Pathol. 2004;28(9):1163–8.
4. Ulbright TM. Germ cell tumors of the gonads: a selective review emphasizing problems in differential diagnosis, newly appreciated, and controversial issues. Mod Pathol. 2005;18(Suppl 2):S61–79.
5. Looijenga LH, et al. Genomic and expression profiling of human spermatocytic seminomas: primary spermatocyte as tumorigenic precursor and DMRT1 as candidate chromosome 9 gene. Cancer Res. 2006;66(1):290–302.
6. Stoop H, et al. Reactivity of germ cell maturation stage-specific markers in spermatocytic seminoma: diagnostic and etiological implications. Lab Invest. 2001;81(7):919–28.
7. Dundr P, et al. Anaplastic variant of spermatocytic seminoma. Pathol Res Pract. 2007;203(8):621–4.
8. Cao D, et al. SALL4 is a novel diagnostic marker for testicular germ cell tumors. Am J Surg Pathol. 2009;33(7):1065–77.
9. Aggarwal N, Parwani AV. Spermatocytic seminoma. Arch Pathol Lab Med. 2009;133(12):1985–8.
10. Menon S, Karpate A, Desai S. Spermatocytic seminoma with rhabdomyosarcomatous differentiation: a case report with a review of the literature. J Cancer Res Ther. 2009;5(3):213–5.
11. Kao CS, et al. Solid pattern yolk sac tumor: a morphologic and immunohistochemical study of 52 cases. Am J Surg Pathol. 2012;36(3):360–7.
12. Zynger DL, et al. Glypican 3 has a higher sensitivity than alpha-fetoprotein for testicular and ovarian yolk sac tumour: immunohistochemical investigation with analysis of histological growth patterns. Histopathology. 2010;56(6):750–7.
13. Ulbright TM. Gonadal teratomas: a review and speculation. Adv Anat Pathol. 2004;11(1):10–23.
14. Michael H, et al. Primitive neuroectodermal tumors arising in testicular germ cell neoplasms. Am J Surg Pathol. 1997;21(8):896–904.
15 Younger C, et al. Molecular evidence supporting the neoplastic nature of some epidermoid cysts of the testis. Arch Pathol Lab Med. 2003;127(7):858–60.
16. Cheng L, et al. Interphase fluorescence in situ hybridization analysis of chromosome 12p abnormalities is useful for distinguishing epidermoid cysts of the testis from pure mature teratoma. Clin Cancer Res. 2006;12(19):5668–72.
17. Ulbright TM, Srigley JR. Dermoid cyst of the testis: a study of five postpubertal cases, including a pilomatrixoma-like variant, with evidence supporting its separate classification from mature testicular teratoma. Am J Surg Pathol. 2001;25(6):788–93.
18. Zhang C, et al. Evidence supporting the existence of benign teratomas of the postpubertal testis: a clinical, histopathologic, and molecular genetic analysis of 25 cases. Am J Surg Pathol. 2013;37(6):827–35.

19. Kendall TJ, et al. Case series: adult testicular dermoid tumours–mature teratoma or pre-pubertal teratoma? Int Urol Nephrol. 2006;38(3–4):643–6.
20. Balzer BL, Ulbright TM. Spontaneous regression of testicular germ cell tumors: an analysis of 42 cases. Am J Surg Pathol. 2006;30(7):858–65.
21. Ulbright TM, Amin MB, Young RH. Intratubular large cell hyalinizing sertoli cell neoplasia of the testis: a report of 8 cases of a distinctive lesion of the Peutz-Jeghers syndrome. Am J Surg Pathol. 2007;31(6):827–35.
22. Stratakis CA, Kirschner LS, Carney JA. Clinical and molecular features of the Carney complex: diagnostic criteria and recommendations for patient evaluation. J Clin Endocrinol Metab. 2001;86(9):4041–6.
23. Partalis N, et al. Juvenile granulosa cell tumor arising from intra-abdominal testis in newborn: case report and review of the literature. Urology. 2012;79(5):1152–4.
24. Henley JD, Young RH, Ulbright TM. Malignant sertoli cell tumors of the testis: a study of 13 examples of a neoplasm frequently misinterpreted as seminoma. Am J Surg Pathol. 2002;26(5):541–50.
25. Knape P, et al. Testicular adrenal rest tumors (TART) in adult men with classic congenital adrenal hyperplasia (CAH). Urologe A. 2008;47(12):1596–7, 1599–602.
26. Ashley RA, et al. Clinical and pathological features associated with the testicular tumor of the adrenogenital syndrome. J Urol. 2007;177(2):546–9; discussion 549.
27. Wang Z, et al. Histopathological and immunophenotypic features of testicular tumour of the adrenogenital syndrome. Histopathology. 2011;58(7):1013–8.

Clinical Implications of the Different Histologic Subtypes of Testicular Tumors

38

Timothy Gilligan

Introduction

As discussed in previous chapters, there are numerous histological subtypes of testis cancer. The vast majority of testis cancers are germ cell tumors, which are divided clinically into pure seminomas and germ cell tumors with nonseminoma elements (nonseminomatous germ cell tumors). The other four germ cell tumor histologies are embryonal carcinoma, teratoma, choriocarcinoma, and yolk sac tumors. In women and children, teratomas are divided into mature and immature categories, and this distinction has not been shown to have prognostic significance in adolescent and adult males, and therefore, teratomatous elements in testis cancers and in extragonadal germ cell tumors in this population are generally reported simply as teratomas with the exception of pure mature teratomas of the mediastinum, which are managed differently from other primary mediastinal nonseminomatous germ cell tumors. Spermatocytic seminomas are rare and are thought to be benign tumors with minimal if any metastatic potential. Sex-cord stromal tumors comprise less than 5 % of testis tumors and include Leydig cell tumors, Sertoli cell tumors, and granulosa cell tumors. Gonadoblastomas consist of a mixture of seminoma-like germ cell tumors and sex-cord tumors with Sertoli differentiation [1]. Adenocarcinoma of the rete testis is a rare, aggressive malignant neoplasm of the collecting system of the testis. In this chapter, the prognostic and management implications of the different histologic types of testicular germ cell tumors will be discussed.

T. Gilligan (✉)
Taussig Cancer Institute, Cleveland Clinic, Mail Code R359500 Euclid Avenue, Cleveland, OH 44195, USA
e-mail: gilligt@ccf.org

Germ Cell Tumors

Seminomas

Seminomas are generally less aggressive than nonseminomatous germ cell tumors. Among men with clinical stage I testicular germ cell tumors that are managed with surveillance following inguinal orchiectomy, the relapse rate is about 17 % for pure seminomas compared to 25–30 % for nonseminomatous tumors [2]. This difference has also been reported in the setting of metastatic disease. In the outcomes analysis performed by the International Germ Cell Cancer Consensus Group in 1997, men with germ cell tumors with metastases to the liver, bone, or other nonpulmonary organs had a 5-year survival of 72 % if the tumor was pure seminomas compared to 48 % if the cancer was a nonseminomatous tumor [3]. Among seminomas, spermatocytic seminomas are a very rare subtype with a distinct histopathological, genetic, and clinical profile as discussed in previous chapters [4]. Spermatocytic seminomas are generally seen in older men and do not have metastatic potential unless sarcomatous transformation is seen. Orchiectomy alone

C. Magi-Galluzzi, C. G. Przybycin (eds.), *Genitourinary Pathology*, DOI 10.1007/978-1-4939-2044-0_38,

without chemotherapy, radiation therapy, or additional surgery is thus appropriate treatment for men with these tumors.

Pure seminomas do have metastatic potential and management paradigms reflect this. Among men with stage I disease, risk stratification can be performed based on the size of the tumor and the presence or absence of invasion of the rete testis. An international pooled analysis of 638 men reported that the risk of relapse was 32% for men with tumors larger than 4 cm and rete testis invasion, 16% for men with one of these risk factors, and 12% for those with neither [5]. The low risk of relapse has been prospectively confirmed in studies by the Spanish Germ Cell Cancer Cooperative Group. For instance, among 153 low-risk and intermediate-risk clinical stage I patients managed with surveillance following orchiectomy, the 3-year disease-free survival rate was 93.5% among patients with no risk factors, 83.7% among men with tumors larger than 4 cm, and 78.3% for those with rete testis invasion; in this study, high-risk men whose tumors were bigger than 4 cm and also invaded the rete testis were treated with carboplatin chemotherapy [6]. The presence or absence of lymphovascular invasion is also associated with risk of relapse in univariable analysis, but not when controlling for tumor size and rete testis invasion. Because the risk of relapse is only about 30% even for high-risk patients and the risk of dying of the cancer is less than one percent, many experts prefer surveillance for all clinical stage I seminoma patients, while others favor a risk-adapted approach so that only high-risk patients are treated either with carboplatin chemotherapy or with radiation therapy.

Embryonal Carcinoma

Embryonal carcinoma (EC) has long been recognized as a more aggressive cancer with a higher rate of relapse for stage I and stage II disease. Many studies over the past 25 years have reported that among men with stage I testis cancer, EC is associated with a higher risk of relapse if the patient is managed either with postorchiectomy surveillance or with retroperitoneal lymph node dissection (RPLND). Although the first major studies to relate this reported that the presence of EC was associated with a higher risk of relapse in stage I patients, subsequent analyses reported an association between the risk of relapse and the proportion or volume of the tumor that consisted of EC. Men who have both lymphovascular invasion (LVI) and preponderance of EC have been reported to be at particularly high risk of having occult metastatic disease.

One challenge in interpreting these findings is the fact that different studies have used different endpoints. Surveillance studies that have used relapse as an endpoint have reported only a modest association between EC and that endpoint. In contrast, much stronger associations have been reported between tumors consisting predominantly of EC, on the one hand, and a finding of lymph node involvement by the tumor in patients undergoing an RPLND. For instance, a study of 223 men undergoing postorchiectomy surveillance for clinical stage I nonseminomatous testicular germ cell tumors reported that the risk of relapse at 3-year follow-up was only 33% among men with a predominance of EC, but this group could be divided into high- and low-risk subgroups: 55% risk of relapse if there was both LVI and a predominance of EC and only a 16% risk of relapse if there was a predominance of EC but no LVI [7]. In contrast, surgical series have reported much higher rates of retroperitoneal lymph node positivity in patients with a predominance of EC, although with varying definitions of predominance. In these series, the association of EC and LVI limited the contribution of EC as an independent variable. In one series of 149 men with clinical stage I nonseminomatous tumors undergoing RPLND, of 48 men with more than 80% EC, 42 also had LVI, and among 77 with less than 45% EC, 71 did not have LVI. Of the six who were LVI positive but had less than 45% EC, 3 (50%) had pathological stage II disease, so the absence of EC predominance only predicted a low risk of relapse if LVI was absent. Of those with 46–79% EC, seven of nine without LVI were pathological stage I, while 15 of 15 with LVI were pathological stage II. It was only when more than 80% of the tumor was EC that it became predictive of a majority of men without LVI (four out of six) having pathological stage II disease [8].

Indiana University reported that a predominance of EC (defined as the presence of more EC than any other histology) was more clinically relevant. Among 226 patients undergoing RPLND with pathological stage I disease, the subsequent relapse rate was about 20% if either LVI or EC predominance was present and 29% if both were present compared to a relapse risk of less than 7% if neither risk factor was present. Similarly, among 292 patients with clinical stage I disease undergoing RPLND, the risk of pathological stage II disease was 39% if LVI was present, 32% if EC was predominant, and 47% if both risk factors were present. However, the difference in risk for one versus two risk factors was not statistically significant in either of these two analyses [9]. Memorial Sloan Kettering Cancer Center reported their findings in patients with clinical stage I pure EC, which showed that 19 of 26 men (73%) had retroperitoneal nodal metastases, including 13 of 18 (72%) with LVI and six of eight (75%) without LVI [10].

The significance of these findings remains unclear. Relevant clinical questions are whether a predominance of EC should be used to decide how to manage patients with clinical stage I or pathological stage II patients. Because the rates of nodal metastases and relapse following RPLND are both higher in patients with EC predominance, should these patients be managed instead with primary chemotherapy rather than nodal dissection or surveillance? For instance, if half or more of patients with pure EC or both LVI and EC predominance will have lymph node metastases discovered at RPLND and most such patients will elect to undergo two cycles of adjuvant chemotherapy, would it be preferable to simply give them one or two cycles of primary chemotherapy in lieu of RPLND? And if such patients have a 50% or higher risk of relapse if placed on surveillance, might such men prefer to be treated now with a relatively brief course of chemotherapy and minimize the likelihood of needing additional treatment in the future rather than live with a high likelihood of having to put their lives on hold at some unpredictable point in the subsequent few years in order to undergo a longer course of chemotherapy in the event of a relapse? In current practice, most recent studies have based such risk stratification on the presence or absence of LVI and have not included EC. So at this time, EC is not generally taken into account when making treatment decisions for patients with testicular cancer but does have some prognostic implications with regard to risk of relapse and nodal metastases among men with clinical stage I disease.

Teratoma

Men with pure teratomas of the testis have a lower risk of metastatic disease and relapse compared to other germ cell tumors, but such tumors are rare. Investigators in southwestern France reported that among 1000 cases of testis cancer, only 17 were pure teratoma, eight of whom had clinical stage I disease, while nine had metastatic disease present at diagnosis. All patients were alive and without evidence of the cancer at a mean follow-up of 10 years [11].

Indiana University identified 41 patients with pure teratoma of the testis, including 18 with clinical stage I disease, four patients with borderline evidence of early stage II disease, three with stage IIA disease, and 16 with disseminate disease (stages IIC-III) [12]. Among patients with clinical stage I disease, 16% had pathological stage II disease discovered at RPLND. Among the ten clinical stage I–II patients found to have pathological stage II disease at RPLND, four had only teratoma in retroperitoneal nodes, four had both teratoma and other germ cell tumor elements, and two had nonteratomatous germ cell tumors. Most patients with pathological stage II disease thus had elements of nonteratomatous germ cell tumors in their retroperitoneal nodes. Of the 25 patients with clinical stage I–IIA disease, relapse-free survival was 84% and all 25 were alive and without evidence of disease at the time of the analysis. Relapse-free survival was 100% among patients with pathological stage I disease, but only 60 % in patients with pathological stage II disease. Among the 16 patients with advanced stage disease, there were two relapses (12.5 %) after treatment with chemotherapy followed by resection of residual masses. One of these was successfully salvaged with chemotherapy and resection, but the other refused additional treatment. One of the 16 died of angiosarcoma, but there were no deaths from germ cell tumors, and 14 of the 16 were alive and without evidence of cancer at the time of the analysis.

Memorial Sloan-Kettering reported their experience with 29 men who underwent primary ($n=11$) or postchemotherapy ($n=18$) RPLND [13]. Lymphovascular invasion was identified in none of the 11 primary RPLND patients and in 3 (17 %) of the patients undergoing postchemotherapy RPLND. Seven of the 11 patients undergoing primary RPLND had clinical stage I disease and 2 (29 %) were found to have nodal disease, one with teratoma and one with seminoma. Of four patients with clinical stage IIA disease, three had nodal involvement, including two with teratoma and one with embryonal carcinoma. There were no relapses among the seven patients with follow-up data (median of 90.4 months). Among the postchemotherapy patients, 9 (50 %) had teratoma, 8 (44 %) had fibrosis, and 1 (5.6 %) had yolk sac tumor, essentially the same rate that has been reported generally for nonseminomatous germ cell tumors. At a median follow-up of 40 months, there was one relapse among the nine patients with teratoma, 22 months after the resection; patient died of his disease 3 years after the relapse. Among the patients with fibrosis, two were lost to follow-up, and one of the remaining six relapsed in the retroperitoneum outside the RPLND template and he was cured with a second RPLND. The patient with yolk sac tumor remained relapse free at the time of the report.

These series provide evidence that pure teratomas of the testis have substantial metastatic potential and that the metastatic disease often contains nonteratomatous germ cell tumor elements. These data support the practice of treating pure teratomas similarly to other nonseminomatous germ cell tumors.

Choriocarcinomas

Choriocarcinomas of the testis have several important distinctive characteristics that are relevant to clinical management: poor prognosis, early metastasis to organs other than the lungs, metastasis to unusual sites, and a tendency to hemorrhage. It is essential to note that choriocarcinoma germ cell tumors, regardless of whether they are gonadal or extragonadal and whether they occur in men or women, are different with regard to their molecular biology, prognosis, and treatment from gestational trophoblastic choriocarcinomas. This section is about germ cell tumors only.

Although the histopathological finding of choriocarcinoma does not directly affect risk stratification and staging of germ cell tumors, choriocarcinomas are associated with highly elevated serum beta-hCG (BHCG), the level of which is used to risk-stratify and stage disseminated germ cell tumors. Choriocarcinomas are aggressive tumors that tend to metastasize widely and qualify as poor-risk cancers on that basis in addition to having BHCG levels in the poor risk range. Choriocarcinomas metastasize hematogenously and metastasize early. Testicular cancers that are pure or predominantly choriocarcinoma are almost always stage III at the time of diagnosis. As noted above, they spread to locations that are unusual for other germ cell tumors, such as the brain, skin, eye (choroid), and digestive tract. Fortunately, they are rare, representing less than one percent of germ cell tumors in men.

Choriocarcinomas are highly vascular tumors that typically have areas of hemorrhage and necrosis. There are numerous case reports of clinically significant hemorrhage in the gastrointestinal tract, lungs, and brain, many of which have been fatal or life threatening. Bleeding events typically occur either very shortly after starting chemotherapy or in patients with rapidly progressing metastatic disease. Choriocarcinoma has also been associated with case reports of tumor lysis syndrome. These risks provide a rationale for initiating chemotherapy in an inpatient setting, so that complications can be treated promptly.

Choriocarcinomas are also associated with hormonal disorders that result from highly elevated BHCG levels. HCG, luteinizing hormone (LH), follicle-stimulating hormone (FSH), and thyroid-stimulating hormone (TSH) are heterodimeric glycoproteins that share identical alpha subunits, and HCG and LH have very similar beta subunits and stimulate the same receptor. At very high levels, BHCG can stimulate the receptors of these other glycoproteins, and stimulation of Leydig cells can result in hyperthyroidism and increased androgen production. The most common manifestation of this is gynecomastia due to peripheral conversion of androgens into estrogen [4]. Hyperprolactinemia has also been reported.

One single-institution case series from Mexico City reported that among 1010 orchiectomies performed between 1999 and 2011, six were pure and nine were predominantly choriocarcinoma. All fifteen had lymphovascular invasion in the primary tumor, nine had liver metastases, three had brain metastases, and three had GI tract involvement, and one each had involvement of the eye and skin. All had poor-risk disseminated disease (stage IIIC) on the basis of a serum BHCG greater than 50,000 IU/L, and 13 of the 15 also had nonpulmonary organ involvement. With regard to outcomes, 11 died, one was alive with disease, and one was lost to follow-up. Both patients whose disease was limited to the lungs and lymph nodes were alive in complete remission with at least 60-month follow-up [14]. A review of published reports described 106 cases of choriocarcinoma in men between 1995 and 2006. Primary sites included testis ($n=35$), mediastinum, pineal body, gastrointestinal tract, lung, and retroperitoneum, but burned out primary testis or mediastinal germ cell tumors could not be excluded. In this series, 81 of 98 (83 %) evaluable patients had metastatic disease, 37 % of patients died within 2 months of diagnosis, only 30 % of patients experienced long-term survival, and mean survival time was 7.7 months [15].

Yolk Sac Tumors

Pure yolk sac tumors represent over 60 % of prepubertal testis tumors, but are rare among postpubertal germ cell tumors in men, representing about 1 % of cases [4, 16, 17]. Yolk sac tumors are a relatively common component of testicular mixed germ cell tumors in adolescent and adult males. In primary germ cell tumors of the mediastinum, which primarily occur in young adult males, yolk sac tumors are more common than embryonal carcinomas and choriocarcinomas combined. A large case series from the Armed Forces Institute of Pathology reported that among 322 cases, 38 were yolk sac tumors, compared with six embryonal carcinomas and eight choriocarcinomas, and most mixed germ cell tumors had yolk sac tumor components [18]. The increased frequency and proportion of yolk sac tumor elements in mediastinal nonseminomatous tumors in relation to retroperitoneal and testicular germ cell tumors is reflected in an analysis of 635 consecutive extragonadal germ cell tumor patients that reported that serum alpha-fetoprotein (AFP) was elevated in 74 % of patients with mediastinal tumors with a median elevation of 2548 ng/ml compared to 51 % of patients with retroperitoneal germ cell tumors with a median elevation of 25 ng/ml [19]. In contrast, BHCG was elevated in 38 and 74 % of patients with mediastinal and retroperitoneal germ cell tumors with median values of 5 and 335 IU/L, respectively.

Although yolk sac tumors are commonly described as aggressive tumors, they have not been associated with a poor prognosis. The presence of yolk sac tumor elements in clinical stage I testis cancer has prospectively been confirmed to be associated with a lower risk of relapse, but this finding is most likely an artifact due to the fact that yolk sac tumors consistently produce AFP and can therefore be staged more accurately: For tumors that produce detectable levels of serum tumor markers, the presence of micrometastases can be detected serologically [20]. A population-based analysis using data from the U.S. Surveillance, Epidemiology, and End Results Program (SEER) between 1973 and 2003 reported that most patients with yolk sac tumors had clinically localized disease and 5-year survival for yolk sac tumors of the testis was 89%. In contrast, extragonadal yolk sac tumors and ovarian yolk sac tumors had 5-year survival rate of 67 and 81%, respectively [21].

Conclusion

The clinical management of the different subtypes of testicular germ cell tumors is differentiated mainly on the basis of the presence or absence of nonseminomatous elements and, for disseminated disease, the level of serum tumor markers, the site of metastatic lesions, and (for nonseminomas) the site of the primary tumor (mediastinal nonseminomatous tumors other than mature teratomas have a poor prognosis). Seminomas are less aggressive tumors with a better prognosis. Among nonseminomatous tumors, embryonal carcinomas and choriocarcinomas are associated with a greater tendency to metastasize, but the main prognostic feature for early stage disease remains lymphovascular invasion.

References

1. Stephenson AJ, Gilligan T. Neoplasms of the testis. In: Wein AJ, Kavoussi LR, Novick AC, Partin AW, Peters CA, editors. Campbell-walshurology. 10th ed. Philadelphia: Elsevier Saunders; 2012. pp. 837–70.
2. Tan A, Gilligan T. Controversies in the management of early-stage germ cell tumors. Curr Oncol Rep. 2009;11(3):235–43.
3. International Germ Cell Cancer Collaborative Group. International germ cell consensus classification: a prognostic factor-based staging system for metastatic germ cell cancers. J Clin Oncol. 1997;15(2):594–603.
4. Ulbright TM. Germ cell tumors of the gonads: a selective review emphasizing problems in differential diagnosis, newly appreciated, and controversial issues. Mod Pathol. 2005;18(Suppl 2):S61–79.
5. Warde P, Specht L, Horwich A, Oliver T, Panzarella T, Gospodarowicz M, et al. Prognostic factors for relapse in stage I seminoma managed by surveillance: a pooled analysis. J Clin Oncol. 2002;20(22):4448–52.
6. Aparicio J, Maroto P, Garcia Del Muro X, Guma J, Sanchez-Munoz A, Margeli M, et al. Risk-adapted treatment in clinical stage I testicular seminoma: the third Spanish germ cell cancer group study. J Clin Oncol. 2011;29(35):4677–81.
7. Kollmannsberger C, Moore C, Chi KN, Murray N, Daneshmand S, Gleave M, et al. Non-risk-adapted surveillance for patients with stage I nonseminomatous testicular germ-cell tumors: diminishing treatment-related morbidity while maintaining efficacy. Ann Oncol. 2010;21(6):1296–301.
8. Heidenreich A, Sesterhenn IA, Mostofi FK, Moul JW. Prognostic risk factors that identify patients with clinical stage I nonseminomatous germ cell tumors at low risk and high risk for metastasis.Cancer. 1998;83(5):1002–11.
9. Hermans BP, Sweeney CJ, Foster RS, Einhorn LE, Donohue JP. Risk of systemic metastases in clinical stage I nonseminoma germ cell testis tumor managed by retroperitoneal lymph node dissection. J Urol. 2000;163(6):1721–4.
10. Pohar KS, Rabbani F, Bosl GJ, Motzer RJ, Bajorin D, Sheinfeld J. Results of retroperitoneal lymph node dissection for clinical stage I and II pure embryonal carcinoma of the testis.[comment]. J Urol. 2003;170(4 Pt 1):1155–8.
11. Labarthe P, Khedis M, Chevreau C, Mazerolles C, Thoulouzan M, Durand X, et al. Management of pure teratoma of the testis in adult, results of a multicenter study over 15 years. Prog Urol. 2008;18(13):1075–81. Prise en charge du teratomepurtesticulairepostpubertaire a propos d'uneseriemulticentriquesur 15 ans.
12. Leibovitch I, Foster RS, Ulbright TM, Donohue JP. Adult primary pure teratoma of the testis. The Indiana experience. Cancer. 1995;75(9):2244–50.
13. Rabbani F, Farivar-Mohseni H, Leon A, Motzer RJ, Bosl GJ, Sheinfeld J. Clinical outcome after retroperitoneal lymphadenectomy of patients with pure testicular teratoma. Urology. 2003;62(6):1092–6.
14. Alvarado-Cabrero I, Hernandez-Toriz N, Paner GP. Clinicopathologic analysis of choriocarcinoma as a pure or predominant component of germ cell tumor of the testis. Am J Surg Pathol. 2014;38(1):111–8.
15. Yokoi K, Tanaka N, Furukawa K, Ishikawa N, Seya T, Horiba K, et al. Male choriocarcinoma with metastasis to the jejunum: a case report and review of the literature. J Nippon Med Sch. 2008;75(2):116–21.
16. Ross JH, Rybicki L, Kay R. Clinical behavior and a contemporary management algorithm for prepubertal testis tumors: a summary of the prepubertaltestis tumor registry. J Urol. 2002;168(4 Pt 2):1675–8; discussion 8–9.
17. Cao D, Humphrey PA. Yolk sac tumor of the testis. J Urol. 2011;186(4):1475–6.
18. Moran CA, Suster S, Koss MN. Primary germ cell tumors of the mediastinum: III. Yolk sac tumor, embryonal carcinoma, choriocarcinoma, and combined nonteratomatous germ cell tumors of the mediastinum—a clinicopathologic and immunohistochemical study of 64 cases. Cancer. 1997;80(4):699–707.
19. Bokemeyer C, Nichols CR, Droz JP, Schmoll HJ, Horwich A, Gerl A, et al. Extragonadal germ cell tumors of the mediastinum and retroperitoneum: results from an international analysis. J Clin Oncol. 2002;20(7):1864–73.

20. Read G, Stenning SP, Cullen MH, Parkinson MC, Horwich A, Kaye SB, et al. Medical research council prospective study of surveillance for stage I testicular teratoma. Medical research council testicular tumors working party. J Clin Oncol. 1992;10(11):1762–8.

21. Shah JP, Kumar S, Bryant CS, Ali-Fehmi R, Malone JM Jr., Deppe G, et al. A population-based analysis of 788 cases of yolk sac tumors: a comparison of males and females. Int J Cancer. 2008;123(11):2671–5.

Familial Syndromes Associated with Testicular Tumors

39

Jesse K. McKenney, Claudio Lizarralde and Cristina Magi-Galluzzi

Introduction

Testicular cancer is most common in white men with a 75% lower incidence reported in African-American men [1]. Extensive analysis, in which family history was assessed, has shown that familial risk for testicular cancer is among the highest reported for any human cancer. A recent large case–control study of familial cancer reported that the testicular cancer risk is increased 4.63-fold when a father, 8.30-fold when a brother, and 5.23-fold when a son of an affected man, respectively, had testicular cancer, compared to no familial testicular cancer [2]. In addition, a 37- to 76.5-fold elevated risk of germ cell tumors (GCT) has been reported in dizygotic/monozygotic twin brothers of men with GCT [3].

Numerous observational, case report, epidemiological, and segregation studies have provided first level of evidence supporting a genetic basis for familial testicular cancer. Nevertheless, it is important to emphasize that genes are not the only factors that cluster in families, and separating other variables such as shared environmental and occupational exposures, patterns of behavior, and diet from genetic causes can be difficult.

Linkage studies have identified several rare tumor syndromes whose phenotypes include testicular cancer, such as Peutz–Jeghers and Carney complex.

See Table 39.1 for a summary of familial syndromes and genes associated with testicular tumors.

Familial Germ Cell Tumors

Germ cell tumors (GCT), the most common testicular cancer, are broadly categorized as seminomas and nonseminomatous GCT (NSGCT). The incidence of GCT has increased significantly during the last 40 years, predominantly in white men, in association with a simultaneous increase in cryptorchidism, hypospadia, and infertility [1].

Familial testicular GCT, defined as those diagnosed in at least two blood relatives, occurs in 1–2% of all cases of testicular GCT. The evidence of the existence of a true familial form of GCT is mainly supported by several years of segregation studies, which suggest an autosomal recessive mode of inheritance [4], and more recently, linkage analyses have identified several genomic regions of modest interest on chromosomes 5, 6, and 12. However, no high-penetrance cancer susceptibility gene has been mapped yet [3–5].

The Y chromosome, which cannot be analyzed by genetic linkage, carries a number of testis- and

C. Magi-Galluzzi (✉) · C. Lizarralde · J. K. McKenney
Department of Pathology, Cleveland Clinic, Robert J. Tomsich Pathology and Laboratory Medicine Institute, Cleveland, OH, USA
e-mail: magic@ccf.org

C. Lizarralde
e-mail: claudiolizarralde@hotmail.comva

J. K. McKenney
e-mail: mckennj@ccf.org

C. Magi-Galluzzi, C. G. Przybycin (eds.), *Genitourinary Pathology,* DOI 10.1007/978-1-4939-2044-0_39,

Table 39.1 Syndromes and genes associated with testicular tumors

Familial syndrome	Gene localization	Candidate gene/locus	Gene function	Testicular lesion/s
Familial germ cell tumors	12q22 5q31	*KITLG* *SPRY4*	Inhibitors of the MAPK signaling pathway	GCT
Peutz–Jeghers	19q13.3	*LKB1 (STK11)*	Negatively regulates organ growth	ITLCHSCN LCSCT
Carney complex	17q22–24 2p16	*PRKAR1A*	Cell growth	LCSCT Leydig cell tumor Adrenocortical rests
Familial adenomatous polyposis	5q21 1p	*APC* *MUTYH*	Cell division regulation DNA repair	Yolk sac tumor Sertoli cell tumor GCT
Cowden disease	10q23	*PTEN*	Cell cycle regulation	Lipomatosis testis Germ cell tumors
Bannayan–Riley–Ruvalcaba syndrome	10q23	*PTEN*	Cell cycle regulation	Lipomatosis testis Seminoma
Gorlin syndrome	9q22.3	*PTCH (PTCH1)*	Formation of embryonic structures	Thecoma
Von Hippel–Lindau disease	3p25–26	*VHL*	Cell growth	Epididymal cystadenoma
Hereditary hemochromatosis	6p22	*HFE*	Iron metabolism	Seminoma
Li-Fraumeni syndrome	17p13.1	*P53*	Genome stability	Mixed GCT Teratoma
Neurofibromatosis type 1	17q11.2	*NF1*	Glial growth regulation	Seminoma Mixed GCT Teratoma
Adrenogenital syndrome	6p21.3 8q22	*CYP21A2* *CYP11B1*	Steroidogenic pathways	TART TART

ITLCHSCN intratubular large cell hyalinizing Sertoli cell neoplasia, *LCSCT* large cell calcifying Sertoli cell tumor, *GCT* germ cell tumors, *TSG* tumor suppressor gene, *TART* testicular adrenal rest tumor

germ cell-specific genes. In 2005, the potential role of the Y chromosome *gr/gr* deletion as a familial testicular GCT risk factor was analyzed. This hypothesized association was based on the clear link between male infertility, whose most commonly identified genetic cause is the gr/gr deletion, and testicular GCT. The presence of gr/gr deletion was associated with a twofold increased risk of testicular GCT and more strongly with seminoma [4]. In 2008, a study of the gene *DND1* in 263 patients showed that, whether it is disease-causing or not, mutations in *DND1* make, at most, a very small contribution to testicular GCT susceptibility in adults and adolescents [5]. More recently, germline mutations in phosphodiesterase 11A (*PDE11A*) were analyzed, concluding that a strong but not perfect concordance between the presence of a testicular tumor and the presence of a mutation existed [4, 5].

Although the genetic basis of familial GCT remains still unknown, two recent genomewide association studies (GWAS) have identified the 12q22 locus as a GCT susceptibility locus in both seminomas and NSGCTs [6, 7]. The 12q22 locus contains *KITLG* (also known as stem cell factor or steel), which encodes the ligand for the membrane-bound receptor tyrosine kinase, c-KIT. It has been postulated that *KITLG* may explain the association on chromosome 12, since intratubular germ cell neoplasia cells, seminoma cells, and primordial germ cells all are known to express c-KIT in a membranous pattern by immunohistochemistry techniques. A second association was identified at 5q31, downstream of SPRY4, a negative regulator of the RAS–ERK–MAPK pathway [8]. A functional association between *KIT* and *SPRY4* has been suggested by tumor studies of imatinib-treated gastrointestinal stromal tumors [9].

Peutz–Jeghers Syndrome

Peutz–Jeghers syndrome is a hereditary autosomal dominant disorder associated with considerable morbidity and decreased life expectancy. It is the most common form of hamartomatous polyposis with a reported prevalence of between 1 in 29,000 and 1 in 200,000. Peutz–Jeghers syndrome clinical hallmarks are intestinal hamartomatous polyposis and melanin pigmentation of skin and mucous membranes [1].

Genetically, Peutz–Jeghers syndrome is characterized by mutations in *LKB1* (also known as *STK11*), a tumor suppressor gene located on the short arm of chromosome 19 (19p13.3). Patients are predisposed to multiple neoplasms. The most common malignancies are small intestinal, colorectal, stomach, and pancreatic adenocarcinomas. In the gynecologic tract, the best-known tumors are ovarian sex cord tumor with annular tubules and adenoma malignum of uterine cervix. In male patients, testicular lesions are less well characterized, but tend to develop during childhood and are associated with estrogenic manifestations, notably gynecomastia. An association with testicular tumors, particularly Sertoli cell tumors, sex cord tumors with annular tubules, and aromatase-producing sex cord tumors, is also reported [10].

The main testicular sex cord stromal tumors described in Peutz–Jeghers syndrome are intratubular large cell hyalinizing Sertoli cell neoplasia and large cell calcifying Sertoli cell tumor. Intratubular large cell hyalinizing Sertoli cell neoplasia is a neoplastic process usually confined to the seminiferous tubules, although it may occasionally progress to invasive Sertoli cell tumor with or without associated calcification. Large cell calcifying Sertoli cell tumor is related to inherited genetic syndromes such as Peutz–Jeghers syndrome and Carney complex in up to 40% of the cases; however, only a small fraction of syndromic patients (<27% of Peutz–Jeghers patients) develop invasive large cell calcifying Sertoli cell tumor [11].

Carney Complex

Carney complex is an autosomal dominant condition characterized by hyperpigmentation of the skin (lentiginosis), myxomas of the heart and skin, endocrine tumors or overactivity, and schwannomas. It is most commonly caused by inactivating mutations of the regulatory subunit 1A of the protein kinase A (PKA) or cAMP-dependent protein kinase (PRKAR1A). The *PRKAR1A* gene, on chromosome 17q22-q24, may function as a tumor-suppressor gene. Inactivating germline mutations of the *PRKAR1A* gene are found in 70% of patients with Carney complex. Germline, protein-truncating mutations of phosphodiesterase type 11A (PDE11A) have been described to predispose to a variety of endocrine tumors, including adrenal and testicular tumors [12]. Less commonly, the molecular pathogenesis of Carney complex is a variety of genetic changes at chromosome 2p16. Despite dissimilar genetics, there appears to be no phenotypic difference between *PRKAR1A* and chromosome 2p16 mutations [13].

In the series described by Carney, nine patients presented with testicular tumors: large cell calcifying Sertoli cell tumor, Leydig cell tumor, adrenocortical rest tumor, or a combination of these. Large cell calcifying Sertoli tumors are the most common lesions and develop in approximately 30% of patients within the first decade and in virtually all carriers by adulthood. Large cell calcifying Sertoli tumors may occur alone or may be associated with Leydig cell tumor, Leydig cell hyperplasia, or adrenal cortical rest components [14].

Sex cord stromal tumors in Carney complex have an apparent indolent natural history with low metastatic potential. Orchiectomy has been standard treatment in the past; however, large cell calcifying Sertoli cell tumors of the testes are overwhelmingly clinically benign, and unless there are significant hormonal changes or complicating symptoms, surveillance may be a preferred management strategy [15]. In patients with Carney complex, enlargement of a solitary testicular tumor to greater than 4 cm is suspicious of malignancy and orchiectomy is typically pursued. Although most unilateral solitary large cell calcifying Sertoli tumors behave in a benign fashion, those exhibiting extratesticular growth and occurring in older patients (mean age 39 years) warrant orchiectomy because of the risk of malignancy [14]. Some authors have suggested that large cell calcifying Sertoli tumors in Carney complex have more benign clinical outcomes when compared with those in Peutz–Jeghers syndrome [15].

Impaired fertility, defective sperm, and oligospermia have been reported in men with Carney complex. The pathway that leads to infertility seems independent of the presence of testicular sex cord neoplasms, but the presence of a relationship is still unclear [16]. Clinical testing is available for *PRKAR1A,* and sequencing detects approximately 55 % of mutations. Many different mutations have been reported in the *PRKAR1A* gene, and in almost all cases, the sequence change leads to a premature stop codon [17]. More than two thirds of patients with Carney complex inherit the mutation from a parent, but approximately 30 % of mutations occur de novo [18].

Familial Adenomatous Polyposis Syndrome

Familial adenomatous polyposis (FAP) is a disease classically characterized by the development of hundreds to thousands of adenomatous polyps in rectum and colon during the second decade of life. Almost all patients will develop colorectal cancer. It can have different inheritance patterns and different genetic causes. Attenuated FAP is a less severe form of FAP, marked by the presence of <100 polyps and a later onset of colorectal cancer. FAP is caused by autosomal dominantly inherited mutations in the *APC* (adenomatous polyposis coli) gene, a tumor suppressor gene that controls beta-catenin turnover in the Wnt pathway. The *APC* gene is localized on chromosome 5q21. De novo occurrence is reported in 30–40 % of the patients. Mutations are detected in 85 % of classical FAP families, while only 20–30 % of attenuated FAP cases will exhibit a germline *APC* mutation. *MYH/MUTYH*, on chromosome 1p, is the second FAP-related gene and is involved with base-excision repair of DNA damaged by oxidative stress. *MUTYH* mutations are inherited in an autosomal recessive fashion and account for 10–20 % of classical FAP cases without an *APC* mutation and for 30 % of attenuated FAP cases [19].

The prevalence of concomitant testicular and colorectal cancer in the same patient is rare. Recent studies have suggested that the protein *APC* plays an important role in cell adhesion and migration, which is intricately linked with its tumor-promoting activities. Tanwar et al. have shown that *APC* is also essential for maintaining the integrity of the seminiferous epithelium [20]. Epigenetic studies suggest the involvement of the *APC* gene in testicular yolk sac tumor of infants. Loss of heterozygosity at 5q21, where the *APC* gene is localized, was detected in at least three of nine testicular yolk sac tumors. Promoter methylation was detected in seven of ten infantile yolk sac tumors; of the seven cases showing methylation, three also harbored loss of heterozygosity at 5q21. These data indicate that inactivation of the *APC* gene, by allelic loss and/or promoter methylation, is related to the occurrence of infantile yolk sac tumors [21].

A case of bilateral Sertoli cell tumor in a FAP patient has been reported. The bilaterality and overexpression of beta-catenin in this tumor strongly suggests an association between these two events. Also, testicular germ cell tumors have been reported in two siblings in the context of an attenuated FAP linked to mutations in *MUTYH* [22].

PTEN Hamartoma Tumor Syndromes: Cowden Disease and Bannayan–Riley–Ruvalcaba Syndrome

Cowden Disease

Cowden disease or multiple hamartoma syndrome, is an uncommon autosomal dominant inherited disorder characterized by multiple hamartomas and by an increased predisposition to breast carcinoma, follicular carcinoma of the thyroid, and endometrial carcinoma [23]. Cowden disease results, most commonly (80 %), from a mutation in the *PTEN* gene on arm 10q23. This mutation leads to characteristic features including macrocephaly, intestinal hamartomatous polyps, benign skin tumors, and dysplastic gangliocytoma of the cerebellum (Lhermitte-Duclos disease).

Testicular lesions are not uncommon in Cowden disease, and both benign and malignant tumors have been reported in these patients. The first case, described by Lindsay et al. [24], was a Cowden disease patient with presumable fat-containing hamartomas in both testes diagnosed by MRI, suggesting the possible association between these benign lesions and Cowden disease. Another case of testicular hamartoma, concomitant with an adenomatoid tumor of the epididymis, was described in a 26-year-old patient with Cowden disease. Although histological confirmation was performed, neither morphological description nor photomicrographs were provided by the authors [25].

In the largest series to date, Woodhouse et al. [26] investigated the possibility of subnormal fertility in eight males with Cowden disease by ultrasound scan. An incidental finding in seven of these patients was diagnosed as testicular lipomatosis. Four of these cases were biopsied and reported as "interstitial lipomatosis consisting of nests of adipocytes within the testicular interstitium with no intratubular calcification or intratubular germ cell neoplasia." The authors proposed testicular lipomatosis as a novel entity based on a distinctive ultrasound appearance and as a pathognomic lesion for Cowden disease that could be used as a major criterion for the diagnosis since it has not been described outside the context of Cowden disease.

Two cases of germ cell tumors have been described in Cowden disease patients: a seminoma [27] and a mixed germ cell tumor composed by embryonal carcinoma, mature teratoma, and yolk sac tumor [28].

Bannayan–Riley–Ruvalcaba Syndrome

Bannayan–Riley–Ruvalcaba syndrome is a rare, usually autosomal dominant disease associated with PTEN hamartoma tumor syndrome, and it is clinically diagnosed in the presence of the triad of macrocephaly, genital lentiginosis, and intestinal polyposis. The syndrome results from a germline mutation in PTEN tumor suppressor gene on chromosome 10q23. Patients with Bannayan–Riley–Ruvalcaba syndrome have been reported to have an increased incidence of benign tumors, especially lipomas and hemangiomas [29]. In 2008, Walker et al. reported a case of testicular seminoma in a background of testicular lipomatosis in a 31-year-old patient [30].

Nevoid Basal Cell Carcinoma Syndrome (Gorlin Syndrome)

Gorlin syndrome (GS) is an autosomal dominantly inherited disorder characterized by malformations of the skin, nerves, eyes, and bone, with frequent loss of heterozygosity at 9q22.3 or abnormalities in the *PTCH (PTCH1)* gene. It is associated with multiple basal cell carcinomas, medulloblastoma, and multiple odontogenic keratocysts. Many women with this syndrome also develop ovarian thecoma or fibroma at a mean age of 30 years [31]. Thecoma is an extremely rare tumor in the testis, and only two cases have been reported to date, one of them in the context of Gorlin syndrome [31].

Von Hipple-Lindau Disease

Von Hippel–Lindau (VHL) disease is an autosomal dominantly inherited multisystem family cancer syndrome, predisposing to retinal and central nervous system hemangioblastomas, clear cell renal cell carcinomas, pheochromocytomas, pancreatic islet cell tumors, and endolymphatic sac tumors. In addition, renal, pancreatic, and epididymal cysts occur [32]. Patients with VHL disease carry a germline mutation of the *VHL* gene, on chromosome 3p25–26.

After hemangioblastoma, which is often the index tumor of the syndrome, the epididymis may represent the most frequently involved site in male patients, since epididymal cystadenomas have been reported in 17–50% of male VHL patients [32]. Gaslker et al. studied ten VHL patients and concluded that epididymal cystadenomas evolve from a variety of microscopic epithelial tumourlets and are confined to the efferent ductular system. The pathogenesis of epididymal cystadenomas, and whether these lesions arise as a result of *VHL* gene inactivation, remains unknown [32].

Hereditary Hemochromatosis

Hereditary hemochromatosis is an inherited autosomal recessive disorder of iron metabolism resulting in inappropriately elevated intestinal iron absorption leading to a progressive iron accumulation in a variety of organs, such as the liver, pancreas, heart, skin, pituitary, joints, and testes. It predominantly affects Caucasian individuals of northern European origin. Genetically, it is caused by a mutation in the hemochromatosis gene *(HFE),* located on chromosome 6p22. Two main *HFE* defects have been described: C282Y and H63D. Gunel-Ozcan et al. have reported that *HFE* H63D mutation seems to be an important risk factor for impaired sperm motility and is clinically associated with male infertility. One year later, a case of seminoma was reported in the context of hereditary hemochromatosis showing homozygosity for the C282Y mutation of *HFE* gene. The authors hypothesized a parallelism between excess iron deposition in the liver leading to cirrhosis and hepatocellular carcinoma to excess iron deposition in the testes leading to testicular atrophy and possible testicular cancer [33].

Li-Fraumeni Syndrome

Li–Fraumeni syndrome is an autosomal dominant hereditary disorder associated with greatly increased susceptibility to malignant neoplasms. The syndrome is linked to germline mutations of the *p53* tumor suppressor gene on chromosome 17p13.1. The classical Li–Fraumeni syndrome is a clinical diagnosis according to the following criteria: a proband with a sarcoma before the age of 45 years, a first-degree relative with any cancer before the age of 45 years, and one additional first- or second-degree relative in the same lineage with any cancer before the age of 60 years or a sarcoma at any age. Patients with Li-Fraumeni syndrome are particularly prone to carcinomas of the breast and adrenal cortex, sarcomas of the soft tissues and bone, acute leukemias, and brain tumors.

Some data suggest that carriers of germline *TP53* mutations may be predisposed to other forms of cancer such as melanoma, carcinomas of the lung, prostate and pancreas, as well as gonadal germ cell tumors [34]. Although testicular tumors were not described in original Li-Fraumeni families, in 1989, Hartley et al. reported the occurrence of five testicular germ cell tumors in relatives of children with bone or soft tissue sarcomas and proposed that germ cell tumors may be an uncommon manifestation of the genetic predisposition to cancer that exists in the Li-Fraumeni cancer family syndrome [35]. Later, Scott et al. reported a classical Li-Fraumeni patient who developed multiple tumors, after presenting with a teratoma of the testis [36]. Recently, Stechet and colleagues reported a case of a 20-month-old boy who presented with a testicular Leydig cell tumor and 6 years later developed a primitive neuroectodermal brain tumor. A novel splice site mutation of the *TP53* gene was found in the proband, his father and younger sister, but only the proband has so far developed malignancy. Although the clinical phenotype in the boy was suggestive of Li-Fraumeni syndrome, the family did not strictly conform to the canonical definition [34].

Neurofibromatosis Type 1 (von Recklinghausen's Disease)

The term neurofibromatosis is used for a group of genetic disorders that primarily affect the cell growth of neural tissues. There are two forms of neurofibromatosis: type 1 and type 2. Peripheral neurofibromatosis type 1 (NF1), also known as von Recklinghausen's disease, is a neurodermal dysplasia and the most common type of neurofibromatosis, estimated to represent 90% of all cases. NF1 is an autosomal dominant condition caused by a spectrum of mutations affecting the *NF1* gene located on chromosome 17q11.2 and characterized by the presence of cutaneous neurofibromas, café au lait spots of the skin, and pigmented iris hamartomas.

The most common neurofibromatosis-associated malignancies derive from neurogenic tissues, although several malignancies originating from non-neurogenic tissue have been also described. In 1988, Groot-Loonen et al. documented a patient with neurofibromatosis and a mixed germ cell tumor of the testis; in 1990, Hilton and colleagues reported a case of testicular teratoma in a patient with peripheral neurofibromatosis. Recently, Kume and colleagues reported a case of bilateral testicular cancer associated with neurofibromatosis type 1, where the patient presented with an embryonal carcinoma of the right testis at age 15 and developed a seminoma of the left testis 10 years later [37]. Since loss of heterozygosity was not seen in intron 26 of the NF1 gene, the pathogenesis of the testicular tumors remains unclear.

Adrenogenital Syndrome

Adrenogenital syndrome, also known as congenital adrenal hyperplasia (CAH), describes a family of autosomal recessive disorders characterized by enzyme defects in the steroidogenic pathways leading to glucocorticoid, and in most cases, mineralocorticoid deficiency [38]. Ninety percent of CAH cases have a defect in 21-α hydroxylase enzyme, caused by severe mutations in the *CYP21A2* gene, located on chromosome 6p21.3 [39]. Steroid 11β-hydroxylase deficiency, caused by mutations in the *CYP11B1* gene on chromosome 8q22, is the second most common cause of CAH and accounts for approximately 5% of cases. This form of CAH is characterized by hypertension and signs of androgen excess [40].

In CAH, cortisol production is reduced via negative feedback and adrenocorticotropic hormone (ACTH) synthesis is increased. Chronic excessive ACTH stimulation may result in hyperplasia of ACTH-sensitive tissues in adrenal glands and other sites such as the testes, causing testicular masses known as "testicular adrenal rest tumors" (TARTs) [41, 42].

TARTs are extremely difficult to differentiate from Leydig cell tumors since both are composed of steroid-secreting cells and could lead to precocious puberty and testicular masses. However, unlike Leydig cell tumors, TARTs never contain Reinke crystalloids, are often bilateral, and most respond to steroid suppressive therapy [41]. TARTs are always benign, although compression of the seminiferous tubules may lead to obstructive azoospermia, irreversible damage of the surrounding testicular tissue, and consequent infertility [42].

References

1. Gallagher DJ, Feifer A, Coleman JA. Genitourinary cancer predisposition syndromes. Hematol Oncol Clin North Am. 2010;24(5):861–83.
2. Nordsborg RB, Meliker JR, Wohlfahrt J, Melbye M, Raaschou-Nielsen O. Cancer in first-degree relatives and risk of testicular cancer in Denmark. Int J Cancer. 2011;129(10):2485–91.
3. LutkeHolzik MF, Rapley EA, Hoekstra HJ, Sleijfer DT, Nolte IM, Sijmons RH. Genetic predisposition to testicular germ-cell tumours. Lancet Oncol. 2004;5(6):363–71.
4. Greene MH, Kratz CP, Mai PL, Mueller C, Peters JA, Bratslavsky G, et al. Familial testicular germ cell tumors in adults: 2010 summary of genetic risk factors and clinical phenotype. Endocr Relat Cancer. 2010;17(2):R109–21.
5. Kratz CP, Mai PL, Greene MH. Familial testicular germ cell tumours. Best Prac Res Clin Endocrinol Metab. 2010;24(3):503–13.
6. Kanetsky PA, Mitra N, Vardhanabhuti S, Li M, Vaughn DJ, Letrero R, et al. Common variation in KITLG and at 5q31.3 predisposes to testicular germ cell cancer. Nat Genet. 2009;41(7):811–5.
7. Rapley EA, Turnbull C, Al Olama AA, Dermitzakis ET, Linger R, Huddart RA, et al. A genome-wide association study of testicular germ cell tumor. Nat Genet. 2009;41(7):807–10.
8. Sasaki A, Taketomi T, Kato R, Saeki K, Nonami A, Sasaki M, et al. Mammalian Sprouty4 suppresses Ras-independent ERK activation by binding to Raf1. Nat Cell Biol. 2003;5(5):427–32.

9. Frolov A, Chahwan S, Ochs M, Arnoletti JP, Pan ZZ, Favorova O, et al. Response markers and the molecular mechanisms of action of Gleevec in gastrointestinal stromal tumors. Mol Cancer Ther. 2003;2(8):699–709.
10. Ulbright TM, Amin MB, Young RH. Intratubular large cell hyalinizingsertoli cell neoplasia of the testis: a report of 8 cases of a distinctive lesion of the Peutz-Jeghers syndrome. Am J Surg Pathol. 2007;31(6):827–35.
11. Kaluzny A, Matuszewski M, Wojtylak S, Krajka K, Cichy W, Plawski A, et al. Organ-sparing surgery of the bilateral testicular large cell calcifying sertoli cell tumor in patient with atypical Peutz-Jeghers syndrome. Int Urol Nephrol. 2012;44(4):1045–8.
12. Libe R, Horvath A, Vezzosi D, Fratticci A, Coste J, Perlemoine K, et al. Frequent phosphodiesterase 11A gene (PDE11A) defects in patients with Carney complex (CNC) caused by PRKAR1A mutations: PDE11A may contribute to adrenal and testicular tumors in CNC as a modifier of the phenotype. J Clin Endocrinol Metab. 2011;96(1):E208–14.
13. Stratakis CA, Kirschner LS, Carney JA. Clinical and molecular features of the Carney complex: diagnostic criteria and recommendations for patient evaluation. J Clin Endocrinol Metab. 2001;86(9):4041–6.
14. Washecka R, Dresner MI, Honda SA. Testicular tumors in Carney's complex. J Urol. 2002; 167(3):1299–302.
15. Gourgari E, Saloustros E, Stratakis CA. Large-cell calcifying Sertoli cell tumors of the testes in pediatrics. Curr Opin Pediatr. 2012;24(4):518–22.
16. Wieacker P, Stratakis CA, Horvath A, Klose S, Nickel I, Buhtz P, et al. Male infertility as a component of Carney complex. Andrologia. 2007;39(5):196–7.
17. Losada Grande EJ, Al Kassam Martinez D, Gonzalez Boillos M. Carney complex. Endocrinol Nutr. 2011;58(6):308–14.
18. Boikos SA, Stratakis CA. Carney complex: the first 20 years. Curr Opin Oncol. 2007;19(1):24–9.
19. Claes K, Dahan K, Tejpar S, De Paepe A, Bonduelle M, Abramowicz M, et al. The genetics of familial adenomatous polyposis (FAP) and MutYH-associated polyposis (MAP). Acta Gastroenterol Belg. 2011;74(3):421–6.
20. Tanwar PS, Zhang L, Teixeira JM. Adenomatous polyposis coli (APC) is essential for maintaining the integrity of the seminiferous epithelium. Mol Endocrinol. 2011;25(10):1725–39.
21. Kato N, Shibuya H, Fukase M, Tamura G, Motoyama T. Involvement of adenomatous polyposis coli (APC) gene in testicular yolk sac tumor of infants. Hum Pathol. 2006;37(1):48–53.
22. Castillejo A, Sanchez-Heras AB, Jover R, Castillejo MI, Guarinos C, Oltra S, et al. Recurrent testicular germ cell tumors in a family with MYH-associated polyposis. J Clin Oncol. 2012;30(23):e216–7.
23. Calva D, Howe JR. Hamartomatous polyposis syndromes. Surg Clin North Am. 2008;88(4):779–817, vii.
24. Lindsay C, Boardman L, Farrell M. Testicular hamartomas in cowden disease. J Clin Ultrasound. 2003;31(9):481–3.
25. Rasalkar DD, Paunipagar BK. Testicular hamartomas and epididymal tumor in a cowden disease: a case report. Case Rep Med. 2010;2010:135029.
26. Woodhouse JB, Delahunt B, English SF, Fraser HH, Ferguson MM. Testicular lipomatosis in Cowden's syndrome. Mod Pathol. 2005;18(9):1151–6.
27. Mazereeuw-Hautier J, Assouere MN, Moreau-Cabarrot A, Longy M, Bonafe JL. Cowden's syndrome: possible association with testicular seminoma. Br J Dermatol. 2004;150(2):378–9.
28. Devi M, Leonard N, Silverman S, Al-Qahtani M, Girgis R. Testicular mixed germ cell tumor in an adolescent with cowden disease. Oncology. 2007;72(3–4):194–6.
29. Hendriks YM, Verhallen JT, van derSmagt JJ, Kant SG, Hilhorst Y, Hoefsloot L, et al. Bannayan-Riley-Ruvalcaba syndrome: further delineation of the phenotype and management of PTEN mutation-positive cases. Fam Cancer. 2003;2(2):79–85.
30. Walker RN, Murphy TJ, Wilkerson ML. Testicular hamartomas in a patient with Bannayan-Riley-Ruvalcaba syndrome. J Ultrasound Med. 2008;27(8):1245–8.
31. Ueda M, Kanematsu A, Nishiyama H, Yoshimura K, Watanabe K, Yorifuji T, et al. Testicular thecoma in an 11-year-old boy with nevoid basal-cell carcinoma syndrome (Gorlin syndrome). J Pediatr Surg. 2010;45(3):E1–3.
32. Glasker S, Tran MG, Shively SB, Ikejiri B, Lonser RR, Maxwell PH, et al. Epididymalcystadenomas and epithelial tumourlets: effects of VHL deficiency on the human epididymis. J Pathol. 2006;210(1): 32–41.
33. Onitilo AA, Engel JM, Sajjad SM. The possible role of hemochromatosis in testicular cancer. Med Hypotheses. 2011;77(2):179–81.
34. Stecher CW, Gronbaek K, Hasle H. A novel splice mutation in the TP53 gene associated with Leydig cell tumor and primitive neuroectodermal tumor. Pediatr Blood Cancer. 2008;50(3):701–3.
35. Hartley AL, Birch JM, Kelsey AM, Marsden HB, Harris M, Teare MD. Are germ cell tumors part of the Li-Fraumeni cancer family syndrome? Cancer Genet Cytogenet. 1989;42(2):221–6.
36. Scott RJ, Krummenacher F, Mary JL, Weber W, Spycher M, Muller H. Hereditary p53 mutation in a patient with multiple tumors: significance for genetic counseling. Schweiz Med Wochenschr. 1993;123(25):1287–92. Vererbbare p53-Mutation bei einem Patienten mit Mehrfachtumoren: Bedeutung fur die genetische Beratung. ger.
37. Kume H, Tachikawa T, Teramoto S, Isurugi K, Kitamura T. Bilateral testicular tumour in neurofibromatosis type 1. Lancet. 2001;357(9253):395–6.
38. Gessl A, Lemmens-Gruber R, Kautzky-Willer A. Adrenal disorders. Handb Exp Pharmacol. 2012;214:341–59.

39. Speiser PW, White PC. Congenital adrenal hyperplasia. N Engl J Med. 2003;349(8):776–88.
40. White PC. Congenital adrenal hyperplasias. Best Pract Res Clin Endocrinol Metab. 2001;15(1):17–41.
41. Rich MA, Keating MA. Leydig cell tumors and tumors associated with congenital adrenal hyperplasia. Urol Clin North Am. 2000;27(3):519–28, x.
42. Claahsen-vander Grinten HL, Otten BJ, Stikkelbroeck MM, Sweep FC, Hermus AR. Testicular adrenal rest tumours in congenital adrenal hyperplasia. Best Pract Res Clin Endocrinol Metab. 2009;23(2):209–20.

40 Molecular and Immunohistochemical Markers of Diagnostic and Prognostic Value in Testicular Tumors

Victor E. Reuter

Introduction

Primary testicular neoplasms are rare with less than 10,000 new cases reported each year in the USA. Once a testicular mass is resected, it is imperative to establish an accurate diagnosis since the most common tumors are mostly curable as long as the therapeutic approach is directed to the specific tumor type. Testicular germ cell tumors (GCTs) have a very good prognosis, even in the presence of metastatic disease, due to their exquisite sensitivity to cisplatinum-based chemotherapy. However, the therapeutic approach to clinical stage 1 primary testicular GCTs will vary significantly based on the pathological diagnosis rendered. In cases of pure seminoma, following orchiectomy, the patients are either placed on surveillance or given low-dose radiation therapy. No pathological features in the primary tumor, including lymphovascular invasion and rete testis involvement, have been validated to predict progression or are utilized to drive subsequent therapy. In mixed GCTs, lymphovascular invasion and the percentage of embryonal carcinoma (EC) have been independently associated with an increased risk of disease progression in multiple studies. For this reason in many institutions, particularly in Europe, these patients will be given a modified protocol of systemic chemotherapy while, in others, a primary retroperitoneal lymph node dissection will be the treatment of choice. Sex cord-stromal tumors are primarily a surgical disease since no systemic therapies have shown significant efficacy. The hallmarks to cure include early detection and surgical removal of all existing disease. Prognostic factors are morphology based since no molecular markers have been identified to predict prognosis or response to therapy.

Germ Cell Tumors

Given the relative rarity of testicular GCTs and their vast morphological heterogeneity, it is understandable that pathologists in routine clinical practice resort to ancillary studies, particularly immunohistochemistry, to establish the correct diagnosis. Another very important clinical scenario where the pathologic diagnosis is critically important is when evaluating retroperitoneal and mediastinal masses (midline masses of unknown origin), particularly in younger patients. While these masses may very well represent sarcoma or lymphoma, for example, GCTs should always enter in the differential diagnosis (Fig. 40.1a–d). Fortunately, there are multiple assays that can help us to establish the histogenesis of the lesion. Unfortunately, the rarity of the disease, the complex morphologies that can be present as well as the abundance of markers that have been published through the years as helpful in distinguishing between various entities have led to overdependence and overuse of ancillary studies

V. E. Reuter (✉)
Department of Pathology, Memorial Sloan Kettering Cancer Center, New York, NY, USA
e-mail: reuterv@mskcc.org

C. Magi-Galluzzi, C. G. Przybycin (eds.), *Genitourinary Pathology,* DOI 10.1007/978-1-4939-2044-0_40,

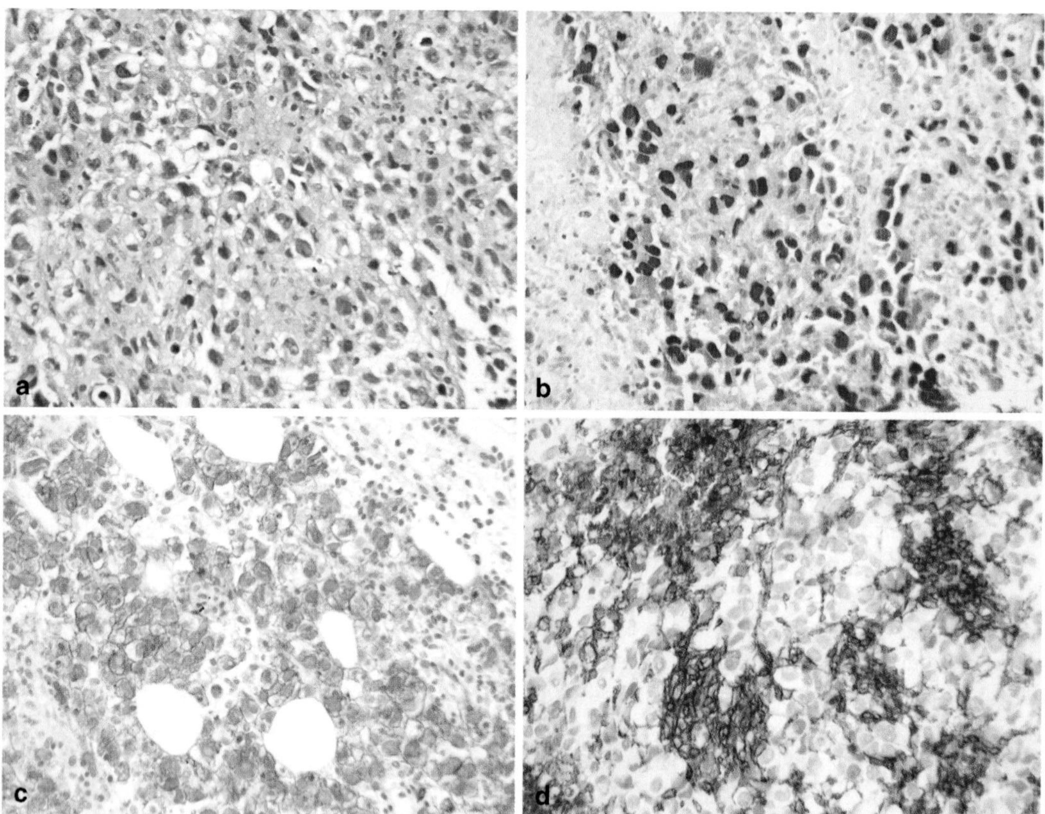

Fig. 40.1 Seminoma in a needle biopsy of the retroperitoneum. **a** H&E stain. **b** OCT3/4 showing nuclear immunoreactivity. **c** CD117 showing cytoplasmic/membranous staining. **d** CD20 staining surrounding lymphocytes

with its predictable negative impact on healthcare costs. The purpose of this chapter is to review the assays that are most useful in arriving at the correct diagnosis, incorporating novel markers that have entered the clinical laboratory in recent years, and limiting/eliminating the use of markers that are either of limited utility or have been supplanted by newer assays with better performance characteristics. As is the case in virtually all tumors, there is no single marker that is 100 % specific or sensitive for any given tumor type. For this reason, markers should always be used in a panel, but this panel should be directed to the specific differential diagnosis under consideration.

Molecular Markers of Germ Cell Lineage

Through the years, a modest but significant amount of work has gone into understanding the molecular pathogenesis of testicular GCTs, the genomic differences among various tumor types, and the genes that are differentially expressed in chemotherapy-sensitive as well as chemotherapy-resistant tumors [1–3].

However, none of these findings are used clinically, either to establish a precise diagnosis (subclassification) or to choose therapy. At this time, the key to selecting proper therapy lies on an accurate pathological diagnosis, assessment of pathologic risk factors, state-of-the-art imaging, and serum tumor markers.

Testicular GCTs can be divided into three groups (infantile/prepubertal, adolescent/young adult, and spermatocytic seminoma (SS)), each with its own constellation of clinical histology, molecular, and clinical feature [4–7]. They originate from germ cells at different stages of development. Tumors arising in prepubertal gonads are either teratomas or yolk sac tumors (YSTs),

Table 40.1 Molecular characterization of testicular germ cell tumors (GCTs)

i(12p) is the most common genetic abnormality seen in testicular germ cell tumors
Presence of i(12p) is characteristic but not entirely specific for germ cell tumor origin
Presence of i(12p) is of diagnostic utility but does not predict histologic type, prognosis or response to therapy
i(12p) is best identified by karyotype analysis
Presence of i(12p) may be analyzed by fluorescent in situ hybridization (FISH) in formalin-fixed, paraffin-embedded tissues, but this assay suffers from less than ideal sensitivity and specificity

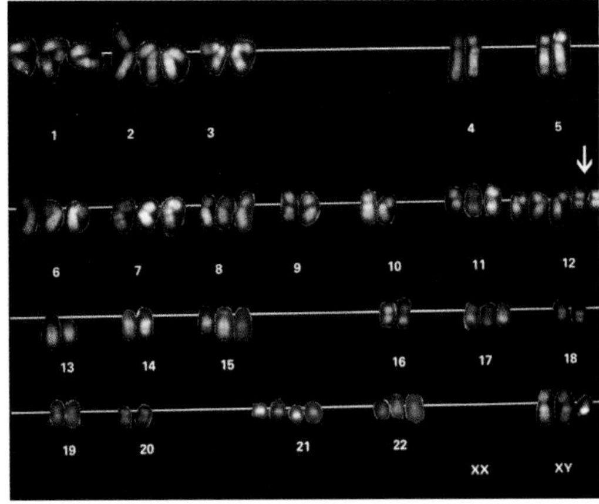

Fig. 40.2 An early karyotype depicting the presence of two copies of isochromosome 12p [i(12p)] (*arrow*). It was these early studies that allowed investigators to define what we now regard as the most common genetic abnormality seen in adult onset testicular germ cell tumors (GCTs)

tend to be diploid, and are not associated with i(12p) nor intratubular germ cell neoplasia unclassified (IGCNU). The annual incidence is approximately 0.12 per 100,000. SS arises in older patients. These benign tumors may be either diploid or aneuploid and have losses of chromosome 9 rather than i(12p). Intratubular SS is commonly encountered but IGCNU is not. Their annual incidence is approximately 0.2 per 100,000. The pathogenesis of prepubertal GCTs and SS is poorly understood.

The most common testicular GCTs arise in postpubertal men and are characterized genetically by the presence of excess genetic material of the short arm of chromosome 12, usually due to one or more copies of i(12p), or other forms of 12p amplification and aneuploidy [8] (Table 40.1). The consistent gain of genetic material from the short arm of chromosome 12 seen in these tumors suggests that it has a crucial role in their development. IGCNU is the precursor to these invasive tumors.

While IGCNU is considered to be the precursor of all GCTs, the stage in germ cells development at which transformation occurs is not known. One model proposed by Skakkebaek and colleagues suggests that fetal gonocytes (primordial germ cells) undergo abnormal cell division (polyploidization) *in utero*, primarily due to environmental factors. These cells undergo abnormal cell division mediated by a kit receptor/kit ligand (stem cell factor) paracrine loop, leading to uncontrolled proliferation of gonocytes. Subsequent invasive growth may be mediated by postnatal and pubertal gonadotrophin stimulation. In this model, i(12p) is seen only after stromal invasion occurs [9]. A second model proposed by Chaganti and colleagues suggests that aberrant chromatid exchange events during meiotic crossing-over may lead to increased 12p copy number and overexpression of cyclin D2 (*CCND2*). In a cell containing unrepaired DNA breaks (recombination associated), overexpressed cyclin D2 may block a p53-dependent apoptotic response and lead to reinitiation of cell cycle and genomic instability. This aberrant, genomically unstable cell is now able to escape the apoptotic effects of p53 and may re-enter the cell cycle as a neoplastic cell. In this model, i(12p) is present in IGCNU [10].

Given the fact that i(12p) or at least excess genetic material of 12p is characteristic of postpubertal GCTs of the testis, it should not come as a surprise that its presence can and has been used as a diagnostic assay. This genetic abnormality is not absolutely pathognomonic of germ cell neoplasia, yet it is a very useful diagnostic tool in selected circumstances due to its rare occurrence in other solid tumors [11–13]. Classically, i(12p) is a feature best seen by karyotype which by definition requires a metaphase spread (Fig. 40.2). However, in daily practice, this assay is rarely

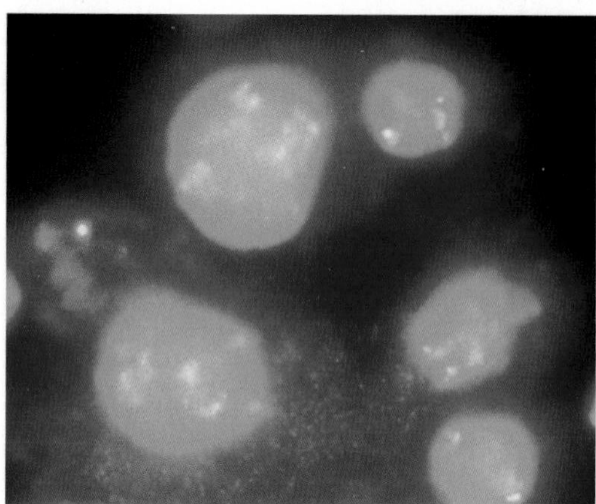

Fig. 40.3 Single-color FISH assay exhibiting large, irregular signals that may represent several copies of i(12p) (*left*). Normal signal can be seen in an adjacent cell (*right*)

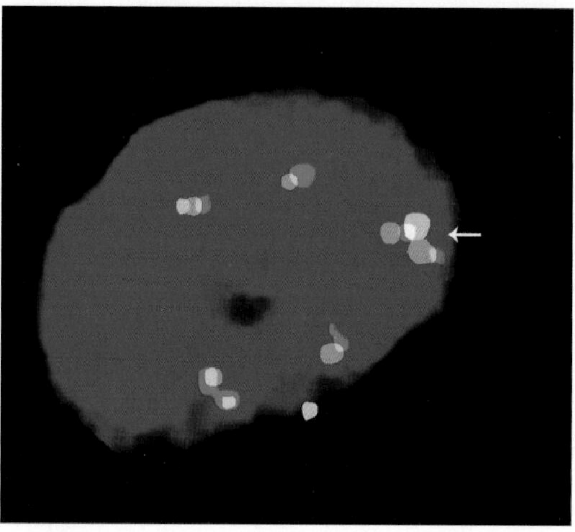

Fig. 40.4 Three-color FISH probe exhibiting i(12p) (*arrow*). The aqua centromeric probe is flanked by *two red–green* probes

performed in solid tumors, given the popularity of modern molecular techniques. Because the possibility of germ cell origin is usually determined after the H&E slides are reviewed, many investigators have used fluorescent in situ hybridization (FISH) to establish the presence of i(12p) in a formalin-fixed, paraffin-embedded (FFPE) tumor-bearing tissue. In fact, multiple papers have been written documenting its utility [14–17] (Figs. 40.3 and 40.4). The most common assay is a library probe covering 12p, sometimes combined with a chromosome 12 centromeric probe. In some cases, a three-color probe is used that includes a portion of 12q. In theory, this approach is more scientifically sound since the goal is to identify excess genetic material of 12p rather than simply chromosomal gains commonly seen in any form of genomically unstable tumors. What all these studies have failed to do is to establish the sensitivity and specificity of their assay. As you can imagine, an assay that depends on the identification of abnormally large, irregular signals in a resting cell can be difficult to evaluate and is prone to problems in interpretation (Figs. 40.3 and 40.4). Now that other molecular assays that can utilize FFPE tissues have entered the diagnostic arena, it is imperative that we develop a more precise assay. One possibility that is being explored is using a single-nucleotide polymorphism (SNP) array, which has the advantage of providing very good copy number data as well chromosome gains and losses. While the price of this assay at the present time is high, the clinical penalty that is paid if this diagnosis is missed certainly merits the financial cost.

Immunohistochemical Markers

Immunohistochemical markers can be a very powerful ancillary tool in classifying GSTs [18]. With experience, the overwhelming majority of tumors can be classified on high-quality H&E slides alone. However, the relative low incidence of these tumors is such that any given pathologist is likely to encounter no more than a handful of cases a year. This fact combined with the wide morphologic spectrum that can be seen in these tumors makes it very likely that the pathologist will be overly dependent on ancillary studies to arrive at a final diagnosis. It is best to first elaborate a differential diagnosis based on morphology and then decide what panel of antibodies should be ordered. Too often, I encounter cases in which virtually every marker associated with any type of GCT has been ordered, even though the differential diagnosis is rather limited. This "shotgun" approach should be avoided.

Intratubular Germ Cell Neoplasia (IGCNU)

IGCNU can be seen adjacent to invasive GCTs in virtually all cases in which residual testicular parenchyma is present [19]. It is present in up to 4 % of cryptorchid patients, up to 5 % of contralateral gonads in patients with unilateral GCT, and up to 1 % of patients biopsied for oligospermic infertility. Its association with testicular GCTs arising in prepubertal patients is still a source of controversy [4, 20, 21]. If present, it certainly does not have the same morphology or immunophenotype than what is seen in postpubertal gonads. Clinically, there are two settings in which it may be critical to confirm the presence of IGCNU: in the evaluation of a testicular biopsy at the time of infertility work up and when evaluating a testicular mass that is difficult to classify.

IGCNU cells contain glycogen and thus are PAS positive, diastase sensitive. Rarely will other intratubular cells, whether spermatogonia, spermatocytes, or Sertoli cells, show similar positivity. Placental-like alkaline phosphatase (PLAP) is one of the isoforms of alkaline phosphatase. PLAP antibodies will stain IGCNU, the majority of seminomas and ECs as well as a smaller percentage of YSTs. Immunoreactivity is seen in virtually all cases of IGCNU, and the staining pattern is usually membranous or cytoplasmic. No other non-neoplastic intratubular cells are immunoreactive for PLAP, but immunoreactivity may be seen in other types of nongerm cell malignancies [22, 23]. Because better markers have been developed over the years, we hardly ever use PLAP in our workup of testicular tumors. C-kit (CD117), a tyrosine kinase receptor expressed on stem cells, is overexpressed in a large percentage of IGCNU as well as seminomas, but not in other GCTs [24]. The staining pattern is cytoplasmic/membranous (Fig. 40.1c). Despite the overexpression of this antigen, CD117 is rarely mutated in these tumors. Care must be taken when interpreting CD117 in IGCNU since spermatogonia may occasionally express this antigen.

Other antibodies which immunoreact with IGCNU but are rarely used in clinical practice include M2A and 43-F [22, 25, 26]. POU5F1 (OCT3/4) is a very interesting marker with great clinical utility [27]. The gene serves as a transcription factor, and its product is expressed in pluripotent mouse and human embryonic stem cells and is down-regulated during differentiation. Since the gene is also required for self-renewal of embryonic stem cells, knocking out the gene is lethal. This antigen is expressed solely in IGCNU, seminoma, and EC, suggesting that these are the types of GCT cells with pluripotency, i.e., with capacity to differentiate. As a transcription factor, staining is localized to the nucleus (Fig. 40.1b).

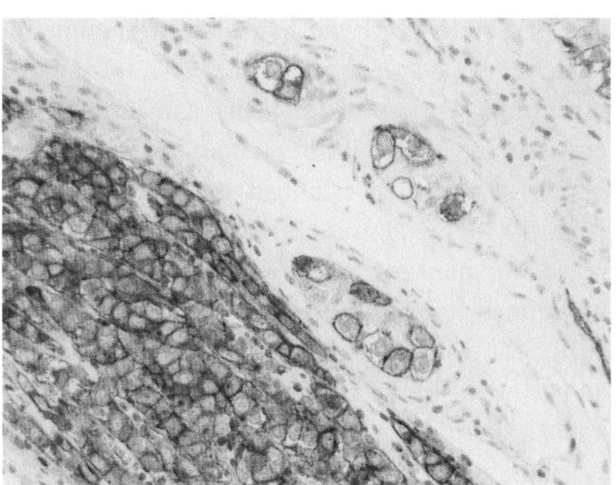

Fig. 40.5 Podoplanin (D2-40) showing strong cytoplasmic/membranous staining in intratubular germ cell neoplasia (*right*) and seminoma (*left*). This stain may be used interchangeably with CD117, but there is no need to perform both

Another transcription factor expressed in IGCNU is SALL4; however, this nuclear marker is expressed in a wider spectrum of GCTs including seminoma, EC, YST, and some glandular elements of teratoma [28]. As such, it is a useful marker in the characterization of GCTs but cannot be used in isolation. Podoplanin (clone D2-40), a transmembrane mucoprotein expressed on fetal germ cells, lymphatic endothelium, and mesotheliums, is an excellent cytoplasmic (membranous) marker with staining restricted to IGCNU and seminoma (Fig. 40.5) [29]. Since the expression patterns for CD117 and D2-40 overlap, there is no need to perform both assays.

There are several situations in which it is critically important to establish the presence or absence of IGCNU and in which immunohistochemistry may be of great utility. These include during the workup of infertility and in the presence of a poorly differentiated testicular neoplasm in order to establish germ cell lineage (Fig. 40.1a–d). However, there is absolutely no reason to perform tests for all of the markers mentioned above. While one antibody may be sufficient, I usually test for two antigens, OCT4 and either CD117 or D2-40. PAS, PLAP, M2A, and 43-F are of no additional clinical utility and I discourage their use. In this situation, SALL-4 adds no additional information to OCT4.

Seminoma

Seminomas are the most common GCTs arising in the male gonad, whether they arise in a pure state or mixed with other morphologic types [30–32]. "Pure" seminoma account for 30% of testicular GCTs and another 15–20% contain syncytiotrophoblasts without other germ cell components. Seminoma cells contain glycogen (PAS positive) and express PLAP, CD117, OCT3/4, and SALL-4 by immunohistochemistry but not cytokeratins, CD30, or inhibin (Table 40.2) [23, 33–37]. In fact, the immunophenotype of seminoma is virtually identical to IGCNU. In our practice, PAS and PLAP are rarely relied upon because of the availability of better discriminating markers. On occasion, weak CD30 cytoplasmic immunoreactivity may be encountered in isolated seminoma cells, a finding that should not warrant a change in diagnosis. It is important to keep in mind that CD30 may be expressed in some hematopoietic cells as well, so attention to nuclear detail is warranted. A minority of seminoma cells may express focal and weak, dot-like, or linear immunoreactivity for cytokeratin AE1/AE3 and CAM 5.2. However, there is never diffuse and strong staining throughout the cytoplasm. Caution must be taken when interpreting cytokeratin markers since syncytiotrophoblasts are usually strongly immunoreactive, as are their mononuclear variants. If one relies on panels of markers, this issue is resolved easily since syncytiotrophoblasts lack immunoreactivity to OCT4, SALL4, D2-40, etc. Like IGCNU, seminoma cells express OCT4 in a nuclear distribution [24, 37]. SALL4 is positive in a nuclear distribution, while CD117 and D2-40 are expressed in a cytoplasmic/membranous distribution, once again similar to ICGNU (Fig. 40.5).

In practical terms, the panel of markers used to establish a diagnosis of seminoma will depend on the differential diagnosis. What is important to remember is that no other invasive GCTs will exhibit diffuse immunoreactivity for CD117 and D2-40, while seminoma shares OCT4 nuclear positivity with EC and SALL4 nuclear immunoreactivity with EC and YST.

Spermatocytic Seminoma

SSs are rare, comprising less than 2% of testicular neoplasms [30]. They represent an entirely separate and distinct clinicopathologic entity from classic seminoma. The peak incidence is in the sixth decade of life (medial 54 years). Patients as old as 87 years and as young as 25 years of age have been affected. This tumor occurs only in the

Table 40.2 Immunohistochemical maker expression in primary testicular germ cell tumors (GCTs)

Marker	IGCNU	Seminoma	Embryonal Ca	Yolk sac tumor
OCT4[a]	Positive	Positive	Positive	Negative
CD117	Positive, membranous	Positive, membranous	Negative (weak/focal positivity can be seen)	Negative (weak/focal positivity can be seen)
D2-40[a]	Positive	Positive	Negative	Negative
CD30[a]	Negative	Negative	Positive	Negative
SALL4	Positive	Positive	Positive	Positive
Glypican 3[a]	Negative	Negative	Negative	Positive
Cytokeratin[b]	Negative[+]	Negative[+]	Positive	Positive

[a] Denotes marker of choice
[b] Either CAM 5.2 or AE1/AE3

male gonad, is not associated with either cryptorchidism, other types of GCTs, or i(12p). Tumor cells do not contain glycogen (negative PAS stain). Immunohistochemical stains for PLAP are negative, although occasional cells may be weakly immunoreactive. Cytokeratin stains are negative, although occasional cells may exhibit dot-like cytoplasmic staining. CD30, OCT4, and podoplanin are negative, while some investigators have reported variable immunoreactivity for CD117 (C-kit) and SALL4 [24, 30, 38].

Embryonal Carcinoma

In its pure form, EC comprise up to 3 % of GCTs, although approximately 40 % of all GCTs contain an EC component. Over 50 % of tumors with either pure or predominant EC components will present with metastatic disease. Pure EC most commonly occurs in patients during the third or fourth decades of life, with an average age of 32 years and is extremely rare in prepubertal children [30]. Up to 10 % of patients present with symptoms related to metastatic disease. Metastases most commonly occur first to retroperitoneal lymph nodes. Twenty percent of patients present with metastatic disease with a smaller percentage also having supradiaphragmatic involvement.

The cells of EC usually show intense and diffuse immunoreactivity for PLAP, OCT4, SALL4, as well as cytokeratins (AE1/AE3 and Cam 5.2) (Fig. 40.6a–d). CD30 (Ber-H2) is a member of the tumor necrosis factor receptor family and has a cytoplasmic membrane and Golgi distribution. It is expressed exclusively in EC (Fig. 40.7). SOX-2 is a transcription factor involved in embryonic development and specifically plays a role in maintenance of pluripotency in undifferentiated embryonic stem cells [37, 39, 40]. It is expressed in a nuclear distribution in the majority of ECs but not seminoma (only isolated cases) or YSTs. While it may serve as an alternative to CD30, the assay is difficult to standardize in a CLIA complicate automated environment so we do not use it clinically. Only about 2 % of ECs react with epithelial membrane antigen (EMA). Staining for CD117 protein generally is negative, although some cells may exhibit low level of staining. β-HCG is demonstrable only in intermingled syncytiotrophoblastic cells [24]. Most AFP-positive foci in ECs probably represent unrecognized foci of YST or early transition to YST. Pertinent negatives include CD117 and D2-40, remembering that the former can rarely stain isolated cells.

Yolk Sac Tumor

YSTs are characterized by multiple patterns of growth that recapitulate the yolk sac, allantois, and extra embryonic mesenchyme. It has a bimodal age distribution: infants and young children and postpubertal males. In children, it commonly presents in its pure form, usually within the first 2 years of life. YSTs account for 75 % of childhood testicular GCTs. In the postpubertal setting, YST rarely presents in a pure form but is present in almost half of mixed GCTs [32, 41]. The incidence of a YST component is higher in primary mediastinal GCTs.

Tumor cells of YST are usually immunoreactive for low molecular weight cytokeratins and α-fetoprotein (AFP), a plasma protein produced by the yolk sac and liver in the fetus. We have found that AFP immunohistochemistry can be difficult to interpret. Staining can be weak, patchy, and it is often associated with a dirty background. While we admit that some of these findings could be laboratory associated, the fact of the matter is that we never perform or interpret this assay in isolation. Because we now have better antibodies, we do not consider this assay to be absolutely necessary. PLAP staining is variable and may be absent. As previously stated, we rarely perform this assay since it lacks discriminatory power. CD117, CD30, and OCT3/4 are usually negative, but SOX2, SALL4, and Glypican 3 are positive [24, 39, 42, 43]. Glypican 3 is a membrane-anchored heparin sulfate which expressed in virtually all YSTs and in the majority of choriocarcinomas (Fig. 40.8). Expression can be seen in the epithelial component of some teratomatous glands and some trophoblastic elements, but it is otherwise limited to YSTs.

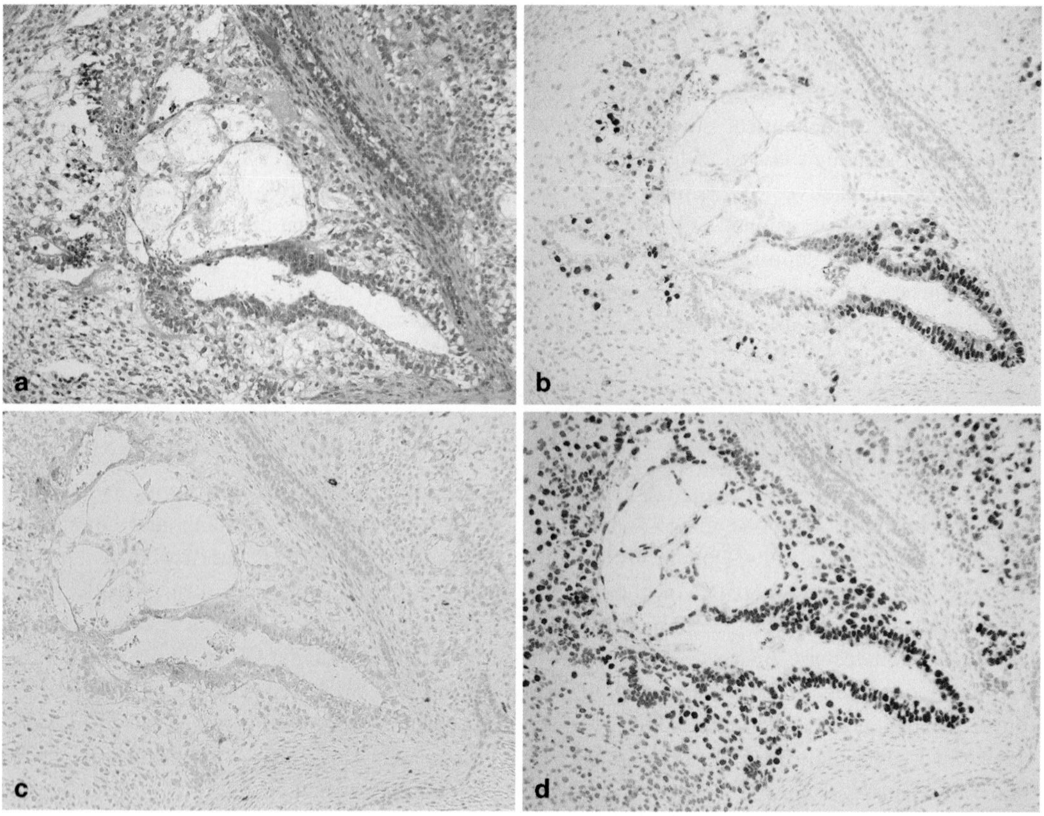

Fig. 40.6 Mixed germ cell tumor (GCT) composed of embryonal carcinoma (EC), yolk sac tumor (YST), and teratoma. **a** H&E stain. **b** OCT3/4 nuclear immunoreactivity is limited to EC. **c** CD117, although usually limited to seminoma, may be weakly positive in EC, as it is here. **d** SALL4 nuclear staining is seen in EC and YST but not in the epithelial teratomatous elements

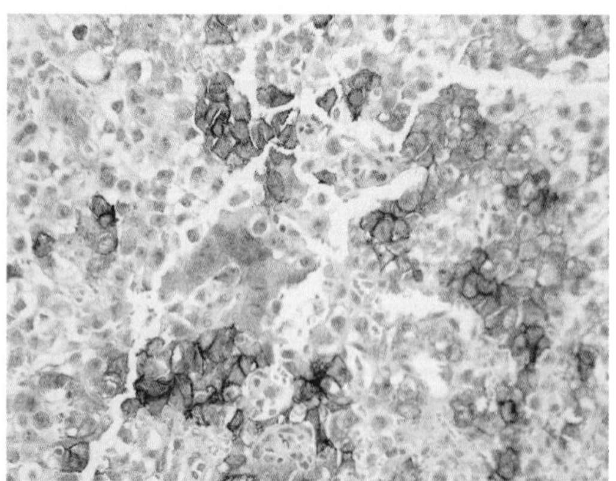

Fig. 40.7 Cytoplasmic staining for CD30 in embryonal carcinoma (EC) while the *adjacent* seminoma cells are negative

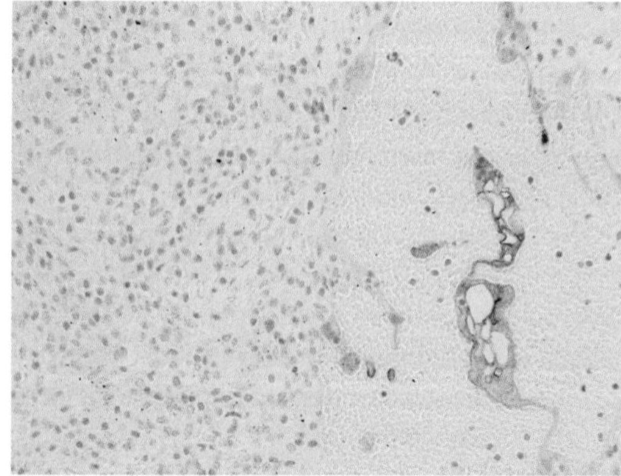

Fig. 40.8 Glypican 3 immunoreactivity in syncytiotrophoblasts *adjacent* to unreactive seminoma

Choriocarcinoma

Choriocarcinoma is composed of syncytiotrophoblastic, cytotrophoblastic, and other trophoblastic cells. It comprises less than 1 % of testicular GCTs in its pure form; however, it may be encountered as a component of a mixed GCT in up to 15 % of cases [30]. In its pure form, these highly malignant tumors occur in the second and third decades of life, are commonly associated with very high levels of serum HCG (usually above 50,000 mIu/mL), and exhibit metastatic disease at the time of initial presentation. In this setting, metastatic disease is found in not only the usual sites for other testicular tumors, but also via hematogenous spread to viscera, including lungs, liver, gastrointestinal tract, spleen, brain, and adrenal glands.

Syncytiotrophoblasts are immunoreactive with ß-hCG as well as inhibin, epithelial EMA, low molecular weight cytokeratins, and Glypican 3. Human chorionic gonadotrophic (hCG) is a dimeric glycoprotein that is produced by placental trophoblastic cells, predominantly the syncytiotrophoblasts. The beta-chain is unique to hCG and thus is the best antigenic marker for it. Essentially all choriocarcinomas are positive for β-hCG, but such reactivity is often limited to syncytiotrophoblasts or intermediate trophoblasts. Cytotrophoblasts are either negative or weakly positive for ß-HCG. PLAP may be positive but staining is variable [30]. Pregnancy-specific β1-glycoprotein and human placental lactogen also are positive in syncytiotrophoblasts and intermediate-sized trophoblasts but are negative in cytotrophoblasts [32, 44].

Teratoma

The term teratoma refers to neoplasms composed of tissues, which have differentiated along any of the three somatic pathways: ectoderm, mesoderm, or endoderm [30, 32, 45]. Tumors composed of only one of these components are regarded as monodermal teratomas. Teratomas may be composed of mature tissues, embryonal-type tissues, or a mixture of both. Historically, they were subclassified as immature and mature forms based on their degree of differentiation. The World Health Organization (WHO) now recommends that these morphologies be considered as a single entity based on their overlapping genetic and clinical features [30].

The immunohistochemical profile of teratomas will depend on the histologic component present. In addition, glandular elements are likely not to be immunoreactive for SALL4 and Glypican 3, although focal staining may be evident for either marker; whether this represents early yolk sac differentiation is unknown. AFP may also be focally positive in glandular elements, which may be associated with the elevation of AFP in the cystic fluid [46].

Sex Cord-Stromal Tumors

The term refers to neoplasms containing Leydig (interstitial) cells, Sertoli cells, granulosa cells, or theca cells. While tumors may be made up of one or a combination of these cell types in varying degrees of differentiation, mixed histologic types are common in the ovary but rarely occur in the male gonad. The terminology used to describe these tumors is confusing and controversial, but it is best to adhere to the classification set forth by the WHO [30]. Sex cord-stromal tumors comprise 4–5 % of primary testicular neoplasms. The morphology of these lesions is less complex that in GCTs, yet they may be difficult to classify and may be confused with other neoplasms, including tumors of germ cell origin, particularly YST and seminoma, or with mesothelioma, adnexal tumors as well as metastatic disease. There is very little known about the molecular underpinnings of this disease, except that some tumors may be associated with syndromes such as Peutz–Jeghers and Carney's syndromes. Approximately 10 % of tumors show malignant behavior. Surgery remains the mainstay of treatment since no form of systemic therapy has shown significant efficacy in treating the disease. To date, there are no molecular markers that can predict clinical outcome or response to treatment.

Table 40.3 Immunohistochemical markers most useful in identifying sex cord-stromal tumors. (Expression of any of these markers may be focal)

Marker	Leydig cell tumor	Sertoli cell tumor	LC calcifying Sertoli cell tumor	Granulosa cell tumor, adult type	Granulosa cell tumor, juvenile type
Inhibin[a]	Positive	Variable[b]	Positive	Positive	Positive
WT-1[a]	Positive	Positive	Positive	Positive	Positive
Calretinin	Positive	Positive	Positive	Positive	Positive
SF-1[a]	Positive	Positive	Positive	Positive	Positive
FOXL2[a]	Negative	Negative	Negative	40 % positive	Unknown
Cytokeratin	Negative	40 % positive	Negative	Usually negative	Positive only in cells lining microcysts

[a] Denotes marker of choice, most likely to be of diagnostic utility
[b] Inhibin positivity is less commonly seen in SCT s as compared to LCTs

Leydig Cell Tumor (LCT)

LCTs are the most common pure testicular sex cord-stromal neoplasms and account for 1–3 % of testicular neoplasms [30, 32, 47]. They may occur at any age, though most common between the third and sixth decades of life. Fifteen to twenty percent of cases will present in prepubertal children. Approximately 10 % will metastasize with metastasis more commonly seen in older patients. LCTs are immunoreactive with inhibin. Inhibin is a glycoprotein belonging to the TGFβ family. It is positive in a cytoplasmic distribution in LCTs as well as other sex cord-stromal tumors. LCTs will also express melan A, calretinin, and vimentin (Table 40.3). Calretinin, a calcium-binding protein, has a very similar staining profile as α-inhibin for the sex cord-stromal tumors. However, while almost all LCTs are positive, only a minority of Sertoli cell tumors (SCTs) is immunoreactive. Cytokeratins and S-100 protein are either negative or only focally positive. CD30, CD117, OCT3/4, and PLAP are negative [30, 40, 48, 49]. Steroidogenic factor 1 (SF-1) is a nuclear transcription factor expressed in testicular Sertoli cells as well as other sex cord-stromal cells [50, 51]. While it appears to be expressed in a high percentage of sex cord-stromal tumors independent of type and eventually may prove to be a better marker than inhibin and calretinin, we need more studies to be performed before we advocate its routine use in lieu of the other markers.

Sertoli Cell Tumor: Usual Type and Its Variants

SCTs are rare, comprising less than 1 % of testicular neoplasms [30, 52]. They may occur at any age and approximately 15 % develop in children, but rarely before the age of 10 years [53]. SCTs are immunoreactive for SF-1 and vimentin, while staining for cytokeratin, inhibin, and calretinin is variable. Cytokeratins and EMA are more likely to be expressed in LCT than in other types of sex cord-stromal tumors. Calretinin cannot be used in isolation since it will also be expressed in adenomatoid tumor and mesothelioma. Markers typically seen in GCTs are negative [30]. The immunophenotype of the sclerosing variant of SCT as well as the large cell calcifying Sertoli cell tumor expresses the same immunophenotype as the usual type, even though the morphology of the latter is quite distinct (Table 40.3).

Granulosa Cell Tumor

There are two subtypes of granulosa cell tumor, adult and juvenile, similar to what is seen in the ovary. The adult variant of granulosa cell tumor very rarely develops in the testis with less than 30 bonafide cases reported in the literature [47, 54, 55]. They have been described in males between the ages of 21 and 73 years and usually present as a testicular mass which may have been present for several years.

Juvenile granulosa cell tumors are the most common sex cord-stromal tumor of the infantile

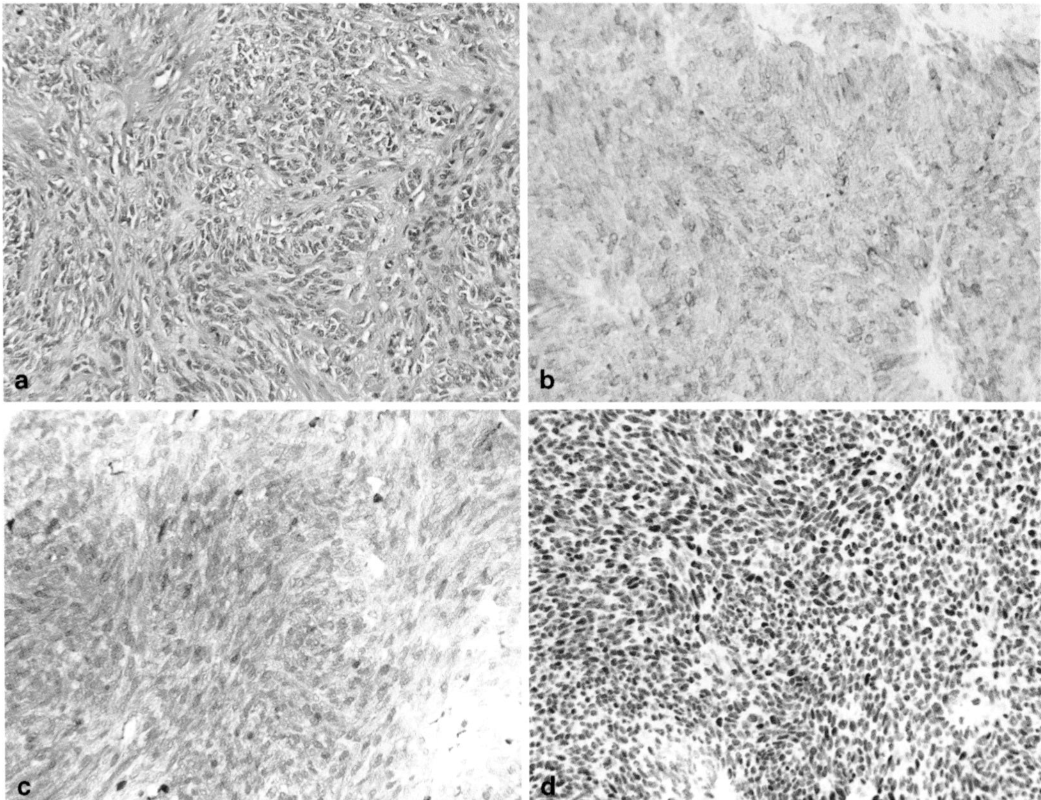

Fig. 40.9 Granulosa cell tumor. **a** H&E stain. **b** Inhibin. **c** Calretinin. **d** FoxL1 exhibits strong and diffuse nuclear immunoreactivity

testis [32, 56, 57]. They are usually encountered in the first 6 months of life, with one isolated case reported in a 21-month old and another in a 4-year old. Two cases have developed in undescended testes. Juvenile granulosa cell tumors may arise in patients with an abnormal karyotype and ambiguous genitalia.

The immunophenotype of granulosa cell tumors is similar to other gonadal stromal tumors. The cells of the adult type will express inhibin, WT-1, and SF-1. FOXL2 is a recently described marker which is expressed in most ovarian granulosa cell tumors. Although there is limited data in testicular primaries, it appears that up 40% will be positive while other types of gonadal stromal tumors are negative (Fig. 40.9a–d) [58, 59]. In the juvenile variant, the cell lining the microcysts may be cytokeratin positive while the surrounding stromal cells are positive for inhibin.

A Rational Approach to the Workup of Testicular Tumors

In the preceding paragraphs, we have given a comprehensive list of all markers that have been used in the classification of testicular neoplasms. Clearly, it is impractical and borderline irresponsible to indiscriminately order these assays without taking into consideration the differential diagnosis suggested by the clinical scenario and the morphological features of the tumor. There are several scenarios in which a pathologist is likely to require ancillary studies.

Is This Metastatic Tumor of Germ Cell Origin?

As always, a good clinical history and attention to the morphology of the tumor is paramount. If

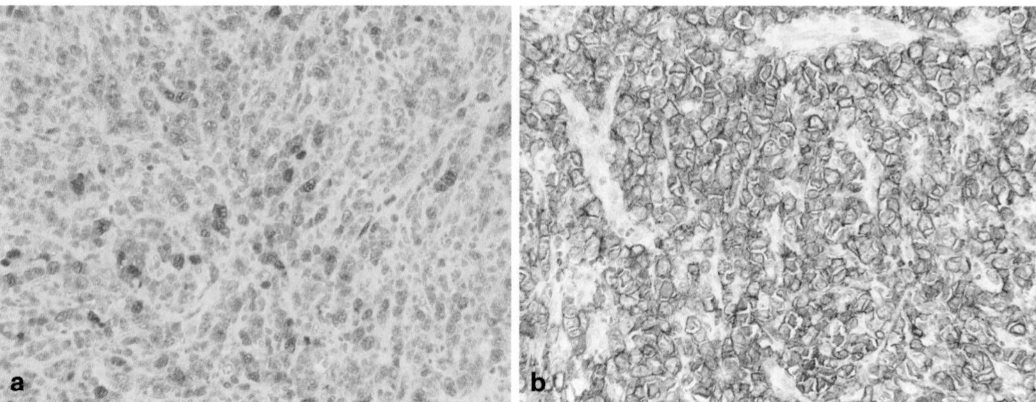

Fig. 40.10 Malignant lymphoma involving the testis. Notice nuclear expression of OCT3/4 (**a**) and CD20 (**b**)

fresh tumor is available, the most specific manner to establish the presence of i(12p) is by karyotype. If only FFPE tissue is available, one can submit the sample for FISH analysis, with the caveat that this assay is neither entirely sensitive nor specific. If immunohistochemical workup is required, a panel consisting of OCT4, D2-40, CD30, and Glypican 3 should suffice.

Is This Testicular Tumor of Germ Cell Origin?

If testicular parenchyma is present, it is important to evaluate for the presence of IGCNU. If any doubt exists, OCT3/4, together with either D2-40 or CD117, will help to identify the neoplastic cells (Table 40.2). Within the invasive tumor, the stem cell marker OCT3/4 is positive in seminoma and EC, but may very rarely be expressed in other primitive tumors; we have seen nuclear immunoreactivity is a few carcinomas as well as in an anaplastic lymphoma (Fig. 40.10a,b). Besides OCT3/4, seminoma should be positive for CD117 and D2-40 and negative for CD30. EC is positive for OCT3/4 and CD30 but negative for CD117, D2-40, and Glypican 3. YST lacks immunoreactivity for OCT3/4, CD-30, CD117, and D2-40, but is positive for AFP and Glypican 3. We find SALL4 to be of limited utility in this differential diagnosis.

Interestingly, the morphology of YSTs can be even more varied in a setting of prior systemic therapy or in late recurrences. In this situation, there is some evidence that Glypican 3 is the best way to identify YST lineage, and even to distinguish if one is dealing with a secondary somatic malignancy of germ cell origin or an unusual morphologic manifestation of YST. While this may be true, one must remember that the epithelial lining of some teratomas can express both AFP and Glypican 3.

Is This Testicular Tumor of Sex Cord-Stromal Origin?

As strictly defined, intratubular germ cell neoplasia will be absent. All variants should be negative for the traditional germ cell markers (OCT3/4, SALL4, D2-40, CD117, CD30, Glypican 3); however, there is generally no need to perform all these assays (Table 40.3). Absence of SALL4 and Glypican 3 should suffice. In this setting, SALL4 may be better than OCT3/4 simply because its expression covers a wider distribution than OCT3/4 that would be expected to be negative in YSTs. Positive markers will vary somewhat between different types of sex cord-stromal tumor being considered, but all should express inhibin, WT-1, calretinin, and SF-1. Cytokeratin is of limited utility but is more likely to be expressed in SCTs. FOXL2 expression appears to be limited to granulosa cell tumors.

Is This Tumor Arising in the Testicular Adnexa (Rete Testis, Epididymis) or the Mesothelial Lining?

Tumors that arise from the testicular adnexa are usually adenocarcinomas. Given their embryological origins, they are likely to express PAX8 as well as other markers typical for adenocarcinomas, such as CK7 and CEA. An unusual variant thought to arise from Müllerian rests will express PAX8 as well as estrogen receptor (ER). Mesotheliomas arising in the tunica vaginalis may involve the testicular parenchyma. These tumors express the same immunophenotype as mesotheliomas arising at any other site, including calretinin, and WT1, but not PAX8. None of these tumors should express markers associated with GCT lineage although the overlap with sex cord-stromal tumors, particularly calretinin in mesotheliomas, should be kept in mind.

Is This Tumor a Lymphoma?

Malignant lymphomarepresents up to 5% of testicular neoplasms. It is the most common bilateral tumor (either synchronous or metachronous) and the most common testicular tumor in men above the age of 60 [60]. The majority of patients have localized disease, but in a third of cases, testicular involvement is part of either regional or systemic disease. Lymphomas will express hematopoietic markers in accordance with their line of differentiation. They will not express cytokeratin or PLAP. We have seen a single large cell lymphoma with focal nuclear immunoreactivity for OCT3/4, but other GCT markers are negative while CD20 is positive (Fig. 40.10a, b). It is worth remembering that anaplastic large cell lymphoma is likely to express CD30, similar to EC and that we have encountered one case of anaplastic lymphoma with nuclear reactivity for the stem cell marker OCT3/4.

Primary leukemic tumors (granulocytic/myeloid sarcoma) of the testis are very rare [61]. Leukemic infiltration of the testis is most commonly seen on biopsy specimens in patents being evaluated for relapse after systemic therapy [62, 63]. However, it may be seen at autopsy in up to 65–30% of patients with acute leukemia and chronic leukemia, respectively. Symptomatic enlargement of the gonad is encountered in 5% of cases. On microscopy, leukemic cells infiltrate between the seminiferous tubules and rarely extend into the seminiferous tubule itself. Marker expression will include MPO, lysozyme, CD68, and CD117, although the precise expression pattern will depend on the precise cell lineage. Common germ cell markers will be negative.

Is This Tumor Metastatic Disease?

Metastasis to the testis from solid tumors is rare and usually presents in patients with known primary disease elsewhere and known metastatic disease. It is typically encountered in patients beyond the age of 50 years. The most common primary sites include prostate, colon, kidney, and melanoma [64]. In children, the most common tumors to metastasize to the testis include neuroblastoma and rhabdomyosarcoma [65–67]. In difficult cases, an immunohistochemical panel which includes a broad spectrum of entities may be required, but there is no substitute for a detailed clinical history.

References

1. Cavallo F, Graziani G, Antinozzi C, Feldman DR, Houldsworth J, Bosl GJ, Chaganti RS, Moynahan ME, Jasin M, Barchi M. Reduced proficiency in homologous recombination underlies the high sensitivity of embryonal carcinoma testicular germ cell tumors to cisplatin and poly (adp-ribose) polymerase inhibition. PLoS One. 2012;7:e51563.
2. Korkola JE, Houldsworth J, Feldman DR, Olshen AB, Qin LX, Patil S, Reuter VE, Bosl GJ, Chaganti RS. Identification and validation of a gene expression signature that predicts outcome in adult men with germ cell tumors. J Clin Oncol. 2009;27:5240–7.
3. Korkola JE, Houldsworth J, Bosl GJ, Chaganti RS. Molecular events in germ cell tumours: linking chromosome-12 gain, acquisition of pluripotency and response to cisplatin. BJU Int. 2009;104:1334–8.
4. Looijenga LH, Oosterhuis JW. Pathogenesis of testicular germ cell tumours. Rev Reprod. 1999;4:90–100.

5. Oosterhuis JW, Looijenga LH. Current views on the pathogenesis of testicular germ cell tumours and perspectives for future research: highlights of the 5th copenhagen workshop on carcinoma in situ and cancer of the testis. APMIS. 2003;111:280–9.
6. Houldsworth J, Korkola JE, Bosl GJ, Chaganti RS. Biology and genetics of adult male germ cell tumors. J Clin Oncol. 2006;24:5512–8.
7. Looijenga LH, Stoop H, Biermann K. Testicular cancer: biology and biomarkers. Virchows Archiv. 2014;464:301–13.
8. Chaganti RS, Houldsworth J. Genetics and biology of adult human male germ cell tumors. Cancer Res. 2000;60:1475–82.
9. Skakkebaek NE, Rajpert-De Meyts E, Jorgensen N, Carlsen E, Petersen PM, Giwercman A, Andersen AG, Jensen TK, Andersson AM, Muller J. Germ cell cancer and disorders of spermatogenesis: an environmental connection? APMIS. 1998;106:3–11; discussion 12.
10. Chaganti RS, Houldsworth J. The cytogenetic theory of the pathogenesis of human adult male germ cell tumors. Review article. APMIS. 1998;106:80–83; discussion 83–84.
11. Bosl GJ, Dmitrovsky E, Reuter VE, Samaniego F, Rodriguez E, Geller NL, Chaganti RS. Isochromosome of the short arm of chromosome 12: clinically useful markers for male germ cell tumors. J Natl Cancer Inst. 1989;81:1874–8.
12. Motzer RJ, Rodriguez E, Reuter VE, Samaniego F, Dmitrovsky E, Bajorin DF, Pfister DG, Parsa NZ, Chaganti RS, Bosl GJ. Genetic analysis as an aid in diagnosis for patients with midline carcinomas of uncertain histologies. J Natl Cancer Inst. 1991;83:341–6.
13. Mukherjee AB, Murty VV, Rodriguez E, Reuter VE, Bosl GJ, Chaganti RS. Detection and analysis of origin of i(12p), a diagnostic marker of human male germ cell tumors, by fluorescence in situ hybridization. Genes Chromosomes Cancer. 1991;3:300–7.
14. Suijkerbuijk RF, Looijenga L, de Jong B, Oosterhuis JW, Cassiman JJ, Geurts van Kessel A. Verification of isochromosome 12p and identification of other chromosome 12 aberrations in gonadal and extragonadal human germ cell tumors by bicolor double fluorescence in situ hybridization. Cancer Genet Cytogenet. 1992;63:8–16.
15. Kernek KM, Brunelli M, Ulbright TM, Eble JN, Martignoni G, Zhang S, Michael H, Cummings OW, Cheng L. Fluorescence in situ hybridization analysis of chromosome 12p in paraffin-embedded tissue is useful for establishing germ cell origin of metastatic tumors. Mod Pathol. 2004;17:1309–13.
16. Motzer RJ, Amsterdam A, Prieto V, Sheinfeld J, Murty VV, Mazumdar M, Bosl GJ, Chaganti RS, Reuter VE. Teratoma with malignant transformation: diverse malignant histologies arising in men with germ cell tumors. J Urol. 1998;159:133–8.
17. Kum JB, Ulbright TM, Williamson SR, Wang M, Zhang S, Foster RS, Grignon DJ, Eble JN, Beck SD, Cheng L. Molecular genetic evidence supporting the origin of somatic-type malignancy and teratoma from the same progenitor cell. Am J Surg Pathol. 2012;36:1849–56.
18. Ulbright TM, Tickoo SK, Berney DM, Srigley JR. Members of the IIiDUPG. Best practices recommendations in the application of immunohistochemistry in testicular tumors: report from the international society of urological pathology consensus conference. Am J Surg Pathol. 2014;38(8):e50–9.
19. Dieckmann KP, Skakkebaek NE. Carcinoma in situ of the testis: review of biological and clinical features. Int J Cancer. 1999;83:815–22.
20. Manivel JC, Simonton S, Wold LE, Dehner LP. Absence of intratubular germ cell neoplasia in testicular yolk sac tumors in children. A histochemical and immunohistochemical study. Arch Pathol Lab Med. 1988;112:641–5.
21. Hu LM, Phillipson J, Barsky SH. Intratubular germ cell neoplasia in infantile yolk sac tumor. Verification by tandem repeat sequence in situ hybridization. Diagn Mol Pathol. 1992;1:118–28.
22. Giwercman A, Cantell L, Marks A. Placental-like alkaline phosphatase as a marker of carcinoma-in-situ of the testis. Comparison with monoclonal antibodies m2a and 43-9f. APMIS. 1991;99:586–94.
23. Wick MR, Swanson PE, Manivel JC. Placental-like alkaline phosphatase reactivity in human tumors: an immunohistochemical study of 520 cases. Hum Pathol. 1987;18:946–54.
24. Leroy X, Augusto D, Leteurtre E, Gosselin B. Cd30 and cd117 (c-kit) used in combination are useful for distinguishing embryonal carcinoma from seminoma. J Histochem Cytochem. 2002;50:283–5.
25. Giwercman A, Lindenberg S, Kimber SJ, Andersson T, Muller J, Skakkebaek NE. Monoclonal antibody 43-9f as a sensitive immunohistochemical marker of carcinoma in situ of human testis. Cancer. 1990;65:1135–42.
26. Marks A, Sutherland DR, Bailey D, Iglesias J, Law J, Lei M, Yeger H, Banerjee D, Baumal R. Characterization and distribution of an oncofetal antigen (m2a antigen) expressed on testicular germ cell tumours. Br J Cancer. 1999;80:569–78.
27. Looijenga LH, Stoop H, de Leeuw HP, de Gouveia Brazao CA, Gillis AJ, van Roozendaal KE, van Zoelen EJ, Weber RF, Wolffenbuttel KP, van Dekken H, Honecker F, Bokemeyer C, Perlman EJ, Schneider DT, Kononen J, Sauter G, Oosterhuis JW. Pou5f1 (oct3/4) identifies cells with pluripotent potential in human germ cell tumors. Cancer Res. 2003;63:2244–50.
28. Cao D, Guo S, Allan RW, Molberg KH, Peng Y. Sall4 is a novel sensitive and specific marker of ovarian primitive germ cell tumors and is particularly useful in distinguishing yolk sac tumor from clear cell carcinoma. Am J Surg Pathol. 2009;33:894–904.
29. Lau SK, Weiss LM, Chu PG. D2-40 immunohistochemistry in the differential diagnosis of seminoma and embryonal carcinoma: a comparative

immunohistochemical study with kit (cd117) and cd30. Mod Pathol. 2007;20:320–5.
30. Eble J, Sauter G, Epstein J, Sesterhenn I. Pathology and genetics of tumours of the urinary system and male genital organs. Lyon: IARC Press; 2004.
31. Ulbright T, Berney DM. Testicular and paratesticular tumors. In: Mills SE, editor. Diagnostic surgical pathology. Philadelphia: Lippincott Williams & Wilkins; 2010. pp. 1944–2004.
32. Ulbright TM, Amin MB, Young RH. Tumours of the testis, adnexa, spermatic cord, and scrotum. In: Rosai J, editor. Atlas of tumor pathology. Washington, DC: Armed Forces Institute of Pathology; 1999. pp. 59–181.
33. Battifora H, Sheibani K, Tubbs RR, Kopinski MI, Sun TT. Antikeratin antibodies in tumor diagnosis. Distinction between seminoma and embryonal carcinoma. Cancer. 1984;54:843–8.
34. Eglen DE, Ulbright TM. The differential diagnosis of yolk sac tumor and seminoma.Usefulness of cytokeratin, alpha-fetoprotein, and alpha-1-antitrypsin immunoperoxidase reactions. Am J Clin Pathol. 1987;88:328–32.
35. Jacobsen GK, Jacobsen M. Alpha-fetoprotein (afp) and human chorionic gonadotropin (hcg) in testicular germ cell tumours. A prospective immunohistochemical study. Acta Pathol Microbiol Immunol Scand A. 1983;91:165–76.
36. Jacobsen GK, Norgaard-Pedersen B. Placental alkaline phosphatase in testicular germ cell tumours and in carcinoma-in-situ of the testis. An immunohistochemical study. Acta Pathol Microbiol Immunol Scand A. 1984;92:323–9.
37. Jones TD, Ulbright TM, Eble JN, Baldridge LA, Cheng L. Oct4 staining in testicular tumors: a sensitive and specific marker for seminoma and embryonal carcinoma. Am J Surg Pathol. 2004;28:935–40.
38. Kraggerud SM, Berner A, Bryne M, Pettersen EO, Fossa SD. Spermatocytic seminoma as compared to classical seminoma: an immunohistochemical and DNA flow cytometric study. APMIS. 1999;107: 297–302.
39. Gopalan A, Dhall D, Olgac S, Fine SW, Korkola JE, Houldsworth J, Chaganti RS, Bosl GJ, Reuter VE, Tickoo SK. Testicular mixed germ cell tumors: a morphological and immunohistochemical study using stem cell markers, oct3/4, sox2 and gdf3, with emphasis on morphologically difficult-to-classify areas. Mod Pathol. 2009;22:1066–74.
40. Emerson RE, Ulbright TM. The use of immunohistochemistry in the differential diagnosis of tumors of the testis and paratestis. Semin Diagn Pathol. 2005;22:33–50.
41. Talerman A. Endodermal sinus (yolk sac) tumor elements in testicular germ-cell tumors in adults: comparison of prospective and retrospective studies. Cancer. 1980;46:1213–7.
42. Emerson RE, Ulbright TM. Intratubular germ cell neoplasia of the testis and its associated cancers: the use of novel biomarkers. Pathology. 2010;42:344–55.
43. Wang F, Liu A, Peng Y, Rakheja D, Wei L, Xue D, Allan RW, Molberg KH, Li J, Cao D. Diagnostic utility of sall4 in extragonadal yolk sac tumors: an immunohistochemical study of 59 cases with comparison to placental-like alkaline phosphatase, alpha-fetoprotein, and glypican-3. Am J Surg Pathol. 2009;33(10):1529–39.
44. Manivel JC, Niehans G, Wick MR, Dehner LP. Intermediate trophoblast in germ cell neoplasms. Am J Surg Pathol. 1987;11:693–701.
45. Ulbright TM. Testicular and paratesticular tumors. In: SternbergSS, editor. Diagnostic surgical pathology. Philadelphia: Lippincott, Williams and Wilkens; 1999. pp. 1973–2004.
46. Beck SD, Patel MI, Sheinfeld J. Tumor marker levels in post-chemotherapy cystic masses: clinical implications for patients with germ cell tumors. J Urol. 2004;171:168–71.
47. Cheville JC. Classification and pathology of testicular germ cell and sex cord-stromal tumors. Urol Clin North Am. 1999;26:595–609.
48. Augusto D, Leteurtre E, De La Taille A, Gosselin B, Leroy X. Calretinin: a valuable marker of normal and neoplastic leydig cells of the testis. Appl Immunohistochem Mol Morphol. 2002;10:159–62.
49. Zheng W, Senturk BZ, Parkash V. Inhibin immunohistochemical staining: a practical approach for the surgical pathologist in the diagnoses of ovarian sex cord-stromal tumors. Adv Anat Pathol. 2003;10: 27–38.
50. Zhao C, Barner R, Vinh TN, McManus K, Dabbs D, Vang R. Sf-1 is a diagnostically useful immunohistochemical marker and comparable to other sex cord-stromal tumor markers for the differential diagnosis of ovarian sertoli cell tumor. Int J Gynecol Pathol. 2008;27:507–14.
51. Sangoi AR, McKenney JK, Brooks JD, Higgins JP. Evaluation of sf-1 expression in testicular germ cell tumors: a tissue microarray study of 127 cases. Appl Immunohistochem Mol Morphol. 2013;21:318–21.
52. Young RH, Koelliker DD, Scully RE. Sertoli cell tumors of the testis, not otherwise specified: a clinicopathologic analysis of 60 cases. Am J Surg Pathol. 1998;22:709–21.
53. Kaplan GW, Cromie WJ, Kelalis PP, Silber I, Tank ES Jr. Gonadal stromal tumors: a report of the prepubertal testicular tumor registry. J Urol. 1986;136:300–2.
54. Jimenez-Quintero LP, Ro JY, Zavala-Pompa A, Amin MB, Tetu B, Ordonez NG, Ayala AG. Granulosa cell tumor of the adult testis: a clinicopathologic study of seven cases and a review of the literature. Hum Pathol. 1993;24:1120–5.
55. Wang BY, Rabinowitz DS, Granato RC Sr., Unger PD. Gonadal tumor with granulosa cell tumor features in an adult testis. Ann Diagn Pathol. 2002;6:56–60.
56. Lawrence WD, Young RH, Scully RE. Juvenile granulosa cell tumor of the infantile testis.A report of 14 cases. Am J Surg Pathol. 1985;9:87–94.

57. Young RH, Lawrence WD, Scully RE. Juvenile granulosa cell tumor—another neoplasm associated with abnormal chromosomes and ambiguous genitalia. A report of three cases. Am J Surg Pathol. 1985;9:737–43.
58. Kommoss S, Gilks CB, Penzel R, Herpel E, Mackenzie R, Huntsman D, Schirmacher P, Anglesio M, Schmidt D, Kommoss F. A current perspective on the pathological assessment of foxl2 in adult-type granulosa cell tumours of the ovary. Histopathology. 2014;64:380–8.
59. Lima JF, Jin L, de Araujo AR, Erikson-Johnson MR, Oliveira AM, Sebo TJ, Keeney GL, Medeiros F. Foxl2 mutations in granulosa cell tumors occurring in males. Arch Pathol Lab Med. 2012;136:825–8.
60. Ferry JA, Harris NL, Young RH, Coen J, Zietman A, Scully RE. Malignant lymphoma of the testis, epididymis, and spermatic cord.A clinicopathologic study of 69 cases with immunophenotypic analysis. Am J Surg Pathol. 1994;18:376–90.
61. Valbuena JR, Admirand JH, Lin P, Medeiros LJ. Myeloid sarcoma involving the testis. Am J Clin Pathol. 2005;124:445–52.
62. Askin FB, Land VJ, Sullivan MP, Ragab AH, Steuber CP, Dyment PG, Talbert J, Moore T. Occult testicular leukemia: testicular biopsy at three years continuous complete remission of childhood leukemia: a southwest oncology group study. Cancer. 1981;47:470–5.
63. Reid H, Marsden HB. Gonadal infiltration in children with leukaemia and lymphoma. J Clin Pathol. 1980;33:722–9.
64. Amin MB. Selected other problematic testicular and paratesticular lesions: rete testis neoplasms and pseudotumors, mesothelial lesions and secondary tumors. Mod Pathol. 2005;18(Suppl2):S131–45.
65. Dutt N, Bates AW, Baithun SI. Secondary neoplasms of the male genital tract with different patterns of involvement in adults and children. Histopathology. 2000;37:323–31.
66. Backhaus BO, Kaefer M, Engum SA, Davis MM. Contralateral testicular metastasis in paratesticular rhabdomyosarcoma. J Urol. 2000;164:1709–10.
67. Simon T, Hero B, Berthold F. Testicular and paratesticular involvement by metastatic neuroblastoma. Cancer. 2000;88:2636–41.

Intraoperative Consultation for Testicular Tumors: Challenges and Implications for Treatment

41

Hiroshi Miyamoto and Steven S. Shen

Introduction

More than 90 % of testicular neoplasms originate from germ cells. Physical examination, scrotal ultrasound, and measurement of serum markers, such as lactate dehydrogenase, α-fetoprotein, and human chorionic gonadotropin, define the nature of most testicular masses. Thus, clinical suspicion for testicular neoplasm on the basis of the current methods of diagnosis, without a cytologic or tissue diagnosis, usually results in prompt radical orchiectomy. Indeed, it is not appropriate to perform fine-needle aspiration and needle core biopsy of the testis because of the risk of implanting malignant cells in the scrotum. It is therefore uncommon for the pathologist to get involved in defining the nature of testicular tumors prior to orchiectomy. Of note is that an increasing number of cases have been treated with partial orchiectomy (testis-sparing surgery) [1, 2] that may require intraoperative frozen section assessment (FSA).

S. S. Shen (✉)
Department of Pathology and Genomic Medicine, Houston Methodist Hospital, Houston, TX, USA
e-mail: stevenshen@houstonmethodist.org

H. Miyamoto
Departments of Pathology and Urology, The Johns Hopkins Medical Institutions, Baltimore, MD, USA
e-mail: hmiyamo1@jhmi.edu

Common Indications for Intraoperative Consultation

- Gross and/or histopathologic diagnosis for testicular/paratesticular lesions (e.g., non-neoplastic process, epidermoid cyst/dermoid cyst, teratoma, non-teratomatous germ cell tumor, lymphoma)
- Surgical margin status during partial orchiectomy
- Histopathologic diagnosis of retroperitoneal lymph node dissection specimen

Assessment of Testicular Lesions for Potential Organ-Sparing Surgery

When intraoperative consultation is requested in the context of a histopathologic diagnosis of testicular masses, macroscopic examination may be all that should be done, as there are often no immediate management issues at stake. However, there are exceptions in which intraoperative FSA for testicular mass plays a significant role particularly in obviating radical orchiectomy.

- Fibrous pseudotumor: Testicular/paratesticular fibrous pseudotumors believed to be reactive lesions resulting from trauma, hydrocele, or infection may exhibit three distinct histologic appearances: (1) "plaque-like" consisting of dense fibrosis with minimal inflammation; (2) "inflammatory sclerotic" consisting of dense fibrosis with significant inflammation; and (3)

C. Magi-Galluzzi, C. G. Przybycin (eds.), *Genitourinary Pathology*, DOI 10.1007/978-1-4939-2044-0_41,

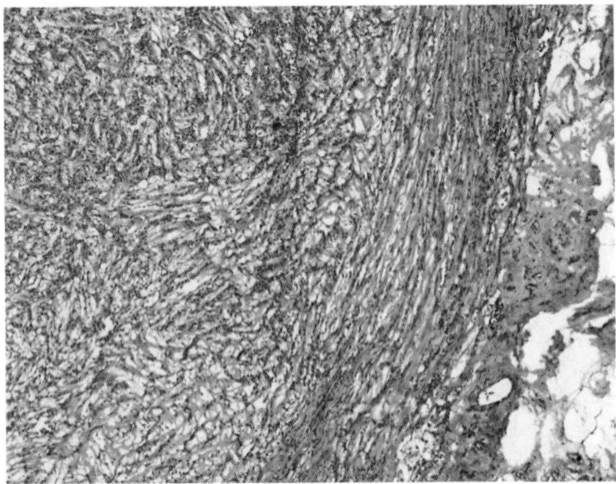

Fig. 41.1 Frozen section of an adenomatoid tumor with cords of tumor cells and fibrotic background mimicking an adenocarcinoma. Original magnification × 100

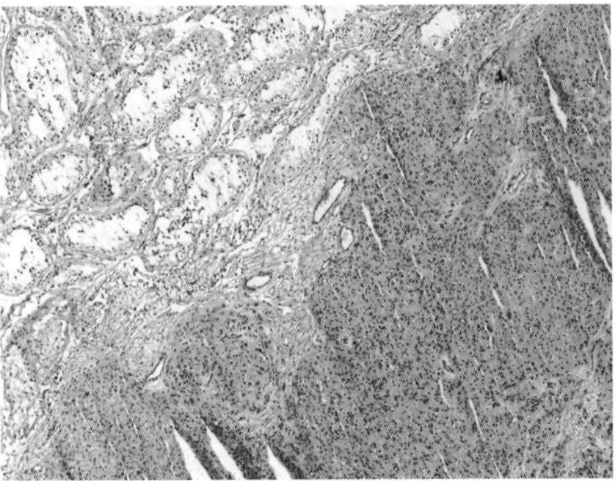

Fig. 41.2 Frozen section of a Leydig cell tumor showing well-circumscribed tumor composed of cells with abundant eosinophilic cytoplasm, large round nuclei, and frequent small nucleoli. Original magnification × 40

"myofibroblastic" consisting of tissue-culture-like cells with numerous capillaries and sparse inflammation [3]. They can clinically mimic neoplasms, and many patients have undergone radical orchiectomy for suspicion of malignancy. Considering this reactive process is often localized and occurs in young males, testicular-sparing surgery should be considered a possibility. Nonetheless, in some of the cases with diffuse process, accurate frozen section diagnosis still failed to prevent radical orchiectomy mainly due to questionable testicular viability [4].

- Adenomatoid tumor: Adenomatoid tumor is a benign neoplasm of mesothelial origin (or may be a peculiar form of nodular mesothelial hyperplasia) most commonly found in the epididymis. It usually presents as a small (up to 5 cm), solid, firm, well-circumscribed mass occasionally containing cysts. It can encroach the testicular or adnexal structures clinically and histologically may mimic a malignant proliferation (Fig. 41.1). An accurate FSA allows for testicular-sparing surgery.
- "Benign" tumors: Most of small masses often detected incidentally (e.g., scrotal ultrasonography) are benign. In the management of these tumors, radical orchiectomy may not be necessary. Neoplasms generally with a benign course suitable for testicular-sparing surgery include Leydig cell tumor (Fig. 41.2), Sertoli cell tumor (Fig. 41.3), epidermoid cyst/dermoid cyst, and teratoma in prepubertal patients. In our experience, there have been situations where an equivocal or incorrect frozen section diagnoses, such as "suspicious for epidermoid cyst" and "mature teratoma" for epidermoid cysts (on permanent section), resulted in radical orchiectomy [5]. Therefore, clear and effective communication between the surgeon and pathologist is always essential.

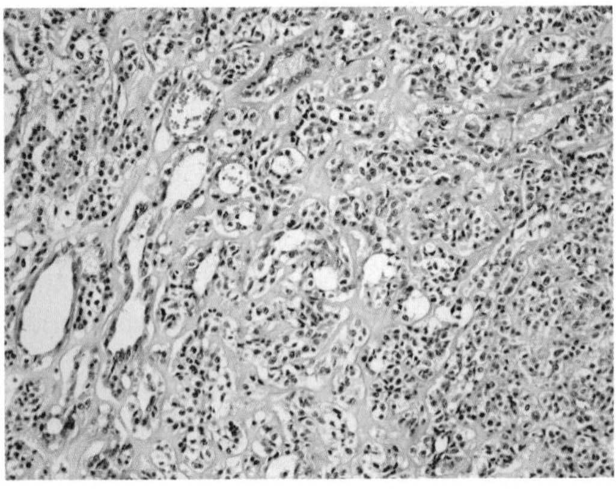

Fig. 41.3 Frozen section of a Sertoli cell tumor showing nests and tubules lined by uniform cells with clear and vacuolated cytoplasm and paucicellular stroma. Original magnification × 100

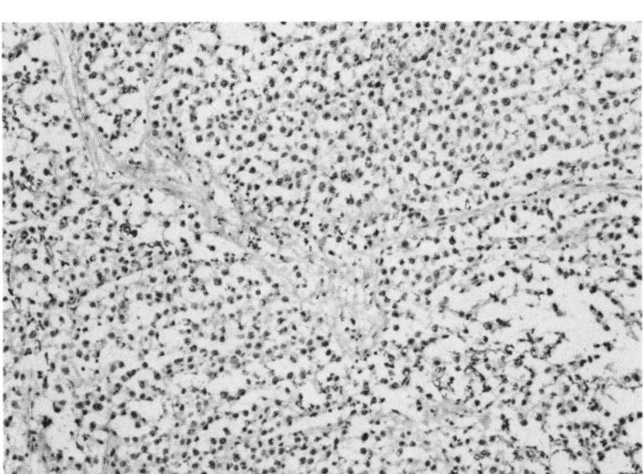

Fig. 41.4 Frozen section of a classic seminoma showing monotonous, evenly spaced tumor cells with abundant clear cytoplasm. Noticed is also the presence of fibrovascular septae filled with lymphocytic infiltrate. Original magnification × 100

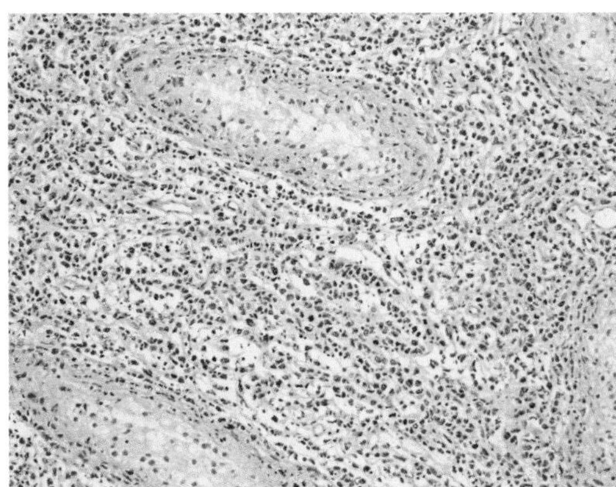

Fig. 41.5 Frozen section of a malignant lymphoma showing diffuse interstitial infiltrate of discohesive tumor cells. Original magnification × 100

- Malignant germ cell tumors: It is very unusual to consider partial orchiectomy for the treatment of malignant germ cell tumors. Patients with palpable masses and hormone-related manifestation such as elevated serum markers and gynecomastia are not typically candidates for testicular-sparing surgery. However, it may be an option in some highly selected patients who have a small mass (less than 2 cm in size) in a solitary testicle or bilateral concurrent testicular tumors and a desire for fertility or avoidance of androgen supplementation [1, 2]. When a partial orchiectomy specimen is submitted for intraoperative consultation, it is important to include adjacent normal-appearing testicular parenchyma in FSA in order to detect potentially multifocal intratubular germ cell neoplasia. Other reported pitfalls of FSA of germ cell tumors include distinctions between squamous metaplasia in a hydrocele or epididymal lesions vs. teratoma, granulomatous process vs. seminoma (Fig. 41.4), and mixed germ cell tumor (when sampled focally) vs. pure seminoma [6].
- Lymphoma: Lymphoma is the most common testicular malignancy in elderly men and frequently involves both testicles. Most of primary testicular lymphomas display a B-cell immunophenotype (e.g., large B-cell lymphoma) (Fig. 41.5). However, T-cell or follicular lymphomas involving the testis have also been reported [7, 8]. Systemic chemotherapy remains the standard treatment for testicular lymphomas, but the blood–testis barrier is known to impede the delivery of chemotherapeutic agents to the testis. Thus, radical orchiectomy is beneficial in providing tissue for diagnosis and removing a potential sanctuary site for tumor cells. Accordingly, frozen section diagnosis of lymphoma/lymphoid proliferation in a biopsy specimen does not readily abstain from proceeding with radical orchiectomy, while it is helpful in reserving fresh tumor from the orchiectomy specimen for flow cytometry and molecular genetics analyses.

Margin Evaluation During Partial Orchiectomy

It is usually unnecessary to perform an FSA of the spermatic cord margin during radical orchiectomy for testicular germ cell tumor, because a positive margin is extremely rare in current practice. However, partial orchiectomy specimen is occasionally submitted for intraoperative consultation for evaluating surgical margins. As mentioned previously, organ-sparing surgery could be suitable for those patients with small benign lesions or rarely for those highly selective patients with malignant tumor. In evaluating the surgical margin for those potentially germ cell tumors, special attention needs to be paid to the presence of intratubular germ cell neoplasia in the grossly unremarkable parenchyma in addition to invasive tumor.

Assessment of Retroperitoneal Lymph Node Dissection in Patients with Testicular Neoplasm

Retroperitoneal lymph node dissection is performed not only for accurate staging but also for therapeutic purposes in patients with nonseminomatous testicular cancer with or without receiving chemotherapy. Residual metastatic seminoma may also be resected after radiotherapy in selected cases. The spread of germ cell tumors to the retroperitoneal nodes generally proceeds in an orderly anatomic fashion. Therefore, intraoperative FSA is used particularly at the margins of the anatomic dissection to guide the extent of node dissection.

If multiple lymph nodes are submitted, the largest or grossly suspicious one should be submitted for FSA. The FSA report needs to indicate the type of germ cell tumor and the relative amount of each component. The findings of totally necrotic and/or fibrotic tissue on FSA in cases following chemotherapy should be reported as a provisional diagnosis, since the permanent sections may reveal focal viable tumor cells. Therefore, the number and selection of tissue for frozen section are both important for an accurate diagnosis. Metastatic tumors may show a variety of histologic features, not only germ cell tumor such as teratoma, embryonal carcinoma (Fig. 41.6), yolk sac tumor, or seminoma, but also components of carcinomatous or sarcomatous transformation. The histologic findings provide important information for choice of additional chemotherapy and prognostication.

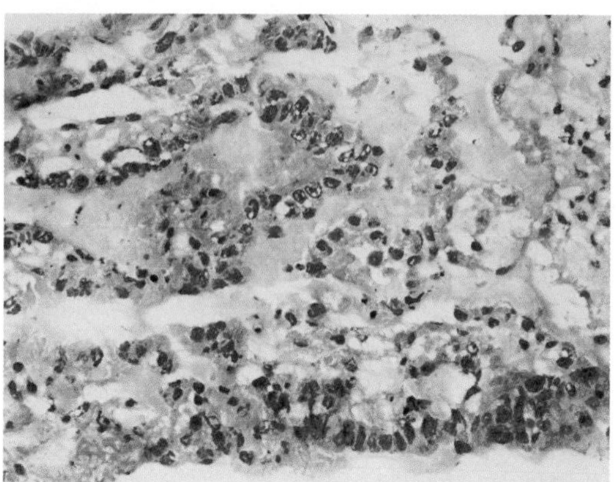

Fig. 41.6 Frozen section of a pelvic lymph node showing focal embryonal carcinoma. Original magnification ×200

References

1. Bazzi WM, Raheem OA, Stroup SP, Kane CJ, Derweesh IH, Downs TM. Partial orchiectomy and testis intratubular germ cell neoplasia: world literature review. Urol Ann. 2011;3(3):115–8.
2. Brunocilla E, Gentile G, Schiavina R, et al. Testis-sparing surgery for the conservative management of small testicular masses: an update. Anticancer Res. 2013;33(11):5205–10.
3. Miyamoto H, Montgomery EA, Epstein JI. Paratesticular fibrous pseudotumor: a morphologic and immunohistochemical study of 13 cases. Am J Surg Pathol. 2010;34(4):569–74.
4. Gordetsky J, Findeis-Hosey J, Erturk E, Messing EM, Yao JL, Miyamoto H. Role of frozen section analysis of testicular/paratesticular fibrous pseudotumours: a five-case experience. Can Urol Assoc J. 2011;5(4):E47–51.
5. Subik MK, Gordetsky J, Yao JL, diSant'Agnese PA, Miyamoto H. Frozen section assessment in testicular and paratesticular lesions suspicious for malignancy: its role in preventing unnecessary orchiectomy. Hum Pathol. 2012;43(9):1514–9.
6. Winstanley AM, Mikuz G, Debruyne F, Schulman CC, Parkinson MC, European Association of Pathologists UDiF. Handling and reporting of biopsy and surgical specimens of testicular cancer. Eur Urol. 2004;45(5):564–73.
7. Cheah CY, Wirth A, Seymour JF. Primary testicular lymphoma. Blood. 2014;123(4):486–93.
8. Vural F, Cagirgan S, Saydam G, Hekimgil M, Soyer NA, Tombuloglu M. Primary testicular lymphoma. J Natl Med Assoc. 2007;99(11):1277–82.

Genetic and Epigenetic Alterations in Testicular Tumors

42

Pallavi A. Patil and Cristina Magi-Galluzzi

Introduction

Testicular germ cell tumors (TGCT) originate from the malignant counterpart of primordial germ cells/gonocytes. Various studies have suggested an inherited predisposition to the development of these tumors, based on the increased risks associated with a positive family history, the higher frequency of bilaterality in familial cases, and the ethnic and racial differences. However, no high-penetrance susceptibility gene has yet been identified, suggesting a genetic architecture in which multiple loci contribute to testicular germ cell tumors susceptibility.

The only recurrent cytogenetic alteration detected in TGCTs is the gain of the short arm of chromosome 12, mostly as isochromosomes.

Candidate gene studies have identified two loci of interest, that is, the Y-chromosome gr/gr deletion and the PDE11A gene, while recent genome-wide association studies have identified at least three genes involved in the KITLG/KIT signaling pathway (KITLG, SPRY4 and BAK1).

Although DNA hypermethylation plays a crucial role in tumorigenesis, aberrant de novo methylation of tumor suppressor genes or tumor-related genes is a rare event in TGCT, particularly in seminomas, although there have been reports on differentially methylated genes among seminomatous and non-seminomatous TGCTs.

MicroRNAs and Piwi-interacting RNAs are increasingly seen as important elements in both gonadal development and spermatogenesis and their pathologies.

Recent expression profiling studies of TGCTs along with advances in embryonic stem-cell research have contributed to our markedly improved understanding of the pathogenesis of testicular cancer. However, many questions remain unanswered and among them probably the most important one concerns the etiology of TGCTs and the relative roles of genetic versus environmental or lifestyle factors.

Genetic Alterations in Testicular Tumors

Though relatively rare, testicular (and extragonadal) germ cell tumors are the most common solid tumors in young men aged 18–35 years and represent the leading cause of cancer-related morbidity and mortality in this group.

Adult male TGTCs arise from malignant transformation of the same precursor, a totipotent germ cell [1], called carcinoma in situ (CIS)/intratubular germ cell neoplasia or testicular intraepithelial neoplasia (ITGCN). The process starts prenatally, is often associated with some degree of gonadal dysgenesis, and involves the

C. Magi-Galluzzi (✉) · P. A. Patil
Department of Pathology, Cleveland Clinic, Robert J. Tomsich Pathology and Laboratory Medicine Institute, Cleveland, OH, USA
e-mail: magic@ccf.org

P. A. Patil
e-mail: Patilp2@ccf.org

C. Magi-Galluzzi, C. G. Przybycin (eds.), *Genitourinary Pathology,* DOI 10.1007/978-1-4939-2044-0_42,

acquisition of specific genetic aberrations and subsequent epigenetic alterations [2]. Evidence from morphological, epidemiological, immunohistochemical, and gene expression profiling studies indicates that the ITGCN cell is derived from a gonocyte or primordial germ cell [3]. ITGCN and seminomatous cells are characterized by expression of OCT3/4 and NANOG, all identified as transcription factors related to pluripotency in embryonic stem cells.

Family history of TGCT is one of the strongest and most consistent risk factors for this tumor. Approximately 1.4% of newly diagnosed TGCT patients report a positive family history of TGCT. Bilateral testicular germ cell tumors are more likely to occur in familial aggregations than in sporadic cases. Studies have estimated that brothers of affected cases have an eight-to tenfold increased relative risk compared with the general population and fathers/sons of TGCT cases have a four- to sixfold higher risk [4]. These high familial risks suggest that inherited susceptibility and/or environmental factors that cluster in families may play a substantial role in the etiology of a significant portion of TGCT cases. Genome-wide screens subsequently provided evidence of a TGCT susceptibility gene on chromosome Xq27 (TGCT1) that might also predispose to cryptorchidism. However, this putative gene has yet to be identified, and other TGCT susceptibility genes probably exist [5]. Although the familial relative risk of TGCT is considerably higher than for most other cancers, the absolute risk is comparatively low (lifetime risk approximately 1/230 in Caucasian men). Since no specific high-penetrance susceptibility gene has been identified, it is likely that the combined contribution of multiple common alleles, each conferring modest risk, might underlie familial testicular cancer [6].

ITGCN, seminomas, and all variants of nonseminomatous germ cell tumors (NSGCT) are characterized by marked aneuploidy in nearly all cases as well as specific chromosome gains and losses. The only recurrent cytogenetic alteration is the gain of the short arm of chromosome 12, mostly as isochromosomes [7, 8]. Specifically, isochromosome 12p is the most common alteration (~80%), with duplication of 12p and amplification of shorter stretches of 12p being much less common. While seminomas show high-level amplification of 12p, gain of proximal 17q and loss of 10q have been detected in NSGCTs [9]. Interestingly, ITGCN without adjacent invasive TGCT does not contain isochromosome 12p in most studies, which suggests that isochromosome 12p is not required for the development of ITGCN [10]. It is believed that the gain of 12p is important in tumor progression and occurs subsequent to aneuploidy. This gain appears to be multifunctional in germ cell tumorigenesis on the basis of the observed overexpression of several candidate genes [including KITLG, NANOG (and its pseudogenes), KRAS2, BCAT1, and CCND2] mapped to this region involved in maintenance of pluripotency and oncogenesis.

Further studies are required before we fully understand the role of chromosome 12p in TGCT carcinogenesis.

Compared to chromosomal abnormalities, specific gene mutations in TGCTs are less frequent. The most frequent single genes affected in TGCTs are KIT, K-RAS, N-RAS, and B-RAF [11]. Eight percent of TGCTs have mutations in KIT, 5% in K-RAS, 3% in N-RAS, 8% in MADH4, and 1% in STK10. Somatic mutations have also been identified in TP53, MET, SNF1LK, and PTEN [12]. Copy number changes are relatively common in TGCT, and point mutations are relatively rare when compared with other cancer types.

Seminomatous and NSGCTs are much more frequent in the testis than in the ovary, which suggests a link to the Y chromosome. This idea is strengthened by the fact that patients with disorders of sex development (DSD) are at risk for development of TGCTs.

The Y chromosome carries a number of testis- and germ cell-specific genes. The region of interest on the Y chromosome is the so-called male-specific Y (MSY) region, which contains high density of genes from nine families, each gene existing in multiple (2–35), near-identical copies [13]. Genes within the MSY are expressed predominantly or exclusively in the testis and are believed to contribute to the development and proliferation of germ cells.

Candidate association studies in sporadic TGCT have detected a Y chromosome 1.6-Mb deletion (designated gr/gr), previously implicated in spermatogenic failure and subfertility, in 3.0 % of TGCT patients with a family history, 2 % of TGCT cases without a family history, and 1.3 % of unaffected male controls, demonstrating that the deletion confers an approximately twofold risk of TGCT [14]. The association between gr/gr and TGCT is stronger for seminomas than for NSGCTs. However, because of its low frequency and modest risk, this microdeletion accounts for approximately 0.5 % of the excess familial risk of TGCT.

Genetic susceptibility conditioning familial TGCTs has been established, confirming mutations or single nucleotide polymorphisms (SNPs) affecting some genes involved in normal germ cell differentiation such as KITLG, SPRY4, PDE11A, and BAK1 [15].

Genome-wide association studies (GWAS) [16–18] utilizing TGCT samples from the UK have recently identified eight SNPs at six loci: 12q21 (KITLG), 5q31 (SPRY4), 6p21 (BAK1), 5p15 (TERT-CLPTM1L), 9p24 (DMRT1), and 12p13 (ATF7IP). The loci at 5q31, 9p24, and 12q21 were independently reported with consistent effect by Kanetsky et al. in their GWAS comprising cases of TGCT from the USA [19]. KITLG, SPRY4, and BAK1 are all involved in the KITLG/KIT signaling pathway. KITLG/ KIT system regulates survival, proliferation, and migration of germ cells [20], and germ line homozygous null mutations of either gene in mice cause infertility due to failure of progenitor germ cell development. SPRY4 is an inhibitor of the mitogen-activated protein kinase pathway that is activated by the KITLG/KIT pathway. BAK1 encodes a protein that promotes apoptosis by binding to and antagonizing the apoptosis repressor activity of BCL2 and other antiapoptotic proteins. BAK1 expression in TCGT is repressed by the KITLG/KIT pathway, and the interaction of BAK1 with antiapoptotic proteins is implicated in germ-cell apoptosis that occurs in response to the blockade of KITLG/KIT pathway [21]. TERT and ATF7IP relate to a pathway of telomerase regulation: TERT encodes telomerase while ATF7IP regulates expression of TERT and its partner TERC. DMRT1 relates to a pathway of sex determination [18].

Since frequencies of risk alleles at 12q21 are much lower in the African population than in the Caucasian, the 12q21 locus may, in part, account for the different frequency of TGCT observed between ethnic groups [22].

Although these SNPs may be biologically significant, these six loci together with gr/gr deletion account only for approximately 15 % of the excess familial risk of TGCT. The remaining 85 % of genetic predisposition is yet unexplained and requires further investigation [18].

Epigenetics of Testicular Tumors

The term "epigenetics" refers to heritable changes in gene function that occur without any change in the DNA sequence. Epigenetics is regulation of gene expression and can be essentially transmitted to daughter cells formed after meiosis or mitosis [23] and possibly also through generations. Environmental factors can affect epigenetic processes. So far, three main epigenetic mechanisms are known: DNA methylation, chromatin remodeling, and microRNA regulation. Of those, DNA methylation is the best known and most thoroughly studied epigenetic mechanism [24].

Methylation

DNA methylation, a key component of the epigenome involved in regulating gene expression, is initially acquired in the germ line at millions of sites across the genome. Hypermethylation of CpG islands (sequences rich in CpG) associated with silencing of tumor suppressor genes or tumor-related genes is a common hallmark of human cancer. TGCTs have distinctive DNA methylation profiles that differ from those of somatic tissue-derived cancers or somatic tissues [25]. TGCTs exhibit greater degree of hypomethylation compared to other cancers [26].

TGCT methylation patterns are similar to those exhibited by primordial germ cells [27].

Seminomas are basically devoid of DNA methylation and NSGCTs in general have methylation levels comparable with other tumor tissues. In general, DNA methylation seems to increase with differentiation, and among NSGCTs, undifferentiated embryonal carcinomas harbor the lowest levels of DNA promoter hypermethylation, whereas well-differentiated teratomas display the highest [28].

So far, a limited number of tumor suppressor genes have been found inactivated by DNA promoter hypermethylation in more than a minor percentage of TGCTs, including MGMT, SCGB3A1, RASSF1A, HIC1, and PRSS21. RASSF1A methylation has been detected in 40 % of seminomas and 83 % of NSCGT components. These findings are consistent with a multistep model in which RASSF1A methylation occurs early in TGCT tumorigenesis and additional epigenetic events characterize progression from seminoma to NSGCT [29]. PRSS21 (testisin gene at 16p13), a serine protease abundantly expressed only in normal testes, is thought to be a tumor suppressor gene silenced by aberrant methylation in TGCTs [30]. CpG sites in the 5′ untranslated region proved to be relevant to testisin gene silencing when methylated. It has been demonstrated that the median normalized index of methylation is 8.6 times higher in TGCTs than in normal testicular samples, and significantly higher in NSGCTs than in seminomas.

LINE1 and Alu are two major DNA repetitive elements, which consist of interspersed and tandem repeats. LINE1 is a long group of interspersed nucleotide elements that constitutes at least 18 % of the human genome. The Alu repetitive element is the most abundant short interspersed nucleotide element in the human genome and accounts for about 10 % of the entire genome [24]. Alu and LINE1 elements are normally heavily methylated and contain much of the CpG methylation found in normal human tissues. However, both LINE1 and Alu repeats are extensively unmethylated in seminomas, whereas in NSGCTs the LINE1 sequence is extensively unmethylated, but Alu elements are methylated, confirming a difference in degree of methylation between seminomatous and NSGCT.

Imprinting defects, DNA hypomethylation of testis/cancer associated genes, and presence of unmethylated XIST (X inactive specific transcript) are frequent in TGCTs [28]. TGCTs contain supernumerical X chromosomes in a hypomethylated state at the 5′ end. XIST is expressed exclusively from the inactive form of the X chromosome and is thought to be involved in the inactivation process of female X chromosomes. XIST gene expression has been found in seminomas (83 %) but less frequently in NSGCTs (25 %) [31].

Genomic imprinting is an epigenetic mechanism causing functional differences between paternal and maternal genomes and playing an essential role in mammalian developmental process. Differential methylation of cytosine residues in CpG dinucleotides in critical regions of imprinted genes is part of the process that differentiates paternal and maternal alleles. Maternally expressed H19 is one of the best-characterized imprinted genes: the 5′ region of H19 is methylated in paternal and unmethylated in maternal alleles [24]. Fetal spermatogonia are predominantly unmethylated at differentially methylated regions of H19, whereas adult germ cells of testis show significant methylation at this region [32]. These phenomena are regarded as "DNA reprogramming," which are observed genome-wide in germ cells or preimplantation embryos. Both seminomatous and NSGCTs show predominant unmethylation or biallelic unmethylation at the 5′-region of H19, suggesting that TGCTs show consistent demethylation at the imprinting domain, analogous to the situation in fetal germ cells.

Chromatin Remodeling

Primordial germ cells and gonocytes are known to undergo extensive epigenetic reprogramming. Recent data in mice have demonstrated that suppression of somatic differentiation programs in primordial germ cells is mediated by a complex of two proteins, Blimp1 (B-lymphocyte induced maturation protein-1) and Prmt5 (protein arginine methyltransferase-5). BLIMP1 and PRMT5 complex mediates symmetrical methylation of histones H2A and H4 at arginine 3, which are involved in somatic differentiation programs and are thought to repress the HOX genes, resulting in widespread epigenetic modification leading to transcriptional repression [33]. In a recent study, Eckert and colleagues have detected BLIMP1, PRMT5, and arginine dimethylation of histones H2A and H4 in human male gonocytes at weeks 12–19 of gestation, indicating a role of this mechanism in human fetal germ cell development as well. Moreover, BLIMP1/PRMT5 and histone H2A/H4 arginine 3 dimethylation has been identified in ITGCN and most seminomas, while being downregulated in NSGCTs [34].

MicroRNA Regulation

Small non-coding regulatory RNAs have emerged as pivotal posttranscriptional modulators of gene expression and are involved in diverse processes of cell differentiation and development. In particular, microRNAs (miRNAs) and Piwi-interacting RNAs (piRNAs) are increasingly seen as important elements in both gonadal development and spermatogenesis and their pathologies [35].

miRNAs are small non-coding RNAs (≈22 nt long) that act as potent modulators of gene expression by targeting 3′ UTR regions of mRNAs inducing their cleavage or translational repression [23]. Deregulation of miRNAs can affect the regulation of expression of mRNA targets, generating complex mechanisms of alterations with pathological consequences in testis development and function.

Recent studies have indicated that miRNA regulation may play a role in TGCTs development. Oncogenic miRNA clusters miR-372 and -373 seem to contribute to testicular cancer development by disabling the p53 pathway [36]. The cluster miR-17-92 may promote development of tumors through prevention of apoptosis [37]. Expression of miR-372 has been detected in 28/32 seminomas and 14/21 NSGCT with no expression in spermatocytic seminomas or normal testis. In NSGCT, miR-372 expression seemed to correlate with larger embryonal carcinoma component [36]. Quantitative reverse transcriptase-PCR (qRT-PCR) studies have shown differential expression of several miRNAs between normal tissue and TGCTs [38]. miR-371–3 cluster is highly overexpressed in seminomas, embryonal carcinomas, and yolk sac tumors; miR-371–3 and -302a–d are the most differentiating miRNAs between different TGCTs subgroups [39].

piRNAs are short RNA molecules (24–32 nt long) that are processed in a DICER/DROSHA-independent manner and associated with PIWI proteins [23]. piRNA with PIWI proteins regulates epigenetic (heterochromatin) and posttranscription (mRNA) events [40]. piRNA maintains germ cell function and stability of genome by silencing transposable elements and interacts with DNA methylation during spermatogenesis [23]. Reduced piRNA expression with PIWI protein gene silencing by hypermethylation has been found in seminomas and NSGCTs [41].

References

1. McCluggage WG, Shanks JH, Arthur K, Banerjee SS. Cellular proliferation and nuclear ploidy assessments augment established prognostic factors in predicting malignancy in testicular Leydig cell tumours. Histopathology. 1998;33(4):361–8.
2. Mosharafa AA, Foster RS, Bihrle R, Koch MO, Ulbright TM, Einhorn LH, et al. Does retroperitoneal lymph node dissection have a curative role for patients with sex cord-stromal testicular tumors? Cancer. 2003;98(4):753–7.
3. Sonne SB, Almstrup K, Dalgaard M, Juncker AS, Edsgard D, Ruban L, et al. Analysis of gene expression profiles of microdissected cell populations indicates that testicular carcinoma in situ is an arrested gonocyte. Cancer Res. 2009;69(12):5241–50.
4. Hemminki K, Li X. Familial risk in testicular cancer as a clue to a heritable and environmental aetiology. Br J Cancer. 2004;90(9):1765–70.
5. Lutke Holzik MF, Rapley EA, Hoekstra HJ, Sleijfer DT, Nolte IM, Sijmons RH. Genetic predisposition to testicular germ-cell tumours. Lancet Oncol. 2004;5(6):363–71.
6. Kratzer SS, Ulbright TM, Talerman A, Srigley JR, Roth LM, Wahle GR, et al. Large cell calcifying Sertoli cell tumor of the testis: contrasting features of six malignant and six benign tumors and a review of the literature. Am J Surg Pathol. 1997;21(11):1271–80.

7. von Eyben FE. Chromosomes, genes, and development of testicular germ cell tumors. Cancer Genet Cytogenet. 2004;151(2):93–138.
8. Houldsworth J, Korkola JE, Bosl GJ, Chaganti RS. Biology and genetics of adult male germ cell tumors. J Clin Oncol. 2006;24(35):5512–8.
9. Mohamed GH, Gelfond JA, Nicolas MM, Brand TC, Sarvis JA, Leach RJ, et al. Genomic characterization of testis cancer: association of alterations with outcome of clinical stage 1 mixed germ cell nonseminomatous germ cell tumor of the testis. Urology. 2012;80(2):485 e1–5.
10. Ottesen AM, Skakkebaek NE, Lundsteen C, Leffers H, Larsen J, Rajpert-De Meyts E. High-resolution comparative genomic hybridization detects extra chromosome arm 12p material in most cases of carcinoma in situ adjacent to overt germ cell tumors, but not before the invasive tumor development. Genes Chromosomes Cancer. 2003;38(2):117–25.
11. Sheikine Y, Genega E, Melamed J, Lee P, Reuter VE, Ye H. Molecular genetics of testicular germ cell tumors. Am J Cancer Res. 2012;2(2):153–67.
12. Forbes S, Clements J, Dawson E, Bamford S, Webb T, Dogan A, et al. Cosmic 2005. Br J Cancer. 2006;94(2):318–22.
13. Skaletsky H, Kuroda-Kawaguchi T, Minx PJ, Cordum HS, Hillier L, Brown LG, et al. The male-specific region of the human Y chromosome is a mosaic of discrete sequence classes. Nature. 2003;423(6942):825–37.
14. Nathanson KL, Kanetsky PA, Hawes R, Vaughn DJ, Letrero R, Tucker K, et al. The Y deletion gr/gr and susceptibility to testicular germ cell tumor. Am J Hum Genet. 2005;77(6):1034–43.
15. Greene MH, Kratz CP, Mai PL, Mueller C, Peters JA, Bratslavsky G, et al. Familial testicular germ cell tumors in adults: 2010 summary of genetic risk factors and clinical phenotype. Endocr Relat Cancer. 2010;17(2):R109–21.
16. Rapley EA, Turnbull C, Al Olama AA, Dermitzakis ET, Linger R, Huddart RA, et al. A genome-wide association study of testicular germ cell tumor. Nat Genet. 2009;41(7):807–10.
17. Turnbull C, Rapley EA, Seal S, Pernet D, Renwick A, Hughes D, et al. Variants near DMRT1, TERT and ATF7IP are associated with testicular germ cell cancer. Nat Genet. 2010;42(7):604–7.
18. Turnbull C, Rahman N. Genome-wide association studies provide new insights into the genetic basis of testicular germ-cell tumour. Int J Androl. 2011;34(4 Pt 2):e86–96; discussion e-7.
19. Kanetsky PA, Mitra N, Vardhanabhuti S, Li M, Vaughn DJ, Letrero R, et al. Common variation in KITLG and at 5q31.3 predisposes to testicular germ cell cancer. Nat Genet. 2009;41(7):811–5.
20. Boldajipour B, Raz E. What is left behind—quality control in germ cell migration. Sci STKE. 2007;2007(383):pe16.
21. Yan W, Samson M, Jegou B, Toppari J. Bcl-w forms complexes with Bax and Bak, and elevated ratios of Bax/Bcl-w and Bak/Bcl-w correspond to spermatogonial and spermatocyte apoptosis in the testis. Mol Endocrinol. 2000;14(5):682–99.
22. International HapMap C, Frazer KA, Ballinger DG, Cox DR, Hinds DA, Stuve LL, et al. A second generation human haplotype map of over 3.1 million SNPs. Nature. 2007;449(7164):851–61.
23. Del-Mazo J, Brieno-Enriquez MA, Garcia-Lopez J, Lopez-Fernandez LA, De-Felici M. Endocrine disruptors, gene deregulation and male germ cell tumors. Int J Dev Biol. 2013;57(2–4):225–39.
24. Okamoto K. Epigenetics: a way to understand the origin and biology of testicular germ cell tumors. Int J Urol. 2012;19(6):504–11.
25. Wood L, Kollmannsberger C, Jewett M, Chung P, Hotte S, O'Malley M, et al. Canadian consensus guidelines for the management of testicular germ cell cancer. Can Urol Assoc J. 2010;4(2):e19–38.
26. Ushida H, Kawakami T, Minami K, Chano T, Okabe H, Okada Y, et al. Methylation profile of DNA repetitive elements in human testicular germ cell tumor. Mol Carcinog. 2012;51(9):711–22.
27. Okamoto K, Kawakami T. Epigenetic profile of testicular germ cell tumours. Int J Androl. 2007;30(4):385–92; discussion 92.
28. Rosen A, Jayram G, Drazer M, Eggener SE. Global trends in testicular cancer incidence and mortality. Eur Urol. 2011;60(2):374–9.
29. Honorio S, Agathanggelou A, Wernert N, Rothe M, Maher ER, Latif F. Frequent epigenetic inactivation of the RASSF1A tumour suppressor gene in testicular tumours and distinct methylation profiles of seminoma and nonseminoma testicular germ cell tumours. Oncogene. 2003;22(3):461–6.
30. Kempkensteffen C, Christoph F, Weikert S, Krause H, Kollermann J, Schostak M, et al. Epigenetic silencing of the putative tumor suppressor gene testisin in testicular germ cell tumors. J Cancer Res Clin Oncol. 2006;132(12):765–70.
31. Kawakami T, Okamoto K, Sugihara H, Hattori T, Reeve AE, Ogawa O, et al. The roles of supernumerical X chromosomes and XIST expression in testicular germ cell tumors. J Urol. 2003;169(4):1546–52.
32. Kerjean A, Dupont JM, Vasseur C, Le Tessier D, Cuisset L, Paldi A, et al. Establishment of the paternal methylation imprint of the human H19 and MEST/PEG1 genes during spermatogenesis. Hum Mol Genet. 2000;9(14):2183–7.
33. Ancelin K, Lange UC, Hajkova P, Schneider R, Bannister AJ, Kouzarides T, et al. Blimp1 associates with Prmt5 and directs histone arginine methylation in mouse germ cells. Nat Cell Biol. 2006;8(6):623–30.
34. Eckert D, Biermann K, Nettersheim D, Gillis AJ, Steger K, Jack HM, et al. Expression of BLIMP1/PRMT5 and concurrent histone H2A/H4 arginine 3 dimethylation in fetal germ cells, CIS/IGCNU and germ cell tumors. BMC Dev Biol. 2008;8:106.
35. Hayashi K, Chuva de Sousa Lopes SM, Kaneda M, Tang F, Hajkova P, Lao K, et al. MicroRNA

biogenesis is required for mouse primordial germ cell development and spermatogenesis. PLoS One. 2008;3(3):e1738.

36. Voorhoeve PM, le Sage C, Schrier M, Gillis AJ, Stoop H, Nagel R, et al. A genetic screen implicates miRNA-372 and miRNA-373 as oncogenes in testicular germ cell tumors. Cell. 2006;124(6): 1169–81.
37. Novotny GW, Nielsen JE, Sonne SB, Skakkebaek NE, Rajpert-De Meyts E, Leffers H. Analysis of gene expression in normal and neoplastic human testis: new roles of RNA. Int J Androl. 2007;30(4):316–26; discussion 26–7.
38. Palmer RD, Murray MJ, Saini HK, van Dongen S, Abreu-Goodger C, Muralidhar B, et al. Malignant germ cell tumors display common microRNA profiles resulting in global changes in expression of messenger RNA targets. Cancer Res. 2010;70(7):2911–23.
39. Gillis AJ, Stoop HJ, Hersmus R, Oosterhuis JW, Sun Y, Chen C, et al. High-throughput microRNAome analysis in human germ cell tumours. J Pathol. 2007;213(3):319–28.
40. Juliano C, Wang J, Lin H. Uniting germline and stem cells: the function of Piwi proteins and the piRNA pathway in diverse organisms. Annu Rev Genet. 2011;45:447–69.
41. Ferreira HJ, Heyn H, Garcia Del Muro X, Vidal A, Larriba S, Munoz C, et al. Epigenetic loss of the PIWI/piRNA machinery in human testicular tumorigenesis. Epigenetics. 2013;9(1):113–8.

Index

Symbols
α-Methylacyl-CoA racemase (AMACR), 123

A
Ablation, 57, 344, 401, 418
Adenocarcinoma, 13, 14, 20, 21
  pseudohyperplastic, 21
Adenomatoid tumor, 436, 495, 510, 518
Adrenogenital
  syndrome, 439, 454, 480, 497
Adult, 174, 213, 293, 324, 410, 492, 510
  malignancies, 341
  renal tumors, 285
Anaplastic seminoma, 473
Anatomy
  microscopic, 173, 176, 271
  of testis, 435, 437
  prostatic, 4, 7, 8, 11
Androgen receptor (AR), 118, 151, 164
Anterior, 3, 277
  fibromuscular stroma, 5
  prostatic tumors, 8

B
Biopsy, 8, 9, 10, 26, 94, 103, 250, 362
  core, 38
  needle core, 74
  of rectum, 39
  prostatic needle, 82
  seminal vesicle, 83
  transperineal, 9
  transrectal, 8
Bladder, 6, 7, 35, 72, 86, 173, 174, 175, 203, 207
  cancer, 241
    epigenetics of, 255
  diverticula, 183, 184
  neck invasion, 59
  urinary, 71, 72, 176

C
Cancer
  epigenetic alteratioms in prostate, 160
  grading irradiated, 50
  staging of testis, 439
Carcinoma in situ (CIS), 70, 190, 193, 196, 203, 235, 254, 438
Carney complex, 455, 456, 478, 493, 494
Central zone, 3, 6, 10, 88
  prostatic, 9
Chemotherapy, 83, 85, 86, 88, 213, 264, 466, 467, 520
  adjuvant, 84
  neoadjuvant, 80, 81, 261
  testicular specimens after, 463
Choriocarcinoma, 216, 443, 452, 453, 466, 486, 487, 509
Chromatin remodeling, 255, 523, 524, 525
  gene, 409
  genes, 398
  regulation of, 152
Chromophobe RCC, 280, 285, 286, 288, 290, 329, 347, 350, 377, 384, 411, 423
Classification, 196, 285
  histoanatomic, 8
  molecular, 156
Clear cell papillary carcinoma, 290, 321
Clear cell RCC, 278, 286, 288, 289, 290, 293, 306, 315, 319, 323, 329, 331, 345, 346, 348, 350, 365, 377, 398
Clinical correlates, 349
Copy number alterations, 149, 166
Cord, 436, 439
  fibrous, 174
  slender, 275
  spermatic, 435, 442, 519
  testicular, 443
Cystic renal mass
  assessment of, 403
Cytogenetics, 409, 413
Cytology, 80, 193, 217, 265, 471, 472
  clear cell, 419, 421, 422, 423
  eosinophilic cell, 423, 424
  urine, 189, 241, 242, 256, 261, 262, 264, 266

D
Decision modeling, 104, 109
Dermoid cysts, 459, 476
Diagnosis, 8, 24, 26, 46, 53, 84, 85, 86, 87, 128
  cancer, 52, 94
  differential, 323, 324, 328, 336

C. Magi-Galluzzi, C. G. Przybycin (eds.), *Genitourinary Pathology,* DOI 10.1007/978-1-4939-2044-0,

of colorectal adenocarcinoma, 72
pathologic, 93
Divergent
clinicopathological, 383
differentiation, 205, 207
histology, 254
DNA methylation, 160, 161, 162, 255, 408, 523, 524
alterations, 166
Dysgenesis, 435, 521
Dysplasia, 189, 193, 204, 475
cervical, 191
urothelial, 190, 191

E
Easily misdiagnosed tumors, 478, 479, 480
Ectopic, 216, 422, 439
Elac2-, 114
Embryology, 173, 433, 434, 435
Embryonal carcinoma (EC), 441, 443, 450, 466, 473, 477, 484, 485, 486, 507, 525
percentage of, 443
Enhancer of Zeste Homolog 2 (EZH2), 138, 164, 166
Epidermoid cyst, 436, 454, 459, 476
Epigenetic, 166, 257, 407, 525
alterations, 160, 256
of bladder cancer, 255
of testicular tumors, 523
regulation, 254, 409
silencing, 119, 257
Epithelial, 174
atypia, 11
briding, 10
cuboidal, 292
hyperplasia, 184
neoplasms, 266
tumors, 419
ERG antibody, 126, 128, 136

F
Familial, 113, 341
familial adenomatous polyposis (FAP), 494
gastric cancer, 118
germ cell tumors (GCT), 491, 492, 493
oncytoma, 381
syndrome, 377
tumors, 344
Fluorescent in situ hybridization (FISH), 136, 153, 239, 242, 267, 328, 334, 422, 504
Frozen section assessment (FSA), 247, 402, 517
Fusions, 254
gene, 70, 126, 130, 136, 330

G
Genetic alterations, 119
in urothelial carcinoma, 253, 254, 255
Germ cell tumors (GCT), 216, 385, 434, 439, 442, 444, 447, 450, 453, 483, 488
gonadal, 496
invasive, 448
malignant, 519
mediastinal, 487
non-seminomatous, 483, 484, 486
postpubertal, 487
regression in, 477
retroperitoneal, 487
testicular, 521
Germ cell tumors (GCTs), 501, 502, 509
testicular, 501, 505
Gleason, 7, 8, 10, 13, 14, 17, 23, 26, 29, 47, 57, 100
grading, 13, 19, 26, 27, 28, 30, 46, 48
Glutathione s-Transferase π 1 (GSTP1), 131, 161, 162
Gorlin
syndrome (GS), 458, 495
Grade, 7, 11, 13, 24, 55, 56, 195
Gleason, 25, 27, 48, 49, 155
histologic, 202
prostatectomy, 46
Granulosa cell tumor, 457, 483, 510
adult type, 457, 458, 478
juvenlie, 511
juvlenile type, 457
ovarian, 511

H
Hereditary, 113, 114, 398
hemochromatosis, 496
leiomyomatosis, 349, 424
retinablastoma, 231, 233
syndrome, 373, 376, 378, 379, 381
types, 373
Histology, 7, 8, 47, 56, 193, 195
Histone modification, 152, 154, 160, 162, 164, 256, 408
Hoxb13, 114, 115

I
Image-guided, 417
Immunohistochemistry (IHC), 13, 17, 125, 128, 133, 235, 290, 294, 333, 334, 336, 466, 479, 492, 501, 507
International Society of Urologic Pathology (ISUP), 14, 17, 18, 23, 25, 47, 55, 286, 315
Intertubular seminoma, 472
Intratubular large cell hyalinizing sertoli cell neoplasia (ITLCHSCN), 455, 456, 477
Intratubular large cell hyalinizing Sertoli cell neoplasia (ITLCHSCN), 493

J
Juvenile granulosa cell tumor, 457, 478, 510

K
Kidney, 72, 173, 271, 273, 274, 281, 291, 300, 326, 336, 513
arterial supply to, 276, 277

cancer, 349, 355, 363, 373, 381
non-neoplastic, 311, 319
parenchyma, 380
polycystic, 380
tumor, 335

L
Lamina propria, 173, 176, 177, 178, 179, 181, 182, 184, 197, 201, 253
Large cell calcifying Sertoli cell tumor, 455, 456, 478, 493, 510
Leydig cell tumor (LCT), 438, 454, 480, 483, 493, 497, 510
malignant, 454, 455
Li-fraumeni
syndrome, 496
Lymph node dissection (LND), 13, 50, 60, 80, 86, 147, 227, 251, 282, 310, 402
retropritoneal, 337, 344
Lymph node metastasis, 24, 41, 42, 54, 60, 61, 97, 147, 217, 280, 291, 310, 326, 331, 410
Lymphoma, 117, 250, 342, 385, 417, 426, 472, 501, 519
anaplastic, 512
malignant, 513
Lymphovascular invasion (LVI), 39, 40, 41, 59, 61, 203, 208, 229, 455, 484, 487, 501
Lynch syndrome (LS), 231, 232

M
Malignant Sertoli Cell Tumors Which Resemble Seminoma, 478, 479
Management, 13, 29, 41, 87, 126, 156, 484
clinical, 26, 45, 50, 417
non-surgical, 427
surgical, 85, 417
Mesenchymal, 68, 74, 84
atypical, 467
nonvascular, 130
Metastasis, 13, 29, 42, 136, 147, 165
Methylation, 131, 135
differential, 524
DNA, 162
Microrna (miRNA), 138, 160
expression, 409, 525
regulation, 257, 523
Molecular, 54, 57, 223
analyses, 8
biology, 241
biomakers, 253
classification, 156
criteria, 156
epidemiological, 113
markers, 223, 501, 509
oncogenic, 134
technique, 239
Morphologic entities, 79
Morphology, 54, 71, 178, 207, 217, 334
basaloid, 239
cancer, 29
micropapillary, 212
nuclear, 473
plasmacytoid, 212
predominant, 7
rhabdoid, 213
skin-like, 476
squamous, 206
tubular, 472
typical, 390
Msr1-, 114
Muscularis mucosae, 180, 181, 182, 184, 240
Muscularis propria, 7, 173, 176, 179, 180, 181, 182, 183, 184, 211, 240, 250, 261

N
Needle biopsy, 8, 9, 10
extraprostatic extension on, 11
Nephroblastoma, 274, 467
Nephroureterectomy, 228, 229, 257, 404, 405
Nested, 177, 179
architecture, 334
urothelial carcinoma, 207, 208, 209, 210
Neurofibromatosis, 496
Nomograms, 96, 108, 147, 365
for other clinical states, 107
Kattan, 13, 27
limitations of, 109, 110
post-prostatectomy, 83
prognostic, 25
progostic, 57
Non-conventional
bioinformatics, 126
Nondermoid benign teratomas, 476
Non-neoplastic kidney, 311, 319
Non-seminomatous germ cell tumors (NSGCTs), 439, 443
Nonseminomatous germ cell tumors (NSGCTs)
unusual variants of, 474, 475
Non-seminomatous tumors, 483, 484, 487, 488

P
Papillary, 10, 20, 48, 79, 178
architecture, 195
clusters, 265
ductal carcinoma, 65
neoplasia, 196
RCC, 280, 286, 288, 289, 290, 292, 295, 307, 315, 323, 407, 419, 422, 425
urothelial carcinoma, 194, 195, 203, 209, 218, 241, 267, 405
urothelial neoplasia, 193
Papillary urothelial neoplasm of low malignant potential (PUNLMP), 193

Papilloma, 179; 196, 197
  urothelial, 197
Partial cystectomy, 247, 249, 250
Partial nephrectomy, 274, 317, 344, 349, 401, 403
Partial orchiectomy, 456, 517, 519
Pathologic correlates, 353
Pathologic staging, 184, 282, 439
Pathology, 30, 101, 211
  genitourinary, 193
  report, 35, 42, 56, 211, 315
  surgical, 4, 9, 83, 317, 319
Percutaneous, 344, 417, 418
Perinephric fat, 271, 272, 282, 294, 302, 309
  peripheral, 306
Perinephricfat
  peripheral, 276
Peripheral zone (PZ), 3, 5, 10, 83
Peutz-jeghers, 455, 456, 477
Peutz–Jeghers
  syndrome, 493, 494
Plasmacytoid, 205, 212, 213, 251
Primary, 15, 16, 24, 25, 69
  colonic tumor, 86
  epithelial, 71
  periurethral ducts, 82
Primitive neuroectodermal tumor (PNET), 475
Prognosis, 11, 26, 29, 30, 33, 37, 41, 56, 67
Prognostic
  factors, 61, 311, 356, 357
  models, 356, 358, 360
Proportional hazards models, 97
Prostate, 36
  anterior, 7
  cancer, 7, 8, 9, 10, 34, 61, 65, 83, 84, 100, 113
  cancer biomarkers, 123
  glandular, 3, 36
  posterolateral, 5
Prostate Cancer Antigen-3 (PCA3), 131, 132
Prostatectomy, 4, 7, 9, 24, 147
  radical, 146, 147, 161
Prostate neoplasm, 65
Prostate-specific antigen (PSA), 9, 35, 93, 145
Prostatic adenocarcinoma, 13, 38, 65, 67, 68, 69, 88, 236, 439

R

Radiation therapy, 26, 46, 50, 58, 68, 84, 93, 484
Radical cystectomy, 86, 203, 211, 227, 228
Radical nephrectomy, 272, 281, 317, 344, 348, 349, 361, 402
Radical orchiectomy, 517, 518, 519
Radical prostatectomy, 4, 7, 8, 9, 10, 35, 41, 46, 48, 56, 57, 83, 96, 99, 100, 101, 109, 110, 145, 146, 161
  rising PSA after, 107
Radiotherapy, 13, 29, 83, 93, 109, 520
  external beam, 103, 110
  external-beam, 99
Regression, 151, 316
  in germ cell tumors, 477
  logistic, 94, 97
  transcriptional, 119
Renal biopsy, 418
Renal cell carcinoma, 123, 214, 266
Renal cell carcinoma (RCC), 271, 272, 292, 299, 316, 326, 341
  chromophobe, 290, 291
  grading of, 285, 286
  multilocular cystic, 288
  papillary, 289
  thyroid-like follicular, 294
Renal lymphatics, 280, 281, 282
Renal mass, 308, 343, 344, 398, 418
Renal sinus, 273, 274, 305
Renal sinus vein, 274, 277, 308
Renal tumors, 271, 285, 295, 373, 379, 385, 390, 403, 412
Renal vein, 276, 277, 278, 279, 282, 302, 307, 309
Reporting
  pathology
    for prostrate cancer, 45
  recommendations for prostate cancer variants, 48
  recommendations for special Gleason grading scenarios, 16
  recommendations for special gleason grading scenarios on needle biopsy specimens, 49
  stage in cystectomy specimens, 203
  subtypes/variants of carcinoma, 203
Retrograde venous invasion (RVI), 307, 308
Retroperitoneal lymph node dissection (RPLND), 337, 344, 463, 484, 520
Rhabdoid, 213, 328
RNaseL-, 114

S

Sarcomatoid, 68, 215, 239, 247, 316, 402, 426
Seminal vesicle, 6, 9, 38, 59, 439
Seminoma variants, 450, 471
Sertoli cell tumor, 455, 456, 479, 512
Sex cord–stromal tumors, 477, 479
Solid variant yolk sac tumor, 474
Somatic mutations, 118, 119, 149, 160
Spermatocytic seminoma, 448, 450, 471, 473, 474, 483, 506, 525
Spermatogenesis, 434, 438, 448, 475, 476, 525
SPINK1, 134, 137, 157
Sporadic, 113, 116, 231, 380, 523
Surgical margin, 517, 519
Surveillance, 13, 29, 132, 343, 444, 501
Survival outcome, 26, 29, 228, 229, 357

T

Template, 9, 202, 319, 486
Teratoma, 453, 467, 475, 476, 485, 509
Testicular adrenal rest tumors (TART), 479, 497

Testicular cancer, 357, 358, 447
Testicular neoplasms, 454, 457, 459, 501, 517
Testicular/paratesticular fibrous pseudotumor, 517
Testicular Tumors of the Adrenogenital Syndrome, 479
Testis
  anatomy of, 435, 437
  cancer
    staging of, 439
  miscellaneous tumor of
    carcinoid tumor, 459
    metaststic tumor, 459
TMPRSS2
  ERG gene fusions, 136
TNM stage, 307, 361
Transformation
  adenocarcinomatous, 468
  nephroblastomatous, 468, 469
  primitive neuroectodermal, 468
  sarcomatous, 468
  somatic, 467
  vs. immature teratoma, 467
Transition zone (TZ), 3, 5, 6, 7, 9
Transurethral resection, 7, 13, 17, 34, 46, 65, 83, 266
Treatment paradigms, 344, 345
Treatment response, 161, 231, 356, 360, 361
Tubular and signet ring seminoma, 473
Tubulocystic carcinoma, 292, 293, 324, 326
Tumor necrosis, 286, 288, 291, 299, 307, 315, 507
Tumor-Node-Metastasis (TNM), 300, 301, 302, 310, 311
Tumor size, 56, 288, 301, 303, 365, 484
Tumor stage, 134, 136, 156, 300, 365
Tumor syndromes, 491, 495

U
Unusual variants, 251, 471
Ureteral neoplasms, 174, 175, 183, 232, 265, 405
Urine-based markers, 242
Urothelial atypia, 189, 190, 193, 265
Urothelial carcinoma (UC), 21, 67, 68, 70, 72, 79, 86, 173, 191, 204, 205
UroVysion, 242, 266

V
Vancouver classification, 425
Variants, 20, 204, 208, 471, 474, 510
Venous invasion, 276, 283, 307, 308, 309
Von Hippel–Lindau (VHL) disease, 495, 496

W
WHO classification, 324, 329, 475

Y
Yolk sac tumor, 450, 454, 466, 487, 525
  solid variant, 474, 475